Examination
and History Taking

Fourth Edition

Barbara Bates, M.D.

Lecturer in Medicine, Department of Medicine
University of Pennsylvania School of Medicine

Lecturer in Nursing
University of Pennsylvania School of Nursing
Philadelphia, Pennsylvania

J.B. Lippincott Company   Philadelphia

London   Mexico City   New York   St. Louis   São Paulo   Sydney

Sponsoring Editor: Patricia L. Cleary
Production Editor: Rosanne Hallowell
Manuscript Editor: Mary Norris
Indexer: Kathleen Garcia
Design Director: Tracy Baldwin
Designer/Coordinator: Don Shenkle
Production Manager: J. Corey Gray
Production Coordinator: Charlene Squibb
Compositor: Progressive Typographers
Printer/Binder: R.R. Donnelley & Sons Company, Inc.
Color Insert Printer: Princeton Polychrome

Fourth Edition

6   5   4   3   2

Library of Congress Cataloging-in-Publication Data

Bates, Barbara, 1928–
  A guide to physical examination and history taking.
  Rev. ed. of: A guide to physical examination.
3rd ed. ©1983.
  Bibliography: p.
  Includes index.
  1. Physical diagnosis.   2. Children — Medical
examinations.   I. Hoekelman, Robert A.   II. Bates,
Barbara, 1928–   . Guide to physical examination.
III. Title.   [DNLM: 1. Physical Examination.
WB 205 B329g]
RC76.B37   1987   616.07'54   86-15226
ISBN 0-397-54623-8

HARPER INTERNATIONAL EDITION
ISBN 0-06-350127-9

A Guide to
Physical Examination
and History Taking

A Guide to
Physical

With a section on the
pediatric examination *by*
Robert A. Hoekelman, M.D.

Professor and Chairman, Department of Pediatrics
University of Rochester School of Medicine and Dentistry

Professor of Nursing
University of Rochester School of Nursing
Rochester, New York

Illustrations *by*
Robert Wabnitz *and Staff*
University of Rochester School of Medicine
Susan Shapiro Brenman, M.S.
Medical Illustrator

*To our readers and colleagues, whose questions
and suggestions have contributed so much
to the book and with whom we have enjoyed
an interprofessional dialogue*

Acknowledgments

We are again pleased to acknowledge the contributions of colleagues in several disciplines. For their suggestions, advice, critiques, and contributions we want to thank Carol A. Brink, R.N., MPH, Cynthia W. Clark, R.N., M.S.N., Arthur S. Hengerer, M.D., Anita B. Lasswell, M.S., R.D., Lissa McAnarney, M.D., Bernadine Z. Paulshock, M.D., Gail Smithwick, R.N., M.S.N., Claire A. Washington, R.N., M.S.N., and Rosalyn J. Watts, R.N., Ed.D. Susan C. Day, M.D., deserves special credit for reviewing all the chapters relevant to adults, asking hard questions, and making numerous valuable suggestions.

Susan Shapiro Brenman, M.S., medical illustrator, has continued to add importantly to the artistic quality of the book. Art Siegel, director of the Biomedical Communications Facility, School of Medicine, University of Pennsylvania, took the new photographs.

In Pennsylvania Elizabeth Popper produced a long and complicated manuscript, while in Rochester Sydney Sutherland provided editorial assistance and Lana Wright prepared the manuscript. Once more we have appreciated and enjoyed the contributions of Mary Norris, manuscript editor. Her keen eye for detail and her skill in making tactful suggestions added both form and substance to the final version.

Finally we would like to thank David T. Miller for nurturing the previous editions of the book and the staff of J.B. Lippincott Company for coping so well with this one.

Contents

List of Color Plates and Tables

Color Plates

Tables

Chapter 2
An Approach to Symptoms

Chapter 3
Mental Status

Chapter 5
The General Survey

Chapter 6
The Skin

Chapter 7
The Head and Neck

Chapter 8
The Thorax and Lungs

Chapter 9
The Cardiovascular System

Chapter 10
The Breasts and Axillae

Chapter 11
The Abdomen

Color tabs identify tables at the end of respective chapters

2

3

6

7

8

9

10

11

12

13

14

15

16

17

18

Introduction

A Guide to Physical Examination and History Taking is designed for students in health care who are learning to talk with patients, to examine them, and to understand and assess their problems. The first three chapters deal with interviewing, the health history, common and important symptoms, and the assessment of mental status. Then, in chapters devoted to body regions or body systems, the book reviews the relevant anatomy and physiology, describes the sequence and techniques of physical examination, and helps the student to identify selected abnormalities. Two final chapters deal with clinical thinking and organizing the patient's record.

We assume that the learners have had basic courses in human anatomy and physiology. The anatomic and physiologic sections in this book are designed to help students apply their knowledge to interpreting symptoms, examining the human body, and understanding physical signs.

Throughout the book we have tried to emphasize common or important problems, in contrast to the infrequent or esoteric. An occasional physical sign has been included despite its rarity because it enjoys a solid niche in classic physical diagnosis.

We assume that students will learn their examination skills by first practicing on other adults. Most of the anatomy and physiology, some of the techniques, and many of the abnormalities are common to both adults and children. Dr. Hoekelman's chapter on the examination of infants and children describes variations as they occur in the younger age groups together with signs or conditions that are unique to them.

THE FOURTH EDITION

The single biggest change in the fourth edition is the introduction of a new Chapter 2, "An Approach to Symptoms." It defines the technical terms for common and important symptoms, suggests specific ways of asking about them, and outlines some of their mechanisms and causes. In a manner analogous to that used in the chapters on physical examination, the various disorders and diseases that may cause symptoms appear both in the right columns and in tables at the end of this chapter. We hope that this addition will enhance students' understanding of their patients' symptoms, improve the efficiency of their interviewing, and help them in making assessments.

The chapter on mental status has been moved so that it now follows the new Chapter 2. It thus continues and completes the topic of talking with patients. Assessment of speech and consciousness has been moved out of "The Nervous System" into this chapter, where it fits more appropriately.

Among other changes, the chapter "The Cardiovascular System" has been renamed, rearranged, expanded, and partly rewritten. In "The Skin," the assessment of skin color has been expanded, and height/weight tables have reappeared in "The General Survey." Height/weight charts may now be found in the chapter on infants and children, and materials on the Denver Developmental Screening Test and guidelines for the supervision of child health have also been added there. We have made numerous smaller changes in virtually every chapter, trying to clarify difficult topics and keep the content current. The bibliography has been reorganized to make it easier to use and a bit more interesting.

Extensive changes and additions have been made in the illustrations, most notably in the chapters on the head and neck, the abdomen, and the musculoskeletal system. Encouraged by readers' requests, we have added color photographs of eardrums and selected skin tumors.

Simplifications and deletions partly balance the expansions. We are now recommending only one method of inspecting the inside of the nose, leaving the nostril-spreading type of nasal speculum, together with the head mirror and reflected light that it properly requires, to the specialist. The suggested techniques of palpating the thyroid gland have been simplified, as have the areas on the thorax now recommended for assessing tactile fremitus, percussing the chest, and listening to the lungs. Special maneuvers relevant to the knee examination and to sacroiliac pain have been omitted. Their proper evaluation now seems to exceed the basic skills reasonably expected of students.

Past users of this guide should also note the changed definition of accommodation (p. 151) and the more accurate placement of the costovertebral angle (p. 332).

SUGGESTIONS FOR USING THE BOOK

History taking and physical examination may be learned separately or together. Most sections of Chapter 2, "An Approach to Symptoms," have counterparts in the later chapters on physical examination, and correlations between these two areas are useful. Students and faculty who choose to make such correlations should take note of where the history and examination do not quite match. Symptoms described under "The Chest" pertain to the chapters on both the thorax and lungs and the cardiovascular system. The symptoms of the urinary tract, moreover, relate unavoidably to chapters on the abdomen, the anus, rectum, and prostate, and both the male and female genitalia.

When learning the physical examination, students should first review the sections on anatomy and physiology and familiarize themselves with the techniques. Next, they should try to practice their new skills on partners, under faculty supervision. The sections on techniques appear by themselves, without interruption, so that they will fit well into such a practice setting. We hope the book has not grown too heavy to rest reasonably comfortably on a partner's lap. After working through each body system and performing one or more comprehensive examinations, students should be ready, again with supervision, to examine some patients.

Skimming the tables of abnormalities helps to give the readers some ideas as to what they should be looking for and why they are asking certain questions. Students should not, however, try to memorize the details that are presented there. The best time to learn about abnormalities and diseases is when a patient (real or described) appears with a problem. The student should then try to analyze the problem with this book and pursue the subject as necessary in other relevant clinical texts.

As students proceed through the body systems and regions, they should periodically refer to Chapter 4, "Physical Examination: Approach and Overview," and to Chapter 20, "The Patient's Record." They will thus learn how to fit their new techniques into a comprehensive physical examination and how to record their findings. Reviewing Chapter 19, "Clinical Thinking: From Data to Plan," will help them to think about and analyze the data that they are learning to collect.

RELATED LEARNING MATERIALS

A Visual Guide to Physical Examination, 2nd edition, is a series of 12 sound motion pictures that demonstrates the examination procedures. It is available from J.B. Lippincott Company.

Clinical Assessment: A Guide for Study and Practice by Gloria A. Hagopian, R.N., Ed.D., Debra P. Hymovich, R.N., Ph.D., F.A.A.N., and Joan E. Lynaugh, R.N., Ph.D., F.A.A.N. (J.B. Lippincott Company, 1987) is a case-oriented study guide that helps students apply their new knowledge to realistic situations. An instructor's manual is available.

EQUIPMENT

Equipment necessary for a physical examination includes the following:

1. An ophthalmoscope and an otoscope (The latter should have appropriate specula for the ears and ideally a short, wide [9 mm] nasal speculum, with magnification, for the nose.)
2. A flashlight
3. Tongue depressors
4. A ruler and flexible tape measure, preferably marked in centimeters
5. A thermometer
6. A watch with a second hand
7. A sphygmomanometer
8. A stethoscope with the following characteristics:
   a. Snugly fitting and comfortable ear tips, achieved through properly sized tips, an angle that approximates that of the ear canal, and an appropriately tight spring in the connecting metal band
   b. Thick-walled tubing as short as feasible in order to maximize the transmission of sound: about 30 cm (12 inches) if possible and no longer than 38 cm (15 inches)
   c. A bell and a diaphragm with a good changeover mechanism
9. Gloves ⎱ For vaginal and rectal examination
10. Lubricant ⎰
11. Vaginal specula
12. A reflex hammer
13. Tuning forks, one of 128 cps and one of 512 cps or possibly 1024 cps
14. Safety pins
15. Cotton
16. Two test tubes (needed only for selected neurologic examinations)
17. Paper and pen or pencil

Chapter 1
Interviewing and the Health History

Barbara Bates and Robert A. Hoekelman

Talking with patients and obtaining their health histories are usually the first and often the most important parts of the health care process. Here you *gather the information necessary* to form tentative diagnoses. You *begin a relationship* that will help your patients trust and confide in you. By talking with you *patients may learn something about themselves,* such as how an illness relates to recent changes in their lives. You share in that learning. Finally, both you and the patient can *start to define your therapeutic goals.*

The purposes of this chapter are (1) to orient you to the structure and purposes of the health history, (2) to identify the items that a comprehensive history includes, (3) to guide you in the basic principles of interviewing, including the variations appropriate to the patient's age, and (4) to suggest some methods that may help you in coping with specific problems as you talk with patients. Chapter 2 deals with interviewing strategies that are useful in approaching and understanding specific bodily symptoms. Chapter 3 continues this approach as it applies to emotional symptoms and mental status.

To obtain a comprehensive history you need to learn both the kind of information to gather and how to get it. The first two sections of this chapter deal with the first of these two tasks.

THE STRUCTURE AND PURPOSES OF A HEALTH HISTORY

The traditional health history has several parts, each with a specific purpose. Together they give structure to your data collection and to your final record, but they do not dictate the exact sequence of the interview. Certain introductory materials in the health history typically precede the account of the patient's story. The *date* is always important, and in rapidly changing circumstances the time should be added. *Identifying data,* such as age, sex, race or ethnic origin, birthplace, and occupation, serve not only to establish who the patient is but also to give you some tentative suggestions as to what kind of person you are talking to and even what the likely problems might be. When patients do not initiate their own visits, the *source of referral* becomes important. It indicates to the responsible clinician that a written report may be necessary, and it helps you to understand the patient's possible motivations. Persons seen at the request of school authorities or an insurance company may have different goals than those who come at their own discretion. The *source of the history*, whether it be the patient, family, friends, police, a letter of referral, or the past medical record, also deserves comment. It helps you assess the value and possible biases of the information. Under some circumstances it is also helpful to comment on the probable *reliability* of the source of your data. Reliability varies with knowledge, memory, trust, and motivation, among other factors, and is a judgment made at the end of the interaction, not at the beginning.

The main part of the history starts with the patient's *chief complaints*. These are the one or more symptoms or other concerns for which the patient is seeking care or advice. The *present illness* amplifies the chief complaints and gives a full, clear, chronological account of how each of the symptoms developed and what events were related to them. The *past history* explores prior illnesses, injuries, and medical interventions while the *current health status* focuses on the present state of health and on environmental conditions, personal habits, and health-related measures that may impinge on it.

The *family history* helps you to assess the patient's risks of developing certain diseases and may also suggest what the patient might be worrying about. Further, a pattern of familial illness may emerge that will prove useful in the care of related persons. The *psychosocial history* sometimes suggests some contributory factors in the patient's illness and helps you to evaluate the patient's sources of support, likely reactions to illness, coping mechanisms, strengths, and concerns. It helps you in getting to know your patient as a person. In the *review of systems* you ask about common symptoms in each major body system and thus try to identify problems that the patient did not mention spontaneously.

THE CONTENT OF A COMPREHENSIVE HISTORY

The items in a comprehensive history necessarily vary with the patient's age, sex, and illness, with the clinician's specialty and available time, and with the goals of the visit. Under many circumstances the clinician's efforts are targeted on a specific complaint, such as a sore throat or burning on urination. A limited approach, tailored to the problem, is then indicated. In other circumstances, however, a comprehensive history is needed. By learning and understanding all the items in such a history you can use them to the best advantage, either all together or in clusters, depending on the situation. Two patterns of such a comprehensive history are detailed in the next few pages: one for adults, the other for children.

Technical terms for symptoms appear in these histories. Definitions of these terms, together with ways to ask about the symptoms, are included in Chapter 2.

Comprehensive History: Adult Patient

DATE OF HISTORY

IDENTIFYING DATA, including at least age, sex, race, place of birth, marital status, occupation, and perhaps religion

SOURCE OF REFERRAL, if any

SOURCE OF HISTORY, such as the patient, a relative, a friend, the patient's medical record, or a referral letter

RELIABILITY, if relevant

CHIEF COMPLAINTS, when possible in the patient's own words ("My stomach hurts and I feel awful.")

PRESENT ILLNESS. This is a clear, chronological narrative account of the problems for which the patient is seeking care. It should include the onset of the problem, the setting in which it developed, its manifestations, and its treatments. The principal symptoms should be described in terms of (1) location, (2) quality, (3) quantity or severity, (4) timing (*i.e.,* onset, duration, and frequency), (5) setting, (6) factors that have aggravated or relieved these symptoms, and (7) associated manifestations. Relevant data from the patient's chart, such as laboratory reports, also belong in the present illness, as do significant negatives (*i.e.,* the absence of certain symptoms that will aid in differential diagnosis).

A present illness should also include patients' responses to their own symptoms and incapacities. What are the underlying worries that have led to seeking professional attention? ("I think I may have appendicitis.") And why is that a worry? ("My Uncle Charlie died of a ruptured appendix.") Further, what impacts has the illness had on the patient's life? This question is especially important in understanding a patient with chronic illness. "How has the backache, shortness of breath, or whatever, affected your ability to work? . . . your life at home? . . . your social activities? . . . your role as a parent? . . . your role as a husband, or wife? . . . the way you feel about yourself as a man, or a woman? . . . your sexual activities?"

PAST HISTORY

General State of Health as the patient perceives it

Childhood Illnesses, such as measles, rubella, mumps, whooping cough, chicken pox, rheumatic fever, scarlet fever, polio

Adult Illnesses

Psychiatric Illnesses

Accidents and Injuries

Operations

Hospitalizations, not already described

CURRENT HEALTH STATUS. Although some of the variables grouped under this heading have past as well as current components, they all have potential impact on current health and possible health-related interventions.

Allergies

Immunizations, such as tetanus, pertussis, diphtheria, polio, measles, rubella, mumps, influenza, hepatitis B, and *Hemophilus influenzae,* type b

Screening Tests appropriate to the patient's age, such as hematocrits, urinalyses, tuberculin tests, Pap smears, mammograms, stools for occult blood, and cholesterol tests, together with the results and the dates they were last performed

Environmental Hazards, including those in the home, school, and workplace

Use of Safety Measures, such as seat belts and other methods related to specific hazards

Exercise and Leisure Activities

Sleep Patterns, including times that the person goes to bed and awakens, daytime naps, and any difficulties in falling asleep or staying asleep

Diet, including all the dietary intake for a recent 24-hour period, and any dietary restrictions or supplements. Be specific in your questions. "Take yesterday, for example. Starting from when you woke up, what did you eat or drink first? . . . then what? . . . and then?" Ask specifically about coffee, tea, cola drinks, and other caffeine-containing beverages.

Current Medications, including home remedies, nonprescription drugs, and medicines borrowed from family or friends. When a patient seems likely to be taking one or more medications, survey one 24-hour period in detail. "Let's look at yesterday. Starting from when you woke up, what was the first medicine you took? How much? How often in the day did you take it? What are you taking it for? What other medicines . . . ?"

Tobacco, including the type, amount, and duration of use, *e.g.,* cigarettes, a pack a day for 12 years

Alcohol, Drugs, and Related Substances. See p. 16 for suggested methods of inquiry.

FAMILY HISTORY

The age and health, or age and cause of death, of each immediate family member (*i.e.,* parents, siblings, spouse, and children). Data on grandparents or grandchildren may also be useful.

The occurrence within the family of any of the following conditions: diabetes, tuberculosis, heart disease, high blood pressure, stroke, kidney disease, cancer, arthritis, anemia, headaches, epilepsy, mental illness, or symptoms like those of the patient.

PSYCHOSOCIAL HISTORY. This is an outline or narrative description that captures the important and relevant information about the patient as a person:

Home Situation and Significant Others. "Who lives at home with you? Tell me a little about them . . . and about your friends."

Daily Life, from the time of arising to bedtime. "What is a typical day like? What do you do first? . . . Next?"

Important Experiences, including upbringing, schooling, military service, job history, financial situation, marriage, recreation, retirement

Religious Beliefs relevant to perceptions of health, illness, and treatment

The Patient's Outlook on the present and outlook for the future

REVIEW OF SYSTEMS

General. Usual weight, recent weight change, weakness, fatigue, fever.

Skin. Rashes, lumps, sores, itching, dryness, color change, changes in hair or nails.

Head. Headache, head injury.

Eyes. Vision, glasses or contact lenses, last eye examination, pain, redness, excessive tearing, double vision, glaucoma, cataracts.

Ears. Hearing, tinnitus, vertigo, earaches, infection, discharge.

Nose and Sinuses. Frequent colds; nasal stuffiness, discharge, or itching; hay fever, nosebleeds, sinus trouble.

Mouth and Throat. Condition of teeth and gums, bleeding gums, last dental examination, sore tongue, frequent sore throats, hoarseness.

Neck. Lumps in the neck, "swollen glands," goiter, pain or stiffness in the neck.

Breasts. Lumps, pain or discomfort, nipple discharge, self-examination.

Respiratory. Cough, sputum (color, quantity), hemoptysis, wheezing, asthma, bronchitis, emphysema, pneumonia, tuberculosis, pleurisy; last chest x-ray film.

Cardiac. Heart trouble, high blood pressure, rheumatic fever, heart murmurs; chest pain or discomfort, palpitations; dyspnea, orthopnea, paroxysmal nocturnal dyspnea, edema; past electrocardiogram or other heart tests.

Gastrointestinal. Trouble swallowing, heartburn, appetite, nausea, vomiting, regurgitation, vomiting of blood, indigestion. Frequency of bowel movements, color and size of stools, change in bowel habits, rectal bleeding or black tarry stools, hemorrhoids, constipation, diarrhea. Abdominal pain, food intolerance, excessive belching or passing of gas. Jaundice, liver or gallbladder trouble, hepatitis.

Urinary. Frequency of urination, polyuria, nocturia, burning or pain on urination, hematuria, urgency, reduced caliber or force of the urinary stream, hesitancy, incontinence; urinary infections, stones.

Genitoreproductive

Male. Hernias, discharge from or sores on the penis, testicular pain or masses, history of venereal diseases and their treatments. Sexual interest, function, satisfaction, and problems; sexual orientation if relevant.

Female. Age at menarche; regularity, frequency, and duration of periods; amount of bleeding, bleeding between periods or after intercourse, last menstrual period; dysmenorrhea, premenstrual tension; age at menopause, menopausal symptoms, postmenopausal bleeding. Discharge, itching, sores, lumps, venereal diseases and treatments. Number of pregnancies, number of deliveries, number of abortions (spontaneous and induced); complications of pregnancy; birth control methods. Sexual interest, function, satisfaction; any problems, including dyspareunia.

Peripheral Vascular. Intermittent claudication, leg cramps, varicose veins, thrombophlebitis.

Musculoskeletal. Muscle or joint pains, stiffness, arthritis, gout, backache. If present, describe location and symptoms (*e.g.,* swelling, redness, pain, tenderness, stiffness, weakness, limitation of motion or activity).

Neurologic. Fainting, blackouts, seizures, weakness, paralysis, numbness, tingling, tremors or other involuntary movements.

Hematologic. Anemia, easy bruising or bleeding, past transfusions and possible reactions.

Endocrine. Thyroid trouble, heat or cold intolerance, excessive sweating; diabetes, excessive thirst or hunger, polyuria.

Psychiatric. Nervousness, tension, mood including depression; memory.

Comprehensive History: Child Patient

In addition to the obvious age-related differences between histories of children and of adults, there are present and past historical data specifically pertinent to the assessment of infants, children, and adolescents. These relate particularly to the patient's chronological age and stage of development. The child's history, then, follows the same outline as the adult's history, with certain additions that are presented here.

IDENTIFYING DATA. Data and place of birth. Nickname, particularly for those between 2 and 10 years of age. First names of parents (and last name of each, if different), their occupations, and where they may be reached during work hours.

CHIEF COMPLAINTS. Make clear whether these are concerns of the patient, the parent(s), or both. In some instances a third party, such as a schoolteacher, may have expressed concerns about the child.

PRESENT ILLNESS. Should include how each member of the family responds to the patient's symptoms, their concerns about them, and whether the patient achieves any secondary gains from the illness.

PAST HISTORY

Birth History. Particularly important during the first 2 years of life and for neurological and developmental problems. Hospital records should be reviewed if preliminary information from the parent(s) indicates significant difficulties before, during, or after delivery.

Prenatal. Maternal health before and during pregnancy, including nutrition and specific illnesses related to or complicated by pregnancy; doses and duration of all drugs taken during pregnancy; weight gain; vaginal bleeding; duration of pregnancy; parental attitudes concerning the pregnancy and parenthood in general and this child in particular.

Natal. Nature of labor and delivery, including degree of difficulty, analgesia used, and complications encountered; birth order if a multiple birth; birth weight.

Neonatal. Onset of respirations; resuscitation efforts; Apgar scores (see pp. 531–532) and estimation of gestational age. Specific problems with feeding, respiratory distress, cyanosis, jaundice, anemia, convulsions, congenital anomalies, or infection. Mother's health postpartum; separation of mother and infant and reasons for; initial maternal reaction to her baby and the nature of bonding. Patterns of crying and sleeping, and of urination and defecation.

Feeding History. Particularly important during the first 2 years of life and in dealing with problems of under- and overnutrition.

Infancy. Breast feeding—frequency and duration of feeds, use of complementary or supplementary artificial feedings, difficulties encountered, timing and method of weaning. *Artificial feeding*—type, concentration, amount, and frequency of feeds, difficulties (regurgitation, colic, diarrhea) encountered, timing and method of weaning. *Vitamin and iron supplements*—type, amount given, frequency, and duration. *Solid foods*—types and amounts of baby foods given, when introduced, infant's response, introduction of junior and table foods, self-feeding, parental and infant responses to feeding process.

Childhood. Eating habits—likes and dislikes, specific types and amounts of food eaten, parental attitudes toward eating in general and toward this child's under- or overeating, parental response to feeding problems (if present). A *diet diary* kept over a 7- to 14-day period may be required for an accurate assessment of food intake in childhood feeding problems.

Growth and Developmental History. Particularly important during infancy and childhood and in dealing with problems of delayed physical growth, psychomotor and intellectual retardation, and behavioral disturbances.

Physical Growth. Actual (or approximate) weight and height at birth and at 1, 2, 5, and 10 years; history of any slow or rapid gains or losses; tooth eruption and loss pattern.

Developmental Milestones. Ages at which patient held up head while in a prone position, rolled over from front to back and back to front, sat with support and alone, stood with support and alone, walked with support and alone, said first word, combinations of words, and sentences, tied own shoes, dressed without help.

Social Development. Sleep—amount and patterns during day and at night, bedtime routines, type of bed and its location; nightmares, terrors, and somnambulation. *Toileting*—methods of training used, when bladder and bowel control attained, occurrence of accidents or of enuresis or encopresis, parental attitudes, terms used within the family for urination and defecation (important to know when a young child is admitted to hospital). *Speech*—hesitation, stuttering, baby talk, lisping, estimate of number of words in vocabulary. *Habits*—bed rocking, head banging, tics, thumb sucking, nailbiting, pica, ritualistic behavior. *Discipline*—parental assessment of child's temperament and response to discipline; methods used, success or failure, negativism, temper tantrums, withdrawal, aggressive behavior. *Schooling*—experience with day care, nursery school, and kindergarten; age and adjustment upon entry; current parental and child satisfaction; academic achievement; school's concerns. *Sexuality*—relations with members of opposite sex; inquisitiveness regarding conception, pregnancy, and girl–boy differences; parental responses to child's questions and the sex education they have offered regarding masturbation, menstruation, nocturnal emissions, development of secondary sexual characteristics, and sexual urges; dating patterns. *Personality*—degree of independence; relationship with parents, siblings, and peers; group and independent activities and interests, congeniality, special friends (real or imaginary); major assets and skills; self-image.

Childhood Illnesses. In addition to specific illnesses experienced, mention of any recent exposures to childhood illnesses should be made here.

Operations
Accidents and Injuries } The reactions of the child and parents to these
Hospitalizations events should be ascertained.

CURRENT HEALTH STATUS

Allergies. Particular attention should be given to those allergies that are more prevalent during infancy and childhood—eczema, urticaria, perennial allergic rhinitis, and insect hypersensitivity.

Immunizations. Specific dates of administration of each vaccine should be recorded so that an ongoing booster program can be maintained throughout childhood and adolescence. Any untoward reactions to specific vaccines should also be recorded.

Screening Procedures. The dates and results of any screening tests performed should be recorded. These include, for all children, vision, hearing, and tuberculin tests, urinalyses, hematocrits, tests for phenylketonuria, galactosemia, and other genetic–metabolic disorders, and, for certain high-risk populations, sickle cell, blood lead, alpha$_1$-antitrypsin deficiency, and other tests that may be indicated.

FAMILY HISTORY. The education attained, job history, emotional health, and family background of each parent or parent substitute. The family socioeconomic circumstances, including income, type of dwelling, and neighborhood in which the family lives. Parental work schedules; family cohesiveness and interdependence; support available from relatives, friends, and neighbors; the ethnic and cultural milieu in which the family lives. Parental expectations, and attitudes toward the patient in relation to siblings. (All or portions of this information may be recorded in the present illness section, if pertinent to it, or under psychosocial history.) Consanguinity of the parents should be ascertained (by inquiring if they are "related by blood").

Once you know what kind of information to gather, you should lay that knowledge aside temporarily lest it come between you and the patient. At least at the start of the interview, and often at other times, you should be guided primarily by what the patient says and does rather than by a printed form or a rigid format.

SETTING THE STAGE FOR THE INTERVIEW

REVIEWING THE CHART. Before seeing the patient, quickly review the chart. Note the identifying data. Age, sex, race, marital status, address, occupation, and religion give you important glimpses into the patient's likely life experiences and may even guide your diagnostic hypotheses. If the patient has been referred from elsewhere, you should know both the source and the goals of referral. Reviewing the medical chart may give you invaluable information about past diagnoses and treatments, although it should not prevent you from developing new approaches or ideas.

THE ENVIRONMENT. Although you may have to talk with the patient under difficult circumstances — for example, in a four-bed room or in the corridor of a busy emergency department — a proper environment will improve communication. Your relationship may begin with the patient's first telephone call to clinic or office. If the response projects courtesy, interest, and a desire to be helpful, if the patient can be seen reasonably promptly, if you are punctual for the appointment, you are setting the stage for a trusting relationship.

These early stages in the patient–clinician communication, including the proper use of names and titles, are the critical determinants of patients' "reflexive self-concept" (what they think you think of them). If this is high, patients are more likely to be satisfied and more likely to cooperate with your diagnostic and therapeutic recommendations. If it is low, it may not matter what you say or do later in the visit in terms of gaining their trust and cooperation.

The environment itself tells the patient something about your interest. Is the setting quiet? Does it afford privacy? Are you free from interruptions? There should be places where both you and the patient can sit down in clear view of each other, preferably at eye level. Leaning against the far wall, inching toward the door, or shifting around uncomfortably from foot to foot discourages the patient's attempts at communication. So do arrangements that indicate inequality of power or even disrespect, such as greeting and interviewing a woman while she is lying supine, positioned for a pelvic examination.

Your distance from the patient should probably be several feet, not so close as to be uncomfortably intimate nor too distant for easy conversation. Patients may be able to talk with you more easily when sitting next to ur desk, rather than peering over it as if over a barrier. When patients ·r greater social distance they are telling you something about themselves, psychologically or perhaps culturally. Lighting also makes a difference. Beware of sitting between patients and a bright light or window. Although your view may be fine, the patient must squint uncomfortably toward your silhouette. You unwittingly conduct an interrogation, not a helping interview.

Finally, your clothing may also affect the ease with which you establish a relationship. There are few rules here except that you should be clean, reasonably neat, and dressed appropriately for the patients you wish to serve. Conservative dress and white coat, for example, are suitable for talking with most adults, whereas casual dress without uniform may be preferable when dealing with children or young people. You may feel that you should dress to express yourself rather than to respond to the wishes of others. You should be aware of the effects of your own appearance, however, and not blame the patient for adverse consequences. Compromises are usually possible.

APPROACH TO THE PRESENT ILLNESS

GREETING THE PATIENT. You are now ready to make your approach, greet the patient by name, and give your undivided attention. Shake hands if you feel comfortable doing so. Unless you are talking with a child or adolescent or unless you already know the patient well, use the appropriate title—for example, Mr. O'Neill or Mrs. Washington. Use of first names or terms of endearment with unfamiliar adults and use of "Granny" for an aged woman or "Mother" for a child's parent tend to depersonalize and demean. Introduce yourself by name. If there is any ambiguity in your role, such as your status as a student, explain your relation to the patient's care.

THE PATIENT'S COMFORT. Be alert to the patient's comfort. In office or clinic, there should be a suitable place for coats and belongings other than the patient's own lap. In the hospital inquire how the patient is feeling and whether your visit now is convenient. Watch for indications of discomfort such as poor positioning, evidence of pain or anxiety, or signs of the need to urinate. An improved position in bed or a short delay so that the patient can say goodbye to visitors or make a trip to the bathroom may be the shortest route to a good history.

OPENING QUESTIONS. Now you are ready to find out why the patient is here—the chief complaints, if any, and the present illness. (Occasionally a patient may come for a checkup or may wish to discuss a health-related matter without having either complaint or illness.) Begin your interview with a general question that allows full freedom of response—for example, "What brings you here?" or "What seems to be the trouble?" After the patient answers, inquire again, or even several times, "Anything else?" When the patient has finished, encourage further description by saying "Tell me about it," or, if there seems to be more than one problem, ask about one of them. "Tell me about the headaches" or ". . . about what bothers you most." As the patient answers, pick up the thread of the history and follow wherever it leads.

FOLLOWING THE PATIENT'S LEADS. Not all histories are complicated. Many patients want help with relatively straightforward medical problems. Others, however, have illnesses with complex psychosocial and pathophysiological causes, and may have complicated feelings about themselves, their illnesses, potential treatments, and those who are trying to help them. At the start you cannot tell one kind of patient from another. In order to do so your interviewing technique must allow patients to recount their own stories spontaneously. If you intervene verbally too soon, if you ask specific questions prematurely, you risk trampling on the very evidence you are seeking. Your role, however, is not passive. You should listen actively and watch for clues to important symptoms, emotions, events, and relationships. You can then guide the patient into telling you more about these areas. Methods of helping and guiding patients without diverting them from their own accounts include facilitation, reflection, clarification, empathic responses, confrontation, interpretation, and questions that elicit feelings. Your demeanor throughout is also important.

Facilitation. You use facilitation when by posture, actions, or words you encourage the patient to say more but do not specify the topic. Silence itself, when attentive yet relaxed, is facilitative. Leaning forward, making eye contact, saying "Mm-hmm" or "Go on" or "I'm listening," all help the patient to continue.

Reflection. Closely akin to facilitation is reflection, a repetition of the patient's words that encourages the patient to give you more details. Reflection may be useful in eliciting both facts and feelings, as in the following example:

> *Patient:*   The pain got worse and began to spread. (Pause)
> *Response:*   It spread?
> *Patient:*   Yes, it went to my shoulder and down my left arm to the fingers. It was so bad that I thought I was going to die. (Pause)
> *Response:*   You thought you were going to die?
> *Patient:*   Yes. It was just like the pain my father had when he had his heart attack, and I was afraid the same thing was happening to me.

Here a reflective technique has helped you to discover not only the location and severity of the pain, but also its meaning to the patient. There was no risk of biasing the story or interrupting the patient's train of thought.

Clarification. Sometimes the patient's words are ambiguous or the associations are unclear. If you are to understand their meaning you must request clarification, as in "Tell me what you meant by a 'cold'," or "You said you were behaving just like your mother. What did you mean?"

Empathic Responses. As patients talk with you, they may express — with or without words — feelings about which they are embarrassed, ashamed, or otherwise reticent. These feelings may well be crucial to understanding their illnesses or planning treatment. If you can recognize and respond to them in a way that shows understanding and acceptance, you show empathy for the patients, make them feel more secure, and encourage them to continue. Empathic responses may be as simple as "I understand." Other examples include, "You must have been very upset," or "That must have been very depressing for you." Empathic responses may also be nonverbal — for example, offering a tissue to a crying patient or gently placing your hand on an arm to convey understanding. In using an empathic response, be sure that you are responding correctly to what the patient has already expressed. If you have acknowledged how upset a patient must have been at the death of a parent, when in fact the death relieved the patient from a longstanding financial and emotional burden, you have seriously misunderstood your patient and possibly blocked further communication on the subject.

Confrontation. While an empathic response acknowledges expressed feelings, confrontation points out to patients something about their own words or behaviors. If you observe clues of anger, anxiety, or depression, for example, confrontation may help to bring these feelings out in the open. "Your hands are trembling whenever you talk about that," or "You say you don't care but there are tears in your eyes." Confrontation may also be useful when the patient's story has been inconsistent. "You say you don't know what brings on your stomach pains, yet whenever you've had them you were feeling picked on."

Interpretation. Interpretation goes a step beyond confrontation. Here you make an inference, rather than a simple observation. "Nothing has been right for you today. You seem fed up with the hospital." "You are asking a lot of questions about the x-rays. Are you worried about them?" In interpreting a patient's words or behavior, you take some risk of making the wrong inference and impeding further communication. When used wisely, however, an interpretation can both demonstrate empathy and increase understanding.

Asking About Feelings. Rather than making an inference or reflecting a feeling, you may simply ask patients how they feel, or felt, about something such as symptoms or events. Unless you let them know that you are interested in feelings as well as in facts, they may withhold the feelings and you may miss important insights.

YOUR GENERAL DEMEANOR. Just as you have been observing the patient throughout the early portions of the interview, so too has the patient been watching you. Consciously or not, you have been sending messages through both your words and your behavior. You should be sensitive to those messages and control them insofar as you can. Posture, gestures, eye contact, and words can all express interest, attention, acceptance, and understanding. The skilled interviewer seems calm and unhurried, even when time is limited. Reactions that betray disgust, disapproval, embarrassment, impatience, or boredom block communication, as do behaviors that condescend, stereotype, or make sport of the patient. Although negative reactions such as these are normal and often quite understandable, they should not be expressed. Guard against them not only when talking with the patient but also when discussing the patient with your colleagues or instructors, either at the bedside or in the hall.

Beginning practitioners may have special problems in dealing with their own limited knowledge; all practitioners confront this problem at least occasionally. When you do not know the answer to a patient's direct question, it is usually best to be honest about it and say so but add that you will try to find out the answer. Clearly acknowledging your status as a student may help you out of otherwise awkward situations.

DIRECT QUESTIONS. Using the nondirective techniques described thus far, you will usually be able to obtain a general idea of the patient's principal problems. You can encourage a chronological account by such questions as "What then?" or "What happened next?" Most of the time, however, you will need further specific information. Fill in the details with direct questions. If the patient's present illness involves pain, for example, you must determine the following:

1. Its location. Where is it? Does it radiate?

2. Its quality. What is it like?

3. Its quantity or severity. How bad is it?

4. Its timing. When did it start? How long does it last? How often does it come?

5. The setting in which it occurs, including environmental factors, personal activities, emotional reactions, or other circumstances that may have contributed to the illness

6. Factors that make it better or worse

7. Associated manifestations

Most other symptoms can be described in the same terms.

Several principles apply to the use of direct questions. They should *proceed from the general to the specific.* A possible sequence, for example, might be "What was your chest pain like? Where did you feel it? Show me. Did it stay right there or did it travel anywhere? . . . to which fingers?"

Direct questions *should not be leading questions.* If a patient says "yes" to "Did your stools look like tar?" you must always wonder if the description ~~i~~e patient's or yours. A better wording is "What color were your ~~?~~" Leading questions often give misleading answers. A classic exam-
~~e~~verything all right at home?"

When possible, ask questions that *require a graded response* rather than a "yes" or "no" answer. "How many stairs can you climb before stopping for breath?" is better than "Do you get short of breath climbing stairs?"

Sometimes patients seem quite unable to describe their symptoms without help. To minimize bias here, *offer multiple choice answers.* "Is your pain aching, sharp, pressing, burning, shooting, or what?" Almost any direct question can provide at least two possible answers. "Do you bring up any phlegm with your cough, or not?"

Ask one question at a time. "Any tuberculosis, pleurisy, asthma, bronchitis, pneumonia?" may lead to a negative answer out of sheer confusion.

Finally, *use language that is understandable and appropriate* to the patient. Although you might ask a trained health professional about dyspnea, the more customary term is shortness of breath. When talking with an Appalachian coal miner, on the other hand, it may help to use the colloquial "smothering spells." Appropriate words for technical terms are given in Chapter 2.

THE REST OF THE STORY

By now you should be able to synthesize a chronological narrative of the present illness, using the patient's spontaneous account and answers to direct questions. You are ready to proceed to the rest of the history. For most of it direct questions will constitute your major technique. Stay alert, however, for important medical or emotional material, and be prepared to revert to a nondirective style whenever indicated. While taking a family history, for example, you may learn of a parent's death or a child's illness. Here is a good opportunity to find out what it meant to the patient. "How was it for you then?" or "What were your feelings at the time?" The review of systems may also uncover material that requires as full an exploration as the present illness. Keep your technique flexible.

TAKING A HISTORY ON SENSITIVE TOPICS. Beginning students always have difficulties talking with patients about topics that are emotionally laden or culturally sensitive. At first the list of such subjects may be long, including sexual activities, death and dying, the financial concerns of patients, their racial and ethnic experiences, family interactions, domestic violence, psychiatric illnesses, physical deformities, and the functions of the urinary tract and bowel. Probably most of us continue to feel a little uncomfortable in a few areas. Many adult patients, if given a good opportunity, however, respond fairly easily to questions in these areas, and you will often learn of important factors that have contributed to their illnesses. A woman's evening headaches are related to sexual problems with her husband, a man's abdominal pain worsens whenever his employer makes racial slurs, or a person's blood pressure is still high because the prescriptions were too expensive to renew.

There are several ways of becoming more comfortable in difficult areas: special courses, professional and general reading, and your own life experiences. Use them all. Further, familiarize yourself with some opening questions on sensitive topics, such as those suggested in Chapter 2, and learn the additional kinds of data you need in order to make the desired assessments. Whenever possible, listen to experienced clinicians as they discuss such subjects with patients, and then try some of the difficult areas yourself. The range of topics that you can explore with comfort will widen progressively, sometimes to your surprise.

ASKING ABOUT ALCOHOL AND DRUGS. One difficult area for many clinicians is asking patients about their uses of alcohol and illicit drugs. Yet alcohol and drugs are often directly related to the patient's symptoms, and tolerance to and dependence upon a substance may importantly affect future management. It is not your role to pass judgment on the use of these substances, but it is your job (if the patient is willing) to gather the data with which to make a correct assessment and plan treatment. A nonjudgmental demeanor will also help patients discuss their practices with you.

Questions about alcohol and other drugs follow naturally after questions about coffee and cigarettes. Ask specifically about beer, wine, liquor, and prescription drugs (such as for sleep, "nerves," or dieting), and then proceed on to marijuana and other illicit drugs. "Have you ever tried cocaine? . . . or heroin? . . . or any other drugs like those? What are you currently using?"

As in other parts of the history, it is often helpful to use questions that ask for graded responses rather than simple "yes" or "no" answers. Thus, "How many marijuana cigarettes do you smoke in a day?" is often better than "Do you smoke marijuana?" Try to get specific, unambiguous answers about the amounts used, expressed in ounces, shotglasses, or other clear terms. "Social drinking" and "only one or two beers a day" both have wide ranges of meaning. Each beer, for example, might be 32 ounces, not the 12 ounces you might have assumed. The terms that people use for illicit drugs and for methods of taking them change over time and vary regionally. When patients use terms that you do not understand, ask for clarification.

Asking about family use of these substances is another fruitful approach. Patients may feel less threatened by sharing family information with you. After they have tested you and found your response nonjudgmental and concerned, they may feel more comfortable sharing their own personal patterns of use.

PHYSICAL VIOLENCE. Talking about a patient's or a family's use of alcohol or drugs often gives a good opportunity to inquire about physical violence. "When he comes home drunk like that, does he ever hit (beat, \you? . . . or the children? What does he do? What do you do?" Or, ou've had a lot to drink, do you ever get into fights? . . . take it out on your family? . . . hit them sometimes? What happens?" Whenever a child or an adult has a poorly explained injury, you also need to ask about violence. In cases of suspected child abuse, you might proceed as follows: "Most parents get very upset when their baby cries or their child has been naughty. How do *you* feel when *your* baby cries? What do you do when your baby won't stop crying? What sort of discipline do you use when your child has done something wrong? Are you ever afraid you might hurt your child?"

TRANSITIONS. As you move from one part of the history to another, it helps to orient the patient with brief transitional phrases. "Now I'd like to ask some questions about your past health," or ". . . about your family's health."

CLOSING. After you have completed your questions, return the initiative briefly to the patient: "Is there anything else we should talk about?" or "Have we omitted anything?" You may want to recapitulate part of the present illness to be sure of a common understanding. Finally, make clear to the patient what to do or what to expect next. "I will step out for a few minutes. Please get completely undressed and put on this gown. I would like to examine you."

NOTE-TAKING. Since no one can remember all the details of a comprehensive history, you need to take notes. Most patients are accustomed to note-taking but some may seem uncomfortable with it. If so, explore their concerns and explain your desire to make an accurate record. With practice you may be able to record most of the past history, current health status, family history, and review of systems in final form as you talk with the patient, especially if you have the help of a written questionnaire. Note-taking should not divert your attention from the patient, however, nor should a written form prevent you from following a patient's leads. While eliciting the present illness, the psychosocial history, or other complex portions of the patient's account, do not attempt to write your final report. Instead, jot down short phrases, words, and dates that will aid your memory later. When the patient is talking about sensitive or disturbing material it is best not to take notes at all.

PATIENTS AT DIFFERENT AGES

As people develop, have families, and age, they provide you with special opportunities and require certain adaptations in your interviewing style.

TALKING WITH PARENTS. In obtaining histories on infants and children, you gather all or at least part of your information from a third party, the parent(s) or legal guardian. Children under 5 years of age usually add no relevant historical data. As children grow older, however, you can get information of increasing value and reliability by interviewing them directly. Special ways of enhancing your interviews with children and adolescents are described in subsequent sections. This section deals with parents. Here your techniques are basically the same as in interviewing adult patients, with some special modifications.

Parents, of course, in describing what they perceive to be their child's symptoms, are speaking in the context of their underlying assumptions about and perceptions of the child. Although the observations are often accurate, they are subject to parental biases and needs. A mother, for example, may think of her ability to keep her children healthy as one important measure of her adequacy in mothering. When you ask her questions about her child's health you are, in a sense, testing her capabilities as a mother, and you should evaluate her responses in that context. There is a lot at stake for most parents as they try to cope with the problems of their children, so they need health practitioners who are supportive rather than judgmental or critical. Comments like, "Why didn't you bring him in sooner?" or "Why, in heaven's name, did you do that?" will not improve your rapport with a worried parent whose infant or child is acutely ill.

Refer to the infant or child by name rather than by "him," "her," or "the baby." When the mother's marital status is not immediately clear, you may avoid embarrassment in asking about the father by saying "Is Jane's father in good health?" rather than "Is your husband in good health?" Address the parents as "Mr. or Mrs. Smith" rather than by their first names or, heaven forbid, "Mother" or "Father." First names may be used with permission when you have established a reasonably longstanding relationship. You should be prepared, however, for the parent who calls you by your first name.

In interviewing parents, open-ended questions are usually more productive than direct questions. In the realm of psychosocial issues and problems, however, you must more often than not use explicit direct questions, since parents rarely introduce these subjects spontaneously even when given the opportunity with open-ended approaches. This may be especially likely for parents of lower socioeconomic status.

Finally, you need to recognize that the chief complaint may not relate at all to the apparent reason the parent has brought the child to see you. The complaint may serve as a "ticket of admission" to care, through which, if the circumstances are right, the parent may bring up another concern that, by itself, is not viewed as a "legitimate" reason for seeking care. Try to create an atmosphere that will allow the parents to express all their concerns. If necessary, ask questions that will facilitate the process.

Are there any other problems with Johnny that you would like to tell me about?

What did you hope that I would be able to do for you when you came today?

Is there anything special you would like me to explain to you about Jody?

Is there anything else bothering you about the other children, your husband (wife), or yourself that you'd like to talk about?

TALKING WITH CHILDREN. For the most part, pediatric practitioners conduct interviews with both the parent and the child present. This is convenient but presents some disadvantages as well as some distinct advantages. The history you obtain in the child's presence may be less accurate and couched in more limited terms than when you interview the parent(s) alone. When sensitive areas are not fully explored because the child is present, you will need to interview the parent at a later time (often at the end of the visit when the child has left the room) to clarify certain points or to fill in missing data.

The interview with the child present, on the other hand, offers an opportunity to observe parent–child interactions and the child's capacity for self-amusement while the parent is engaged in conversation. These observations may provide a clearer picture of the relationship between parent and child (and between parents if both are present) than can the answers to any number of questions.

For the younger child, this interlude may help to dispel fears of the practitioner or of the visit and allow for a smooth transition from the interview to the examination.

The older child will be able to add significantly to the history and can describe more accurately the severity of the symptoms and the child's own level of concern regarding them. You can sometimes improve the accuracy of your information by interviewing the child without the parent.

Take care to avoid "talking down" to children, for they are sensitive to affectations of speech and condescending behaviors.

TALKING WITH ADOLESCENTS. Many adults find talking with an adolescent difficult and frustrating because the adolescent often does not answer questions in an "adult" manner and may appear laconic and disdainful. This need not be the case. Adolescents, like most other people, will usually respond positively to anyone who demonstrates a genuine interest in them, not as "cases" but as people. That interest must be established early and then sustained if communication is to be effective. Adolescents tend to "open up" when the focus of the interview is on themselves and not on their problems. Thus, a good way to begin the interview with adolescents is to chat informally about their friends, school, hobbies, and family.

Adolescents seek health care on their own initiative or at the suggestion or insistence of their parents. They may come alone or with at least one parent. In the latter case, it is best to explain to both parent and adolescent that health care at this stage of one's individual development requires some degree of confidentiality. This requires speaking to the adolescent alone after obtaining past medical and social information from the parent(s). A confidential relationship is not based on "keeping secrets"; it is based on mutual respect. If it becomes necessary for the adolescent's own sake or for the sake of others to share confidential information, it is important to include the adolescent in that process.

In a preceding section of this chapter, certain techniques of promoting good communication are discussed. For the adolescent, some of these approaches may be threatening. Reflection is a technique that should be avoided with the younger, cognitively immature adolescent, since it requires thinking skills not yet acquired. The use of silence in an attempt to get the patient to talk is rarely successful with adolescents, who usually do not have sufficient self-assurance to respond appropriately to this form of facilitation. Confrontation, rather than "bringing feelings out in the open," may cause an anxious adolescent to retreat into silence. Closely related to this is the technique of asking about feelings. Adolescents often find discussing their feelings with adults very difficult.

These caveats need not deter you from talking with adolescents. Most adolescents will talk to someone they respect and accept when given the opportunity in a friendly, informal atmosphere. You are more likely to succeed as a professional if you "play it straight," act your age, and do not stretch too far in trying to bridge the generation gap.

AGING PATIENTS. At the other end of the life cycle, aging patients also pose special opportunities and special problems. They face relatively high risks for a number of conditions, such as decreased vision and hearing, memory loss, and depression. They often have chronic illnesses, with their associated discomforts and difficulties in getting about, and have usually experienced important losses including the deaths of family members or friends and diminutions in vigor, physical attractiveness, status, power, or income. Be especially alert for problems such as these, but be sure not to stereotype the aging patient. Many older persons adapt well to change, continue to grow and learn, and maintain a high morale.

From middle age on people become increasingly aware of their personal aging and begin to measure their lives in terms of the years left rather than the years lived. It is normal for older people to reminisce about the past and to reflect upon previous experience, including joys, regrets, and conflicts. Listening to this process of life review can give you important insights into your patients and may help them work through some of their painful feelings.

Try to determine the patients' priorities and goals. Learn how they have handled crises in the past. Because they may pursue similar adaptive patterns in the present situation, this knowledge will help you plan with them. Because aging patients have longer histories and may tell them more slowly, they often require extra time. Do not try to accomplish everything in one visit.

Many interviewers face special problems within themselves in relating to older patients. They may feel helpless in curing the ills of the aged, and their views toward aging people may be distorted by their own feelings toward parents and grandparents. They may fear their own old age and want to avoid reminders of it. Be alert to your own feelings.

SPECIAL PROBLEMS

Regardless of patient age, certain behaviors and special situations may particularly vex the practitioner.

SILENCE. Neophyte interviewers may grow uncomfortable during periods of silence, feeling somehow obligated to keep the conversation going. They need not feel so. Silences have many meanings and many uses. When recounting their present illnesses, patients frequently fall silent for short periods in order to collect their thoughts or remember details. An attentive silence on the interviewer's part is usually the best response here, sometimes followed by brief encouragement to continue. During periods of silence be particularly alert to nonverbal signs of distress. Patients may fall silent because they are having difficulty controlling their emotions. If so, these are almost invariably significant feelings that are best expressed. A gentle confrontation may help: "You seem to be having trouble talking about this." Depressed patients or those with organic brain syndrome may have lost their usual spontaneity of expression, give short answers to questions, and fall silent quickly after each one. If you sense one of these problems, shift your inquiry to an exploratory mental status examination (see pp. 99–108).

At times, a patient's silence results from interviewer error or insensitivity. Are you asking too many direct questions in rapid sequence? The patient may simply have yielded the initiative to you and taken the passive role you seem to expect. Have you offended the patient in any way—for example, by signs of disapproval or criticism? Have you failed to recognize an overwhelming symptom such as pain, nausea, dyspnea, or the need to urinate or defecate? If so, you may need to abbreviate the interview considerably or return after the patient has been relieved.

OVERTALKATIVE PATIENTS. The garrulous, rambling patient may be just as difficult as the silent one, and possibly more so. Faced with limited time and the perceived need to "get the whole story," the interviewer may grow impatient, even exasperated. Although there are no perfect solutions for this problem, several techniques are helpful. First, you may need to lower your own goals and accept less than a comprehensive history. It may be unobtainable. Second, give the patient free rein for the first 5 or 10 minutes of the interview. You will then have the chance to observe the patient's pattern of speech. Does the patient seem obsessively detailed or unduly anxious? Is there a flight of ideas or a disorganization of thought processes that suggests a psychotic disorder? Third, try to focus the account on what you judge to be most important. Show interest and ask questions in those areas. Facilitate sparingly. Interrupt if you must, but courteously. A brief summary may help you change the topic while letting the patient know that you have both heard and understood. "As I understand it, your chest pains come frequently, last a long time, and do not necessarily stay in any one place. Now tell me about your breathing." Finally, do not let your impatience show. If you have used up the allotted time or, more likely, gone over it, explain that to the patient and arrange for a second meeting. Setting a time limit for the next appointment may be helpful. "I know we have much more to talk about. Can you come again next week? We will have a full half hour then."

PATIENTS WITH MULTIPLE SYMPTOMS. Some patients seem to have every symptom that you mention. They have an "essentially positive review of systems." Although it is conceivable that such a patient has multiple organic illnesses, serious emotional problems are much more likely. In such cases it will profit little to explore each symptom in detail. Guide the interview into a psychosocial assessment instead.

ANXIOUS PATIENTS. Anxiety is a frequent and natural reaction to sickness, to therapy, and to the health-care system itself. For some patients anxiety has importantly colored their reactions to life stress and may have contributed to their illnesses. Be sensitive to nonverbal and verbal clues.

For example, anxious patients may sit tensely, fidgeting with their fingers or clothes. They may sigh frequently, lick their dry lips, sweat more than average, or actually tremble. Carotid pulsations may betray a rapid heart rate. Some anxious patients fall silent, unable to speak freely or confide. Others try to cover their feelings with words, busily avoiding their own basic problems. When you sense an underlying anxiety, encourage such patients to talk about their feelings.

REASSURANCE. When you are talking with anxious patients, it is tempting to reassure them: "Don't worry. Everything is going to be all right." This approach is usually counterproductive. Unless you and the patient have had a chance to explore the nature of the anxiety, you may well be giving reassurance about the wrong thing. Moreover, premature reassurance blocks further communication. Since admitting anxiety exposes a weakness, it requires encouragement, not a coverup. The first step to effective reassurance involves identifying and accepting the patient's feelings. This promotes a feeling of security. The final steps come much later in the health-care process, after you have completed the interview, the physical examination, and perhaps some laboratory studies. Then you can interpret for the patient what is happening and deal openly with the real concerns.

ANGER AND HOSTILITY. Patients have reasons to be angry: they are ill, they have suffered loss, they lack their accustomed control over their own lives, they feel relatively powerless in the health-care system. They may direct this anger toward you. It is possible that you have justly earned their hostility. Were you late for your appointment, inconsiderate, insensitive, or angry yourself? If so, recognize the fact and try to make amends. More often, however, patients are displacing their anger onto the clinician as a symbol of all that is wrong. Allow them to get it off their chests. Accept their feelings without getting angry in return. Beware of joining such patients in their hostility toward another part of the clinic or hospital, even when you privately harbor similar feelings. After such patients have calmed down, you may be able to identify specific steps that will help in the future. Rational solutions to emotional problems are not always possible, however, and people need time to resolve their angry feelings.

THE OBSTREPEROUS INEBRIATE. Few patients can disrupt the clinic or emergency room more quickly than acutely intoxicated persons who are angry, belligerent, and uncontrolled. Before interviewing such patients, it is wise to alert the security force of the hospital. As you make your approach greet patients by name and title, introduce yourself, and offer a handshake. In this situation it is especially important to appear accepting, not challenging. To do this, avoid all but the briefest eye contact and keep your posture relaxed and nonthreatening, your hands loosely open rather than clenched into fists. Do not try to make the patients lower their voices or stop cursing at you or the staff, but listen carefully and try to understand what they are saying. Since some such persons feel trapped in small rooms it is usually best to talk with them in an open area, and you are likely to feel more comfortable there, too. In addition, an offer of food, coffee, or a cigarette may help to quiet the agitated person and bring some calm to the stormy scene.

CRYING. Like anger, crying is an important clue to emotions. Rarely should it be suppressed. If the patient seems on the verge of tears, gentle confrontation or an empathic response may simply allow crying. Quiet acceptance is then appropriate. Offer a tissue; wait for recovery; perhaps make a facilitating or supportive remark: "It's good to get it out." Most patients will soon compose themselves and, if properly accepted, will feel better and capable of continuing the discussion.

DEPRESSION. Masquerading as fatigue, weight loss, insomnia, or mysterious aches and pains, depression is one of the commonest problems in clinical medicine, and is commonly missed or ignored. Be alert for it, identify it, and explore its manifestations. Be sure you know how bad it is. Just as you would evaluate the severity of angina pectoris, you must evaluate the severity of depression. Both are potentially lethal. You need not fear that asking about suicide will suggest it to the patient. For appropriate questions about depression, see Chapter 3.

SEXUALLY ATTRACTIVE OR SEDUCTIVE PATIENTS. Practitioners of both sexes may occasionally find themselves attracted to their patients. If you become aware of such feelings, accept them as normal human responses but prevent them from affecting your behavior. Keep your relationship with the patient within professional bounds.

Occasionally patients may be frankly seductive or may make sexual advances. Calmly, but firmly, you should make clear that your relationship is professional, not personal. You may also wish to review your own image. Have you been overly warm with the patient? expressed your affection physically? sought his or her emotional support? Has your dress or demeanor been unconsciously seductive? Avoid these problems when you can.

CONFUSING BEHAVIORS OR HISTORIES. At times you may find yourself baffled, frustrated, and confused in your interaction with the patient. The history is vague and difficult to understand; ideas are poorly related to one another; and language is hard to follow. Even though you word your questions carefully, you seem unable to get clear answers. The patient's manner of relating to you may also seem peculiar: distant, aloof, inappropriate, or bizarre. Symptoms may be described in bizarre terms: "My fingernails feel too heavy," or "My stomach knots up like a snake." These characteristics should alert you to possible mental illnesses, such as schizophrenia. With the usual nondirective techniques you may be able to get more information about the unusual qualities of the symptoms. You should also include in your interview an assessment of the patient's mental status, with special attention to mood, thought, and perceptions (see pp. 101–104).

Many psychotic patients are functioning, with varying degrees of success, in the community. Such patients are frequently capable of telling you freely about their diagnoses, their symptoms, their hospitalizations, and their current medications. You should feel comfortable inquiring about these without embarrassment or circumlocution.

Schizophrenia is not the only cause of confusing histories. Some patients have underlying disorders of cognitive function—disorders generally classified as organic brain syndromes, such as delirium or dementia. Be particularly alert for delirium when dealing with an acutely ill or intoxicated patient, and for dementia when dealing with an elderly patient. Patients with these problems may be unable to give clear histories. They are vague and inconsistent about symptoms or events and unable to report when and how things happened. They may be inattentive to your questions and hesitant in their answers. Occasionally such patients may confabulate, that is, make up part of their histories in order to fill in the gaps in their memories. When you suspect an organic brain syndrome, do not spend too much time trying to get a detailed history. You will only tire and frustrate the patient as well as yourself. Switch your inquiry instead to an evaluation of mental status, checking particularly on level of consciousness, orientation, and memory (see pp. 99 and 104–105). You can work the initial questions smoothly into the interview. "When was your last appointment in the clinic? Let's see, then, that was about how long ago?" "Your address now is? . . . and your phone number?" Responses can all be checked against the chart (presuming, of course, that the chart is accurate).

PATIENTS WITH LIMITED INTELLIGENCE. Patients of moderately limited intelligence can usually give adequate histories. You may, in fact, overlook their limitations and thereby make mistakes, such as omitting their dysfunction from a disability evaluation or giving instructions they cannot understand. If you suspect such a problem, pay special attention to the patients' schooling. How far did they go in school? Why did they drop out? How were they doing at the time? What kinds of courses are (were) they taking? High school seniors of normal intelligence are not usually taking simple arithmetic. If your patient is, you can make a smooth transition into a mental status examination, including simple calculations, vocabulary, information, and tests of abstract reasoning (see pp. 106–107).

When patients suffer from severe mental retardation, you will have to obtain their history from family or friends. By showing interest in the patients themselves, however, and by engaging them in simple conversation, try to establish a personal relationship.

LITERACY. Although it is not synonymous with intelligence, literacy should sometimes be assessed, especially before giving written instructions. Some patients who cannot read because of a language barrier, learning disorder, or poor vision will admit it on direct questioning. Others, however, will deny it. You can check, as if testing their vision, by asking them to read some words or sentences for you.

LANGUAGE BARRIERS. Nothing will more surely convince you that a history is essential than having to do without one. When you cannot communicate with your patient because you speak different languages, take every possible step to find a translator. A few broken words and gestures are no substitute. The ideal translator is a neutral, objective person who is familiar with both languages. When family members or friends try to help, they are more likely to distort meanings and may also present problems in confidentiality to both the patient and the interviewer. Many translators try to speed the process by telescoping a long communication into a few words. Try to make clear at the beginning that you need the translator to translate everything, not to interpret or summarize. Make your questions clear and short. You can also help the translator by outlining the goals for each segment of your history.

When available, written bilingual questionnaires are invaluable, especially for the review of systems. Before using one, however, be sure patients can read in their own language or can get help with the questionnaire.

THE HEARING-IMPAIRED. Communicating with people whose hearing is severely impaired presents many of the same problems as does communicating with a patient who speaks a different language. Here, again, written questionnaires are a great help. Although very time-consuming, handwritten questions and answers may be the only solution. If the patient knows sign language, make every effort to find a translator who speaks, hears, and can use it. When such patients have partial hearing impairment or can read lips, face them directly, in good light. Speak slowly and in a relatively low-pitched voice. Do not let your voice trail off at the ends of sentences, avoid covering your mouth, and use gestures to reinforce your words. If the patient has a "good" ear, arrange the seating to take advantage of it. A person who has a hearing aid should, of course, wear it. Supplement any oral instructions with writing.

BLIND PATIENTS. When talking with a blind patient, be especially careful to announce yourself and explain who and what you are. Taking the patient's hand may help to establish contact and indicate where you are. If the room is unfamiliar, orient the patient to it and explain what is there and whether anyone else is present. Remember to respond vocally to such patients when they speak, since facilitative postures and gestures will not work. At the same time guard against raising your voice unnecessarily.

FATALLY ILL PATIENTS. In communicating with fatally ill or dying patients, most interviewers face problems within themselves — their own discomforts, anxieties, and desires to avoid the subject or even avoid the patients themselves. With the help of reading and discussion, you will need to work through your own feelings. As in any clinical situation, it is helpful to know what reactions the patient is likely to have. Kübler-Ross has described five stages in a patient's response to impending death: denial and isolation, anger, bargaining, depression or preparatory grief, and acceptance. Regardless of the stage, your approach is basically the same. Be alert to the feelings of such patients and to cues that they want to talk about them. Help them to bring out their concerns with nondirective techniques. Make openings for them to ask questions: "I wonder if you have any concerns about the operation? . . . your illness? . . . how it will be when you go home?" Explore these concerns and provide whatever information the patients are asking for. Be wary of inappropriate reassurance. If you can explore and accept the patients' feelings, if you can answer the patients' questions, if you can assure and demonstrate your ability to stay with the patients throughout the illness, reassurance will grow where it really matters — within the patients themselves.

Fatally ill or dying patients rarely want to talk about their illnesses all the time, nor do they wish to confide in everyone they meet. Give such patients opportunities to talk, and listen receptively, but if the patient prefers to keep the conversation on a lighter plane you need not feel like a failure. Remember that illness — even a terminal one — is only one small part of personhood. A smile, a touch, an inquiry after a family member, a comment on the day's ballgame, or even some gentle kidding all recognize and reinforce other parts of the patient's individuality and help to sustain the living person. To communicate appropriately you have to get to know the patient: that is part of the helping process.

TALKING WITH FAMILIES OR FRIENDS. Some patients are totally unable to give their own histories. Others may be unable to describe parts of them such as their behavior during a convulsion. Under these circumstances you must try to find a third person from whom to get the story. At times, although you may think you have a reasonably comprehensive knowledge of the patient, other sources may offer surprising and important information. A spouse, for example, may report significant family strains, depressive symptoms, or drinking habits that the patient has denied. When you suspect such discrepancies, look for opportunities to get additional information from persons other than the patient.

When you decide to seek information from a third person, it is usually wise to get the patient's approval. Assure such patients that you will keep confidential what they have already told you, or get their permission to share certain information. Data from other persons must also be held in confidence.

The basic principles of interviewing apply to your conversations with relatives or friends. Find a private place to talk. Leaning against opposite sides of a hospital corridor is not conducive to good communication. Introduce yourself, state your purpose, inquire how they are feeling under the circumstances, and recognize and acknowledge their concerns. As you listen to their versions of the history, be alert for clues as to the quality of their relationships with the patient. These may color their credibility or give you helpful ideas in planning the patient's care.

RESPONDING TO PATIENTS' QUESTIONS. Patients' questions may seek simple factual information. More often, however, they express feelings or concerns. Try to elicit these feelings or delve further, lest you offer a misguided answer.

> *Patient:* What are the effects of this blood pressure medicine?
> *Response:* There are several effects. Why do you ask?
> *Patient:* (Pause) Well, I was reading up on it in a friend's book. I read it could make me impotent.

Similar caution is indicated when patients seek advice for personal problems. Should the patient quit a stressful job, for example, or move to Arizona, or have an abortion? Before responding, find out what approaches he or she has considered, what pros and cons there might be to the possible solutions. A chance to talk through the problem with you is usually much more valuable than any possible answer you could give.

Finally, when the patient is asking for specific information about the diagnosis, progress, or treatment plan, answer when you can but be careful that your responses do not conflict with those provided by others. When you are unsure of the answer, offer to find out if you can. Alternatively, you can suggest that the patient ask Dr. X because Dr. X knows more about the case or is making that decision. Beware, however, of using this approach simply to avoid a difficult issue. If you carry the primary patient responsibility yourself, share your opinions and plans and the patient's prognosis with other members of the health team so that each in turn can communicate with the patient effectively.

Chapter 2
An Approach to Symptoms

While Chapter 1 deals with the general methods of interviewing, this chapter tailors those methods to common or important symptoms. It (1) defines the technical terms for these symptoms, (2) suggests ways of asking about them, and (3) outlines some of their most common mechanisms and causes.

Technical terms, of course, are not intended for use with most patients. As a clinician you must learn, however, to translate the patient's observations into words such as tinnitus, hemoptysis, or nocturia. In this way you can accumulate knowledge systematically, apply it to clinical problems, and communicate clearly with other professionals.

Data to gather about symptoms appear in bold-faced type. Specific questions are suggested, especially in difficult or sensitive areas. When no suggestions are made, identify the seven attributes of the symptom, as described in Chapter 1, and use the general principles of interviewing that you have already learned.

Your growing skill in asking questions will depend in part on your understanding of what symptoms and their various attributes may mean. The symptoms are organized according to the likely bodily systems or structures involved, and some of the mechanisms that help to explain them are described. Interpretive comments on the meaning of certain symptoms appear in the right-hand columns, together with examples of specific abnormalities that may cause them. Tables at the end of the chapter compare various disorders and diseases according to their symptoms. Where assessment of symptoms depends heavily on physical examination, reference is made to later chapters.

No table, of course, exhausts all the possible explanations for symptoms, nor can any table, which is necessarily oversimplified, capture the infinite variety of human perceptions and experience. Real patients seldom match a textbook in every detail.

One of the qualities that is difficult for one person to communicate to another is color. A chart that includes the various colors of sputum, urine, and feces is often helpful in getting an accurate history. You can easily make such a chart by cutting rectangles out of the colored pages of a magazine and taping them to a small card. Colors should range from white to yellowish and light green for sputum; from pale to deep yellow, orange, pink, reddish, and brown for urine; and from gray and light tan to brown and black for feces. The bright and dark red colors of blood should also be included. These colors can be arranged into one scheme from which the patient can select the closest match.

Symptoms and Approaches to Them

GENERAL SYMPTOMS

Changes in *body weight* result from quantitative changes in either the body tissues or the body fluids. *Weight gain* occurs when caloric intake exceeds caloric expenditure over a period of time, and typically appears as increased body fat. Weight gain may also result, however, from an abnormal accumulation of body fluids. When the retention of fluid is relatively mild it may not be visible, but as several pounds of it accumulate it usually appears as edema.

Rapid changes in weight (over a few days) suggest changes in body fluids, not tissues.

See Table 15-3, Mechanisms and Patterns of Edema, pp. 422–423.

Weight loss is an important symptom that has many causes. Mechanisms include one or more of the following: decreased intake of food for reasons that include anorexia, dysphagia, vomiting, and insufficient supplies of food; defective absorption of nutrients through the gastrointestinal tract; increased metabolic requirements; and loss of nutrients through the urine, feces, or injured skin.

A person may also lose weight when a fluid-retaining state improves or responds to treatment. Moreover, the greater part of the weight lost when a person starts on a low-calorie diet is fluid.

Causes of weight loss include gastrointestinal diseases; endocrine disorders (diabetes mellitus, hyperthyroidism, adrenal insufficiency); chronic infections; malignancies; chronic cardiac, pulmonary, or renal failure; depression; and anorexia nervosa.

Good opening questions include "How often do you check your weight? Has it changed in the past year? . . . in what manner? Why has it changed, do you think? What would you like to weigh?" If weight change in either direction appears to be a problem, try to ascertain the amount of change, its timing, the setting in which it occurred, and any associated symptoms.

In the *overweight patient*, for example, when did the weight gain begin? Was the patient heavy as an infant or a child? Using milestones appropriate to the patient's age, inquire about the weight at the time of birth, on entrance to kindergarten, on graduation from high school or college, on discharge from the service, at marriage, following each pregnancy, at menopause, and on retirement. What was going on in the patient's life during the periods of weight gain? Has the patient tried to lose weight? How? With what results?

When the problem is *weight loss*, try to determine whether the intake of food has diminished proportionately or whether it has remained normal or even increased.

Weight loss with a relatively high food intake suggests diabetes mellitus, hyperthyroidism, or malabsorption. Consider also binge eating (bulimia) with clandestine vomiting.

Symptoms associated with the weight loss often suggest its likely cause. So does a good psychosocial history. Who cooks and shops for the patient? Where and with whom does the patient eat? Are there any

Poverty, old age, social isolation, physical disability, emotional or mental impairment,

difficulties in getting, storing, preparing, or chewing the food? Does the patient restrict certain foods for medical, religious, or other reasons?

Throughout the history, moreover, be alert for manifestations of malnutrition. Symptoms here are often subtle and nonspecific: weakness, easy fatigability, cold intolerance, flaky dermatitis, and ankle swelling, among other examples. A good dietary history is of course mandatory.

Like weight loss, *fatigue* is a relatively nonspecific symptom with many causes. It refers to a sense of weariness or loss of energy that patients describe in various ways. "I've lost my pep. . . . I just feel blah. . . . I'm all in. . . . I can hardly get through the day. . . . By the time I get to the office I feel as though I've done a day's work." Because fatigue is a normal response to hard work, sustained stress, or grief you must consider the context in which it occurs, but fatigue that is unexplained by such factors becomes a symptom.

In infants and children fatigue is not expressed verbally but is manifested by withdrawal from normal activities, irritability, loss of interest in the surroundings, and excessive sleeping.

Use open-ended questions to explore the attributes of the patient's fatigue, and get as clear an idea as possible as to what the patient is experiencing. Important clues to the cause of the problem often lie in a good psychosocial history, review of systems, and exploration of sleep patterns.

Weakness is different from fatigue. It denotes a demonstrable loss of muscular power and will be discussed later with other neurologic symptoms (see pp. 57–58).

Fever refers to an abnormal elevation in body temperature (see pp. 132–133). **Ask about it when the patient has an acute or chronic illness. Find out whether the patient has measured the temperature with a thermometer. Has the patient felt feverish or unusually hot, noted excessive sweating, or felt chilly and cold? Try to distinguish between subjective *chilliness* and a *shaking chill* in which the body shivers and the teeth chatter.**

Feelings of coldness, gooseflesh, and shivering accompany a rising temperature, while hot feelings and sweats accompany defervescence. The normal temperature rises during the day and falls during the night. When fever exaggerates this swing, *night sweats* occur. Malaise, headache, and pain in the muscles and joints often accompany fever.

lack of teeth, ill-fitting dentures, and alcoholism increase the likelihood of malnutrition.

Fatigue is a common symptom of depression and anxiety states, but consider also infections (such as hepatitis, infectious mononucleosis, and tuberculosis); endocrine disorders (hypothyroidism, adrenal insufficiency, diabetes mellitus, and panhypopituitarism); heart failure; chronic disease of the lungs, kidneys, or liver; electrolyte imbalance; moderate to severe anemia; malignancies; nutritional deficits; rheumatoid arthritis; Parkinson's disease; medications; and drug withdrawal.

Weakness, especially if localized in a neuroanatomic pattern, suggests a disorder of the nervous system or muscles.

Recurrent shaking chills suggest more extreme swings in temperature.

Feelings of heat and sweating also accompany menopause.

Fever has many causes. **Focus your questions on the timing of the illness and its associated symptoms. Become familiar with patterns of infectious diseases to which your patient may have been subject, and inquire about travel, contacts with sick persons, or other unusual exposures. Inquire about medications.** They may cause fever, while antipyretics such as aspirin or acetaminophen may mask it or in febrile patients may produce exaggerated swings in temperature with associated shaking chills.

THE SKIN

Start your inquiry about the patient's skin with a few open-ended questions: "Have you noticed any changes in your skin? . . . your hair? . . . your nails? Have you had any rashes? . . . sores? . . . lumps? . . . itching? . . . any moles that have changed in appearance? Where? When?" Further questions are usually best deferred until your physical examination when you can see what the patient is talking about.

See Chapter 6, The Skin, and pp. 546–548.

Causes of generalized itching without obvious reason include dry skin, aging, pregnancy, uremia, obstructive jaundice, lymphomas and leukemia, drug reactions, and body lice.

THE HEAD

Headache is an extremely common symptom. Although only a very small fraction of people with headaches harbor life-threatening problems as the cause, the symptom requires careful evaluation. **Get as full a description as possible. After your usual open-ended approach, ask the patient to show you where the discomfort is. Is it one-sided or bilateral? steady or throbbing? The single most important attribute of headache is its chronological pattern. Are you dealing with a new and acute problem, a chronic and recurring one that has not changed very much in its pattern, or a chronic, recurring one that has recently changed in its characteristics or has become progressively severe? Does the pain recur at the same time every day? Associated symptoms and a family history may also give you important clues.**

See Table 2-1, Headaches, pp. 60–63.

Subarachnoid hemorrhage and meningitis cause acute severe headaches. Tension and migraine headaches are the most common kinds of recurring headaches. Changing or progressively severe headaches increase the likelihood of tumor or other demonstrable organic cause.

Inquire specifically about associated nausea and vomiting and about neurologic symptoms. Explore the physical and emotional settings in which the headaches occur.

Nausea and vomiting are common with migraine but also occur with brain tumors.

Ask whether coughing, sneezing, or changing the position of the head affects the headache.

Such maneuvers may increase the pain of brain tumor and acute sinusitis.

THE EYES

"How is your vision?" and **"Have you had any trouble with your eyes?"** conveniently start your inquiry about ocular problems. If the patient has noted a visual disturbance,

Refractive errors most commonly explain gradual blurring. High blood sugar levels may cause blurring.

Has it started suddenly or gradually?	Sudden visual loss suggests retinal detachment, vitreous hemorrhage, or occlusion of the central retinal artery.
Is it troublesome only with close work or only at distances?	Difficulty with close work suggests hyperopia (farsightedness) or presbyopia (aging vision); with distances, myopia (nearsightedness).
Is the entire visual field blurred or only parts of it? Is the defect central or peripheral in the visual field, or does it involve only one side of it?	Slow central loss in nuclear cataract (p. 192), macular degeneration (p. 175); slow peripheral loss in open-angle glaucoma (p. 169); one-sided loss in hemianopsia and quadrantic defects (p. 188)
Are there specks in the vision or spots where the patient cannot see *(scotomas)?* **If so, do they move around in the visual field when the patient shifts gaze, or are they fixed?** **Does the patient wear glasses?**	Moving specks or strands suggest vitreous floaters; fixed defects (scotomas) suggest lesions in the retinas or visual pathways.
Continue with questions about *pain* **in or around the eyes,** *redness,* **and** *excessive tearing or watering.*	See Table 7-5, Red Eyes, p. 191.
Ask about double vision *(diplopia).* **If diplopia is present, find out whether the images are side-by-side (horizontal diplopia) or on top of each other (vertical diplopia).** One kind of horizontal diplopia is physiologic. Hold one finger upright about 6 inches in front of your face, a second at arm's length. When you focus on either finger, the image of the other is double. An occasional patient who notices this phenomenon can be reassured.	Diplopia indicates a weakness or paralysis of one or more extraocular muscles (pp. 152, 195, 556–561). Horizontal diplopia implicates the 3rd or 6th cranial nerve; vertical diplopia, the 3rd or 4th cranial nerve.

THE EARS

Opening questions for the ears are "How is your hearing?" and "Have you had any trouble with your ears?" If the patient has noticed a *hearing loss,* **does it involve one or both ears? Did it start suddenly or gradually? What are the associated symptoms, if any?**	See Table 7-17, Patterns of Hearing Loss, pp. 210–211.
Try to distinguish between two basic types of hearing impairment: conduction loss, which results from problems in the external or middle ear, and sensorineural loss, which results from problems in the inner ear, the cochlear nerve, or its central connections in the brain. **Two questions may be helpful here. Does the patient have special difficulty understanding people as they talk? What difference does a noisy environment make?**	Persons with sensorineural loss have particular trouble understanding speech, often complaining that others mumble. Noisy environments make it worse. In conduction loss, noisy environments may help.

Symptoms associated with hearing loss, such as earache or vertigo, help you to assess the likely causes. In addition, inquire specifically about medications that might contribute to the impairment and ask about sustained exposure to loud noise.

Medications include aminoglycosides, aspirin, quinine, furosemide, and others.

Infants with hearing loss or total deafness are usually suspected of such when their parents note a lack of response to their voices or to environmental sounds. Such concerns deserve thorough investigation. Toddlers with hearing loss often manifest this by a delay in the development of speech.

Tinnitus is a perceived sound that has no external stimulus. It is commonly heard as a musical ringing but may also be heard as a rushing or roaring noise. One or both ears may be involved. Tinnitus may accompany hearing loss of any kind and often remains unexplained. Occasionally popping sounds originate in the temporomandibular joint, or patients become aware of vascular noises from their own necks.

Tinnitus is a common symptom, increasing in frequency with age. When associated with hearing loss and vertigo it suggests Meniere's disease.

Vertigo refers to the false perception that either the patient or the environment is rotating or spinning. These sensations point primarily to a problem in the inner ear, the cochlear nerve, or its central connections in the brain.

See Table 2-2, Vertigo, p. 64.

Vertigo poses a great challenge to the interviewer. **"Are there times when you feel dizzy?" is an appropriate first question,** but patients often have great difficulty describing their sensations. Vertigo is frequently difficult to distinguish from (1) a sense of unsteadiness without the feeling of movement, (2) faintness or an impending loss of consciousness, and (3) a vague light-headedness. **Try to get the story without biasing it. You may need a multiple-choice question. Determine whether or not the patient has felt pulled to the ground or off to one side during the dizziness. Does a change in position alter or provoke the dizziness? Ask about nausea and vomiting, which typically accompany vertigo, and about other associated symptoms. Pay special attention to the timing and course of the problem.**

A feeling of being pulled suggests true vertigo.

Further symptoms relevant to the ears include

Discharge from the ear

Unusually soft wax, debris from inflammation or rash in the ear canal, or discharge through a perforated eardrum secondary to acute or chronic otitis media

Pain in the ear, or *earache*

Inquire about these in your usual manner.

Pain suggests a problem in the external or middle ear but may also be referred from other structures in the mouth, throat, or neck.

THE NOSE AND SINUSES

Rhinorrhea refers to a nasal discharge and is often associated with *nasal stuffiness,* a sense of obstruction. These symptoms frequently occur together with *sneezing,* watery eyes, and discomfort in the throat. *Itching* may also be felt in the eyes, nose, and throat. **Assess the chronology of the illness. Does it occur for a week or so, especially when common colds and related syndromes are prevalent, or does it occur seasonally when pollens are in the air? Is it associated with specific contacts or environments? What remedies has the patient used? for how long? and how well do they work?**

Causes include viral infections, allergic rhinitis ("hay fever"), and vasomotor rhinitis. Itching favors an allergic cause.

Relation to seasons or environmental contacts suggests allergy.

Excessive use of decongestants can worsen the symptoms.

Inquire about drugs that might cause stuffiness.

Oral contraceptives, reserpine, guanethidine, and alcohol

Are there other symptoms associated with the nasal ones, such as pain and tenderness in the face, local headache, or fever?

These together suggest sinusitis.

Is the patient's nasal stuffiness limited to one side? If so, you are dealing with a different set of possible problems that require careful physical examination.

Consider a deviated nasal septum, foreign body, or tumor.

Epistaxis means bleeding from the nose. The blood usually originates from the nose itself but may come from a paranasal sinus or the nasopharynx. There is usually no difficulty in getting a history of epistaxis. When the patient is lying down, however, or when the bleeding originates in posterior structures, blood may pass into the throat rather than out the nostrils. You must then differentiate it from coughing or regurgitating blood. **Try to determine the site of the bleeding, its severity, and associated symptoms. Is it a recurrent problem, and has there been easy bruising or bleeding elsewhere in the body?**

Local causes of epistaxis include trauma (especially nose-picking), inflammation, drying and crusting of the nasal mucosa, tumors, and foreign bodies.

Bleeding disorders may contribute to epistaxis.

THE MOUTH, THROAT, AND NECK

Bleeding from the gums is a common symptom, most often noted when brushing the teeth. **Inquire about local lesions and any tendency to bleed or bruise elsewhere.**

Most often caused by gingivitis (p. 216)

A sore tongue may be caused by local lesions as well as by general conditions.

Aphthous ulcers (p. 215); sore smooth tongue of nutritional deficiency (p. 218)

Sore throat is a frequent complaint, usually developing as part of an acute illness with other upper respiratory symptoms.

See Table 7-23, Abnormalities of the Pharynx (p. 219).

Hoarseness refers to an altered quality of the voice that is often described as husky, rough, or harsh. The pitch may be lower than before. Hoarseness most often results from disease of the larynx, but may also develop when

Overuse of the voice (as in cheering) and acute infections are the most likely causes.

extralaryngeal lesions press on the nerves that supply it. **Inquire about overuse of the voice, allergy, smoking or other inhaled irritants, and any associated symptoms. Distinguish between an acute and a chronic problem.** Hoarseness lasting two or more weeks usually makes visual examination of the larynx advisable.

Causes of chronic hoarseness include smoking, allergy, voice abuse, hypothyroidism, chronic infections such as tuberculosis, and tumors.

"Have you noticed any 'swollen glands' or lumps in your neck?" is a useful question, even though "glands" is not the proper technical term for lymph nodes. Ask about an enlarged thyroid gland or *goiter* (al-though symptoms of thyroid dysfunction will be discussed later in the chapter). You may also wish to include *pain or stiffness in the neck* here, but these are discussed with the musculoskeletal system.

Enlarged, tender lymph nodes commonly accompany pharyngitis. Increased, decreased, or normal thyroid function may accompany a goiter.

THE BREASTS

Questions about a woman's breasts may be included in the history or deferred to the physical examination. **Inquire about *pain or discomfort, lumps,* and any *discharge from the nipples.* Has the patient ever examined her own breasts? How often does she do it?** Approximately 50% of women have palpable lumps or nodularity in their breasts. Premenstrual enlargement and tenderness are common.

Lumps may be physiologic or pathologic. They include cysts, benign tumors, and cancers. See Table 10-3, Differentiation of Common Breast Nodules (p. 327).

THE CHEST

Pain or discomfort in the chest frequently raises concern about heart disease, but it commonly originates in other structures as well.

See Table 2-3, Chest Pain, pp. 66–67.

Chief among the sources of chest pain are:

The myocardium

Myocardial infarction, angina pectoris

The aorta

Dissecting aneurysm

The trachea and large bronchi

Tracheobronchitis

The parietal pleura

Pleurisy, pericarditis

The esophagus

Reflux esophagitis, esophageal spasm

The chest wall, including the musculoskeletal system and the skin

Costochondritis, herpes zoster

Extrathoracic structures, such as the neck, gallbladder, and stomach

Cervical arthritis, biliary colic

Lung tissue itself has no pain fibers, and if lung conditions such as pneumonia or pulmonary infarction cause pain, they usually do so by inflammation of the adjacent parietal pleura. Muscle strain produced by coughing may also be responsible. The pericardium has few pain fibers, and the pain of pericarditis usually arises from inflammation of adjacent parietal

Anxiety is the most common cause of chest pain in children. Among organic causes, costochondritis is most frequent.

pleura. Chest pain commonly accompanies anxiety but its mechanism remains obscure.

Your initial questions should be as broad as possible. "Do you have discomfort or unpleasant feelings in your chest?" As you proceed to get the full history, ask the patient to show you exactly where the discomfort is, and watch for any gestures used to describe it. Follow your usual style of questioning. All seven attributes of this symptom may be helpful in differentiating among the various causes of chest pain.

A clenched fist over the sternum suggests angina pectoris; a finger pointing to a small area "over my heart" suggests a noncardiac origin; a hand moving up and down from epigastrium to neck suggests heartburn.

Palpitations refer to an unpleasant awareness of the heartbeat. Patients report their sensations in various terms such as skipping, jumping, throbbing, racing, fluttering, pounding, or stopping of the heart. Palpitations may result from an irregular heartbeat, from rapid acceleration or slowing of the heart, or from increased forcefulness of cardiac contraction, but the perception also depends on patients' sensitivities to their own bodily sensations. Palpitations do not necessarily mean heart disease at all, and the most serious arrhythmias, such as ventricular tachycardia, often do not produce palpitations.

Transient skips and flipflops suggest premature contractions; persisting irregularity, atrial fibrillation. A rapid regular beating of sudden onset and cessation suggests paroxysmal tachycardia.

You may ask directly about palpitations, but if the patient does not understand your question, reword it. "Are you sometimes aware of your heartbeat? What is it like?" Ask the patient to show you how it feels by tapping out the rhythm with a hand or finger. Was it fast or slow? regular or irregular? How long did it last? If there was an episode of rapid heart action, did it start and stop suddenly or gradually?

See Tables 9-1 to 9-3 for the differentiation of selected heart rates and rhythms (pp. 293–296).

You may wish to teach selected patients how to make serial measurements of their pulse rates should they have further episodes.

A rapid regular rate of less than 120 per minute is usually sinus tachycardia.

Dyspnea refers to a nonpainful but uncomfortable awareness of breathing that is inappropriate to the circumstances. Only the patient can report dyspnea. An observer may notice abnormally rapid or deep breathing, but these cannot be equated with the subjective sensation. Dyspnea commonly results from cardiac or bronchopulmonary disease but also frequently accompanies anxiety.

See Table 2-4, Dyspnea, pp. 68–69.

Ask if the patient has had any difficulty in breathing. Dyspneic patients may describe shortness of breath, a smothering feeling, inability to get enough air, or difficulty in taking a deep enough breath. **Ask when the symptom occurs, at rest or with exercise, and how much effort produces it.** Because of variations in age, body weight, and physical fitness there is no absolute scale on which to quantify dyspnea, but **try to determine its severity according to the patient's everyday activities. How many steps can the patient climb without pausing for breath? or how many flights of stairs? How about work? carrying the groceries? mop-**

Episodic dyspnea that occurs at rest as well as with exercise suggests anxiety with hyperventilation. Such patients often report that they cannot get a deep enough breath. Deep sighs are frequently observed.

ping the floor or making a bed? Has the symptom altered the patient's activities? How? Qualitative descriptions are not often helpful in assessing the nature of dyspnea, but carefully determine the timing, setting, associated symptoms, and factors that aggravate it or relieve it.**

Orthopnea is dyspnea that occurs lying down and improves when sitting up. It is classically quantified according to the number of pillows on which the patient sleeps, or the fact that the patient prefers to sleep sitting up. There are traps, however, in this evaluation. Be sure the patient uses the extra pillows or sleeps in a sitting position because of dyspnea, not for other reasons such as habit.

Orthopnea suggests left ventricular failure or mitral stenosis but may also accompany obstructive lung disease.

Paroxysmal nocturnal dyspnea describes episodes of sudden dyspnea and orthopnea that waken a patient from sleep, usually one or two hours after going to bed. The patient typically sits up, stands up, or goes to a window for air. Wheezing and cough may be associated. The episode usually subsides spontaneously but may recur at about the same time on subsequent nights.

Paroxysmal nocturnal dyspnea suggests left ventricular failure or mitral stenosis and may be mimicked by nocturnal asthmatic attacks.

Wheezes refer to musical respiratory sounds that may be audible both to the patient and to others.

Wheezing suggests partial airway obstruction.

Edema refers to the accumulation of excessive fluid in the interstitial spaces, and appears as swelling. Although questions about edema are typically included in the chest history, it has many other causes and may signify local problems as well as more general ones. **Focus your questions on the distribution and timing of the swelling, and explore the associated symptoms and the setting in which it occurs. "Have you had any swelling anywhere? Where? . . . anywhere else? When does it occur? Is it worse in the morning or at night? Do your shoes get tight? Do the rings on your fingers get too tight? Are your eyelids puffy or swollen in the morning? Have you had to let your belt out? Have your clothes gotten too tight around your middle?"** Because several liters of extra fluid may accumulate in a person's body before overt edema appears, it is useful to ask the patient who tends to retain fluid to record daily morning weights.

See Table 15-3, Mechanisms and Patterns of Edema, pp. 422–423.

Dependent edema refers to edema in the lowest body parts, usually the feet and legs. Consider peripheral, cardiac, and other causes. Puffy eyelids and tight rings, when associated with edema elsewhere, suggest renal disease or hypoalbuminemia. An enlarged waistline may indicate *ascites* (fluid in the peritoneal cavity), but may also simply be fat.

Cough is a frequent symptom that varies in significance from the trivial to the ominous. A person may cough voluntarily, but more typically cough is a reflex response to stimuli that irritate receptors in the larynx, trachea, or large bronchi. These stimuli include both external agents such as irritating dusts, foreign bodies, and even extremely hot or cold air, and internal substances such as mucus, pus, and blood. Inflammation of the respiratory mucosa, and pressure or tension on the air passages as from a tumor or enlarged peribronchial lymph node, may also cause coughing. Although cough typically signals a problem in the respiratory tract, the underlying cause may also be cardiovascular.

See Table 2-5, Cough, p. 70.

Cough is an important symptom of left-sided heart failure.

"Do you have a cough?" may be an adequate opening question, but for some patients, especially those who smoke, a morning cough has be-

come so habitual that they fail to mention it. Further questions here are "Do you have to clear your throat in the morning?" and "Do you have a cigarette cough?" Determine the timing of the cough. Is it a new symptom or more chronic? How frequent is it? When does it occur? Is it seasonal? Are there factors that seem to precipitate or aggravate it? Has a chronic cough changed in any way?

Assess the cough qualitatively by whether it is dry or productive of *sputum* (phlegm). Because some patients, especially women, may swallow their sputum, you may have difficulty here. If possible, however, try to get a description of the volume of the sputum and its color, odor, and consistency. Many patients have difficulty in describing the volume of their sputum. A multiple-choice question may be helpful in eliciting a rough estimate. "How much do you think you cough up in 24 hours: a teaspoon, tablespoon, quarter cup, half cup, cupful, or what?" If the patient coughs in your presence, offer a tissue and ask the patient to cough any phlegm into it so that you can inspect it. A specimen from deep in the chest is desirable. **Symptoms associated with the cough often lead you to its cause.**

Mucoid sputum is translucent, white, or gray. Purulent sputum is yellowish or greenish. Mucopurulent sputum has components of both. Large volumes of purulent sputum suggest bronchiectasis or lung abscess.

Hemoptysis refers to the coughing or "spitting up" of blood, which may vary from blood-streaked phlegm to pure blood. **Ask if the patient has ever coughed up either of these. Assess the volume of blood produced together with other attributes of the sputum. Focus your further questions on the setting in which the hemoptysis occurred and the associated symptoms.**

See Table 2-6, Hemoptysis, pp. 71–72. Hemoptysis is a rare and usually terminal event in infants, children, and adolescents, seen most often in older children with cystic fibrosis.

Before labelling this symptom you should try to determine by history and examination the origin of the bleeding. If the blood or blood-streaked material appears without coughing, it may originate in the mouth or pharynx. If it is vomited rather than coughed it probably originates in the gastrointestinal tract. Blood from either the nasopharynx or gastrointestinal tract, however, is occasionally aspirated and then coughed out.

Blood originating in the stomach is usually darker than that from the respiratory tract and may be mixed with food particles.

THE GASTROINTESTINAL TRACT

Dysphagia refers to difficulty in swallowing, the sense that food or liquid is sticking, hesitating, or "won't go down right." Although pain may be associated with dysphagia, the term itself does not imply pain. The sensation of a lump in the throat or in the retrosternal area, unassociated with swallowing, is not true dysphagia. Dysphagia may result from disorders of the mouth and pharynx that interfere with the early phases of swallowing, but difficulties at a lower level point to a disorder of the esophagus.

See Table 2-7, Dysphagia, p. 73.

Ask the patient to show you where the dysphagia is felt.

Where dysphagia is felt may suggest the location of an esophageal lesion, but disorders of the lower esophagus may cause symptoms higher up.

Timing is helpful in assessing dysphagia. When did it start? Is it intermittent or persistent? Is it progressing, and if so, how quickly?

Determine what precipitates it: relatively solid foods such as meat, softer foods such as ground meat and mashed potatoes, or hot or cold liquids. Has the pattern changed? What are the associated symptoms and medical conditions?

Dysphagia with solid foods but not liquids suggests a mechanical narrowing of the esophagus; dysphagia especially related to swallowing cold liquids suggests a disorder of esophageal muscle.

Indigestion is a common complaint that generally refers to distress associated with eating, but people use the term for many different symptoms. Find out just what your patient means. Possibilities include:

1. *Heartburn,* a sense of burning or warmth that is felt retrosternally and may radiate from the epigastrium to the neck. It has nothing to do with the heart. When severe, however, it may raise the question of heart disease, in both your mind and that of the patient. Pay particular attention to what brings it on and what relieves it.

Heartburn points to reflux of gastric acid into the esophagus and is often precipitated by a heavy meal, lying down, or bending forward. Ingested alcohol, citrus juices, or aspirin may also cause it. When it is chronic, consider reflux esophagitis. See Table 2-3, Chest Pain, pp. 66–67.

2. *Excessive gas,* as manifested by frequent belching, abdominal bloating or distention, or flatus (the passage of gas by rectum). Inquire about specific foods that seem to produce these symptoms. Start with open-ended questions here, but be sure to discover any relationship to the ingestion of milk or milk products. (A deficiency of intestinal lactase commonly causes gaseousness after the ingestion of milk or milk products.) A normal person passes roughly 600 ml of gas per rectum daily.

Swallowing air (aerophagia) is the normal cause of belching but does not cause bloating or excessive flatus. Consider instead gas-producing foods such as legumes, deficiency of intestinal lactase, and irritable bowel syndrome.

3. Unpleasant *abdominal fullness after meals* of normal size or *inability to eat a full meal*

Causes include anticholinergic drugs, obstruction of the gastric outlet, gastric cancer, and gastroparesis (a complication of diabetes mellitus).

4. *Abdominal pain*

5. *Nausea and vomiting*

In order to approach the problem of *abdominal pain,* you should understand its possible mechanisms and clinical patterns. There are three broad categories.

1. *Visceral pain* originates in the abdominal organs. Hollow structures such as the intestine or biliary tree may become painful when they contract unusually forcefully or when they are distended or stretched. Solid organs such as the liver become painful when their capsules are stretched. Visceral pain is rather poorly localized but is typically,

though not necessarily, felt near the midline, at levels that vary according to the structure involved, as illustrated below.

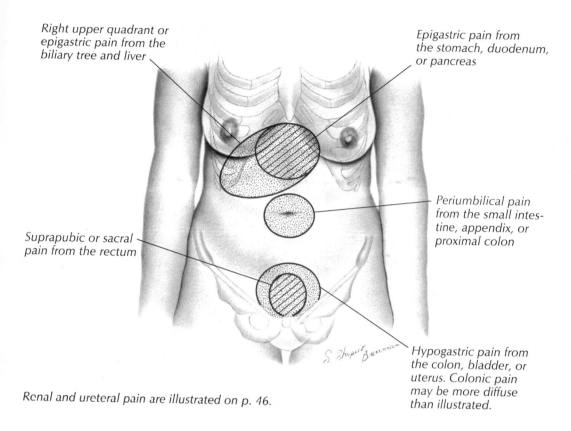

Right upper quadrant or epigastric pain from the biliary tree and liver

Epigastric pain from the stomach, duodenum, or pancreas

Periumbilical pain from the small intestine, appendix, or proximal colon

Suprapubic or sacral pain from the rectum

Hypogastric pain from the colon, bladder, or uterus. Colonic pain may be more diffuse than illustrated.

Renal and ureteral pain are illustrated on p. 46.

Visceral pain varies in quality and may be gnawing, burning, cramping, or aching. When it becomes severe, it may be associated with sweating, pallor, nausea, vomiting, and restlessness.

Acute appendicitis exemplifies both visceral and parietal pain. Early distention of the inflamed appendix produces periumbilical pain, which is gradually replaced by right lower quadrant pain due to inflammation of the adjacent parietal peritoneum.

2. *Parietal pain* originates in the parietal peritoneum and is caused by inflammation. It is a steady, aching pain that is usually more severe than visceral pain and more precisely localized over the involved structure. It is typically aggravated by movement or coughing, and patients with this kind of pain usually prefer to lie still.

3. *Referred pain* is felt in more distant sites that are innervated at approximately the same spinal levels as the disordered structure. Referred pain often develops as the initial pain becomes more intense and thus seems to radiate or travel from the initial site. It may be felt superficially or more deeply, but is usually well localized.

Pain of duodenal or pancreatic origin may be referred to the back; pain from the biliary tree may be referred to the right shoulder or the right posterior chest.

Pain not only may be referred from abdominal organs to nonabdominal sites; it may also be referred to the abdomen from the chest, spine, or pelvis, thus complicating the assessment of abdominal pain.

The pain of pleurisy or acute myocardial infarction may be referred to the upper abdomen.

After you get the history of abdominal pain in the patient's own words, ask the patient to show you just where it is. If clothes intervene, repeat

See Table 2-8, Abdominal Pain, pp. 74–75.

the question during your examination. **Where does the pain start? Does it travel anywhere?**

What is the pain like? If the patient has trouble describing it, try a multiple-choice question. "Is it aching, cramping, burning, gnawing, or what?"

Cramping (colicky) pain suggests a relationship to peristalsis.

How severe is the pain? Is it bearable? Does it interfere with the patient's usual activities? Does it make the patient lie down? Severity of the pain may tell you something about the patient's responses to pain and its impact on the patient's life, but it is not consistently helpful in assessing cause. Sensitivity to abdominal pain varies widely among people and tends to diminish over the later years, thus masking acute abdominal problems in the elderly, especially those in or beyond their 70s.

Careful timing of the pain, on the other hand, is particularly helpful. Did it start suddenly or gradually? When did the pain begin? How long does it last? What is its pattern over a 24-hour period? over the weeks and months? Are you dealing with an acute illness or a chronic or recurring one?

What aggravates or relieves the pain, with special reference to eating, antacids, alcohol, medications (including aspirin-containing and other over-the-counter drugs), emotional factors, and possibly posture? Is the pain related to bodily functions such as defecation, menstruation, and urination?

Citrus fruits may aggravate the pain of reflux esophagitis. Abdominal discomfort with milk ingestion suggests lactase deficiency.

What symptoms are associated with the pain, and in what sequence do they occur?

"How is your appetite?" continues the gastrointestinal history but may also lead into other important areas. *Anorexia* refers to the loss or lack of appetite. Distinguish it from intolerance to certain foods or reluctance to eat anything because of anticipated discomfort. *Nausea*, which patients often describe as "feeling sick to my stomach," may progress to retching and vomiting. *Retching* describes the spasmodic movements of the chest and diaphragm that precede and culminate in *vomiting*—the forceful expulsion of gastric contents out through the mouth.

Anorexia, nausea, and vomiting accompany gastrointestinal disorders and many other conditions such as pregnancy, responses to prescribed or other drugs, diabetic acidosis, adrenal insufficiency, hypercalcemia, uremia, liver disease, emotional states, and (though without nausea) anorexia/bulimia nervosa.

Regurgitation, the raising of esophageal or gastric contents in the absence of nausea or retching, has implications quite different from vomiting.

Regurgitation may occur when the esophagus is narrowed or when the gastroesophageal sphincter is incompetent.

Assess these symptoms in the usual manner. Ask about any vomitus or regurgitated material, and inspect it yourself if possible. What color is it? What does the vomitus smell like? How much has there been? Ask specifically about blood in the vomitus and try to estimate its amount.

Gastric juice is clear or mucoid. Small amounts of yellowish or greenish bile are common and have no special significance. Brownish or blackish vomitus with small particles that look like coffee grounds suggests blood that has been altered by gastric acid. Either this (when confirmed by chemical testing) or red blood is termed *hematemesis.*

Common causes of hematemesis include duodenal or gastric ulcer, esophageal or gastric varices, and gastritis. A fecal odor suggests obstruction of the ileum or a gastrocolic fistula.

Do the symptoms or setting suggest the complications of vomiting, such as aspiration into the lungs (especially in elderly, debilitated, or obtunded patients), dehydration and electrolyte imbalance (after prolonged vomiting), or significant loss of blood?

Symptoms of blood loss (light-headedness, faintness, syncope) depend on the rate and volume of bleeding and rarely appear before 500 ml or more are lost.

To assess *bowel function,* start with some open-ended questions: "How are your bowel movements? How often do you move your bowels? Do you have any difficulties? Has there been any change in your bowel habits?" The frequency of bowel movements varies in normal adults from about three times a day to twice a week. Changes within these limits, however, may be very significant in an individual patient.

When asking details about the appearance of the stools, it may be helpful to find out if the patient looks at them. You may thus avoid being misled by confusing or negative responses.

Inquire about the color of the stools and ask about any *black stools* (suggesting *melena*) or *red blood in the stools.* If either condition is present, how long has the patient noticed it? How often? If the patient has seen red blood, how much is there? Is it pure blood, mixed in with the stool, or on the surface of it? Is there blood on the toilet paper?

See Table 2-9, Black and Bloody Stools, p. 76.

Patients vary widely in their concepts of constipation and diarrhea. **When a person complains of either symptom, determine his or her meaning of the term. What is the *constipation* like: a decrease in the frequency of bowel movements? the passage of hard and perhaps painful stools? the need to strain unusually hard? a sense of incomplete defecation or pressure in the rectum? What do the stools look like? What remedies has the patient tried? Explore the setting in which the constipation has occurred, with particular reference to medications, emotional stress, the person's ideas of normal bowel habits, and the time and conditions available for defecation.** Occasionally constipation becomes complete, with passage of neither feces nor gas. This is termed *obstipation.*

See Table 2-10, Constipation, p. 77.

Obstipation occurs in intestinal obstruction.

Diarrhea refers to the passage of excessively frequent stools that are usually unformed or watery.

Consistently large diarrheal stools suggest a disorder in the small bowel or proximal colon; small, frequent stools with urgency to pass them suggest a disorder of the left colon or rectum.

Try to determine the size or the volume of the stools as well as their frequency. Are they bulky or small? How often must the patient go to the toilet to pass them?

What are the stools like qualitatively? Are they mushy or watery? What color are they? Do they look greasy or oily? frothy? Do they smell unusually foul? Is mucus, pus, or blood associated?

Large, yellowish or gray, greasy, foul-smelling, and sometimes frothy stools suggest steatorrhea (fatty stools), associated with malabsorption.

Assess the course of the diarrhea over time. Is it acute, chronic, or recurrent? Remember, however, that your patient may be experiencing the first acute episode in a chronic or recurrent illness.

See Table 2-11, Acute Diarrhea (pp. 78–79), and Table 2-12, Chronic and Recurrent Diarrhea (pp. 80–81).

Does diarrhea waken the patient at night?

Nocturnal diarrhea suggests an organic cause.

What seems to aggravate and relieve the diarrhea? Does the patient get relief from a bowel movement, or is there an intense urge, with straining, but little or no result *(tenesmus)*?

Relief by moving the bowels or passing gas suggests a disorder in the left colon or rectum. Tenesmus suggests a problem in the rectum near the anal sphincter.

In what setting has the diarrhea occurred, including travel, emotional stress, or a new medication? Do family members or companions have similar symptoms?

What are the associated symptoms? Does fecal soiling accompany the diarrhea?

In adults, fecal soiling suggests an organic cause.

Jaundice, or icterus, refers to the yellowish discoloration of the skin and eyes by an increased amount of bilirubin, a bile pigment derived chiefly from the breakdown of hemoglobin. Normally liver cells take up this bilirubin, conjugate (or combine) it with other substances so that it becomes water soluble, and then excrete it into the bile. Bile passes normally through the biliary tree into the small intestine. Mechanisms of jaundice include:

Bilirubin in the blood is predominantly unconjugated in jaundice due to any of the first three mechanisms. Causes include hemolytic anemia (increased production) and Gilbert's syndrome.

1. Increased production of bilirubin
2. Decreased uptake of bilirubin by the liver cells
3. Decreased ability of the liver to conjugate the bilirubin, and
4. Decreased excretion of bilirubin into the bile with resulting escape of some bilirubin, now in its conjugated form, back into the blood. The cause may lie *within the liver itself,* as

   a. Hepatocellular jaundice, due to damage to the liver cells, or as
   b. Cholestatic jaundice, a more selective excretory impairment due to damage of liver cells or to damage of intrahepatic bile ducts.

When excretion of bilirubin is impaired, the bilirubin in the blood is predominantly conjugated. Causes include:
   a. Viral hepatitis, cirrhosis
   b. Drug-induced cholestasis (oral contraceptives, methyl testosterone, chlorpromazine) or primary biliary cirrhosis

Alternatively, the cause may lie in *obstruction of the extrahepatic bile ducts.*

Obstruction of the common bile duct by gallstones or cancer of the pancreas

As you interview the jaundiced patient, pay special attention to the associated symptoms and the setting in which the illness occurred.

What color was the urine as the patient became ill? and now? When conjugated bilirubin increases in the blood it may appear in the urine, darkening it into a yellowish brown or tea-like color. Unconjugated bilirubin is not excreted in the urine.

Dark urine stained by bilirubin indicates impaired excretion of bilirubin.

How about the color of the stools? When excretion of bile into the intestine is completely obstructed, the stools become light-colored and gray (or *acholic,* **without bile).**

Acholic stools may occur briefly in viral hepatitis and are common in obstructive jaundice.

Does the skin itch without other obvious explanation?

Itching favors cholestatic or obstructive jaundice.

Is there associated pain? What is its pattern? Have there been past and repeated attacks of pain?

Consider the aching pain of a distended liver capsule; the persistent pain of pancreatic cancer; and episodes of biliary colic.

Are there factors in the patient's setting that increase the risks of liver disease, such as

1. **Hepatitis: travel in areas of poor sanitation, known contacts with jaundiced persons, sexual contacts with carriers of hepatitis B, ingestion of raw clams or oysters, use of inadequately sterilized needles or syringes (as in drug addiction), treatment with blood transfusions or blood products or exposure to them (as in laboratories, dental offices, or dialysis units)**

2. **Cirrhosis and other alcohol-related liver disease. (Interview the patient carefully about the consumption of alcohol.)**

3. **Toxic liver damage, as produced by medications and industrial exposure**

4. **Gallbladder disease or gallbladder surgery that might have contributed to extrahepatic biliary obstruction**

5. **Hereditary disorders (Review the family history.)**

THE URINARY TRACT

Disorders of the urinary tract may cause pain in either the back or the abdomen. *Kidney pain* is felt at or below the costal margin posteriorly, near the costovertebral angle. It may radiate anteriorly toward the umbilicus.

Kidney pain occurs in acute pylonephritis.

Kidney pain is a visceral pain that is usually produced by sudden distention of the renal capsule and is typically dull, aching, and steady. Dramatically different is *ureteral pain (ureteral or renal colic),* a severe colicky pain that often originates in the costovertebral angle and radiates around the trunk into the lower quadrant of the abdomen and possibly on into the upper thigh and testicle or labium. Ureteral pain results from sudden distention of the ureter and associated distention of the renal pelvis.

Renal or ureteral colic is caused by sudden obstruction of a ureter, as by urinary stones or blood clots.

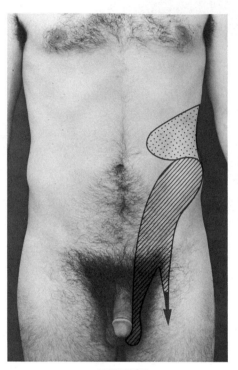
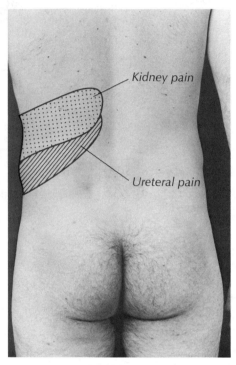

ANTERIOR   **POSTERIOR**

Bladder disorders may cause suprapubic pain. Pain associated with bladder infection, if present at all in the abdomen, is typically dull and steady. Pain associated with sudden overdistention of the bladder is often agonizing, while chronic bladder distention is usually painless. *Prostatic pain* is felt in the perineum and occasionally in the rectum.

Pain of sudden overdistention in acute urinary retention

*Pain on urination** accompanies inflammation or irritation of either the bladder or the urethra and is usually felt as a burning sensation. Men typically feel it in or proximal to the glans penis, while women perceive it in one of two ways: as an internal urethral discomfort, sometimes described as pressure, or as an external burning caused by urine as it flows across irritated or inflamed labia.

Cystitis and urethritis commonly cause painful urination. Consider also stones, foreign bodies or tumors in the bladder, and acute prostatitis.

Internal burning suggests cystitis or urethritis; external burning, vulvovaginitis.

---

* Clinicians often refer to painful urination as *dysuria.* Some authorities, however, prefer to define dysuria as any difficulty in voiding.

Several symptoms other than pain may accompany voiding. *Urinary urgency* is an unusually intense and immediate desire to void. It sometimes leads to involuntary voiding *(urge incontinence)*. In a man with partial obstruction to urinary outflow from the bladder, a cluster of symptoms often develops together: *hesitancy* in starting the urinary stream, *straining* to void, *reduced caliber and force of the urinary stream,* and *dribbling* as he tries to complete the voiding process.

Urinary urgency suggests infection or irritation of the bladder. In men pain on urination without frequency or urgency suggests urethritis.

The most common cause of obstruction to urinary outflow is prostatic enlargement. A urethral stricture may also cause it.

Three terms describe important alterations in the patterns of voiding urine. *Polyuria* refers to a significant increase in 24-hour urinary volume, roughly defined as exceeding 3 liters. It must be distinguished from *urinary frequency*, abnormally frequent voiding. Although urinary frequency may be secondary to polyuria and is then associated with a high volume of urine with each voiding, frequency is often associated instead with relatively small volumes at each passage. *Nocturia* refers to urinary frequency at night, sometimes defined as when the bladder wakens the patient more than once. A change in nocturnal voiding patterns as well as the number of trips to the toilet should be considered in assessing this symptom. Like frequency itself, nocturia may be associated with large or small volumes of urine. *Polydipsia* is an abnormally high intake of water or other fluids and is commonly associated with polyuria.

Polyuria indicates an abnormally high production of urine by the kidneys. Frequency without polyuria (during the day or night) suggests either a disorder of the urinary bladder or impairment to flow at or below the bladder neck.

See Table 2-13, Polyuria, Frequency, and Nocturia, pp. 82–83.

Blood in the urine is an important symptom known as *hematuria* but is often identified only by urinalysis. When visible to the naked eye it is called *gross hematuria.* Blood may give the urine a pinkish or brownish cast or in larger amounts may make it look frankly bloody. Be sure not to mistake menstrual bleeding for hematuria. If urine is reddish, inquire about the ingestion of beets or medications that sometimes discolor the urine. Test the urine with dipstick and microscopic examination before settling on the term hematuria.

Causes of hematuria include cystitis, malignancy of the bladder or kidney stones, and acute glomerulonephritis. Bilirubin, among other endogenous substances, may discolor the urine.

Drugs that discolor the urine include phenolphthalein (common in over-the-counter laxatives) and phenazopyridine (Pyridium).

Urinary incontinence refers to an involuntary loss of urine that has become a social or hygienic problem. It usually points to a disorder in the urinary bladder or urethra, in the structures that support or surround them, or in the neural regulatory mechanisms that control urination.

The normal adult bladder is a hollow muscular organ that can expand to accommodate roughly 300 ml of urine at relatively low pressures. As distention continues it stimulates the smooth muscle of the bladder (the detrusor muscle) to contract, pressure in the bladder rises, and the urge to

Incontinence may result when detrusor contractions are too strong *(urge incontinence)*, when intraurethral pressure is too low

void becomes conscious. If the setting is inconvenient for voiding, higher centers in the brain can inhibit detrusor contractions until the normal bladder capacity of 400 ml to 500 ml is reached. Pressure within the urethra that exceeds that in the bladder holds the accumulating urine within the bladder reservoir and prevents incontinence. Factors contributing to intraurethral pressure include smooth muscle in the urethra (the internal urethral sphincter), the thickness of normal urethral mucosa, and, in women, sufficient muscular support of the bladder and proximal urethra to maintain the proper geometric relations between them. Striated muscle around the urethra can contract voluntarily to interrupt the voiding process.

(stress incontinence), and when the bladder is grossly enlarged because of outlet obstruction *(overflow incontinence)*. Incontinence may also be due to poor general health, to environmental factors *(functional incontinence)*, or to medications. See Table 2-14, Urinary Incontinence, pp. 84–85.

Neuroregulatory control of the bladder functions at several levels. In an infant the bladder empties by a reflex mechanism at the sacral level of the spinal cord. Adult voluntary control of urination depends also on higher centers within the brain and on motor and sensory pathways between the brain and the sacral cord.

General questions for a urinary history include: "Do you have any difficulty passing your urine? How often do you go? Do you get up at night to go? How often? How much do you pass at a time? Is there any pain or burning? Do you have to go so badly that you sometimes have trouble getting to the toilet in time? Do you ever leak any urine? . . . or wet yourself?" If the patient has been incontinent, ask when it happens and how often. Can the patient sense when the bladder is full? and when voiding occurs? Ask women specifically if sudden coughing, sneezing, or laughing makes them lose urine *(stress incontinence)*. Roughly half of even young women who have not borne children report this experience.

Unawareness of a full bladder or of wetness suggests a sensory or mental deficit.

Occasional leakage of small amounts of urine is not necessarily significant.

What color is the urine? Has it ever been reddish, or brownish? If it seems relevant inquire about pain in the abdomen or back, but in the absence of urinary symptoms you may prefer to cover these topics in your gastrointestinal and musculoskeletal histories.

Ask additional questions of middle-aged or elderly men. "Do you have trouble getting your stream started? Do you have to stand closer to the toilet than you used to? Have you noticed a change in the force or size of your stream? Do you have to strain down in order to void? Do you hesitate or stop in the middle of voiding? Do you dribble after you're through?"

The most common cause of these symptoms is obstruction of the bladder outlet due to prostatic hypertrophy.

THE GENITOREPRODUCTIVE SYSTEM — FEMALE

Questions in this section focus on menstruation, pregnancy and related topics, vulvovaginal symptoms, and sexual functions.

For the menstrual history ask the patient how old she was when her monthly, or menstrual, periods began (age at *menarche*). When did her last period start, and if possible, the one before that? How often do the periods come (as measured by the first day of successive periods)? How regular or irregular are they? How long do they last? How heavy is the flow? What color is it? Flow can be roughly assessed by the number of pads or tampons used daily. Because women vary in their assessments of when sanitary equipment should be changed, however, ask the patient whether she usually soaks a pad or tampon, spots it lightly, or what. Further, does she use more than one at a time? Does she have any bleeding between periods? any bleeding after intercourse or after douching?

The dates of previous periods may alert you to possible pregnancy or menstrual irregularities.

Unlike the normal dark red menstrual discharge, excessive flow tends to be bright red and may include "clots" (not true fibrin clots).

Does the patient have any discomfort or pain before or during her periods? If so, what is it like, how long does it last, and does it interfere with her usual activities? Are other symptoms associated? Ask a middle-aged or older woman if she has stopped menstruating. When? Did any symptoms accompany her change? Has she had any bleeding since?

Questions about menarche, menstruation, and menopause may give you excellent opportunities to explore the patient's need for information, her self-image, and her attitude toward her body. When talking with an adolescent girl, for example, opening questions might include: "How did you first learn about monthly periods? How did you feel when they started? Many girls worry when their periods aren't regular or come late. Has anything like that bothered you?" For a middle-aged woman, "How did (do) you feel about not having your periods any more? Has it affected your life in any way?"

Girls in the United States usually begin to menstruate between the ages of 9 and 16 years and often take a year or more before they settle into a reasonably regular pattern. Age at menarche varies with several factors. One is the age at which women in the adolescent's parents' families began to menstruate. Another is race: white girls on the average have earlier menarches than black girls. A third is nutritional status: well nourished girls start to menstruate earlier than those who are poorly nourished. The interval between periods ranges roughly from 24 to 32 days; the flow lasts from 3 to 7 days.

Amenorrhea refers to the absence of periods. Failure to initiate periods is called *primary amenorrhea,* while the cessation of periods after they have been established is termed *secondary amenorrhea.* Pregnancy, lactation, and menopause are physiologic forms of the secondary type. *Oligomenorrhea* refers to infrequent periods, which may also be irregular. This pattern is common for as long as 2 years after menarche and it also occurs before menopause.

Other causes of secondary amenorrhea include low body weight from any cause including malnutrition and anorexia nervosa; stress; chronic illness; and hypothalamic–pituitary–ovarian dysfunctions.

Polymenorrhea means abnormally frequent periods, and *menorrhagia* refers to an increased amount or duration of flow. Bleeding may also occur

Increased frequency, increased flow, or bleeding between

between periods (variously termed *metrorrhagia* or *intermenstrual bleeding*), after intercourse *(postcoital bleeding)*, or after other vaginal contact such as occurs with douches.

Menopause, the cessation of menses, usually occurs between the ages of 45 and 52 years, but the range of normal is wider. *Postmenopausal bleeding* is defined as bleeding that occurs after 6 months without periods. The only symptoms clearly associated with menopause are *hot flushes* (or *flashes*), the sweating associated with them, and sometimes the disturbance of sleep that they may cause.

Dysmenorrhea refers to pain with menstruation and is usually felt as a bearing down, aching, or cramping sensation in the lower abdomen and pelvis. The *premenstrual tension syndrome* (PMS) refers to several symptoms noted by some women during the 4 to 10 days before a period. These include tension, nervousness, irritability, depression, and mood swings; weight gain, abdominal bloating, edema, and tenderness of the breasts; and headaches. Though usually mild, the symptoms may be severe and disabling.

Standard questions related to pregnancies include: "Have you ever been (or how often have you been) pregnant? Have you ever had a miscarriage or an abortion? How often? How many living children do you have?" Inquire about any difficulties with the pregnancies and the timing and circumstances of any abortion (spontaneous or induced). What kind of birth control methods, if any, have the patient and her partner used, and how satisfied is she with them?

If amenorrhea suggests a pregnancy now, inquire about its possibility (history of intercourse) and about common early symptoms: tenderness, tingling, or increased size of the breasts; urinary frequency; nausea and vomiting; easy fatigability; and feelings that the baby is moving (the last usually noted at about 20 weeks). Be alert to the patient's feelings in discussing all these topics and explore them as seems indicated.

The most common vulvovaginal symptoms are *vaginal discharge* and local *itching.* **Follow your usual approach, inquiring about the amount, color, consistency, and odor of any discharge. Ask too about any local *sores* or *lumps* in the vulvar area. Are they painful or not? Because patients vary in their understanding of anatomic terms here, be prepared with some alternative phrasing: "Any itching (or other symptom) near your vagina? . . . between your legs? . . . in your privates?"**

Local symptoms or findings on physical examination may raise the possibility of sexually transmitted diseases. After establishing the

periods may have organic causes or may be dysfunctional. Postcoital bleeding suggests cervical disease (*e.g.,* polyps, cancer) or, in an older woman, atrophic vaginitis.

Postmenopausal bleeding raises the question of endometrial cancer, although it also has other causes.

Amenorrhea followed by heavy bleeding suggests a threatened abortion or dysfunctional uterine bleeding related to lack of ovulation.

See Table 13-4, Inflammations of and Around the Vagina, pp. 392–393.

See Table 13-1, Lesions of the Vulva, p. 388.

usual attributes of any symptoms, inquire about sexual contacts and past history of venereal disease. "Have you ever had herpes? . . . any other problems such as gonorrhea? . . . syphilis? . . . VD? . . . pelvic infections? Are you sexually active? When was the last time you had sexual contact? How many partners have you had in the past two months?"

With these questions, or elsewhere during the interview, you may have already learned a fair amount about the patient's sexual history. If not, a few screening questions are helpful. **"Are you aware of any specific problems in the area of sexuality? For example, have you maintained an interest in (appetite for) sex? Are you able to reach a climax (reach an orgasm or 'come')? Is it important for you to reach a climax? Do you get sexually aroused? Do you lubricate easily (get wet)? Do you stay too dry? Are you satisfied with your sex life as it is now? Has there been any significant change in the last few years? Are you satisfied with your ability to perform sexually? How satisfied do you think your partner is? Do you feel that your partner is satisfied with the frequency of sexual activity?"**

Sexual dysfunction can be classified according to the phase of sexual response: desire, arousal, and orgasm. A woman may lack desire *(inhibited sexual desire)*, she may fail to become aroused and to attain adequate lubrication of her vagina *(inhibited sexual arousal)*, or she may be unable to reach orgasm much or all of the time *(orgasmic dysfunction)*.

In addition to ascertaining the nature of a sexual problem, ask about its onset, severity (persistent or sporadic), setting, and factors, if any, that make it better or worse. What does the patient think is the cause of the problem, what has she tried to do about it, and what does she hope for? The setting of a sexual dysfunction is an important but complicated topic, involving the patient's general health, medications and drugs including alcohol, her partner's and her own knowledge of sexual practices and techniques, her attitudes, values, and fears, the relationship and communication between her and her partner(s), and the environment in which sexual activity takes place.

Ask also about any discomfort or pain on intercourse *(dyspareunia)*. If present, try to localize the symptom. Is it near the outside, occurring at the start of intercourse, or does she feel it further in, when her partner's penis (or other objects) are pushing deeper? *Vaginismus* refers to an involuntary spasm of the muscles surrounding the vaginal orifice that makes penetration during intercourse painful or impossible.

Superficial pain suggests local inflammation, atrophic vaginitis, or inadequate lubrication; deeper pain may be due to pelvic disorders or pressure on a normal ovary. The cause of vaginismus may be physical or psychological.

THE GENITOREPRODUCTIVE SYSTEM — MALE

For men, questions about the genitoreproductive system follow naturally after those dealing with the urinary system. They focus on local symptoms and on sexual function.

Ask about any *discharge from the penis* or any staining of the underwear. If discharge is present, ascertain the amount, its color and consistency, and any associated symptoms. Inquire about *sores* or *growths on the penis* and any *swelling or pain in the scrotum*.

A penile discharge, often with pain on urination, suggests urethritis.

See Table 12-1, Abnormalities of the Penis (p. 368) and Table 12-2, Abnormalities in the Scrotum (pp. 369–370).

These symptoms raise the question of sexually transmitted diseases. **Ask about previous symptoms or a past history of venereal diseases such as herpes, gonorrhea, syphilis, or other problems. Has the patient been exposed to any of these conditions as far as he knows? If so, when? How often?**

Many skin conditions other than sexually transmitted diseases affect the genitalia, and a sexually transmitted disease may be present without symptoms or signs.

The risk of acquiring sexually transmitted diseases increases with the number of sexual partners. The kinds of diseases acquired and their localization within the body, moreover, depend upon the person's sexual practices. Inquiry into these practices is important, therefore, and helps you to focus your later questions and subsequent physical examination. **Start with open-ended questions that do not suggest particular assumptions about sexual practices or preferences. "Can you tell me something about your sexual activity? . . . how often you have sex? . . . your sexual partners? . . . which sexual act you engage in most often?" More directly, "When was your last sexual contact? How many partners have you had in the last two months?"** An explanatory statement may be useful in introducing more specific questions. **"Sexually transmitted diseases can involve any bodily opening where you have sex. It's important for you to tell me which openings you use." And further, as needed, "Do you have oral sex? . . . anal sex?" If the answers to these questions are affirmative, ask about symptoms such as diarrhea, rectal bleeding, anal itching or pain, and sore throat.**

Infections from oral–penile transmission include gonorrhea, *Chlamydia*, syphilis, and herpes. Symptomatic or asymptomatic proctitis caused by one or more microorganisms may follow anal intercourse.

Answers to these questions often clarify the patient's sexual preferences. **If not, "Have you been having sex with women, with men, or with both?" Particularly if the patient has been sexually active with other men, inquire about the acquired immune deficiency syndrome. "Have you had contact with anyone with AIDS? Do you have any concerns or questions about AIDS? Have you taken any precautions such as "safe sex" to avoid AIDS?"***

Inquire about sexual functioning, assessing each phase of the sexual response: desire, arousal, and orgasm. "Are you having any problems with sexual function?" Ask about the desire phase: "Have you maintained an interest in (appetite for) sex?"

To assess the arousal phase, ask, "Are you able to achieve and maintain an erection?" If there seems to be a problem here, ask the patient how

In an *erectile dysfunction* (impotence) a man cannot attain and

---

* "Safe sex," as currently defined, includes limiting the number of sexual partners and avoiding exposure to any of the partner's bodily fluids including blood, semen, saliva, urine, and feces. For further reading on taking a sexual history, see the bibliography.

firm the penis becomes. Is the problem constant or sporadic? Are there circumstances in which erection is normal: with other partners? on awakening during the night or in the morning? with masturbation? Were there any changes in his marriage or life situation at the time when the problem began?

maintain an erection sufficient for penetration. Causes are organic, psychogenic, or both. Consistent dysfunction in all circumstances favors an organic cause. Consider medications, other drugs, diabetes mellitus, arterial insufficiency, and neurologic problems.

Questions relating to ejaculation refer to the phase of orgasm. For ejaculation that is premature (too soon and out of control) ask "About how long does intercourse last? Do you come too soon? Do you feel you have any control over it? Do you think your partner would like intercourse to last longer?" For retarded ejaculations, "Do you sometimes find that you can't come (ejaculate, have an orgasm) even though your erection is all right?" Inquire about the frequency of the problem, medications, and other circumstances in which it developed.

Premature ejaculation is very common, especially in young men.

Retarded ejaculation is less common and usually affects middle-aged and older men. It may be psychogenic, organic, or both.

Further, "Are you satisfied with your sex life as it is now? Has there been any significant change over the last few years? How satisfied do you think your partner is? Do you feel that your partner is satisfied with the frequency of sexual activity?"

As with women, inquire about the onset, severity, and setting of any problem. What does the patient think has caused it, what has he tried to do about it, and what does he hope for?

Most if not all students, like many more experienced clinicians, feel uncomfortable about taking a sexual history. Patients, too, are often embarrassed or reticent, yet many feel relieved when given the chance to express their concerns. The screening questions serve to give patients permission to talk or ask questions if they wish to, but you should not press inquiries on a reluctant patient. Privacy and interpersonal trust are both essential to this interview.

The word "partner" (or "partners") avoids making assumptions about marriage and sexual preference. Listen to how the patient responds. Some men and women with homosexual preferences choose not to discuss them, while others are comfortable with the subject, like to have their special needs recognized, and resent a clinician's quick assumption that they are heterosexual. **In talking with patients whom you have seen before, you can invite a discussion of this and other sexual topics as follows: "Lately many patients have been raising questions about sexual function. Do you happen to have any sex-related questions?"** The patient may say "No," then reflect, and bring up the subject on the next visit.

THE PERIPHERAL VASCULAR SYSTEM

Pain in the arms and legs may arise from the skin, the peripheral vascular system, the musculoskeletal system, or the nervous system. In addition, visceral pain, such as that from myocardial infarction, may be referred to the extremities.

Symptoms associated with the pain often give clues to its vascular nature. *Swelling of the feet and legs*, for example, may signify venous disease, although it has many other causes, and *coldness* and *numbness* often accompany arterial disorders. The *redness, swelling,* and *tenderness* of local inflammation are seen in some vascular disorders as well as in other conditions that may mimic them. In contrast, relatively brief leg cramps that commonly occur at night in otherwise healthy people do not indicate a circulatory problem, and cold hands and feet are so common in healthy people that they have relatively little predictive value.

See Table 2-15, Painful Peripheral Vascular Disorders and Their Mimics, pp. 86–87. Local inflammation in superficial thrombophlebitis, lymphangitis, cellulitis, and erythema nodosum. The origin of the common leg cramp is poorly understood.

For most patients, inquiry about two symptoms suffices for screening: swelling of the feet and legs, and pain or discomfort in the legs. "Do your fingertips change color in the cold? How?" may also be useful.

Severe pallor of the fingers, often followed by cyanosis and then redness, indicates Raynaud's disease or phenomenon.

With middle-aged and older people you should also ask about *intermittent claudication*, a specific pattern of pain that accompanies impairment of arterial flow. "How far can you walk without stopping to rest?" is a good opening question. Then determine what makes the patient stop and how quickly relief is felt.

Aching, cramping, and possibly numbness or severe fatigue that appear with walking and disappear promptly with rest typify intermittent claudication.

THE MUSCULOSKELETAL SYSTEM

"Have you had any *pains in your joints?"* turns the interview explicitly to the musculoskeletal system. An affirmative answer to this question may indicate, however, a problem not only in the joints but also in bones, muscles, and tissues around the joints. **Either now or during the examination ask the patient to show you as clearly as possible where the pain is felt. Where did it start? What then?** Pain originating in the small joints of the hands and feet is more sharply localized than that from the larger joints. Pain from the hip joint is especially deceptive. Although it is typically felt in the groin or the buttock, it is sometimes felt in the anterior thigh or partly or solely in the knee.

Problems in tissues around joints include inflammation of bursae *(bursitis)*, tendons *(tendonitis)*, or tendon sheaths *(tenosynovitis)*, and stretching or tearing of ligaments *(sprains)*.

"Hip pain" felt near the greater trochanter of the femur suggests trochanteric bursitis.

Determine whether the pain has involved one joint or its adjacent tissues or whether several joints have been affected. If the latter, in what pattern has the involvement spread? Has the pain disappeared from the one or more joints initially involved only to migrate to others, or has the initial pain persisted while at the same time progressing to

Pain in only one joint suggests bursitis, tendonitis, monoarticular arthritis, or an injury. Rheumatic fever and early gonococcal arthritis have a migratory

other joints? Is the involvement symmetrical, affecting similar joints on both sides of the body?

pattern of spread; rheumatoid arthritis shows a progressive or additive pattern and is typically symmetrical.

Assess the quality and severity of the pain.

Timing is particularly important. Did the pain develop rapidly over the course of a few hours, or insidiously over weeks or even months? Has the course been one of slow progression, or have there been periods of improvement and worsening? How long has the pain lasted? What is it like over the course of a day? in the morning? and as the day wears on?

Unusually severe and rapidly developing pain in a swollen joint, not explained by injury, suggests acute gouty or septic arthritis. In children osteomyelitis involving bone contiguous to a joint must be considered.

What aggravates and relieves the pain, with special reference to exercise, rest, and treatments? In what setting did the pain develop? Was there an acute injury or excessive use of the body part?

What symptoms are associated? Here there are three relevant categories. First, are there *other symptoms in the involved joint(s)* — **specifically, swelling, stiffness, limitation of motion, tenderness, warmth, or redness?** Pains in the joints without other objective evidence of arthritis such as swelling, tenderness, or warmth are called *arthralgias.* Pains in the muscles are called *myalgias.* **Inquire about** *swelling* **in your usual manner, trying to localize it as accurately as possible.**

See Table 2-16, Patterns of Chronic Pain In or Around the Joints, pp. 88–89.

For *limitation of motion* **ask about activities with which the joint problems have interfered. When relevant, specifically inquire about the patient's ability to walk, stand, lean over, sit, sit up, rise from a sitting position, climb, pinch, grasp, turn a page, open a door or jar, and care for his or her own bodily needs, such as combing the hair, brushing the teeth, feeding, dressing, and washing, including hard-to-reach areas such as the perineum.**

Stiffness is often a more difficult area for question because people use the term in different ways. Stiffness in the musculoskeletal interview refers to the subjective perception of tightness or resistance to movement, the opposite of feeling limber. It is often associated with discomfort or pain. If the patient has not volunteered a sense of stiffness, ask about it. **Two good questions are "What time do you get up in the morning?" and "What time do you feel about as loose as you are going to get?"** Then calculate the duration of the patient's stiffness. Stiffness, together with muscular soreness, is felt by healthy people after unusually strenuous muscular exertion and peaks in intensity around the second day after exertion.

Stiffness after inactivity is common in degenerative joint disease but usually lasts only a few minutes. This is sometimes called *gelling.* Stiffness in rheumatoid arthritis and other inflammatory arthritides often lasts 30 minutes or longer. Stiffness also accompanies the "fibrositis" syndrome and polymyalgia rheumatica.

Tenderness, warmth, and redness are often best detected on examination, but patients can sometimes give you this information and guide you to points of tenderness.

Tenderness, warmth, and redness in a joint suggest acute gout, septic arthritis, or possibly rheumatic fever.

The second category of associated symptoms includes *generalized symptoms* such as *fever, chills, fatigue, anorexia, weight loss,* and *weakness.*

Generalized symptoms are common in rheumatoid and other inflammatory arthritides. High fever and chills suggest an infectious cause.

Third, are there *symptoms elsewhere in the body that give important clues as to the nature of the problem?* These include

> *Skin conditions* such as
>> A butterfly rash on the cheeks

Systemic lupus erythematosus

>> The scaly rash and pitted nails of psoriasis

Psoriatic arthritis

>> A few red macules, papules, pustules, or vesicles on the distal extremities

Gonococcal arthritis

>> Hives

Serum sickness, drug reaction

>> Erosions or scales on the penis and crusted scaling papules on the soles and palms

Reiter's syndrome, which also includes arthritis, urethritis, and conjunctivitis

>> The maculopapular rash of rubella

Arthritis of rubella

>> Clubbing of the fingernails (see p. 145)

Hypertrophic osteoarthropathy

> Red, burning, and itchy eyes *(conjunctivitis)*

Reiter's syndrome

> Preceding *sore throat*

Acute rheumatic fever or gonococcal arthritis

> *Diarrhea* and *abdominal pain*

Arthritis with ulcerative colitis or regional enteritis

> Symptoms of *urethritis*

Reiter's syndrome or possibly gonococcal arthritis

Even if the patient denies joint pains, specifically ask about *backache,* **a very common symptom. Use your usual interviewing method to develop a clear picture of the problem. If pain radiates into the legs, ask about numbness, tingling, or weakness that may be associated.**

See Table 2-17, Low Back Pain, p. 90.

Associated numbness, tingling, or weakness suggests involvement of nerve roots.

Pain in the neck **is also common. Approach it in the same manner. When neck pain is chronic, be alert for manifestations of pressure on the spinal cord: weakness, loss of sensation, and, in late stages, loss of bladder and bowel control.**

See Table 2-18, Pains in the Neck, p. 91.

THE NERVOUS SYSTEM

"Have you ever fainted or passed out?" turns the discussion to *loss of consciousness.* **Get as complete and unbiased a description of the event as you can. Try to determine what seems to have precipitated the**

In young people with temporary loss of consciousness, consider especially vasodepres-

attack(s), what kind of warning, if any, the patient felt before passing out, how long the unconsciousness lasted, and how the patient felt after recovery. Was the patient standing, sitting, or lying down when the attack started? What was the patient's appearance just before and during the attack? Patients may have learned from others about their appearance and activities while they were unconscious, but if the nature of the problem is uncertain try to talk with someone who has observed the event.

sor syncope, hyperventilation, and tonic–clonic (grand mal) seizures. In elderly patients think first of cardiac causes and postural hypotension. When temporary loss of consciousness lasts more than a few minutes, think of hypoglycemia, hypocapnia from hyperventilation, and hysterical fainting.

Syncope refers to the sudden but temporary loss of consciousness that occurs when blood flow to the brain becomes insufficient. It is commonly described as fainting. The symptoms of an impending faint, including muscular weakness, lightheadedness, and other premonitory feelings without actual loss of consciousness, are called *near syncope* or *pre-syncope*. These are assessed in the usual manner. Syncope must be distinguished from generalized seizures—a task sometimes made difficult by the fact that a severe syncopal attack can occasionally produce a few clonic movements and even urinary incontinence. Syncope is not usually associated, however, with a fully developed tonic–clonic (grand mal) seizure or with fecal incontinence.

See Table 2-19, Syncope and Similar Disorders, pp. 92–93.

In contrast to syncope, a tonic–clonic (grand mal) seizure usually starts more quickly, lasts longer, is more likely to involve injury and incontinence, and is followed by a slower recovery.

A *seizure* is a paroxysmal disorder that may or may not involve a loss of consciousness, and may also involve abnormal sensations, movements, feelings, or thought processes. It is caused by a sudden, excessive electrical discharge in the cerebral cortex or its underlying structures. **"Have you ever had any seizures or spells? . . . any fits or convulsions?"** opens the discussion. As with syncope, get as full a description as possible, including precipitating circumstances, warnings, behavior and feelings during the attack, duration of the attack, and feelings after it. Ask about the age at onset, the frequency of seizures, any recent change in frequency, and use of medications. Is there a history of prior head injury or other conditions that may be causally related?

See Table 2-20, Seizure Disorders, pp. 94–95.

To assess motor performance ask about *weakness* **of any part of the body and about** *paralysis,* **an inability to move a part. Did the weakness start slowly or suddenly? Has it progressed and how? What bodily parts are involved? Does the weakness affect one or both sides? What movements are affected? Try to distinguish between distal and proximal weakness. For distal weakness in the arms, inquire about hand movements such as opening a jar or can or using hand tools such as scissors, pliers, or a screwdriver. For distal weakness of the legs, ask about frequent tripping. For proximal weakness ask about combing the hair, trying to reach something on a high shelf, and difficulty in rising from a chair or taking a high step up. Does the person get weaker**

Local weakness may result from abnormalities in the upper motor neurons, the lower motor neurons, the neuromuscular junctions, or the muscles themselves. If it does not follow a neuroanatomic pattern and is unexplained otherwise, consider a conversion reaction. Bilateral, predominantly distal weakness suggests a polyneuropathy;

with repeated effort and improve after rest? Are there associated sensory or other symptoms?

bilateral proximal weakness, a myopathy. Weakness made worse with repeated effort and improved with rest suggests myasthenia gravis and related syndromes.

Tremors and other *involuntary movements* occur with or without additional neurologic manifestations. **Ask about trembling, shakiness, or bodily movements that the patient seems unable to control.**

See Table 17-6, Involuntary Movements, pp. 518–520.

Pain may stem from neurologic causes and is usually reported in other parts of the systems review, such as the head and musculoskeletal system.

Other sensory symptoms include loss of or alteration in sensation. **Ask about numbness, tingling, pins-and-needles sensations, or other peculiar or unpleasant feelings in the body. If a patient reports numbness, try to determine the real meaning—a** *loss of sensation,* **an inability to move the part, or an altered sensation. Use your usual style of questioning, paying particular attention to location.**

Loss of sensation, paresthesias, and dysesthesias occur with lesions involving the peripheral nerves, sensory roots, spinal cord, and higher centers. Paresthesias in the hands and around the mouth commonly accompany hyperventilation.

Paresthesias refer to peculiar sensations of various kinds that have no obvious stimulus. They include tingling, pricking, and feelings of warmth, coldness, and pressure. Paresthesias are what everyone feels when an arm or a leg "goes to sleep" after the compression of a nerve. *Dysesthesias* are distorted sensations in response to a stimulus, and may last longer than the stimulus itself. For example, a person may perceive a light touch or a pinprick as an unpleasant burning or tingling sensation.

Distinct from these symptoms is an almost indescribable *restlessness of the legs* that typically develops at rest and is accompanied by an urge to move about.

These symptoms suggest the common but often overlooked restless legs syndrome. Moving about gives relief.

THE HEMATOLOGIC SYSTEM

The assessment of hematologic disorders depends heavily on physical examination and the laboratory, but symptoms too have some value. Anemia must become moderate or severe before producing symptoms. It then decreases exercise tolerance and leads to dyspnea and palpitations. In persons with atherosclerosis it may decrease the threshold for angina pectoris, intermittent claudication, or transient ischemic attacks. Patients with severe anemia may report a variety of symptoms that may lead you astray: headache, dizziness, vertigo, syncope, anorexia, nausea, intolerance to cold, amenorrhea, menorrhagia, loss of libido, and impotence.

Spontaneous bleeding and bleeding disproportionate to an injury suggest a generalized bleeding disorder. It may be congenital or acquired. Normal

Congenital bleeding disorders, involving the clotting mecha-

hemostasis depends on three mechanisms: (1) vasoconstriction following a vascular injury, (2) formation of a platelet plug, and (3) formation of a fibrin clot. The most common bleeding disorders result from deficits in the last two categories. Platelet plugs are essential for prompt hemostasis, especially in the capillaries of the skin and mucous membranes. Fibrin clots are especially important as a second line of defense, particularly in larger vessels such as arterioles or venules.

nism, are most common in males. The family history is often positive.

A platelet disorder, therefore, is likely to cause capillary bleeding into the skin or mucous membranes. When the bleeding is caused by injury, it tends to occur without delay. In contrast, a clotting disorder tends to result in bleeding deep in the tissues. When caused by injury, it tends to appear several hours later. Bleeding due to a vascular defect tends to resemble that of a platelet disorder and may be associated with it.

Petechiae (see p. 144) in the skin and mucous membranes and small bruises are common in platelet disorders. Large bruises, deep hematomas (local masses of extravasated blood), and hemarthroses (blood in the joints) are seen in clotting disorders.

"Do you bleed or bruise easily?" opens this discussion. Further, "Have you ever bled a lot (or too much) after having a tooth pulled? . . . or after an operation? How about nosebleeds?" If there is a history of bleeding, try to distinguish between a localized problem and a more general bleeding tendency. If the latter is present, determine the sites of bleeding, timing in relation to possible injury, duration, frequency, and severity. Has the patient needed blood transfusions? Ask about medications, including aspirin and "blood thinners," and, if you have not already specifically done so, carefully review the family history for bleeding problems. Are there reasons to suspect a deficiency of vitamin C or K?

Spontaneous bleeding, bleeding with minor trauma, and bleeding in several sites suggest a general disorder.

Inadequate diet, malabsorption

THE ENDOCRINE SYSTEM

The assessment of endocrine function depends not so much on additional symptoms as on pulling together the data already gathered and recognizing the underlying pattern of an endocrine disorder. When you begin to recognize such a pattern, ask about symptoms that you know might be relevant but try to avoid leading the patient. When you suspect Addison's disease, for example, "Have you noticed any change in the color of your skin?" is safer than "Has your skin become darker?"

Obesity, weakness, fatigue, easy bruising, ankle edema, and decreased or absent menstrual periods suggest Cushing's syndrome (adrenal cortical hyperfunction), while weakness, weight loss, nausea, vomiting, darkened skin, and symptoms of postural hypotension suggest Addison's disease (adrenal insufficiency).

There are, however, a few additional symptoms that are important in an endocrine evaluation. These relate primarily to diabetes mellitus and to thyroid dysfunction.

Polyuria, already described in the section on the urinary tract, is a frequent symptom of diabetes mellitus. It is then typically associated with excessive *thirst,* and with *polydipsia* (an increased intake of fluids). *Polyphagia* (an increased food intake) may also occur.

Other symptoms that often accompany the onset of diabetes mellitus include weakness, fatigue, weight loss, and blurred vision.

(Text continues on p. 65)

Table 2-1

Table 2-1 Headaches

PROBLEM	PROCESS	LOCATION	QUALITY AND SEVERITY	TIMING	
				ONSET	DURATION
TENSION HEADACHES	Uncertain, may be related to sustained muscle contraction	Usually bilateral; may be generalized or localized to the back of the head and upper neck or to the frontotemporal area	Mild and aching or a nonpainful tightness and pressure	Gradual	Variable: hours or days, but often weeks or months
MIGRAINE HEADACHES (*"Classic migraine" is distinguished from "common migraine" by visual or neurological symptoms during the half hour before the headache.*)	Dilatation of arteries outside and probably also inside the skull, probably of biochemical origin; often familial	Typically frontal or temporal, one or both sides, but also may be occipital or generalized. "Classic migraine" is typically unilateral.	Throbbing or aching; variable in severity	Fairly rapid, reaching a peak in 1–2 hr	Several hours to 1–2 dy
CLUSTER HEADACHES	Uncertain	One-sided; high in the nose, and behind and over the eye	Steady, severe	Abrupt, often 2–3 hr after falling asleep	Roughly 1–2 hr
HEADACHES WITH EYE DISORDERS					
Errors of refraction (farsightedness and astigmatism, but not nearsightedness)	Probably the sustained contraction of the extraocular muscles, and possibly of the frontal, temporal, and occipital muscles	Around and over the eyes, may radiate to the occipital area	Steady, aching, dull	Gradual	Variable
Acute glaucoma	Sudden increase in intraocular pressure (see pp. 168–169)	In and around one eye	Steady, aching, often severe	Often rapid	Variable, may depend on treatment
HEADACHES WITH ACUTE PARANASAL SINUSITIS	Mucosal inflammation of the paranasal sinuses and their openings	Usually above the eye (frontal sinus) or in the cheekbone area (maxillary sinus), one or both sides	Aching or throbbing, variable in severity	Variable	Often several hours at a time, recurring over days or longer
TRIGEMINAL NEURALGIA	Mechanism variable, often unknown	Cheek, jaws, lips, or gums (second and third divisions of the trigeminal nerve)	Sharp, short, brief, lightninglike jabs; very severe	Abrupt	Each jab is transient, but jabs recur in clusters at intervals of seconds or minutes.

* Blanks appear in these tables when the categories are not applicable or are not usually helpful in assessing the problem.

Table 2-1

Table 2-1   (Cont'd.)

COURSE	ASSOCIATED SYMPTOMS	FACTORS THAT AGGRAVATE OR PROVOKE	FACTORS THAT RELIEVE	CONVENIENT CATEGORIES OF THOUGHT
Often recurrent or persistent over long periods	Symptoms of anxiety, tension, and depression may be present.	Sustained muscular tension, as in driving or typing; emotional stress	Variable	The two most common kinds of headache
Often begins between childhood and early adulthood. Typically recurrent at intervals of weeks, months, or years, usually decreasing with pregnancy and advancing age.	Often nausea and vomiting. A minority of patients have preceding visual disturbances (local flashes of light, blind spots) or neurological symptoms (local weakness, sensory disturbances, and other symptoms).	May be provoked by alcohol or tension. More common premenstrually. Aggravated by noise and bright light.	Quiet, dark room; sleep; pressure on the artery, if early in the course	
Typically clustered in time, with several each day or week and then relief for weeks or months	Unilateral stuffy, runny nose, and reddening and tearing of the eye	During a cluster, may be provoked by alcohol		
Variable	Eye fatigue, "sandy" sensations in the eyes, redness of the conjunctivas	Prolonged use of the eyes, particularly for close work	Rest of the eyes	Face pains
Variable, may depend on treatment	Diminished vision, sometimes nausea and vomiting	Sometimes provoked by drops that dilate the pupils		
Often recurrent in a repetitive daily pattern, such as mornings	Local tenderness, nasal congestion and discharge	May be aggravated by coughing, sneezing, or jarring the head	Nasal decongestants	
Pain may be troublesome for months, then disappear for months, but often recurs. Uncommon at night.	Exhaustion from recurrent pain	Typically triggered by touching certain areas of the lower face or mouth, or by chewing, talking, or brushing the teeth		

(Table continues on next page)

Table 2-1

Table 2-1   (Cont'd.)

PROBLEM	PROCESS	LOCATION	QUALITY AND SEVERITY	TIMING	
				ONSET	DURATION
GIANT CELL ARTERITIS	Chronic inflammation of the cranial arteries, cause unknown, often associated with polymyalgia rheumatica	Localized near the involved artery (most often the temporal, also the occipital); may become generalized	Aching, throbbing, or burning, often severe	Gradual or rapid	Variable
CHRONIC SUBDURAL HEMATOMA	Bleeding into the subdural space after trauma, followed by slow accumulation of fluid that compresses the brain	Variable	Steady, aching	Gradual onset weeks to months after the injury	Often depends on surgical intervention
POSTCONCUSSION SYNDROME	Mechanism unclear	May be localized to the injured area, but not necessarily	Variable	Within a few hours of the injury	Weeks, months, or even years
POSTTRAUMATIC MIGRAINE-LIKE HEADACHE		(See *Migraine Headaches.*)			
MENINGEAL IRRITATION, *as from infection (meningitis) or blood (subarachnoid hemorrhage)*	Inflammation of the meninges and related pain-sensitive structures within the skull	Generalized; particularly severe at the base of the skull	Steady and severe; may be throbbing in meningitis	Fairly rapid (meningitis) or abrupt, peaking in 1–2 min (subarachnoid hemorrhage)	Variable, usually days
BRAIN TUMOR	Displacement of or traction on pain-sensitive arteries and veins or pressure on nerves, all within the skull	Varies with the location of the tumor	Aching, steady, variable in intensity	Variable	Often brief

Table 2-1

Table 2-1 (Cont'd.)

COURSE	ASSOCIATED SYMPTOMS	FACTORS THAT AGGRAVATE OR PROVOKE	FACTORS THAT RELIEVE	CONVENIENT CATEGORIES OF THOUGHT
Recurrent or persistent over weeks to months	Tenderness of the adjacent scalp; fever, malaise, fatigue, and anorexia; muscular aches and stiffness; visual loss or blindness			Consider these three in older adults.
Progressively severe but may be obscured by clouded consciousness	Alterations in consciousness, changes in personality, and hemiparesis (weakness on one side of the body). The injury is often forgotten.			
Tends to diminish over time	Giddiness or vertigo, irritability, restlessness, tenseness, fatigue, and difficulty concentrating	Mental and physical exertion, straining, stooping, emotional excitement, alcohol	Rest	Headaches following head trauma
Persistent single headache in an acute illness	An acute febrile illness (meningitis) or headache and sudden collapse, often with loss of consciousness (hemorrhage). Vomiting and fever may accompany either.			Acute, severe illnesses
Often intermittent, but progressive	Neurological and mental symptoms and nausea and vomiting may develop.	May be aggravated by coughing, sneezing, or sudden movements of the head		An underlying concern of patient and clinician alike

Table 2-2

Table 2-2 Vertigo

PROBLEM	TIMING			HEARING	TINNITUS	OTHER ASSOCIATED SYMPTOMS
	ONSET	DURATION	COURSE			
BENIGN POSITIONAL VERTIGO	Sudden, on rolling over onto the affected side or tilting the head up	Brief, a few seconds to minutes	Persists a few weeks, may recur	Not affected	Absent	Sometimes nausea and vomiting
VESTIBULAR NEURONITIS (*acute labyrinthitis*)	Sudden	Hours to days, up to 2 wk	May recur over 12–18 mo	Not affected	Absent	Nausea, vomiting
MENIERE'S DISEASE	Sudden	Several hours to a day or more	Recurrent	Sensorineural hearing loss that improves and recurs, eventually progresses; one or both sides*	Present, fluctuating*	Nausea, vomiting, pressure or fullness in the affected ear
DRUG TOXICITY	Insidious	May or may not be reversible. Partial adaptation occurs.		May be impaired, both sides	May be present	Nausea, vomiting
TUMOR, PRESSING ON THE 8TH NERVE	Insidious**	Variable	Variable	Impaired, one side	Present	Those of pressure on the 5th, 6th, and 7th cranial nerves

Additional disorders of the brainstem or cerebellum may also cause vertigo. These include ischemia secondary to atherosclerosis, tumors, and multiple sclerosis. Additional neurological symptoms and signs are usually present.

* Hearing impairment, tinnitus, and rotary vertigo do not always develop concurrently. Time is often required to make this diagnosis.
** Persistent unsteadiness rather than vertigo is usual here.

(Text continued from p. 59)

An assessment of thyroid function involves questions concerning *temperature intolerance* and *sweating*. **Opening questions include "Do you prefer hot or cold weather? Do you generally dress more warmly or less warmly than most people? Do you use more blankets or fewer blankets than others at home? Do you sweat (or perspire) more or less than most people?"** As people grow older, they sweat less, tolerate cold less well, and tend to prefer warmer environments.

Intolerance to cold, preferences for warm clothing and many blankets, and decreased sweating suggest hypothyroidism; the opposites suggest hyperthyroidism. For other symptoms see Table 7-24, Thyroid Enlargement and Function (p. 220).

Episodic sweating and heat intolerance often occur during menopause.

SCREENING FOR MENTAL STATUS

In the course of the interview you often identify clues to emotional or other psychiatric problems. It is usually wise to inquire about these when the patient mentions them. A few screening questions about *nervousness, tensions, mood,* and possibly *memory* should be included in most histories. This subject is sufficiently important, however, to warrant its own chapter.

Table 2-3

Table 2-3 Chest Pain

PROBLEM	PROCESS	LOCATION	QUALITY	SEVERITY
ANGINA PECTORIS	Temporary myocardial ischemia, usually secondary to coronary atherosclerosis	Retrosternal or across the anterior chest, sometimes radiating to the shoulders, arms, neck, lower jaw, or upper abdomen	Pressing, squeezing, tight, heavy, occasionally burning	Mild to moderate, sometimes not really painful
MYOCARDIAL INFARCTION	Prolonged myocardial ischemia, resulting in irreversible muscle damage (necrosis)	Same as in angina	Same as in angina	Often but not always severe
PERICARDITIS	1. Irritation of parietal pleura adjacent to the pericardium	Precordial	Sharp, knifelike	Often severe
	2. Mechanism uncertain	Retrosternal, may radiate to the neck and shoulders	Crushing	Severe
DISSECTING AORTIC ANEURYSM	A splitting within the layers of the aortic wall, allowing the passage of blood to dissect a channel	Anterior chest, radiating to the neck, back, or abdomen	Ripping, tearing	Very severe
TRACHEOBRONCHITIS	Inflammation of the trachea and large bronchi	Upper sternal or on either side of the sternum	Burning	Mild to moderate
PLEURAL PAIN	Irritation of the parietal pleura as from acute pleurisy, pneumonia, pulmonary infarction, or neoplasm	Chest wall overlying the process	Sharp, knifelike	Often severe
REFLUX ESOPHAGITIS	Inflammation of the esophageal mucosa by reflux of gastric acid	Retrosternal, may radiate to the back	Burning, may be squeezing	Mild to severe
DIFFUSE ESOPHAGEAL SPASM	Motor dysfunction of the esophageal muscle	Retrosternal, may radiate to the back, arms, and jaw	Sharp or squeezing	Mild to severe
CHEST WALL PAIN	Variable, often uncertain	Often below the left breast or along the costal cartilages, also elsewhere	Stabbing, sticking, or dull, aching	Variable
ANXIETY	Uncertain	Precordial, below the left breast, or across the anterior chest	Stabbing, sticking, or dull, aching	Variable

Table 2-3

Table 2-3 (Cont'd.)

TIMING	FACTORS THAT AGGRAVATE	FACTORS THAT RELIEVE	ASSOCIATED SYMPTOMS
Usually 1–3 min but up to 10 min. Prolonged episodes up to 20 min	Effort, especially in the cold; meals; emotional stress. May occur at rest	Rest, nitroglycerine	Sometimes dyspnea, nausea, sweating
20 min to several hr			Nausea, vomiting, sweating, weakness
Persistent	Breathing, coughing, lying down, sometimes swallowing	Sitting up may relieve it.	Of the underlying illness
Persistent			Of the underlying illness
Persistent, maximal at the onset			Syncope, hemiplegia, paraplegia
Variable	Coughing		Cough
Persistent	Breathing, coughing, movements of the trunk	Lying on the involved side may relieve it.	Of the underlying illness
Variable	Large meal; bending over, lying down	Antacids, sometimes belching	Sometimes regurgitation, dysphagia
Variable	Swallowing of food or cold liquid; emotional stress	Sometimes nitroglycerine	Dysphagia
Fleeting to hours or days	Movement of chest, trunk, arms		Often local tenderness
Fleeting to hours or days	May follow effort, emotional stress		Breathlessness, palpitations, weakness, anxiety

Table 2-4

Table 2-4   Dyspnea

PROBLEM	PROCESS	TIMING
LEFT-SIDED HEART FAILURE *(left ventricular failure or mitral stenosis)*	Elevated pressure in the pulmonary capillary bed with transudation of fluid into the interstitial spaces and alveoli, decreased compliance (increased stiffness) of the lungs, and increased work of breathing	Dyspnea may progress slowly, or suddenly as in acute pulmonary edema.
CHRONIC BRONCHITIS*	Excessive mucus production in the bronchi, followed by chronic obstruction of the airways	Chronic productive cough followed by slowly progressive dyspnea
PULMONARY EMPHYSEMA*	Overdistention of the air spaces distal to the terminal bronchioles with destruction of the alveolar septa and chronic obstruction of the airways	Slowly progressive dyspnea; relatively mild cough later
BRONCHIAL ASTHMA	Airways narrowed by smooth muscle contraction, edema of the bronchial walls, and secretions	Acute episodes, separated by symptom-free periods
DIFFUSE INFILTRATIVE LUNG DISEASES *(such as sarcoidosis, widespread pulmonary neoplasms, and coal workers' pneumoconiosis)*	Abnormal and widespread infiltration of cells, fluid, and collagen into the interstitial spaces. Many causes.	Progressive dyspnea, which varies in its rate of development with the cause
PNEUMONIA	Inflammation of the lung parenchyma from the respiratory bronchioles to the alveoli	An acute illness, the timing of which varies with the etiologic agent
SPONTANEOUS PNEUMOTHORAX	Leakage of air into the pleural space through blebs on the visceral pleura with resulting partial or complete collapse of the lung	Sudden onset of dyspnea
ACUTE PULMONARY EMBOLISM	Sudden occlusion of all or part of the pulmonary arterial tree by a blood clot that usually originates in the deep veins of the legs or pelvis	Sudden onset of dyspnea
ANXIETY WITH HYPERVENTILATION	Overbreathing with resultant respiratory alkalosis and fall in the partial pressure of carbon dioxide in the blood	Episodic, often recurrent

* Chronic bronchitis and emphysema often coexist.

Table 2-4

Table 2-4   (Cont'd.)

FACTORS THAT AGGRAVATE	FACTORS THAT RELIEVE	ASSOCIATED SYMPTOMS	SETTING
Exertion, lying down	Rest, sitting up, though dyspnea may become persistent	Often cough, orthopnea, paroxysmal nocturnal dyspnea; sometimes wheezing	History of heart disease or its predisposing factors
Exertion, inhaled irritants, respiratory infections	Expectoration; rest, though dyspnea may become persistent	Chronic productive cough, recurrent respiratory infections; wheezing may develop	History of smoking, air pollutants, recurrent respiratory infections
Exertion	Rest, though dyspnea may become persistent	Cough, with scant mucoid sputum	History of smoking, air pollutants, sometimes a familial deficiency of alpha$_1$-antitrypsin
Variable, including allergens, irritants, respiratory infections, exercise, and emotion	Separation from aggravating factors	Wheezing, cough	Environmental and emotional conditions
Exertion	Rest, though dyspnea may become persistent	Often weakness, fatigue. Cough less common than in other lung diseases	Variable
		Pleuritic pain, cough, sputum, fever	Variable
		Pleuritic pain	Often a previously healthy young adult
		Often none. Retrosternal oppressive pain if the occlusion is massive. Pleuritic pain, cough, and hemoptysis may follow an embolism if pulmonary infarction ensues. Symptoms of anxiety (see below).	Postpartum or postoperative periods; prolonged bed rest; congestive heart failure, chronic lung disease, and fractures of hip or leg; thrombophlebitis
Often occurs at rest as well as after exercise. An upsetting event may not be evident.	Breathing in and out of a paper or plastic bag sometimes helps the associated symptoms.	Sighing, lightheadedness, numbness or tingling of the hands and feet, palpitations, chest pain	Other manifestations of anxiety may be present.

Table 2-5

Table 2-5   Cough

PROBLEM	COUGH AND SPUTUM	ASSOCIATED SYMPTOMS AND SETTING
ACUTE INFLAMMATIONS		
LARYNGITIS	Dry (without sputum); may become moist and productive of varying amounts of sputum	An acute, relatively minor illness with hoarseness. Often associated with viral syndromes that include sore throat, runny nose and eyes.
TRACHEOBRONCHITIS	Dry; may become productive (as above)	An acute illness, often with burning retrosternal discomfort. Often associated with viral syndromes as described above.
ACUTE EXACERBATION OF CHRONIC BRONCHITIS	Increase in a chronic cough with increased volume of sputum that typically becomes purulent	See *Chronic Bronchitis* below.
MYCOPLASMA AND VIRAL PNEUMONIAS	Dry cough often becoming productive of mucoid sputum	An acute febrile illness, possibly dyspnea
LOBAR PNEUMONIA	Mucoid or purulent sputum often mixed with blood and diffusely pinkish or rusty in color	An acute illness with chills, high fever, dyspnea, and chest pain, often preceded by symptoms of an upper respiratory infection
CHRONIC INFLAMMATIONS		
CHRONIC BRONCHITIS	Mucoid sputum, especially in the mornings; may become purulent during recurrent acute infections	Often longstanding cigarette smoking. Recurrent superimposed infections. Wheezing and dyspnea may develop.
BRONCHIECTASIS	Chronic productive cough with purulent, often copious sputum; may be foul-smelling	Recurrent bronchopulmonary infections common. Sinusitis may coexist.
PULMONARY TUBERCULOSIS	Dry cough, becoming productive of mucoid or purulent sputum	Early, no symptoms. Anorexia, weight loss, fatigue, fever, and night sweats as the disease advances.
FUNGAL INFECTIONS OF THE LUNG	Dry to productive cough	Variable, may resemble tuberculosis
BRONCHIAL ASTHMA	Cough, with thick mucoid sputum especially toward the end of an attack	Episodic wheezing and dyspnea, but occasionally the cough appears alone. There may be a history of allergy.
NEOPLASM		
CANCER OF THE LUNG	Dry to productive. Be alert to a change in a "cigarette cough."	Often longstanding cigarette smoking. Associated manifestations are numerous.
CARDIOVASCULAR DISORDERS		
LEFT VENTRICULAR FAILURE AND MITRAL STENOSIS	Often dry, especially on exertion or at night; may progress to the pink frothy sputum of pulmonary edema or frank hemoptysis	Dyspnea, orthopnea, paroxysmal nocturnal dyspnea
PULMONARY INFARCTION	Dry or productive	Dyspnea, often chest pain
TRAUMA AND PHYSICAL AGENTS		
IRRITATING PARTICLES, CHEMICALS, OR GASES	Variable. There may be a latent period between exposure and symptoms.	Exposure to irritants. Eyes, nose, and throat may be affected.
FOREIGN BODY LODGED IN THE LOWER AIRWAY	Acute: dry. Later: dry or productive	Acute: choking. Later: dyspnea and wheezing. Aspiration of the foreign body may not be recalled.

Table 2-6

Table 2-6 Hemoptysis

PROBLEM	PROCESS	COUGH AND SPUTUM
INFLAMMATIONS		
CHRONIC BRONCHITIS	Excessive mucus production in the bronchi, followed by chronic obstruction of the airways. Superimposed acute infections are common.	Mucoid, mucopurulent, or purulent sputum with blood-streaking or even gross blood
BRONCHIECTASIS	Abnormal dilatation of one or more of the large bronchi, typically complicated by chronic or recurrent infection	Chronic productive cough, often with copious purulent sputum that may be blood-streaked or grossly bloody
PULMONARY TUBERCULOSIS	A chronic infection of the lung(s) caused by *Mycobacterium tuberculosis*	Chronic productive cough with sputum that may be scant and mucoid or copious and purulent. Sputum may be blood-streaked or grossly bloody.
PNEUMONIA	An acute inflammation of the lung parenchyma. Pneumonias associated with hemoptysis are caused most often by *Streptococcus pneumoniae* (pneumococcus) and *Klebsiella pneumoniae*.	*Pneumococcus:* blood-streaked or diffusely pinkish or rusty-colored sputum *Klebsiella:* similar, or may be sticky, red, and jellylike
LUNG ABSCESS	A localized destructive and suppurative process in the lung that may complicate certain pneumonias or follow aspiration during a period of altered consciousness	Moderate to copious amounts of sputum, often bloody and foul-smelling
NEOPLASM		
LUNG CANCER	A malignant neoplasm of the lung	Often a preceding cigarette cough. Sputum often blood-streaked, may be frankly bloody.
CARDIOVASCULAR		
MITRAL STENOSIS	Narrowing of the mitral valve raises the pressure in the left atrium and pulmonary veins. Anastomotic venous channels between the pulmonary and bronchial veins may rupture, with bleeding into the bronchi.	Bright red blood
ACUTE PULMONARY EDEMA SECONDARY TO LEFT VENTRICULAR FAILURE OR MITRAL STENOSIS	Elevated pressure in the pulmonary capillary bed with escape of red cells into the alveoli	Pink frothy sputum
PULMONARY INFARCTION	Necrosis of lung usually following the occlusion of part of the pulmonary arterial tree by an embolus	Sputum may be dark, bright red, or mixed with blood.
TRAUMA		
EXTERNAL TRAUMA TO THE CHEST	Puncture, laceration, or contusion of the lung	Blood-streaked sputum or bright red blood
BLEEDING DISORDERS		
INHERITED OR ACQUIRED BLEEDING DISORDERS	Generalized increased bleeding tendency	Bright red blood

(Table continues on next page)

Table 2-6

Table 2-6 (Cont'd.)

PROBLEM	ASSOCIATED SYMPTOMS MAY INCLUDE	SETTING
INFLAMMATIONS		
CHRONIC BRONCHITIS	Dyspnea, wheezing	Cigarette smoking, air pollutants
BRONCHIECTASIS	Recurrent episodes of bronchopulmonary infection. If advanced, fatigue, weight loss, and fever. Sinusitis may coexist.	Bronchial obstruction, previous suppurative pneumonias, or systemic illnesses such as cystic fibrosis and hypogammaglobulinemia
PULMONARY TUBERCULOSIS	Constitutional symptoms of insidious onset: anorexia, fatigue, weight loss, fever, and night sweats	Now uncommon among American adolescents and young adults. Most cases of active disease now occur in elderly patients, who first became infected when tuberculosis was much more prevalent.
PNEUMONIA	An acute illness with fever, chills, dyspnea, and chest pain	*Pneumococcal pneumonia* often follows acute upper respiratory infections.
		Klebsiella pneumonia is relatively uncommon and typically occurs in middle-aged or older men, often alcoholics.
LUNG ABSCESS	A febrile illness that may develop slowly over weeks or may be acute, like pneumonia	In abscess from aspiration, often a history of altered consciousness, as from drugs or alcohol, epilepsy, or stroke; periodontal disease, gingivitis, and carious teeth are often present.
NEOPLASM		
LUNG CANCER	Many other manifestations, including weight loss and chest pain, but most associated symptoms occur in the late stages of the cancer	Cigarette smoking, also industrial air pollutants
CARDIOVASCULAR		
MITRAL STENOSIS	Dyspnea, orthopnea, and paroxysmal nocturnal dyspnea secondary to the mitral stenosis	Background of rheumatic heart disease. Exercise, excitement, sexual intercourse, and pregnancy may precipitate the hemoptysis.
ACUTE PULMONARY EDEMA SECONDARY TO LEFT VENTRICULAR FAILURE OR MITRAL STENOSIS	Dyspnea, orthopnea, and paroxysmal nocturnal dyspnea; cough, especially at night	Underlying heart disease
PULMONARY INFARCTION	Dyspnea, pleuritic pain, fever, but no chills	Left ventricular failure, mitral stenosis, and chronic obstructive lung disease predispose to infarction after an embolism occurs.
TRAUMA		
EXTERNAL TRAUMA TO THE CHEST	Variable	Trauma
BLEEDING DISORDERS		
INHERITED OR ACQUIRED BLEEDING DISORDERS	Other kinds of bleeding or bruising without an apparently adequate external cause	History of past bleeding; predisposing illnesses of many kinds; anticoagulant therapy. Remember a local bronchopulmonary lesion may coexist.

Table 2-7

Table 2-7 Dysphagia

PROCESS AND PROBLEM	TIMING	FACTORS THAT AGGRAVATE	FACTORS THAT RELIEVE	ASSOCIATED SYMPTOMS AND CONDITIONS
MECHANICAL NARROWING OF THE ESOPHAGEAL LUMEN	Either gradual or sudden in onset. Often worse over time so that the size of the bolus a patient can swallow steadily diminishes.	Particularly solid foods such as meat; with progression, softer foods and liquids	With increasing obstruction, regurgitation of food by self-induced vomiting	Variable with the cause. See below.
ESOPHAGEAL CANCER	Initially intermittent but becomes relentlessly progressive over a few months	See above.	See above.	Weight loss, pain in the chest and back
ESOPHAGEAL STRICTURE, *most often from inflammation produced by reflux of gastric juice*	Slowly progressive. Dysphagia may precede stricture in esophagitis.	See above.	See above.	Long prior history of heartburn, peptic ulcer, or recurrent vomiting
MOTOR DISORDERS AFFECTING THE ESOPHAGEAL MUSCLE *(such as achalasia, diffuse esophageal spasm, and scleroderma)*	Usually gradual in onset. Usually not progressively severe, except possibly in achalasia.	Particularly cold liquids but also solid foods	Repeated swallowing, drinking of warm fluids, throwing back the shoulders and straining down against a closed glottis (Valsalva maneuver)	Variable. Associated chest pain suggests diffuse esophageal spasm but may also occur with achalasia.
MOTOR DISORDERS AFFECTING THE PHARYNGEAL MUSCLES — *difficulty transferring food from the mouth to the esophagus*	Acute or gradual onset depending on the underlying disorder			Aspiration into the lungs or regurgitation of fluid into the nose with attempts to swallow. Neurological evidence of stroke, bulbar palsy, myasthenia gravis, or other neuromuscular conditions.
PAINFUL INFLAMMATIONS OF THE THROAT *(such as severe pharyngitis or retropharyngeal abscess)*	Onset over a few days			An acute illness with a painful, inflamed throat

Table 2-8

Table 2-8 *Abdominal Pain*

PROBLEM	PROCESS	LOCATION	QUALITY
PEPTIC ULCER AND DYSPEPSIA *(These disorders cannot be reliably differentiated by symptoms and signs.)*	Peptic ulcer refers to a demonstrable ulcer, usually in the duodenum or stomach. Dyspepsia causes similar symptoms but no ulceration.	Epigastric, may radiate to the back	Variable: gnawing, burning, boring, aching, pressing, or hungerlike
CANCER OF THE STOMACH	A malignant neoplasm	Epigastric	Variable
ACUTE PANCREATITIS	An acute inflammation of the pancreas	Epigastric, sometimes radiating to the back or other parts of the abdomen; may be poorly localized	Usually steady
CHRONIC PANCREATITIS	Fibrosis of the pancreas secondary to recurrent inflammation	Epigastric, radiating through to the back	Steady, deep
CANCER OF THE PANCREAS	A malignant neoplasm	Epigastric, with pain in either upper quadrant, depending on the location of the cancer; often radiates to the back	Steady, deep
BILIARY COLIC	Sudden obstruction of the cystic duct or common bile duct by a gallstone	Epigastric or right upper quadrant; may radiate to the right scapula and shoulder	Steady, aching; *not* colicky
ACUTE CHOLECYSTITIS	Inflammation of the gallbladder usually triggered by persisting obstruction of the cystic duct by a gallstone	Right upper quadrant or upper abdominal; may radiate to the right scapular area	Steady, aching
ACUTE DIVERTICULITIS	Acute inflammation of a colonic diverticulum, a saclike mucosal outpouching through the colonic muscle	Left lower quadrant	May be cramping at first but becomes steady
ACUTE APPENDICITIS	Acute inflammation of the appendix with distention or obstruction	1. Poorly localized *periumbilical pain* followed usually by 2. *Right lower quadrant pain*	1. Mild but increasing, possibly cramping 2. Steady and more severe
ACUTE MECHANICAL INTESTINAL OBSTRUCTION	Obstruction of the bowel lumen, most commonly caused by (1) adhesions or hernias (small bowel), or (2) cancer or diverticulitis (colon)	1. *Small bowel:* periumbilical or upper abdominal 2. *Colon:* lower abdominal or generalized	1. Cramping 2. Cramping

Table 2-8

Table 2-8 (Cont'd.)

TIMING	FACTORS THAT MAY AGGRAVATE	FACTORS THAT MAY RELIEVE	ASSOCIATED SYMPTOMS AND SETTING
Intermittent. Duodenal ulcer is more likely than gastric ulcer or dyspepsia to cause pain that (1) wakes the patient at night, and (2) occurs intermittently over a few weeks, then disappears for months, and then recurs.	Variable	Food and antacids may bring relief, but not necessarily in any of these disorders and least commonly in gastric ulcer.	Nausea, vomiting, belching, bloating; heartburn (more common in duodenal ulcer); weight loss (more common in gastric ulcer). Dyspepsia is more common in the young (20–29 yr), gastric ulcer in the older (over 50 yr), and duodenal ulcer in those from 30 to 60 yr.
The history of pain is typically shorter than in peptic ulcer. The pain is persistent and slowly progressive.	Often food	*Not* relieved by food or antacids	Anorexia, nausea, easy satiety, weight loss, and sometimes bleeding. Most common in ages 50–70.
Acute onset, persistent pain	Lying supine	Leaning forward with trunk flexed	Nausea, vomiting, abdominal distention, fever. Often a history of previous attacks and of alcohol abuse or gallstones.
Chronic or recurrent course	Alcohol, heavy or fatty meals	Possibly leaning forward with trunk flexed; often intractable	Symptoms of decreased pancreatic functions may appear: diarrhea with fatty stools (steatorrhea) and diabetes mellitus.
Persistent pain; relentlessly progressive illness		Possibly leaning forward with trunk flexed; often intractable	Anorexia, nausea, vomiting, weight loss, and jaundice. Emotional symptoms including depression.
Rapid onset over a few minutes, lasts one to several hours and subsides gradually. Often recurrent.			Anorexia, nausea, vomiting, restlessness
Gradual onset; course longer than biliary colic	Jarring, deep breathing		Anorexia, nausea, vomiting, and lowgrade fever
Often a gradual onset			Fever, constipation. There may be initial brief diarrhea.
1. Lasts roughly 4–6 hr 2. Depends on intervention	1. 2. Movement or cough	1. 2. If it subsides temporarily, suspect perforation of the appendix.	Anorexia, nausea, possibly vomiting, which typically follow the onset of pain
1. Occurs in paroxysms, may decrease over time as bowel mobility is impaired 2. Occurs in paroxysms but typically milder than in small bowel obstruction			1. Vomiting of bile and mucus (with high obstruction) or foul-smelling fecal material (with low obstruction). Obstipation develops. 2. Vomiting late if at all. Obstipation occurs early. Prior symptoms of the underlying cause, such as a change in bowel habits or bleeding.

Table 2-9

Table 2-9 Black and Bloody Stools

PROBLEM	SELECTED CAUSES	ASSOCIATED SYMPTOMS AND SETTING
MELENA, the passage of black, tarry (sticky and shiny) stools. Melena signifies the loss of at least 50–60 ml of blood into the gastrointestinal tract (less in infants and children), usually from the esophagus, stomach, or duodenum. Less commonly, when intestinal transit is slow, the blood may originate in the jejunum, ileum, or ascending colon. In infants melena may result from swallowing blood during the birth process.	Peptic ulcer	Often, but not necessarily, a history of epigastric pain
	Gastritis or stress ulcers	Recent ingestion of alcohol, aspirin, or other anti-inflammatory drugs; recent bodily trauma, severe burns, surgery, or increased intracranial pressure
	Esophageal or gastric varices	Cirrhosis of the liver or other cause of portal hypertension
	Reflux esophagitis	History of heartburn
BLACK, NONSTICKY STOOLS, which usually give negative results when tested for occult blood. (Ingestion of iron or other substances, however, may cause a positive test result in the absence of blood.) These stools have no pathologic significance.	Ingestion of iron, bismuth, licorice, or even commercial chocolate cookies	
RED BLOOD IN THE STOOLS Red blood usually originates in the colon, rectum, or anus, and much less frequently in the jejunum or ileum. Upper gastrointestinal hemorrhage, however, may also cause red stools. The amount of blood lost is then usually large (over a liter). Transit time through the intestinal tract is accordingly rapid, thus giving insufficient time for the blood to turn black.	Cancer of the colon	Often a change in bowel habits
	Benign polyps of the colon	Often no other symptoms
	Diverticula of the colon	Often no other symptoms
	Inflammatory conditions of the colon and rectum	
	Ulcerative colitis	See Table 2-14, Chronic or Recurrent Diarrheas.
	Infectious dysenteries	See Table 2-13, Acute Diarrhea.
	Proctitis in homosexual men (various causes)	Rectal urgency, tenesmus
	Ischemic colitis	Lower abdominal pain, sometimes fever or shock in persons over 50 yr
	Hemorrhoids	Blood on the toilet paper, on the surface of the stool, or dripping into the toilet
	Anal fissure	Blood on the toilet paper or on the surface of the stool; anal pain
REDDISH BUT NONBLOODY STOOLS	The ingestion of beets	Pink urine, which usually precedes the reddish stool

Table 2-10

Table 2-10 Constipation

PROBLEM	PROCESS	SETTING AND ASSOCIATED SYMPTOMS
LIFE ACTIVITIES AND HABITS		
INADEQUATE TIME OR SETTING FOR THE DEFECATION REFLEX	Ignoring the sensation of a full rectum inhibits the defecation reflex.	Hectic schedules, unfamiliar surroundings, bed rest
FALSE EXPECTATIONS OF BOWEL HABITS	Expectations of "regularity" or more frequent stools than a person's norm	Beliefs, treatments, and advertisements that promote the use of laxatives
IRRITABLE BOWEL SYNDROME	A common disorder of bowel motility	Small hard stools, often with mucus. Periods of diarrhea. Cramping abdominal pain. Stress may aggravate.
MECHANICAL OBSTRUCTION		
CANCER OF THE RECTUM OR SIGMOID COLON	Progressive narrowing of the bowel lumen	Change in bowel habits; often diarrhea, abdominal pain, and bleeding. In rectal cancer, tenesmus and pencil-shaped stools.
FECAL IMPACTION	A large, firm, immovable fecal mass, most often in the rectum	Rectal fullness, abdominal pain. Common in debilitated, bedridden, and often elderly patients.
OTHER OBSTRUCTING LESIONS (*such as diverticulitis, volvulus, intussusception, or hernia*)	Narrowing or complete obstruction of the bowel	Colicky abdominal pain, abdominal distention, and in intussusception, often "currant jelly" stools (red blood and mucus)
PAINFUL ANAL LESIONS	Pain may cause spasm of the external sphincter and voluntary inhibition of the defecation reflex.	Anal fissures, painful hemorrhoids, perirectal abscesses
DRUGS	A variety of mechanisms	Opiates, anticholinergics, antacids containing calcium or aluminum, and many others
DEPRESSION	A disorder of mood. See Table 3-3, Distinguishing Features of Depressive Disorders.	Fatigue, feelings of depression, and other somatic symptoms
NEUROLOGIC DISORDERS	Interference with the autonomic innervation of the bowel	Spinal cord injuries, multiple sclerosis, Hirschsprung's disease, and other conditions
METABOLIC CONDITIONS	Interference with bowel motility	Pregnancy, hypothyroidism, hypercalcemia

Table 2-11

Table 2-11 *Acute Diarrhea*

PROBLEM	PROCESS
ACUTE DIARRHEA, OR UNCOMPLICATED GASTROENTERITIS	Viral or bacterial infection, or ingestion of a toxin elaborated by bacteria
PROLONGED DIARRHEA	Acute gastroenteritis may unmask an underlying lactase deficiency or may be followed by transient bacterial overgrowth in the small bowel that prolongs the symptoms. Infection by toxigenic *Escherichia coli* or *Giardia lamblia* may also cause prolonged diarrhea.
DYSENTERY	Invasion of the colonic or rectal mucosa by bacteria (such as *Shigella, Salmonella,* gonococci, and invasive *E. coli*) or by *Entamoeba histolytica* (amebic dysentery)
DRUG-INDUCED DIARRHEA	Pharmacological actions of many drugs, including magnesium-containing antacids, digoxin, broad-spectrum antibiotics, and laxatives
FECAL IMPACTION	Partial obstruction of the rectum by impacted stool, with overflow diarrhea around it

Table 2-11

Table 2-11 *(Cont'd.)*

SYMPTOMS	TIMING	SETTING
Watery diarrhea, lower abdominal cramping pain, nausea, and vomiting, with relatively little or no fever	Sudden onset, lasts 2–5 dy	May occur in epidemics; often a detectable common food source
Same as in acute diarrhea (see above). Intolerance to milk and milk products if the diarrhea is due to lactase deficiency.	Sudden onset, lasts longer than 5 dy	Toxigenic *E. coli* is a common cause of "traveler's diarrhea." *Giardia* may contaminate water supplies.
Lower abdominal cramping pain and often fever. There may be rectal urgency, tenesmus, and blood or pus in the stools, most notably in *Shigella* infections.	An acute illness of variable duration	Travel, contaminated water or food. Gonococci and other organisms may infect the rectum and colon of homosexual men.
Usually a watery diarrhea with relatively little if any pain. Possibly nausea and drug fever.	Variable	Carefully review all over-the-counter and prescribed medications of a patient with unexplained diarrhea.
A sense of rectal fullness, urgency, and tenesmus, with frequent small liquid stools	Variable	Debilitated, bedridden, and often elderly patients who may or may not be able to give a good history. In infants and young children consider Hirschsprung's disease.

Table 2-12

Table 2-12   Chronic or Recurrent Diarrhea

PROBLEM	PROCESS	CHARACTERISTICS OF STOOL
DIARRHEA WITH PERIODS OF CONSTIPATION		
IRRITABLE BOWEL SYNDROME	A disorder of bowel motility	Loose; may show mucus but no blood. Small, hard stools when constipated
CANCER OF THE SIGMOID COLON	Partial obstruction by a malignant neoplasm	May be blood-streaked
NONSPECIFIC DIARRHEAL SYNDROMES		
IRRITABLE BOWEL SYNDROME	A disorder of bowel motility	Loose; may show mucus but no blood
CANCER OF THE SIGMOID COLON	Partial obstruction by a malignant neoplasm	May be blood-streaked
DRUGS *(See Table 2-11, Acute Diarrhea.)*		
INFLAMMATORY DIARRHEAS		
ULCERATIVE COLITIS	Inflammation of the mucosa and submucosa of the rectum and colon with ulceration; cause unknown	From soft to watery, often containing blood
CROHN'S DISEASE OF THE SMALL BOWEL *(regional enteritis)* OR COLON *(granulomatous colitis)*	Chronic inflammation of the bowel wall, typically involving the terminal ileum and/or proximal colon	Small, soft to loose or watery, usually free of gross blood (enteritis) or with less bleeding than ulcerative colitis (colitis)
VOLUMINOUS DIARRHEAS		
MALABSORPTION SYNDROMES	Defective absorption of fat and other substances including fat-soluble vitamins, with excessive excretion of fat (steatorrhea); many causes	Typically bulky, soft, light yellow to gray, mushy, greasy or oily, and sometimes frothy
OSMOTIC DIARRHEAS *Lactose intolerance*	Deficiency of intestinal lactase	Watery diarrhea of large volume
Abuse of osmotic purgatives	Laxative habit, often surreptitious	Watery diarrhea of large volume
SECRETORY DIARRHEAS, *associated with a number of uncommon conditions, such as the Zollinger–Ellison syndrome*	Variable	Watery diarrhea of large volume

Table 2-12

Table 2-12 (Cont'd.)

TIMING	ASSOCIATED SYMPTOMS	PERSONS AT HIGHER RISK
Alternating periods of diarrhea and constipation. Diarrhea rarely wakes the patient at night.	Crampy lower abdominal pain, abdominal distention, flatulence, nausea	Young and middle-aged adults, especially women
Periods of both diarrhea and constipation	Change in usual bowel habits, crampy lower abdominal pain	Middle-aged and older adults, especially over 55 yr
Often worse in the morning. Diarrhea rarely wakes the patient at night.	Crampy lower abdominal pain, abdominal distention, flatulence, nausea	Young and middle-aged adults, especially women
Variable	Change in usual bowel habits, crampy lower abdominal pain	Middle-aged and older adults, especially over 55 yr
Onset ranges from insidious to acute. Typically recurrent, may be persistent. Diarrhea may wake the patient at night.	Crampy lower or generalized abdominal pain, anorexia, weakness, fever	Often young people
Insidious onset, chronic or recurrent. Diarrhea may wake the patient at night.	Crampy periumbilical or right lower quadrant (enteritis) or diffuse (colitis) pain, with anorexia, low fever, and/or weight loss. Perianal or perirectal abscesses and fistulas.	Often young people, especially in the late teens, but also in the middle years. More common in Jews.
Onset of illness typically insidious	Anorexia, weight loss, fatigue, abdominal distention, often crampy lower abdominal pain. Symptoms of nutritional deficiencies such as bleeding (vitamin K), bone pain and fractures (vitamin D), glossitis (vitamin B), and edema (protein).	Variable, depending on cause
Follows the ingestion of milk and milk products; is relieved by fasting	Crampy abdominal pain, abdominal distention, flatulence	Blacks, Asians, Native Americans
Variable	Often none	Persons with anorexia nervosa or bulimia nervosa
Variable	Weight loss, dehydration, nausea, vomiting, and cramping abdominal pain	Variable, depending on cause

Table 2-13

Table 2-13 Polyuria, Frequency, and Nocturia

PROBLEM	MECHANISMS	SELECTED CAUSES	ASSOCIATED SYMPTOMS
POLYURIA	Diminished ability of the kidneys to concentrate the urine	Chronic renal failure, hypokalemia, hypercalcemia	Variable according to the cause. The polyuria and accompanying thirst are relatively mild.
	Excessive excretion of a solute that is poorly reabsorbed by the kidney, most commonly glucose	Diabetes mellitus	Thirst, polydipsia, polyphagia (increased food intake), and fatigue
	Deficiency of antidiuretic hormone or renal unresponsiveness to it	Diabetes insipidus, nephrogenic diabetes insipidus	Thirst and polydipsia, typically very severe and persistent. Nocturia.
	Excessive water intake	Primary (or "psychogenic") polydipsia	Polydipsia, which may be episodic; often, but not necessarily, thirst. Usually no nocturia.
FREQUENCY WITHOUT POLYURIA	Decreased capacity of the bladder		
	Increased bladder sensitivity to stretch because of inflammation	Cystitis, bladder stones, tumor, or foreign body	Burning on urination, urinary urgency, sometimes gross hematuria
	Decreased elasticity of the bladder wall	Infiltration by scar tissue or tumor	Symptoms of associated inflammation (see above) are common.
	Decreased cortical inhibition of bladder contractions	Upper motor neuron disease	Urinary urgency; symptoms of upper motor neuron disease such as weakness and paralysis
	Impaired emptying of the bladder		
	Partial mechanical obstruction of the bladder neck or proximal urethra	Prostatic hypertrophy, urethral stricture	Hesitancy in starting the urinary stream, straining to void, reduced size and force of the stream, and dribbling during or at the end of urination
	Loss of lower motor or sensory nerve supply to the bladder	Neurologic disease affecting the sacral nerves or nerve roots, *e.g.*, diabetic neuropathy	Weakness or sensory defects
	Anxiety	Student examinations among other stressful events; sometimes anxiety over possible incontinence	Possibly other symptoms of anxiety

Table 2-13

Table 2-13   (Cont'd.)

PROBLEM	MECHANISMS	SELECTED CAUSES	ASSOCIATED SYMPTOMS
NOCTURIA			
WITH HIGH VOLUMES	Polyuria (see p. 82)		
	Excessive fluid intake before bedtime	Habit, especially involving alcohol and coffee	
	Fluid-retaining, edematous states. Dependent edema accumulates during the day and is excreted when the patient lies down at night.	Congestive heart failure, nephrotic syndrome, hepatic cirrhosis with ascites, chronic venous insufficiency	Edema and other symptoms of the underlying disorder. Urinary output during the day may be reduced as fluid reaccumulates in the body. See Table 15-3, Mechanisms and Patterns of Edema.
WITH LOW VOLUMES	Frequency without polyuria (see p. 82)		
	Voiding while up at night without a real urge, a "pseudo-frequency"	Insomnia	Variable

Table 2-14

Table 2-14 *Urinary Incontinence*

PROBLEM	MECHANISMS
STRESS INCONTINENCE The urethral sphincter is weakened so that transient increases in intraabdominal pressure raise the bladder pressure to levels that exceed urethral resistance.	In women, most often a weakness of the pelvic floor with inadequate muscular support of the bladder and proximal urethra and a change in the angle between the bladder and urethra. Suggested causes include childbirth and surgery. Local conditions affecting the internal urethral sphincter, such as postmenopausal atrophy of the mucosa and urethral infection, may also contribute.
URGE INCONTINENCE Detrusor contractions are stronger than normal and overcome the normal urethral resistance. The bladder is typically small.	1. Decreased cortical inhibition of detrusor contractions, as by strokes, brain tumors, dementia, and lesions of the spinal cord above the sacral level 2. Hyperexcitability of sensory pathways, caused by, for example, bladder infections, tumors, and fecal impaction 3. Deconditioning of voiding reflexes, caused by, for example, frequent voluntary voiding at low bladder volumes
OVERFLOW INCONTINENCE Detrusor contractions are insufficient to overcome urethral resistance. The bladder is typically large, even after an effort to void.	1. Obstruction of the bladder outlet, as by prostatic hypertrophy or tumor 2. Weakness of the detrusor muscle associated with lower motor neuron disease at the sacral level 3. Impaired bladder sensation that interrupts the reflex arc, as from diabetic neuropathy
FUNCTIONAL INCONTINENCE This is a functional inability to get to the toilet in time because of impaired health or environmental conditions.	Problems in mobility resulting from weakness, arthritis, poor vision, or other conditions. Environmental factors such as an unfamiliar setting, distant bathroom facilities, bedrails, or physical restraints.
INCONTINENCE SECONDARY TO MEDICATIONS Drugs may contribute to any type of incontinence listed.	Sedatives, tranquilizers, anticholinergics, sympathetic blockers, and potent diuretics

Unfortunately elderly patients, who are most likely to experience urinary incontinence, often have more than one kind of dysfunction, and differentiation on clinical grounds may be impossible.

Table 2-14

Table 2-14   (Cont'd.)

SYMPTOMS	PHYSICAL SIGNS
Momentary leakage of small amounts of urine concurrent with stresses such as coughing, laughing, and sneezing	The bladder is not detectable on abdominal examination. Stress incontinence may be demonstrable, especially if the patient is examined before voiding and in a standing position. Atrophic vaginitis may be evident.
Incontinence preceded by an urge to void. The volume tends to be moderate. Urgency; frequency and nocturia with small to moderate volumes If acute inflammation is present, pain on urination Possibly "pseudo-stress incontinence"—voiding 10–20 sec after stresses such as a change of position, going up or down stairs, and possibly coughing, laughing, or sneezing.	The bladder is not detectable on abdominal examination. When cortical inhibition is decreased, signs of upper motor neuron disease or mental deficits are often, though not necessarily, present. When sensory pathways are hyperexcitable, signs of local pelvic problems or a fecal impaction may be present.
A continuous dripping or dribbling incontinence Decreased force of the urinary stream Prior symptoms of partial urinary obstruction or symptoms of neurologic disease may be present.	The bladder is often found enlarged on abdominal examination and may be tender. Other possible signs include prostatic enlargement, signs of lower motor neuron disease, a decrease in sensation including perineal sensation, and diminished to absent reflexes.
Incontinence on the way to the toilet or only in the early morning	The bladder is not detectable on physical examination. Look for physical or environmental clues to the likely cause.
Variable. A careful history and chart review are important.	Variable

Table 2-15

Table 2-15   Painful Peripheral Vascular Disorders and Their Mimics

PROBLEM	PROCESS	LOCATION
ARTERIAL DISORDERS ARTERIOSCLEROSIS OBLITERANS *Intermittent claudication*	Episodic muscular ischemia induced by exercise, due to obstruction of large or middle-sized arteries by atherosclerosis	Usually the calf, but may also be felt in the buttock, hip, thigh, or foot, depending on the level of obstruction
Rest pain	Ischemia even at rest	Distal pain, in the toes or forefoot
ACUTE ARTERIAL OCCLUSION	Embolism or thrombosis, possibly superimposed on arteriosclerosis obliterans	Distal pain, usually involving the foot and leg
VENOUS DISORDERS SUPERFICIAL THROMBOPHLEBITIS	Clot formation and acute inflammation in a superficial vein	Pain in a local area along the course of a superficial vein, most often in the saphenous system
DEEP THROMBOPHLEBITIS	Clot formation in a deep vein	Pain, if present, is usually in the calf, but the process more often is painless.
CHRONIC VENOUS INSUFFICIENCY	Chronic venous engorgement secondary to venous occlusion or incompetency of venous valves	Diffuse aching of the leg(s)
ACUTE LYMPHANGITIS	Acute bacterial infection (usually strepto-coccal) spreading up the lymphatic channels from a portal of entry such as an injured area or an ulcer	An arm or a leg
THROMBOANGIITIS OBLITERANS *(Buerger's disease)*	Inflammatory and thrombotic occlusions of small arteries and also of veins, occurring in smokers	1. Intermittent claudication, particularly in the arch of the foot 2. Pain in the fingers or toes
RAYNAUD'S DISEASE *(and phenomenon)*	Episodic spasm of the small arteries and arterioles, without organic occlusion. When the syndrome is secondary to other conditions (and then called Raynaud's phenomenon) occlusion may occur.	Distal portions of one or more fingers. Pain is usually not prominent unless fingertip ulcers develop. Numbness and tingling are common.
MIMICS* ACUTE CELLULITIS	Acute bacterial infection of the skin and subcutaneous tissues	Arms, legs, or elsewhere
ERYTHEMA NODOSUM	Inflammatory lesions associated with a variety of systemic disorders	Anterior surfaces of both lower legs

* Mistaken primarily for acute superficial thrombophlebitis

Table 2-15

Table 2-15 (Cont'd.)

TIMING	FACTORS THAT AGGRAVATE	FACTORS THAT RELIEVE	ASSOCIATED MANIFESTATIONS
Fairly brief: pain usually forces the patient to rest	Exercise such as walking	Rest usually stops the pain in 1–3 min.	Local fatigue, numbness, diminished pulses, often signs of arterial insufficiency (see p. 420)
Persistent, often worse at night	Elevation of the feet, as in bed	Sitting with legs dependent	Numbness, tingling, signs of arterial insufficiency (see p. 420)
Sudden onset; associated symptoms may occur without pain			Coldness, numbness, weakness, absent distal pulses
An acute episode lasting days or longer			Local redness, swelling, tenderness, a palpable cord, possibly fever
Often hard to determine because of lack of symptoms			Possibly swelling of the foot and calf and local calf tenderness
Chronic, increasing as the day wears on	Prolonged standing	Elevation of the leg(s)	Chronic edema, pigmentation, possibly ulceration (see pp. 420–421)
An acute episode lasting days or longer			Red streak(s) on the skin, with tenderness, enlarged tender lymph nodes, and fever
1. With exercise 2. Chronic, persistent, may be worse at night		Permanent cessation of smoking (but patients seldom stop)	Distal coldness, sweating, numbness, and cyanosis; ulceration and gangrene at the tips of fingers or toes; migratory thrombophlebitis
Relatively brief (minutes) but recurrent	Exposure to cold, emotional upset	Warm environment	Color changes in the distal fingers: severe pallor (essential for the diagnosis) followed by cyanosis and then redness
An acute episode lasting days or longer			A local area of diffuse swelling, redness, and tenderness with enlarged, tender lymph nodes and fever; no palpable cord
Pain associated with a series of lesions over several weeks			Raised, red, tender swellings recurring in crops; often malaise, joint pains, and fever

Table 2-16 Patterns of Chronic Pain In and Around the Joints

PROBLEM	PROCESS	COMMON LOCATIONS	PATTERN OF SPREAD	ONSET	PROGRESSION AND DURATION
RHEUMATOID ARTHRITIS	Chronic inflammation of synovial membranes with secondary erosion of adjacent cartilage, bone, ligaments, and tendons	Hands (proximal interphalangeal and metacarpophalangeal joints), feet (metatarsophalangeal joints), wrists, knees, elbows, and ankles	Symmetrically additive: progresses to other joints while persisting in the initial ones	Usually insidious	Often chronic with remissions and exacerbations
OSTEOARTHRITIS (*degenerative joint disease*)	Degeneration and progressive loss of cartilage within the joints, damage to underlying bone, and the formation of new bone at the margins of the cartilage	Knees, hips, hands (distal interphalangeal and sometimes the proximal interphalangeal joints), cervical and lumbar spine, and wrists (the first carpometacarpal joint); also joints previously injured or diseased	Additive	Usually insidious	Slowly progressive with temporary exacerbations after periods of overuse
GOUTY ARTHRITIS					
ACUTE GOUT	An inflammatory reaction to microcrystals of sodium urate	Base of the big toe (the first metatarsophalangeal joint), and possibly the instep and ankle	Early attacks are usually confined to one joint.	Sudden, often at night, often after injury, surgery, fasting, or excessive food or alcohol intake	Occasional isolated attacks lasting days up to 2 wk; they may increase in frequency and severity, and persisting symptoms may develop
CHRONIC TOPHACEOUS GOUT	Multiple local accumulations of sodium urate in the joints and other tissues (tophi), with chronic and acute inflammation	Feet, ankles, wrists, fingers, and elbows	Additive, not so symmetrical as rheumatoid arthritis	Gradual development of chronicity with repeated attacks	Chronic symptoms with acute exacerbations
POLYMYALGIA RHEUMATICA	A disease of uncertain nature seen in people over 50 yr, especially women; may be associated with giant cell arteritis	Muscles of the neck, shoulders, and upper arms, and sometimes the hips and thighs; symmetrical		Abrupt or insidious	Chronic
THE "FIBROSITIS" SYNDROME	Muscular aching and stiffness with specific, tender "trigger areas." May accompany rheumatoid arthritis. Mechanisms uncertain.	"All over" but especially in the neck, shoulders, elbows, hands, low back, and knees	Shifts unpredictably or worsens in response to immobility, excessive use, or chilling	Variable, may follow an upsetting event	Chronic with "ups and downs"

Table 2-16 (Cont'd.)

ASSOCIATED SYMPTOMS

SWELLING	REDNESS, WARMTH, AND TENDERNESS	STIFFNESS	LIMITATION OF MOTION	GENERALIZED SYMPTOMS
Frequent, in joints or tendon sheaths; also subcutaneous nodules	Tender, often warm, but seldom red	Prominent, often for an hour or more in the mornings, also after inactivity	Often develops	Weakness, fatigue, weight loss, and low fever are common.
Small effusions in the joints may be present, especially in the knees; also bony enlargement	Possibly tender, seldom warm, and rarely red	Frequent but brief (usually 5–10 min), in the morning and after inactivity	Often develops	Usually absent
Present, within and around the involved joint	Hot, red, and exquisitely tender	May appear as chronic symptoms develop	Motion is limited primarily by pain	Fever may be present.
Present, as tophi, in joints, bursae, and subcutaneous tissues	Tenderness, warmth, and redness may be present during exacerbations.	Present	Present	Possibly fever; may also develop symptoms of renal failure and renal stones
None	Muscles often tender, but not warm or red	Prominent, especially in the morning	Usually none, unless a late contracture develops	Malaise, possibly anorexia, weight loss, and fever, but no true weakness
None	Specific tender "trigger areas," often not recognized until examination	Present, especially in the morning	Absent, though stiffness is greater at the extremes of movement	Fatigue, difficulty sleeping

Table 2-17 Low Back Pain

PATTERNS	POSSIBLE CAUSES	POSSIBLE PHYSICAL SIGNS
COMMON LOW BACK PAIN Acute, recurrent, or chronic aching pain in the lumbosacral area, possibly radiating into the posterior thighs but not below the knees and not in a dermatomal distribution. The pain is often precipitated or aggravated by moving, lifting, or prolonged standing and is relieved by rest. Spinal movements are typically limited by pain.	1. The lumbosacral sprain syndrome, presumably related to the faulty mechanics of poor posture, possibly with superimposed injury after lifting, twisting, or other movement. This is by far the most common cause. 2. Congenital disorders of the spine such as spondylolisthesis and transitional vertebrae 3. Spondylosis—degenerative disease of the intervertebral discs with bony spurring. This occurs in the older age groups. 4. Osteoporosis complicated by collapse of a vertebra. This occurs primarily in older women.	1. Local tenderness, muscle spasm, pain on movement of the back, and loss of the normal lumbar lordosis, but no motor or sensory loss or reflex abnormalities 2. In addition to above, a spinous process (L4 or L5) unusually prominent in relation to the one above it 3. Signs as in the lumbosacral sprain syndrome 4. Other signs of osteoporosis: thoracic kyphosis, perhaps percussion tenderness over a spinous process, and fractures elsewhere (as in a hip)
CHRONIC PERSISTENT LOW BACK PAIN WITH STIFFNESS Usually of insidious onset with stiffness worse in the mornings. Spinal range of motion becomes limited.	Ankylosing spondylitis, a chronic inflammatory polyarthritis most common in young men	Loss of the normal lumbar lordosis, muscle spasm, and limitation of both anterior and lateral flexion
LOW BACK PAIN RADIATING BELOW THE KNEE(S) IN A DERMATOMAL DISTRIBUTION In addition to low back pain the patient has *radicular (nerve root)* pain. This is a shooting pain that radiates down one or both legs, usually to below the knee(s) in a dermatomal distribution, often with associated numbness and tingling and possibly local weakness. When compression or stretching of the nerve roots is involved, the pain is worsened by spinal movements such as bending and by sneezing, coughing, or straining.	1. Herniated intervertebral disc with compression of nerve root(s), the most common cause. Unilateral pain usually radiates in the L5 or S1 distribution (see pp. 475–476). 2. Spondylosis, with compression of nerve root(s). This occurs mainly in men over 60 yr. 3. Spinal cord tumor or abscess, with compression of nerves or nerve roots 4. Diabetic mononeuropathy	1, 2, and 3. Pain on straight leg raising and crossed straight leg raising, tenderness of the sciatic nerve, loss of sensation in a dermatomal distribution, local muscular weakness and atrophy, and decreased to absent reflex(es), especially affecting the ankle jerks. Dermatomal signs and reflex changes, however, may be absent when only a single root is compressed. Tumors or abscesses are more likely to compress a greater number of roots and more often produce neurologic deficits. 4. Partial motor and sensory loss in a sciatic distribution
BACK PAIN REFERRED FROM THE ABDOMEN OR PELVIS Usually a deep aching pain. The spinal level of the pain may be helpful in diagnosis. For example: 1. Lower thoracic or upper lumbar pain (from upper abdominal diseases) 2. Lumbar pain (from lower abdominal diseases) 3. Sacral pain (from pelvic diseases) The level of pain may vary with the level of the lesion.	 1. Peptic ulcer, especially with posterior penetration, pancreatitis, pancreatic cancer, acute pyelonephritis 2. Colitis, diverticulitis, retrocecal appendicitis 3. Endometriosis, chronic prostatitis 4. Dissecting aortic aneurysm 5. Retroperitoneal tumor	Range of motion is not usually affected by these conditions, nor are spinal movements painful. 1. Tenderness in the abdomen (pancreatitis) or the costovertebral angle (pyelonephritis), or an abdominal mass and jaundice (pancreatic cancer) 2. Tenderness, abdominal or rectal depending on the cause 3. Nodules on pelvic examination (endometriosis) or abnormalities of the prostate gland (see p. 405) 4. Variable 5. Variable

Table 2-18   Pains in the Neck

Classifications of neck pain vary considerably, partly because pathologic or other presumably definitive criteria are usually lacking. While "simple stiff neck" is very common, for example, people who have it seldom seek care for it.

PATTERNS	POSSIBLE CAUSES	POSSIBLE PHYSICAL SIGNS
"SIMPLE STIFF NECK" Acute, episodic, localized pain in the neck, often appearing on awakening and lasting 1–4 dy. No dermatomal radiation	The mechanisms are not understood.	Local muscular tenderness and pain on certain movements
ACHING NECK A persistent dull aching in the back of the neck, often spreading to the occiput. This is common with postural strain, as with prolonged typing or studying, and may also accompany tension and depression.	Poorly understood; may be related to sustained muscle contraction, as in muscle tension headaches	Local muscular tenderness. When areas of pain and tenderness are also present elsewhere in the body, consider the fibrositis syndrome (see Table 2-16, Patterns of Chronic Pain In and Around the Joints).
"CERVICAL SPRAIN" Acute and often recurrent neck pains that are often more severe and last longer than "simple stiff neck." There may be a precipitating factor such as a whiplash injury, heavy lifting, or a sudden movement, but there is no dermatomal radiation.	Poorly understood	Local tenderness and pain on movement
NECK PAIN WITH DERMATOMAL RADIATION* Neck pain as in "cervical sprain" but with radiation of the pain to the shoulder, back, or arm in a dermatomal distribution. The radicular pain is typically sharp, burning, or tingling in quality.	1. A herniated cervical disc with compression of nerve root(s) 2. Cervical spondylosis—degenerative disease of the intervertebral discs with bony spurring and compression of one or more nerve roots	1 and 2. Muscle tenderness and spasm, a limited range of neck motion, increase in the pain on coughing or straining, and possible sensory loss, weakness, muscular atrophy, and decreased reflexes in the areas involved
NECK PAIN WITH SYMPTOMS SUGGESTING COMPRESSION OF THE CERVICAL SPINAL CORD* Associated here is weakness or paralysis of the legs, often with a decrease in or loss of sensation. These symptoms may occur in addition to the radicular symptoms or by themselves. The neck pain may be mild or even absent.	1. A herniated cervical disc with compression of the spinal cord in the neck 2. Cervical spondylosis with similar compression	1 and 2. Limited range of motion in the neck, weakness or paralysis in the legs of the upper motor neuron type, Babinski responses, loss of position and vibration sense in the legs, and, less commonly, loss of pain and temperature sensation. Radicular signs in the arms may also be present.

* Tumors or abscesses of the cervical spinal cord, though less common, should also be considered.

Table 2-19

Table 2-19 Syncope and Similar Disorders

PROBLEM	MECHANISM	PRECIPITATING FACTORS
VASODEPRESSOR SYNCOPE *(the common faint)*	Sudden peripheral vasodilatation, especially in the skeletal muscles, without a compensatory rise in cardiac output. Blood pressure falls.	A strong emotion such as fear or pain
POSTURAL *(orthostatic)* HYPOTENSION	1. *Inadequate vasoconstrictor reflexes* in both arterioles and veins, with resultant venous pooling and decreased cardiac output	1. Standing up
	2. *Hypovolemia,* a diminished blood volume insufficient to maintain cardiac output and blood pressure, especially in the upright position	2. Standing up after hemorrhage or dehydration
COUGH SYNCOPE	Several possible mechanisms associated with increased intrathoracic pressure	Severe paroxysm of coughing
MICTURITION SYNCOPE	Uncertain	Emptying the bladder after getting out of bed to void
CARDIAC DISORDERS ARRHYTHMIAS	Decreased cardiac output secondary to rhythms that are too fast (usually over 180) or too slow (less than 35–40)	A sudden change in rhythm
AORTIC STENOSIS AND HYPERTROPHIC CARDIOMYOPATHY	Mechanism uncertain	Effort
MYOCARDIAL INFARCTION AND MASSIVE PULMONARY EMBOLISM	Variable	Variable
DISORDERS RESEMBLING SYNCOPE HYPOCAPNIA *(decreased carbon dioxide)* DUE TO HYPERVENTILATION	Constriction of cerebral blood vessels secondary to hypocapnia that is induced by hyperventilation	Possibly a stressful situation
HYPOGLYCEMIA	Secretion of epinephrine in response to a low blood glucose and insufficient glucose to maintain cerebral metabolism	Variable, including fasting
HYSTERICAL FAINTING*	The symbolic expression of an unacceptable idea through bodily language	Stressful situation

* Important diagnostic observations in hysterical fainting include normal skin color and normal vital signs, sometimes bizarre and purposive movements, and occurrence in the presence of others.

Table 2-19

Table 2-19 (Cont'd.)

PREDISPOSING FACTORS	PRODROMAL MANIFESTATIONS	POSTURAL ASSOCIATIONS	RECOVERY
Fatigue, hunger, a hot, humid environment	Pallor, nausea, salivation, sweating, yawning	Usually occurs when standing, possibly when sitting	Prompt return of consciousness when lying down, but pallor, weakness, nausea, and slight confusion may persist for a time
1. Peripheral neuropathies and disorders affecting the autonomic nervous system; drugs such as antihypertensives and vasodilators; prolonged bed rest	1. Often none	1. Occurs soon after the person stands up	1. Prompt return to normal when lying down
2. Bleeding from the GI tract or trauma, potent diuretics, vomiting, diarrhea, polyuria	2. Lightheadedness and palpitations (tachycardia) on standing up	2. Usually occurs soon after the person stands up	2. Improvement on lying down
Chronic bronchitis in a muscular man	Often none except for cough	May occur in any position	Prompt return to normal
Nocturia, usually in elderly or adult men	Often none	Standing to void	Prompt return to normal
Organic heart disease and old age decrease the tolerance to abnormal rhythms.	Often none	May occur in any position	Prompt return to normal unless brain damage has resulted
The cardiac disorders	Often none	Occurs with or after exercise	Usually a prompt return to normal
Variable	Often none	May occur in any position	Variable
A predisposition to anxiety attacks and hyperventilation	Dyspnea, palpitations, chest discomfort, numbness and tingling of the hands and around the mouth lasting for several minutes. Consciousness is often maintained.	May occur in any position	Slow improvement as hyperventilation ceases
Insulin therapy and a variety of metabolic disorders	Sweating, tremor, palpitations, hunger; headache, confusion, abnormal behavior, coma. True syncope is uncommon.	May occur in any position	Variable, depending on severity and treatment
Hysterical personality traits	Variable	A slump to the floor, often from a standing position without injury	Variable, may be prolonged, often with fluctuating responsiveness

Table 2-20

Table 2-20   Seizure Disorders

Partial seizures are those that start with focal manifestations. They may or may not become generalized. They are further divided into *simple partial seizures*, which do not impair consciousness, and *complex partial seizures*, which do. Either of these two may progress into a third type, *partial seizures that become generalized*. Partial seizures of all kinds usually indicate a structural lesion in the cerebral cortex, such as scars, tumors, or infarctions. The quality of such seizures helps the clinician to localize the causative lesion in the brain.

PROBLEM	CLINICAL MANIFESTATIONS	POSTICTAL (POSTSEIZURE) STATE
PARTIAL SEIZURES		
SIMPLE PARTIAL SEIZURES		
With motor symptoms		
Jacksonian	Tonic, then clonic movements that start unilaterally in the hand, foot, or face and then spread to other bodily parts on the same side	Normal
Other motor	Turning of the head and eyes to one side, or tonic and clonic movements of an arm or leg without the Jacksonian spread	Normal
With sensory symptoms	Numbness, tingling; simple visual, auditory, or olfactory hallucinations such as flashing lights, buzzing, or odors	Normal
With autonomic symptoms	A "funny feeling" in the epigastrium, pallor, flushing	Normal
With psychic symptoms	Anxiety or fear; feelings of familiarity (déjà vu) or unreality; flashback experiences; more complex hallucinations	Normal
COMPLEX PARTIAL SEIZURES These may start with simple partial seizures or with impaired consciousness. Automatisms may develop.	The seizure usually starts with autonomic or psychic symptoms. Consciousness is impaired and the person appears confused. Automatisms include automatic motor behaviors such as chewing, smacking the lips, walking about, and unbuttoning clothes; also more complicated and skilled behaviors such as driving a car.	The patient may remember initial autonomic or psychic symptoms (then termed an *aura*) but is amnesic for the rest of the seizure. Temporary confusion and headache may occur.
PARTIAL SEIZURES THAT BECOME GENERALIZED	Partial seizures that become generalized resemble tonic–clonic seizures (see p. 95). Unfortunately the patient may not recall the focal onset, and observers may overlook it.	As in a tonic–clonic seizure. Two attributes indicate a partial seizure that has become generalized: (1) the recollection of an aura, and (2) a unilateral neurologic deficit during the postictal period.

Table 2-20

Table 2-20 (Cont'd.)

Generalized seizures, in contrast to partial ones, begin with either bilateral bodily movements or impairment of consciousness, or both. They suggest a widespread, bilateral cortical disturbance that may be either hereditary or acquired. When generalized seizures of the tonic–clonic (grand mal) variety start in childhood or young adulthood, they are often hereditary. When tonic–clonic seizures begin after the age of 30, suspect either a partial seizure that has become generalized or a general seizure caused by a toxic or metabolic problem. Toxic and metabolic causes include withdrawal from alcohol or other sedative drugs, uremia, hypoglycemia, hyperglycemia, hyponatremia and water intoxication, and bacterial meningitis.

PROBLEM	CLINICAL MANIFESTATIONS	POSTICTAL (POSTSEIZURE) STATE
GENERALIZED SEIZURES		
TONIC–CLONIC (*grand mal*)*	The person loses consciousness suddenly, sometimes with a cry, and the body stiffens into tonic extensor rigidity. Breathing stops and the person becomes cyanotic. A clonic phase of rhythmic muscular contraction follows. Breathing resumes and is often noisy, with excessive salivation. Injury, tongue-biting, and urinary incontinence may occur.	Confusion, drowsiness, fatigue, headache, muscular aching, and sometimes the temporary persistence of bilateral neurologic deficits such as hyperactive reflexes and Babinski responses. The person has amnesia for the seizure and recalls no aura.
ABSENCE	A sudden brief lapse of consciousness, with momentary blinking, staring, or movements of the lips and hands but no falling	Prompt return to normal. The person recalls no aura.
AKINETIC SEIZURE, OR DROP ATTACK	Sudden loss of consciousness with falling but no movements. Injury may occur.	Either a prompt return to normal or a brief period of confusion
MYOCLONUS	Sudden, brief, rapid jerks, involving the trunk or limbs. Associated with a variety of disorders.	Variable

* *Febrile convulsions* that resemble brief tonic–clonic seizures may occur in infants and young children. They are usually benign but occasionally may be the first manifestation of a seizure disorder.

Chapter 3
Mental Status

Components of Mental Function

In every body system clinicians have selected certain readily observable characteristics with which to assess the structure and function of that system, to distinguish a healthy from a pathologic state, and to diagnose disease. While symptoms, heart sounds, pressures, and pulse waves serve these purposes in the cardiovascular system, for example, various components of mental function do so for the mind. Although these components in no way encompass all the aspects of human thought and feeling, they serve as useful clinical tools.

Level of consciousness refers to people's alertness and state of awareness of their environment. *Attention* refers to the ability to focus or concentrate over time on one task or activity. An inattentive or distractible person whose consciousness is clouded will be grossly impaired in giving a history or responding to questions. *Memory,* too, contributes importantly to such responses. A person first must register or record material in the mind—a function usually tested by asking for immediate repetition of material. Information must then be stored or retained in memory. *Recent memory*—a rather loosely defined term—refers to memory over an interval of minutes, hours, or days, while *remote memory* refers to intervals of years. *Orientation* depends on both memory and attention. It refers to people's awareness of who or what they are in relation to time, place, and other people.

A person becomes aware of objects in the environment and their qualities and interrelationships through sensory *perceptions.* While most perceptions are initiated by external stimuli, others, like dreams and hallucinations, arise in the mind itself.

Thought processes refer to the sequence, logic, coherence, and relevance of a person's thought as it leads to selected goals. While thought processes describe how people think, *thought content* refers to what they think about. In contrast, affect and mood describe how people feel. *Affect* is an immediately observable, usually episodic feeling tone expressed through voice, facial expression, or demeanor, while *mood* is a more sustained emotion that may color a person's view of the world. As weather is to climate, so affect is to mood.

People communicate with each other through *language,* a complex symbolic system of expressing, receiving, and comprehending words. Like consciousness, attention, and memory, language is essential to other mental functions; significant impairment here makes assessment of certain other functions difficult or even impossible.

Higher intellectual functions include a person's *vocabulary,* fund of *information,* and capacity to reason abstractly and to make judgments. *Abstract reasoning* refers to the ability to think beyond concrete terms — to grasp, for example, the similarities or differences between terms, or to understand the general meaning of literally worded proverbs. In making *judgments* a person compares and evaluates alternatives for purposes of deciding on a course of action. Inherent in judgment is a set of values that may or may not be based on reality and may or may not conform to societal norms.

None of the functions described in this chapter deals directly with personality, psychodynamics, or personal experiences. These other, very important aspects are explored during the interview. By integrating and correlating all the relevant data the clinician tries to understand the person as a whole.

CHANGES WITH AGE

Although psychological research has demonstrated many alterations in mental function over the normal lifespan, clinical assessment identifies relatively few of these changes.

Adolescence marks a time of continuing intellectual maturation during which a person's fund of information and vocabulary continue to grow — a process that began in childhood. At approximately 12 years of age adolescents begin to think abstractly — to use generalizations, make hypotheses, develop theories, reason logically, and consider future plans, risks, and possibilities. Given intelligence, education, and experience, among other requisites, judgment develops along with an underlying set of values. This maturational process, however, like height, weight, and puberty, varies in its time of onset, pace, and duration and cannot be predicted by chronological age alone. Some individuals never achieve the levels customarily defined as normal adult function.

Most intellectual functions that are tested clinically hold up quite well in the later decades of life. Vocabulary and information, for example, decline relatively little, although they do diminish somewhat. Immediate memory persists well too, although in tests that require reorganization of data, such as repeating numbers backward, older people do less well than younger ones. Memory declines to some extent with age, and elderly people take longer to retrieve information from their minds.

Techniques of Examination

Most of the mental status examination should be done in the context of the interview. As you talk to the patient and listen to the story, you should assess level of consciousness, general appearance and affect, and ability to pay attention, remember, understand, and speak. By noting the patient's vocabulary and general fund of information in the context of cultural and educational background you can often make a rough estimate of intelligence, while the patient's responses to the illness give you insight into judgment. If the patient has unusual thoughts, preoccupations, beliefs, or perceptions, you should explore them as the subject arises. Moreover, if you suspect a problem in orientation or memory, you can check these too as part of the interview. "Let's see, your last clinic appointment was when? . . . and the date today is . . . ?"

For many patients such an evaluation is sufficient. For others, however, you need to go further. All patients with documented or suspected brain lesions, those with psychiatric symptoms, and those in whom family members or friends have reported vague behavioral symptoms need further careful, specific assessment. Patients who seem unable to take their medications properly, whose attention to home or business responsibilities seems to be slipping, and who are losing interest in their usual activities may be showing signs of dementia. The patient who is behaving strangely after surgery or during an acute illness may be delirious. Each problem should be identified as expeditiously as possible. Mental function, moreover, importantly influences a person's ability to find and hold a job and thus may constitute the critical component in evaluating disability.

For these kinds of patients, and others as well, you will need to supplement your interview with questions in specific areas. In doing so, give simple introductory explanations, be tactful, and show the same acceptance and respect for the patient as in other portions of the examination.

Many students feel insecure in performing mental status examinations and are reluctant to do them. They may worry about upsetting patients, invading their privacy, and labeling their thoughts or behavior as pathologic. It may be helpful to discuss these concerns or some of the issues they raise with your instructor or other experienced clinicians. As in other parts of the assessment process your skills and confidence will improve with practice, and rewards will follow. Many patients will appreciate an understanding listener, and some will owe their health, their safety, or even their lives to your attention.

The format that follows should help to organize your observations. Although it includes suggestions concerning technique, it is not intended as a step-by-step guide. When a full examination is indicated, you should be flexible in your approach while thorough in your coverage. In some situations, however, sequence is important. If during your initial interview the patient's consciousness, attention, comprehension of words, or ability to speak seems impaired, assess the problem promptly. A person so impaired cannot give a reliable history and you will not be able to test the higher intellectual functions.

APPEARANCE AND BEHAVIOR

Use here all the relevant observations made throughout the course of your history and examination. Include:

LEVEL OF CONSCIOUSNESS. Is the patient awake and alert? Does the patient seem to understand your questions and respond appropriately and reasonably quickly, or is there a tendency to lose track of the topic and fall silent or even asleep?

If the patient does not respond to your questions, escalate the stimulus in steps by

1. Giving a command to see if the patient can follow it ("Open your eyes. Squeeze my hand.")
2. Calling the patient's name
3. Touching the arm
4. Shaking the shoulder, or
5. Producing pain. For example, you can press the bony ridges above the eyes with your thumb or pinch the side of the neck. Avoid undue roughness that might cause bruising or other injury.

Note both the stimulus required and the patient's response to it, including opening the eyes, other bodily movements, and vocal responses. Observe what happens when the stimulus stops.

See Table 3-1, Levels of Consciousness (p. 109). Loss of consciousness may result from extensive impairment of the cerebral cortex or of arousal mechanisms in the brainstem. The cause may be structural (as in a cerebrovascular accident or a tumor) or metabolic (as in hypoglycemia, hypoxia, and poisoning).

POSTURE AND MOTOR BEHAVIOR. Does the patient lie in bed, or prefer to walk about? Note bodily posture and the patient's ability to relax. Observe the pace, range, and character of movements. Do they seem to be made under voluntary control? Are certain parts immobile? Do posture and motor activity change with topics under discussion or with activities or people around the patient?

Tense posture, restlessness, and fidgetiness of anxiety; crying, pacing, and handwringing of agitated depression; hopeless, slumped posture and slowed movements of depression; bizarre or sustained posture in schizophrenia; singing, dancing and expansive movements of the manic syndrome; oral–facial dyskinesias

DRESS, GROOMING, AND PERSONAL HYGIENE. How is the patient dressed? Is clothing clean, pressed, and properly fastened? How does it compare with clothing worn by people of comparable age and social group? Note the patient's hair, nails, teeth, skin, and, if present, beard. How are they groomed? How do the person's grooming and hygiene

Deterioration in grooming and personal hygiene may occur in depression, schizophrenia, and organic brain syndromes, but always consider the norms of a

compare with other people of comparable age, lifestyle, and socioeconomic group? Compare one side of the body with the other.

person's group. Excessive fastidiousness may be seen in an obsessive–compulsive disorder. One-sided neglect may result from a lesion in the opposite parietal cortex, usually the nondominant side.

FACIAL EXPRESSION. Observe the face, both at rest and when the patient is interacting with others. Watch for variations in expression with topics under discussion. Are they appropriate? Or is the face relatively immobile throughout?

Expressions of anxiety, depression, apathy, anger, elation. Facial immobility of parkinsonism

MANNER, AFFECT, AND RELATIONSHIP TO PERSONS AND THINGS. Using your observations of facial expression, voice, and bodily movements, assess the patient's affect. Does it vary appropriately with topics under discussion? Does one consistent affect prevail, or is the affect labile, blunted, or flat? Does it seem inappropriate or extreme at certain points? If so, how? Note the patient's openness, approachability, and reactions to others and to the surroundings. Does the patient seem to hear or see things that you do not or seem to be conversing with someone who is not there?

Anger, hostility, suspiciousness, or evasiveness of paranoid patients. Elation and euphoria of the manic syndrome. Flat affect and remoteness of schizophrenia. Apathy (dulled affect with detachment and indifference) in organic brain syndromes. Anxiety, depression

SPEECH AND LANGUAGE

Throughout the interview note the characteristics of the patient's speech, including

QUANTITY. Is the patient talkative or relatively silent? Are comments spontaneous or only in response to direct questions?

RATE. Is speech fast or slow?

Slow speech of depression; rapid loud speech in a manic syndrome

VOLUME (loudness)

FLUENCY, which includes not only the rate but also the ability to speak smoothly, clearly, and with appropriate inflections. Be alert to specific abnormal patterns such as:

See Table 3-2, Disorders of Speech, p. 110.

Poor articulation of words. What sounds are especially affected?

Dysarthria

Disturbed rhythm and inflection, such as hesitancy and speaking in a monotone

Monotonous, slow, weak voice in parkinsonism. Hesitancy and searching for words in aphasia

Circumlocutions, in which phrases or sentences are substituted for a word the person cannot think of, as ''what you write with'' for ''pen''

Circumlocutions and paraphasias are noted in aphasic disorders.

Paraphasias, in which words are malformed (''I write with a den''), wrong (''I write with a bar''), or invented (''I write with a dar'')

SPECIAL TESTING FOR APHASIA. If your observations of the patient's spontaneous speech suggest a possible disorder of language *(aphasia),* proceed with further specific testing. When language is seriously im-

Aphasia may lead to incoherent, unintelligible speech and may then be mistaken for a psychotic

paired, taking a history from the patient and assessing cognitive functions may be impossible. Although these additional observations are not part of a routine examination, they will help you to identify and differentiate among the several kinds of aphasias.

illness unless the language deficit is recognized.

Testing for Aphasia

WORD COMPREHENSION	You can test a person's comprehension of spoken language by two methods. First, ask the patient to point to objects in the room or to specify body parts as you name them. "Will you please point to your nose . . . the telephone . . . the bedspread." Second, ask a series of questions that can be answered with "yes" or "no" or with an appropriate head movement. "Are you sitting on a chair? Can dogs fly?"	Word comprehension is impaired in some but not all kinds of aphasia. Deficiencies of vision, hearing, and intellectual capacity may also affect performance.
REPETITION	Ask the patient to repeat items of increasing length and complexity, from monosyllabic words to sentences. Note the fluency and accuracy of the responses.	Repetition is impaired in some but not all kinds of aphasia.
NAMING	Ask the patient to name a series of objects or colors as you point them out. Gradually increase the difficulty of the questions — from "hat" and "red," for example, to "belt buckle" and "purple." Note the fluency and accuracy of the responses.	Naming is impaired in some but not all kinds of aphasia.
READING COMPREHENSION	Write several simple commands, each on a separate paper in large clear print. "CLOSE YOUR EYES" and "RAISE YOUR HAND." A person's prior reading ability and educational experience affect performance here.	Failure in reading comprehension often accompanies failure in word comprehension but each may occur independently.
WRITING	Ask the patient to make up and write a sentence about a topic such as the room, the patient's job, or family. Note whether the sentence makes sense, has a subject and verb, and is correctly spelled.	Writing, like speech, is affected by some forms of aphasia. Motor impairment, such as hemiplegia, may affect performance.

MOOD

You should assess mood during the interview by exploring the patient's own perceptions of it. Find out about the patient's usual mood level and how it has varied with life events. "How did you feel about that?", for example, or, more generally, "How are your spirits?"

If you suspect depression, you must assess its depth and any associated risk of suicide. A series of questions such as the following is useful, proceeding as far as the patient's positive answers warrant.

See Table 3-3, Distinguishing Features of Depressive Disorders (p. 111).

> Do you get pretty discouraged (or depressed or blue)?
> How low do you feel?
> What do you see for yourself in the future?
> Do you ever feel that life isn't worth living? Or that you had just as soon be dead?
> Have you ever thought of doing away with yourself?
> How did (do) you think you would do it?
> What would happen after you were dead?

Although many student clinicians feel uneasy about exploring thoughts of suicide, most patients can discuss their thoughts and feelings about it freely with you, sometimes with considerable relief. By such discussion you demonstrate your interest and concern for what may well be the patient's most serious and threatening problem. By avoiding the issue, you may miss the most important feature of the patient's illness.

THOUGHT PROCESSES, THOUGHT CONTENT, AND PERCEPTIONS

THOUGHT PROCESSES. Assess the logic, relevance, organization, and coherence of the patient's thought processes as they are revealed in words and speech throughout the interview. Does speech progress in a logical manner toward a goal? Here you are using the patient's speech as a window into the patient's mind. Listen for patterns of speech that suggest disorders of thought processes, as outlined in the following table.

Variations and Abnormalities in Thought Processes

CIRCUMSTANTIALITY	Speech characterized by indirection and delay in reaching the point because of unnecessary detail, although the components of the description have a meaningful connection. Many people without mental disorders are circumstantial.	Observed in persons with compulsive personality disorders
LOOSENING OF ASSOCIATIONS	Speech in which a person shifts from one subject to others that are unrelated or only obliquely related without realizing that the subjects are not meaningfully connected	Observed in schizophrenia, manic episodes, and other psychiatric disorders
FLIGHT OF IDEAS	An almost continuous flow of accelerated speech in which a person changes abruptly from topic to topic. Changes are usually based on understandable associations, plays on words, or distracting stimuli, but the ideas do not progress to sensible conversation.	Most frequently noted in manic episodes, but may also be present in organic mental disorders and schizophrenia
NEOLOGISMS	Invented or distorted words, or words with new and highly idiosyncratic meanings	Observed in schizophrenia, other psychotic disorders, and aphasia
INCOHERENCE	Speech that is largely incomprehensible because of illogic, lack of meaningful connections, abrupt changes in topic, or disordered grammar or word use. Both loosening of associations and flight of ideas, when severe, may produce incoherence.	Observed in severely disturbed psychotic persons (usually schizophrenic) and also in persons with aphasia
BLOCKING	Sudden interruption of speech in mid-sentence or before completion of an idea. The person attributes this to losing the thought. Blocking occurs in normal people.	Blocking may be striking in schizophrenia.
CONFABULATION	Fabrication of facts or events in response to questions, to fill in the gaps in an impaired memory	Common in the organic amnestic syndrome
PERSEVERATION	Persistent repetition of words or ideas	Occurs in organic mental disorders, schizophrenia, and other psychotic disorders
ECHOLALIA	Repetition of the words and phrases of others	Occurs in organic mental disorders and schizophrenia
CLANGING	Speech in which a person chooses a word on the basis of sound rather than meaning, as in rhyming and punning speech. For example, "Look at my eyes and nose, wise eyes and rosy nose. Two to one, the ayes have it!"	Clanging occurs in schizophrenia and manic episodes.

THOUGHT CONTENT. You should ascertain most of the information relevant to thought content during the interview. Follow appropriate leads as they occur rather than using stereotyped lists of specific questions. For example, "You mentioned a few minutes ago that a neighbor was responsible for your entire illness. Can you tell me more about that?" Or, in another situation, "What do you think about at times like these?"

You may need to make more specific inquiries. If so, couch them in tactful and accepting terms. "When people are upset like this, they sometimes can't keep certain thoughts out of their minds," or " . . . things seem unreal. Have you experienced anything like this?"

In these ways find out about any of the patterns shown in the following table.

Abnormalities of Thought Content		
COMPULSIONS	Repetitive acts that a person feels driven to perform in order to produce or prevent some future state of affairs, although expectation of such an effect is unrealistic	Compulsions, obsessions, phobias, and anxieties are often associated with neurotic disorders. See Table 3-4, Irrational Anxiety and Avoidance Behaviors (pp. 112–113).
OBSESSIONS	Recurrent, uncontrollable thoughts, images, or impulses that a person considers unacceptable and alien	
PHOBIAS	Persistent, irrational fears, accompanied by a compelling desire to avoid the stimulus	
ANXIETIES	Apprehensions, fears, tensions, or uneasiness that may be focused (phobia) or free-floating (a general sense of ill-defined dread or pending doom)	
FEELINGS OF UNREALITY	A sense that things in the environment are strange, unreal, or remote	Delusions and feelings of unreality or depersonalization are more often associated with psychotic disorders. See Table 3-5, Distinguishing Features of Psychotic Disorders (pp. 114–115).
FEELINGS OF DEPERSONALIZATION	A sense that one's self is different, changed, or unreal, or has lost identity	
DELUSIONS	False, fixed, personal beliefs that are not shared by other members of the person's culture or subculture. Examples include *Delusions of persecution* *Grandiose delusions* *Delusional jealousy* *Delusions of reference* in which a person believes that external events, objects, or people have a particular and unusual personal significance (for example, that the radio or television might be commenting on or giving instructions to the person) *Delusions of being controlled* by an outside force *Somatic delusions* *Systematized delusions,* a single delusion with many elaborations or a cluster of related delusions around a single theme, all systematized into a complex network	

PERCEPTIONS. Inquire about false perceptions in a manner similar to that used for thought content. For example, "When you heard the voice speaking to you, what did it say? How did it make you feel?" Or, "After you've been drinking a lot, do you ever see things that aren't really there?" Or, "Sometimes after major surgery like this, people hear peculiar or frightening things. Have you experienced anything like that?" In these ways find out about the following perception problems.

Abnormalities of Perception

ILLUSIONS	Misinterpretations of real external stimuli
HALLUCINATIONS	Subjective sensory perceptions in the absence of relevant external stimuli. The person may or may not recognize the experiences as false. Hallucinations may be auditory, visual, olfactory, gustatory, tactile, or somatic. (False perceptions associated with dreaming, falling asleep, and awakening are not classified as hallucinations.)

Illusions and hallucinations are usually associated with psychotic disorders such as schizophrenia and delirium. See Table 3-5, Distinguishing Features of Psychotic Disorders (pp. 114–115).

COGNITIVE FUNCTIONS

ORIENTATION. By skillful questioning you can often determine the patient's orientation in the context of the interview. For example, you can ask quite naturally for specific dates and times, the patient's address and telephone number, the names of family members, or the route taken to the hospital. At times — when rechecking the status of a delirious patient, for example — simple, direct questions may be indicated. "Can you tell me what time it is now . . . and what day is it?" In either of these ways, determine the patient's orientation for:

Disorientation occurs especially when memory and attention are impaired, as in organic brain syndromes. See Table 3-6, Distinguishing Features of Organic Brain Syndromes (pp. 116–117).

1. *Time* (*e.g.,* the time of day, day of the week, month, season, date and year, duration of hospitalization)
2. *Place* (*e.g.,* the patient's residence, the name of the hospital, city, and state)
3. *Person* (*e.g.,* the patient's own name, and the names of relatives and professional personnel)

ATTENTION. Tests of attention include

Digit Span. Explain that you would like to test the patient's ability to concentrate, perhaps adding that people tend to have trouble with that when they are in pain, or ill, or feverish, or whatever. Read a series of digits, starting with the shortest set and enunciating each number clearly at a rate of about 1 per second. Ask the patient to repeat them back to you. If the patient makes a mistake, try once more with a series of the same length. Stop after a second failure in a series of any given length. In choosing digits you may use street numbers, zip codes, telephone numbers, and other numerical sequences that are familiar to you, but avoid consecutive numbers, easily recognized dates, and sequences that are possibly familiar to the patient.

Poor performance of digit span is characteristic of organic brain syndromes such as delirium and dementia. Performance is also limited by mental retardation and by performance anxiety.

5,2	5,3,8,7	3,6,7,9,5,2	9,4,7,2,5,6,1,8
9,3	2,1,7,9	4,1,5,3,7,9	3,5,8,1,4,9,7,6
6,1,7	4,7,2,9,3	7,2,4,8,3,5,9	6,1,9,8,2,5,4,3,7
8,4,1	5,3,8,7,1	3,6,1,5,8,4,2	3,8,7,2,4,9,1,6,5

Now (starting again with the shortest series) ask the patient to repeat the numbers to you backwards.

Normally a person should be able to repeat correctly at least five to eight digits forward and four to six backwards.

Serial 7s or Serial 3s. Instruct the patient, "Starting from a hundred, subtract 7, and keep subtracting 7. . . ." Note the effort required and the speed and accuracy of the responses. (Writing down the answers helps you keep up with the arithmetic.) Normally, a person can complete serial 7s in 1½ minutes, with fewer than four errors. If the patient cannot do serial 7s, try 3s or counting backward. Still easier tests are counting forward or reciting the alphabet.

Poor performance may be secondary to organic brain syndromes such as delirium and dementia, but also occurs with mental retardation, lack of education, loss of calculating ability, anxiety, and depression.

MEMORY. Most questions relevant to remote and recent memory can be asked in the context of the interview. Evaluate

Remote Memory (*e.g.,* birthdays, anniversaries, names of schools attended, jobs held, past historical events such as presidents or wars relevant to the patient's past)

Remote memory may be impaired in the late stages of dementia.

Recent Memory (*e.g.,* the events of the day). Ask questions with answers that you can check against other sources so that you will know whether or not the patient is confabulating (making up facts to compensate for a defective memory). These might include the day's weather, today's appointment time in the clinic, and medications or laboratory tests taken during the day.

New Learning Ability. Give the patient three or four words such as "83 Water Street and blue," or "table, flower, green, and hamburger." Ask the patient to repeat them so that you know that the information has been heard and registered. (This step, like digit span, tests registration and immediate recall.) Then proceed to other parts of the examination. After about 3 to 5 minutes ask the patient to repeat the words. Note the accuracy of the response, awareness of whether or not it is correct, and any tendency to confabulate. Normally a person should be able to remember the words.

Recent memory, including new learning ability, is impaired in organic brain syndromes such as dementia, delirium, and the amnestic syndrome. Impairments in attention produced by anxiety, depression, and mental retardation also impair recent memory. See Table 3-6, Distinguishing Features of Organic Brain Syndromes (pp. 116–117).

CONSTRUCTIONAL ABILITY. The task here is to copy figures of increasing complexity onto a piece of blank unlined paper. Show each figure one at a time and ask the patient to copy it as well as possible.

The three diamonds below are rated poor, fair, and good (but not excellent).

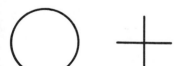 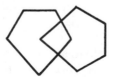 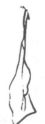 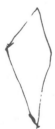 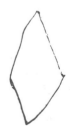

(Strub RL, Black FW: *The Mental Status Examination in Neurology*, 2nd ed, p 107. Philadelphia, FA Davis, 1985)

In another approach, ask the patient to draw a clock face complete with numbers and hands. The example below is rated excellent.

These three clocks are poor, fair, and good.

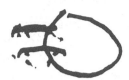 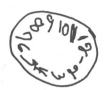

(Strub RL, Black FW: The Mental Status Examination in Neurology, 2nd ed, p 114. Philadelphia, FA Davis, 1985)

If vision and motor ability are intact, poor performance in constructional ability suggests organic brain disease such as dementia or parietal lobe damage. Mental retardation may also impair performance.

HIGHER INTELLECTUAL FUNCTIONS

Information. You can explore a person's fund of information in the context of the interview. Ask a student, for example, about favorite courses, or inquire about a person's work or hobbies, or about current events. More directly, you can ask the patient to name the last five presidents or five big cities in the country. Alternatively, ask a series of specific questions such as the following:

1. How many days are there in a week?
2. What must you do to water to make it boil?
3. How many things are there in a dozen?
4. Name the four seasons of the year?
5. What do we celebrate on the 4th of July?
6. How many pounds are there in a ton?
7. What does the stomach do?
8. What is the capital of Greece?
9. Where does the sun set?
10. Who invented the airplane?
11. Why does oil float on water?
12. What do we get turpentine from?
13. When is Labor Day?
14. How far is it from New York to Chicago?
15. What is a hieroglyphic?
16. What is a barometer?
17. Who wrote "Paradise Lost?"
18. What is a prime number?
19. What is *habeas corpus*?
20. Who discovered the South Pole?

If considered against the patient's cultural and educational background, information is a good indicator of underlying intelligence. It is relatively unaffected by any but the most severe psychiatric disorders and may be helpful in distinguishing mentally retarded adults (whose information is poor) from those with mild or moderate dementia (whose information is relatively good).

Persons of average ability should be able to answer correctly from 8 to 13 of these questions. Take into consideration, however, the patient's cultural and educational background.

Vocabulary. By listening to the patient's speech you can make a judgment about vocabulary. Further, you can ask the patient either to give you the meaning of a series of words or to use each of these words in a sentence. The words should become increasingly difficult, as in the following list:

If considered against the patient's cultural and educational background, vocabulary is probably the best indicator of

1. Apple	9. Tint	17. Seclude
2. Donkey	10. Armory	18. Spangle
3. Diamond	11. Fable	19. Recede
4. Nuisance	12. Nitroglycerine	20. Affliction
5. Join	13. Microscope	21. Chattel
6. Fur	14. Stanza	22. Dilatory
7. Shilling	15. Guillotine	23. Flout
8. Bacon	16. Plural	24. Amanuensis

underlying intelligence. It is relatively unaffected by any but the most severe psychiatric disorders. It may help you to distinguish mentally retarded adults (whose vocabulary is limited) from those with mild or moderate dementia (whose vocabulary is fairly well preserved).

Persons of average intellectual ability should be able to define or use from 8 to 16 of these words. Again, keep in mind the patient's cultural and educational background.

Calculations. Test the patient's ability to do arithmetical calculations, starting at the rote level with simple addition ("What is 4 + 3? . . . 8 + 7?") and multiplication ("What is 5 × 6? . . . 9 × 7?"). The task can be made more difficult by using two-digit numbers ("15 + 12" or "25 × 6") or longer, written examples.

Poor performance may be a useful sign of dementia or may accompany aphasia, but it must be assessed in terms of the patient's intelligence and education.

Abstract Reasoning. The capacity to reason abstractly can be tested in two ways.

Proverbs. Ask the patient what people mean when they use some of the following proverbs:

Concrete responses are often given by persons with mental retardation, delirium, or dementia, but may also be simply a function of little education. Schizophrenics may respond concretely or with personal, bizarre interpretations.

A stitch in time saves nine.
Don't count your chickens before they're hatched.
The proof of the pudding is in the eating.
A rolling stone gathers no moss.
The squeaking wheel gets the grease.

Note the relevance of the answers and their degree of concreteness or abstractness. For example, "You should sew a rip before it gets bigger" is concrete, while "Prompt attention to a problem prevents trouble" is abstract. Average patients should give abstract or semi-abstract responses.

Similarities. Ask the patient to tell you how the following are alike:

1. An orange and an apple
2. A cat and a mouse
3. A child and a dwarf
4. A church and a theater
5. A piano and a violin
6. Paper and coal

Note the accuracy and relevance of the answers and their degree of concreteness or abstractness. For example, "A cat and a mouse are both animals" is abstract, while "A cat chases a mouse" is neither abstract nor relevant to the question.

Judgment. You can usually assess judgment during the interview by noting the patient's responses to family situations, jobs, use of money, and interpersonal conflicts. Note whether decisions and actions are based on reality or, for example, on impulse, wish fulfillment, or disordered thought content. What values seem to underlie the patient's decisions and behavior? Allowing for cultural variations, how do these compare with mature adult standards? Some additional hypothetical questions may help you evaluate the patient's judgment and comprehension of other circumstances. For example,

Judgment may be poor in organic brain disease, mental retardation, and psychotic states.

1. What should you do if you are stopped for speeding?
2. What should you do if you lose a library book?
3. What should you do if you see a train approaching a broken track?
4. What would you do if you found a stamped, addressed, and sealed letter lying in the street?
5. Why are criminals put in prison?

Since judgment is part of the maturational response, it may be variable and unpredictable during adolescence.

A NOTE ON MENTAL ASSESSMENT

As in other portions of the interview and examination, you should vary your focus according to the nature of the patient's problems. The tables on pages 109–117 may help to guide your approach.*

While all human observations are inherently subject to error, assessments of mental status are especially susceptible to bias based on such factors as age, race, sex, class, cultural background, personal appearance, and even body weight. For example, most adults of any age have at some time lost track of the date, forgotten the name of an acquaintance, or allowed a pot to boil dry on the stove. Just because a person is elderly such lapses do not by themselves justify the label of "senility" or organic brain disease. Neither teenage pregnancy nor rejection of medical treatment necessarily means poor judgment; each may well be quite appropriate to the patient's cultural milieu or personal situation. A person who displays anger, suspiciousness, or depression may be responding fittingly to an oppressive, restrictive, or discriminatory environment; it may be society, not the man or woman, that is "abnormal" or inappropriate. A patient, moreover, may remind you of someone such as your parents or grandparents, and your reactions and perceptions may be colored accordingly. As you develop your skills in evaluating mental status, try to be sensitive to sources of bias such as these, monitor your judgments, and modify them as necessary.

* The terminology and differential points used in Tables 3-3 through 3-6 are based primarily on the third edition of *Diagnostic and Statistical Manual of Mental Disorders*, published by the American Psychiatric Association in 1980.

Table 3-1

Table 3-1   Levels of Consciousness

Consciousness varies on a continuum from normal to deep coma. Clinical states of consciousness are classified in various ways, one of which, outlined below, includes normal consciousness, drowsiness, stupor, and coma. Delirium, included in this table, does not fall on this continuum and is distinguished by other characteristics, but it does overlap considerably with the other conditions.

Specific observations about a patient's appearance, behavior, and responses to stimuli are much more valuable clinically than a single word such as "stupor." Such words, though useful in quickly summarizing an assessment, are inevitably ambiguous and preclude evaluation of slight but important changes over time.

NORMAL CONSCIOUSNESS	Normally conscious persons are alert, awake, and aware of both self and the environment, and respond to external stimuli.
DROWSINESS	Drowsy persons are not fully alert to their environment. Consciousness is clouded and attentiveness impaired. They think more slowly and less clearly. Spontaneous movement is diminished. Though responsive to stimuli such as questions or commands, they tend to fall asleep afterward.
STUPOR	Stuporous persons show a marked reduction in mental and physical activity. Vigorous stimuli such as pain are needed to elicit responses, and these responses are markedly reduced, slowed, inadequate, or even absent. They may, for example, consist only of mumbling, groans, or restless movements. Reflex activity is preserved.
COMA	Comatose persons are completely unconscious and cannot be aroused even by painful stimuli. There are no voluntary movements. In light coma some reflex activity is preserved but in deep coma it is lost. For further evaluation of the comatose patient see pp. 508–511.
DELIRIUM	Delirium refers to an acute confusional state in which consciousness is clouded. Delirious persons are not fully aware of all aspects of their environment and have difficulty concentrating. They think less clearly, show a loss of recent memory, and are often disoriented. They may be fearful and agitated, may misinterpret the meaning of sounds or events in their environment, and may experience hallucinations and illusions.

Table 3-2

Table 3-2   Disorders of Speech

Disorders of speech may be divided into three groups: (1) disorders of the voice, (2) disorders of articulation, and (3) disorders involving the production and comprehension of language. In the terms below the prefix dys- implies a less severe impairment than the prefix a- (or an-), but these distinctions are not always made in practice. The term given first is the more commonly used.

Aphonia (dysphonia) refers to a *disorder of the volume, quality, or pitch of the voice* secondary to disease of the larynx or its nerve supply. The voice may be hoarse or reduced to a whisper. Articulation and language itself are unimpaired. Causes include laryngitis, laryngeal tumors, and a unilateral vocal cord paralysis (10th cranial nerve).

Dysarthria (anarthria) refers to *defective articulation* secondary to a motor deficit involving the lips, tongue, palate, or pharynx. Words may be nasal, slurred, or indistinct. There may be special difficulty with consonants formed by the lips (*m, b, p*), the tongue (*d, t, l*), or the pharynx (*k* and hard *g* as in got). Causes include disorders of the upper or lower motor neurons, the cerebellum, the extrapyramidal system, or the muscles.

Aphasia (dysphasia) refers to a *disorder of language* itself. The cause usually lies in the left cerebral cortex. Two of the several kinds of aphasia are compared below.

	BROCA'S (EXPRESSIVE) APHASIA	**WERNICKE'S (RECEPTIVE) APHASIA**
QUALITIES OF SPONTANEOUS SPEECH	Nonfluent; slow, with few words and laborious effort. Inflection and articulation are impaired, but words are meaningful with nouns, transitive verbs, and important adjectives. Small grammatical words are often dropped.	Fluent; often rapid, voluble and effortless. Inflection and articulation are good but sentences lack meaning and words are malformed (paraphasias) or invented (neologisms). Speech may be totally incomprehensible.
COMPREHENSION	Fairly good	Impaired
REPETITION	Impaired (as in spontaneous speech)	Impaired
NAMING	Impaired, though the patient recognizes objects	Impaired
READING COMPREHENSION	Fairly good	Impaired
WRITING	Impaired	Impaired

Table 3-3

Table 3-3 *Distinguishing Features of Depressive Disorders*

SYMPTOMS

Clinical depression is manifested by several of the following:

1. Poor appetite or significant weight loss, or increased appetite or significant weight gain
2. Sleep disturbance (*e.g.,* insomnia, hypersomnia)
3. Fatigue, loss of energy
4. Psychomotor agitation or retardation
5. Loss in interest in stimulating activities
6. Decreased ability to think and concentrate
7. Feelings of worthlessness, self-reproach, or guilt
8. Recurrent thoughts of death or suicide

Four, or preferably five, of the above, occurring nearly every day for at least 2 weeks, constitute a major depression.

HISTORY	POSSIBLE DIAGNOSIS
What preceded the present depressive state?	*Then consider:*
A psychiatric diagnosis	Primary degenerative dementia with depressive features
	Organic affective syndrome
	Psychotic disorder with depression (*e.g.,* schizophrenia)
A serious medical diagnosis	Depression associated with cancer, heart disease, or other life-threatening or life-changing illness
Previous episode(s) of depression lasting at least 2 wk	Major affective disorder—depressive
Previous episode(s) of manic syndrome with or without depressive episodes	Major affective disorder—bipolar (manic–depressive)
Over the past 2 yr numerous episodes of manic and depressive symptoms that were shorter and less severe than in a major depression. No psychotic features	Cyclothymic disorder
Over the past 2 yr (1 yr for adolescents) recurrent or persistent depressive symptoms that were shorter or less severe than in a major depression. No psychotic features	Dysthymic disorder

Table 3-4 Irrational Anxiety and Avoidance Behaviors

	ORGANIC MENTAL DISORDER	PSYCHOTIC DISORDER	SEPARATION ANXIETY DISORDER*	AVOIDANT DISORDER OF CHILDHOOD AND ADOLESCENCE*	OVER-ANXIOUS DISORDER*	AGORAPHOBIA WITH PANIC ATTACKS	AGORAPHOBIA WITHOUT PANIC ATTACKS
Known organic cause?	Yes, see Table 3-6	No	No	No	No	No	No
Psychotic features?		Yes, see Table 3-5	No	No	No	No	No
Excessive anxiety about separation from those to whom person is attached?			Yes, for at least 2 wk	No	No		
Persistent shrinking from contact or familiarity with strangers?				Yes, for at least 6 wk	No		
Generalized, persistent anxiety or worry?					Yes, for at least 6 mo		
Irrational avoidance— of objects or situations?						Yes, fear of being alone or in a public place where escape seems impossible	
of leaving home?						Yes. Fears and avoidance increase to constrict normal life.	
of special social situations, with overconcern about humiliation or embarrassment?							
Recurrent panic attacks?						Yes	No
Obsessions or compulsions?							
Relation of stress to anxiety?							
Repeated reexperiencing of traumatic events?							

* Pay special attention to these three possibilities when the patient is a child or an adolescent.

Table 3-4   (Cont'd.)

SOCIAL PHOBIA	PANIC DISORDER	SIMPLE PHOBIA	OBSESSIVE COMPULSIVE DISORDER	GENERALIZED ANXIETY DISORDER	POST-TRAUMATIC STRESS DISORDER	ADJUSTMENT DISORDER WITH ANXIOUS MOOD
No	No	No	No	No	No	No
No	No	No	No	No	No	No
				Yes, with tension, autonomic symptoms, apprehensive expectations, dysfunctional vigilance		
No	Not specifically	Yes, specific (*e.g.,* dogs, heights)	No	No	No	No
No	Not specifically	No	No	No	No	No
Yes	Not specifically	No	No	No	No	No
	Yes, without consistent stimulus					
			Yes	No	No	No
				Generalized anxiety for at least a month without specific stressor	Unusually severe stress (*e.g.,* rape, combat) preceded symptoms.	Stressor present within 3 months but less severe
					Yes	No

Table 3-5

Table 3-5 Distinguishing Features of Psychotic Disorders*

Psychotic manifestations include delusions, hallucinations, incoherence, a marked loosening of associations, markedly illogical thinking, and bizarre, grossly disorganized, or catatonic behavior.

	ORGANIC BRAIN SYNDROME (e.g., *Delusional, Hallucinosis*)	MALINGERING OR FACTITIOUS DISORDERS	BRIEF REACTIVE PSYCHOSIS
PSYCHOTIC MANIFESTATIONS	Present	Present	Present
KNOWN ORGANIC FACTOR CAUSALLY RELATED	*Present.* See Table 3-6.	Absent	Absent
SYMPTOMS DELIBERATE, PURPOSEFUL, VOLUNTARY	No	*Yes*	No
DURATION			From a few hours to *less than 2 wk*
PROFOUNDLY UPSETTING ENVIRONMENTAL EVENT JUST BEFORE ILLNESS			*Yes*
MOOD AND AFFECT			
DELUSIONS			
HALLUCINATIONS, INCOHERENCE, OR MARKED LOOSENING OF ASSOCIATIONS	Hallucinations, if present, are often visual.		

* Abnormalities are printed in red, key features in italics.

Table 3-5

Table 3-5 (Cont'd.)

MAJOR AFFECTIVE DISORDERS	SCHIZO-AFFECTIVE DISORDER	SCHIZOPHRENIA	PARANOID DISORDERS
Present	Present	Present	Present
Absent	Absent	Absent	Absent
No	No	No	No
		At least 6 mo	
Full depressive or manic syndrome		Blunt, flat, or inappropriate affect, but depressive or manic syndrome is absent, relatively brief, or follows psychotic syndrome	Depression or manic syndrome is absent, relatively brief, or follows psychotic symptoms.
May be present	Differentiation between major affective disorders and schizophrenia cannot be made in these individuals.	*Often present*	*Present, predominantly delusions of persecution or jealousy*
May be present		*Often present;* hallucinations are usually auditory	Not present

Table 3-6

Table 3-6   Distinguishing Features of Organic Brain Syndromes*

	DELIRIUM	DEMENTIA	AMNESTIC SYNDROME
LEVEL OF CONSCIOUSNESS	*Clouded; reduced awareness of environment*	*Not clouded (unless delirium coexists)*	*Not clouded*
MAJOR INTELLECTUAL ABILITIES	General loss	*Significant general loss*	*No significant general loss*
MEMORY	Impaired	Impaired	*Impaired (recent and remote)*
ORIENTATION	Disorientation	May become impaired	Often impaired
THOUGHT PROCESSES AND PERCEPTIONS	Often shows illusions, misinterpretations, hallucinations		May confabulate
MOOD			
PERSONALITY CHANGE		Alteration or accentuation of premorbid traits	
TIME COURSE	Develops over short period, fluctuates; duration usually brief	Varies with cause but often slow and progressive	Varies with cause but often has rapid onset, chronic course
ORGANIC FACTOR JUDGED CAUSAL	Present	Present or presumed	Present
EXAMPLES OF CAUSE	Many, such as drug intoxications, hypoglycemia, postoperative states, systemic infections, chronic renal or liver or pulmonary disease, heart failure	Many, often involving diffuse brain disease such as Alzheimer's disease, cerebrovascular disorders, brain trauma	Head trauma, thiamine deficiency associated with alcohol abuse

* Abnormalities are printed in red, key features in italics.

Table 3-6

Table 3-6   (Cont'd.)

ORGANIC DELUSIONAL SYNDROME	ORGANIC HALLUCINOSIS	ORGANIC AFFECTIVE SYNDROME	ORGANIC PERSONALITY SYNDROME
Not clouded	*Not clouded*	*Not clouded*	*Not clouded*
Intact	*Intact*	*Intact*	*Intact*
Delusions, often persecutory. Hallucinations, if present, not prominent	*Hallucinations*. Delusions, if present, relate to hallucinations.	Delusions and hallucinations, if present, relate to mood and are not predominant.	
		Depressive or *manic*	
			A marked change of behavior such as lability, impaired impulse control, marked apathy, or suspiciousness
Varies with cause	Varies		
Present	Present	Present	Present
Amphetamines, cannabis, hallucinogens; brain damage	Chronic alcohol abuse, sensory deprivation, epilepsy	Depressive—reserpine, methyldopa, other drugs, viral illnesses. Manic—adrenocortical steroids, stimulants.	Most often brain damage of frontal or temporal lobes; toxic and metabolic factors

Chapter 4
Physical Examination: Approach and Overview

Most patients view a physical examination with at least some anxiety. They feel vulnerable, physically exposed, apprehensive about possible pain, and uneasy over what the clinician may find. At the same time, they often appreciate detailed concern for their problems and may even enjoy the attention they receive.

Mindful of such feelings, the skillful clinician is thorough without wasting time, systematic without being rigid, gentle yet not afraid to cause discomfort if this should be required. By listening, looking, touch, or smell, the skillful clinician examines each body part and at the same time senses the whole patient, notes the wince or worried glance, and calms, explains, and reassures.

Early in their experience students, like patients, are apprehensive—uncertain in their ambiguous roles as student-professionals and uneasy with their newfledged competencies. This stage of anxiety is unavoidable. With study, repetitive practice, and time, however, both competence and confidence grow. As a beginning student, you will make notable gains within a few weeks; continuing progress should be a lifetime goal.

Despite inevitable insecurities as you begin to examine patients, you should take command of your own demeanor and affect. Try to look calm, organized, and competent, even when you do not exactly feel that way. If you forget a portion of your examination, as you undoubtedly will, you do not need to get flustered. Simply do that part out of sequence—smoothly. If you have already left the patient, return and ask if you can check one more thing. Avoid expressions of disgust, alarm, distaste, or other negative reactions. They have no place at the bedside, even when you come upon an ominous mass, a deep and smelly ulcer, or even a pubic louse.

As in the interview, be sensitive to the patient's feelings. The patient's facial expression or an apparently casual question such as "Is it okay?" may give you clues to previously unexpressed worries. Ascertain them when you can. Pay attention to the patient's physical comfort as well. Adjust the slant of the bed or examining table according to the patient's needs insofar as it is possible, and use pillows for comfort or blankets for warmth as necessary. Assure as much privacy as possible by using drapes appropriately and closing doors.

As an examiner you too should be comfortable, because awkward positions may impair your perceptions. Adjust the bed to a convenient height, and ask the patient to move toward you if this will help you reach a body part more comfortably.

Good lighting and a quiet environment contribute importantly to what you can see and hear but may be remarkably hard to find in a hospital. Do the best you can. If a nearby patient's television is interfering with your ability to hear the sounds in your patient's chest, ask the neighbor politely to lower the volume. Most people cooperate readily. Remember to thank them when you are through.

As you proceed with your examination, keep the patient informed as to what you intend to do, especially when you anticipate possible embarrassment or discomfort. Patients vary considerably in their knowledge of examination procedures and hence in their need for information. Some people want to know what you are doing when you listen to the lungs or feel for a liver, while others already know or do not care. By words or gestures, be as clear as possible in your instructions. When telling patients what to do, be courteous rather than authoritarian. "I would like to examine your heart now. Would you please lie down" carries a different and better message than "I'm going to examine your heart now. Lie down on the table." Authority stems from competence and personal relationship, not from command.

Clinicians differ in how and when they report their findings to their patients. Beginning students should avoid almost all such interpretive statements because they do not yet carry the primary responsibility for the patient and may give conflicting or erroneous information. As experience and responsibility increase, however, sharing findings with the patient becomes appropriate. If you know or suspect the patient has specific concerns, it may be helpful to make a reassuring comment as you finish examining the relevant area. A steady series of reassuring comments, however, presents at least one potential problem: what to say when you find an unexpected abnormality. You may wish you had maintained judicious silence.

All students, however, should develop one habit with which they can reassure their patients and avoid unnecessary alarm. As a beginner, you may spend much more time with some procedures, such as the ophthalmoscopic examination or cardiac auscultation, than does the experienced clinician. Whenever you realize you are doing this, pause and explain. "I would like to spend a long time examining your heart because I want to listen to each of the heart sounds carefully. It does not mean that I hear anything wrong." Be forthright with the patient about your status as a student. Such openness will clarify your relationship and probably reduce anxieties on both sides.

No dogmatic answers can be given to one common question: How complete should the examination be? The outline that follows describes a fairly comprehensive examination such as you might perform on an adult patient who either is ill or wants a general checkup. For other patients who have symptoms related to specific body systems, a more limited examination may be more appropriate. Here, as in the history, you select the relevant methods to assess the problem as precisely and efficiently as possible. The patient's age, sex, symptoms, and other factors all influence this selection and help you decide what to do. They may even suggest special techniques that are not part of the usual comprehensive examination. Techniques such as these are described in later chapters. The clinical thinking that underlies and guides these variations is discussed in Chapter 20.

The sequence of the comprehensive examination described below is designed to minimize the patient's movements as well as your own. Variations in this sequence are possible, of course, and you may wish to develop a method of your own. Whatever the approach, use it repetitively until you have mastered it and can perform it without omissions. Some students like to write a brief outline of the examination on index cards and use it unobtrusively during their first several examinations. Soon the cards become superfluous.

Under certain circumstances the sequence of the examination must differ from your routine. Some patients, for example, may be unable to sit up in bed or stand. You can then examine the head, neck, and anterior trunk of such persons as they lie supine. Then roll the patient onto each side to listen to the lungs, examine the back, and inspect the skin. Acute problems, such as coma, indicate a different approach from your usual procedures, as discussed in Chapter 17. On repeated examinations of the same person, moreover, you will probably focus on the active problems—no one needs a "complete" examination every day.

This book recommends that students examine a supine patient from the patient's right side, moving to the foot of the bed or to the other side as necessary. Accustoming yourself to working chiefly from one side helps you to master the skills more quickly and promotes the efficiency of your examination, although it admittedly may limit the ease with which you can adapt to unusual circumstances.

The right side has several advantages over the left: the jugular veins on the right are more reliable for estimating venous pressure, the palpating hand rests more comfortably on the apical impulse, the right kidney is more frequently palpable than the left, and examining tables are sometimes placed against one wall to favor this right-handed approach.

Left-handed students will understandably find this position awkward at first but are encouraged to practice it. Unless they are reasonably ambidextrous, however, most will find it easier to use the left hand while percussing or while holding instruments such as an otoscope or a reflex hammer.

You may wish to skim the following outline now to get an overview of the physical examination. Subsequent chapters deal with individual body regions or systems, each considered in isolation. After you have completed the study and practice involved in several chapters, reread this overview to see how each component of the examination fits into an integrated whole.

GENERAL SURVEY. Observe the general state of health, stature and habitus, and sexual development. Weigh the patient, if possible. Note posture, motor activity, and gait; dress, grooming, and personal hygiene; and any odors of body or breath. Watch the patient's facial expressions and note the manner, affect, and reaction to the persons and things in the environment. Listen to the patient's speech and note the state of awareness or level of consciousness.

The survey continues throughout the history and examination.

VITAL SIGNS. Count the pulse and respiratory rate. Measure the blood pressure and, if indicated, the body temperature.

SKIN. Observe the skin and its characteristics. Identify any lesions, noting their location, distribution, arrangement, type, and color. Inspect and palpate the hair and nails. Study the patient's hands.

The patient is sitting on the edge of the bed or examining table, unless this position is contraindicated. You should be standing in front of the patient, moving to either side as you need to.

Begin your assessment of the skin with the exposed areas — the hands, forearms, and face. Continue it as you examine other body regions such as the thorax, abdomen, genitalia, and limbs.

HEAD. Examine the hair, scalp, skull, and face.

EYES. Check visual acuity and, if indicated, the visual fields. Note the position and alignment of the eyes. Inspect the scleras, conjunctivas, and pupils. Test the pupillary reactions to light, and check the extraocular movements. With an ophthalmoscope inspect the ocular fundi.

The room should be darkened for the ophthalmoscopic examination.

EARS. Inspect the auricles, canals, and drums. Check auditory acuity. If acuity is diminished, check lateralization (Weber test) and compare air and bone conduction (Rinne test).

NOSE AND SINUSES. Examine the external nose, nasal mucosa, septum, and turbinates. Palpate for tenderness of the frontal and maxillary sinuses.

MOUTH AND PHARYNX. Inspect the lips, buccal mucosa, gums, teeth, roof of the mouth, tongue, and pharynx.

NECK. Inspect and palpate the cervical nodes. Note any masses or unusual pulsations in the neck. Feel for any deviation of the trachea. Inspect and palpate the thyroid gland.

Move behind the sitting patient to feel the thyroid gland and to examine the back, posterior thorax, and lungs.

BACK. Inspect and palpate the spine and muscles of the back. Check for costovertebral angle tenderness.

POSTERIOR THORAX AND LUNGS. Inspect, palpate, and percuss the chest. Listen to the breath sounds, and identify any added sounds.

BREASTS, AXILLAE, AND EPITROCHLEAR NODES. In a woman, inspect the breasts with her arms relaxed and then elevated, and then with her hands pressed on her hips. In either sex, inspect the axillae and feel for the axillary nodes. Feel for the epitrochlear nodes.

Move to the front again.

By this time you have examined the patient's hands, surveyed the back, and, at least in women, made a fair estimate of the range of motion at the shoulders. Your examination of the anterior thorax will include inspection of additional musculoskeletal structures. Use these observations, together with the patient's history and ease of movement throughout the examination, in deciding whether or not to continue with a full musculoskeletal examination.

If you need to do a more complete musculoskeletal examination, it is convenient to examine the hands, arms, shoulders, neck, and jaw while the patient is still in the sitting position. Inspect and palpate the joints and check their range of motion.

BREASTS. Palpate the breasts, while at the same time continuing your inspection.

The patient is supine. You should stand on the right side of the patient's bed.

ANTERIOR THORAX AND LUNGS. Inspect, palpate, and percuss the chest. Listen to the breath sounds and identify any added sounds.

CARDIOVASCULAR SYSTEM. Inspect and palpate the carotid pulsations. Listen for carotid bruits. Identify the jugular venous pulsations, and measure the jugular venous pressure in relation to the sternal angle.

Inspect and palpate the precordium. Note the location, diameter, amplitude, and duration of the apical impulse. Listen at the apex and the lower sternal border with the bell of a stethoscope. Listen at each auscultatory area with the diaphragm. Listen for physiologic splitting of the second heart sound and for any abnormal heart sounds or murmurs.

Elevate the head of the bed to about 30° for the cardiovascular examination, adjusting it as necessary to see the jugular venous pulsations. The patient should roll partly onto the left side while you listen at the apex. Then have the patient lie back while you listen to the rest of the heart. The patient should sit, leaning forward, and exhale while you listen for the murmur of aortic regurgitation.

ABDOMEN. Inspect, auscultate, and percuss the abdomen. Palpate lightly, then deeply. Try to feel the liver, spleen, and kidneys.

The patient should be supine. Lower the bed to the flat position.

INGUINAL AREA. Feel for the inguinal nodes, and palpate the femoral arteries.

RECTAL EXAMINATION IN MEN. Examine the anus, rectum, and prostate. If the patient cannot stand, examine the genitalia before doing the rectal.

The patient is lying on his left side for the rectal examination.

LEGS. Inspect the legs, noting any evidence of peripheral vascular, musculoskeletal, or neurologic abnormalities. Palpate for edema. Check the dorsalis pedis and posterior tibial pulses. Continue a complete musculoskeletal examination, if this is indicated, by inspecting and palpating the joints and checking their range of motion.

The patient is supine.

MUSCULOSKELETAL SYSTEM. Examine the alignment of the spine and its range of motion, the alignment of the legs, and the feet.

The patient is standing. You should sit on a chair or stool.

PERIPHERAL VASCULAR SYSTEM. Inspect for varicose veins.

GENITALIA AND HERNIAS IN MEN. Examine the penis and scrotal contents and check for hernias.

SCREENING NEUROLOGIC EXAMINATION. Observe the patient's gait and ability to walk heel-to-toe, walk on the toes, walk on the heels, hop in place, and do shallow knee bends. Screen for arm strength and grip.

Then assess sensory function by testing pain and vibration in the hands and feet, light touch on the limbs, and stereognosis in the hands.

The patient is sitting or supine.

Check deep tendon reflexes and the plantar responses.

FULL NEUROLOGIC EXAMINATION. If indicated, go on to a more thorough examination, including:

Motor. Muscle bulk, muscle tone, strength, coordination, and involuntary movements or abnormal positions

Sensory. Pain, temperature, light touch, position, vibration, and discrimination

Abdominal Reflexes

MENTAL STATUS. Check cognitive functions, if indicated and not previously done.

Other portions of the mental status examination are usually completed during the history.

GENITALIA AND RECTAL EXAMINATION IN WOMEN. Examine the external genitalia, vagina, and cervix. Obtain Pap smears. Palpate the uterus and the adnexa. Do a rectovaginal and rectal examination.

The patient is supine in the lithotomy position. You should be seated at first, then standing at the foot of the examining table.

Alternatively, the pelvic and rectal examinations are conveniently done right after the abdominal and inguinal examinations.

When you have completed your examination, tell the patient what to do and what to expect next. If you are examining a hospitalized patient, rearrange the immediate environment to suit the patient. If you initially found the bed rails up, put them back in this position unless you are sure that they are not necessary. Lower the bed so that the patient can get in and out easily without risking falls. When you have finished, wash your hands.

When you record the physical examination, the sequence you use will not be exactly the same as this one. Refer to Chapter 20 for a sample of a patient's record.

Chapter 5
The General Survey

Anatomy and Physiology

Much of the specific anatomy and physiology relevant to the general survey may be found in later chapters. This section deals briefly with the more general topics of body height, weight, and habitus, and will introduce the concept of sexual maturity ratings.

In all these attributes people vary importantly according to the region of the world in which they live, socioeconomic status, nutrition, genetic makeup, early illnesses, gender, and the era in which they were born. The apparent shortening of aging Americans, for example, is partially illusory. Although people do shrink with age, their heights also vary according to the year of their birth. Young adults today on the average have grown taller than their parents, and the parents taller than the grandparents. This section cannot deal with all the variations of "normal" resulting from these many factors, but the clinician should be extremely cautious in applying the norms of one group to a person of another.

HEIGHT, GROWTH, AND HABITUS. Persons grow in height from birth to late adolescence. When the annual gain in height is measured and charted, one can readily discern an *adolescent growth spurt,* which in girls peaks relatively early in puberty, approximately at the age of 12, and in boys relatively late, approximately at the age of 14. Musculoskeletal proportions change during this growth spurt, with variations in degree and timing according to gender. A boy's shoulders, for example, broaden more than a girl's, while a girl's hips widen more than a boy's. These changes are summarized in the illustration on the next page.

Toward the other end of the lifespan other changes occur. People decrease in height, and posture may become somewhat stooped as the thoracic spine becomes more convex and the knees and hips fail to extend fully. Fat tends to concentrate near the hips and lower abdomen and, together with weakening of the abdominal muscles, often produces a potbelly. The figure on page 127 illustrates some of the changes occurring in persons ranging in age from 78 to 94. These and other changes with age are further detailed in subsequent chapters.

SEXUAL MATURITY RATINGS. Changes in an adolescent's reproductive organs and secondary sex characteristics are closely related to the growth

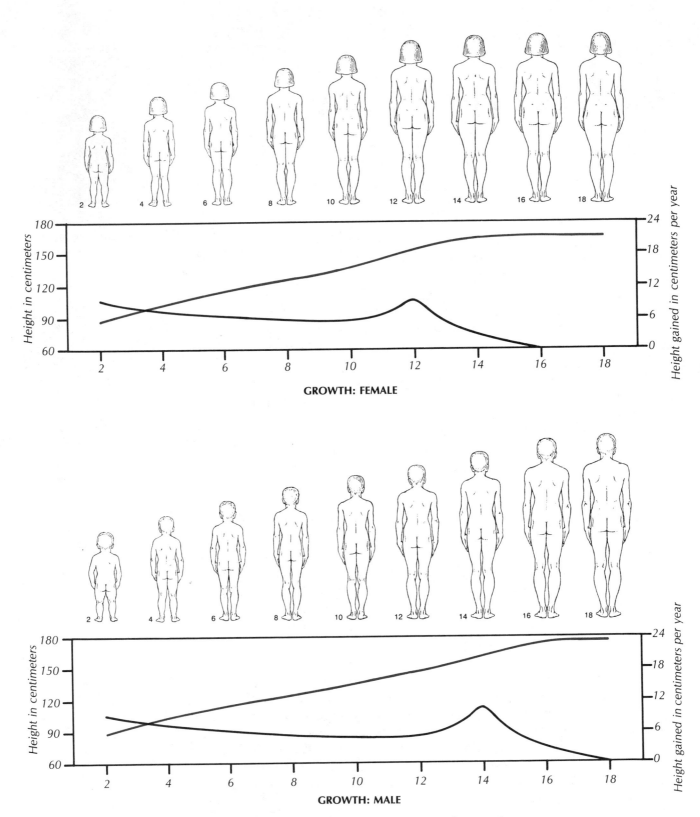

(Modified from Tanner JM: Growing up. Scientific American 229: 36–37, September 1973)

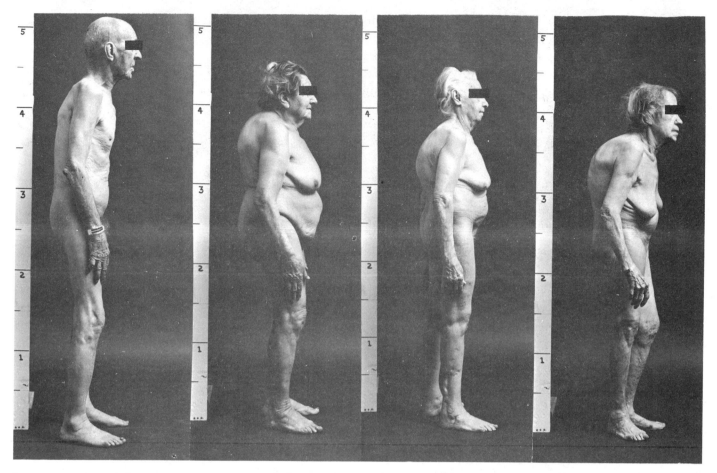

A man, age 82, and three women, ages 78, 79, and 94 respectively. (Rossman I: Clinical Geriatrics, 3rd ed, p 4. Philadelphia, JB Lippincott, 1986)

spurt. Later chapters describe sexual maturity ratings by which the clinician can assess sexual development: in breasts and pubic hair of girls and in genitalia and pubic hair of boys. The interrelationships between these sexual characteristics and the adolescent growth spurt give the clinician a biological yardstick with which to assess an adolescent's growth and development and to identify significant deviations from normal patterns. They also help the clinician to interpret for the adolescent whether growth and sexual maturation are proceeding normally and to predict what further changes may be expected.

During your initial survey of the adolescent patient, you measure only one of these variables — height. You may also make a few preliminary observations of breast and muscular development, pitch of voice, and facial hair. The full meaning of these observations, however, does not emerge until you correlate them with other data: the patient's body habitus, growth pattern over time, muscular development, sexual maturity ratings, psychosexual feelings, attitudes, and knowledge. During the assessment process you will bring these interrelated variables together and try to understand the patient's development and any related problems as well as you can.

WEIGHT. Definitions of appropriate weights for adults remain controversial. They are influenced by aesthetic preferences, cultural attitudes, and medical specialty, among other factors, and there are scientific arguments over the interpretation and applicability of available data. The 1983 Metropolitan figures for height and weight, shown in Table 5-1, are based on actuarial data from 25 insurance companies in the United States and Canada. The weights listed are associated with the lowest mortality rates for men and women between the ages of 25 and 59, during the years from 1954 to 1972.

Body frame, as used in Table 5-2, is determined by *elbow breadth*: the distance between the medial and lateral epicondyles of the elbow (see p. 429), with the forearm flexed to 90° and held in front of the body. The

Table 5-1   Height/Weight Table for Adults
(Weight in Pounds Without Clothes)

HEIGHT WITHOUT SHOES		MEN AGED 25–59 YEARS			WOMEN AGED 25–59 YEARS		
FEET	INCHES	SMALL FRAME	MEDIUM FRAME	LARGE FRAME	SMALL FRAME	MEDIUM FRAME	LARGE FRAME
4	9				99–108	106–118	115–128
4	10				100–110	108–120	117–131
4	11				101–112	110–123	119–134
5	0				103–115	112–126	122–137
5	1	123–129	126–136	133–145	105–118	115–129	125–140
5	2	125–131	128–138	135–148	108–121	118–132	128–144
5	3	127–133	130–140	137–151	111–124	121–135	131–148
5	4	129–135	132–143	139–155	114–127	124–138	134–152
5	5	131–137	134–146	141–159	117–130	127–141	137–156
5	6	133–140	137–149	144–163	120–133	130–144	140–160
5	7	135–143	140–152	147–167	123–136	133–147	143–164
5	8	137–146	143–155	150–171	126–139	136–150	146–167
5	9	139–149	146–158	153–175	129–142	139–153	149–170
5	10	141–152	149–161	156–179	132–145	142–156	152–173
5	11	144–155	152–165	159–183			
6	0	147–159	155–169	163–187			
6	1	150–163	159–173	167–192			
6	2	153–167	162–177	171–197			
6	3	157–171	166–182	176–202			

(Derived from 1983 Metropolitan Height and Weight Tables: Stat Bull Metrop Life Found 64, No. 1: 6–7, 1983)

figures below show elbow breadths calculated for persons of medium frame in five different height groups. Elbow breadths that are greater or smaller than the given ranges for a specific height indicate large and small frames respectively.

Table 5-2   Body Frame According to Height and Elbow Breadth

MEN		WOMEN	
HEIGHT WITHOUT SHOES (in Feet & Inches)	ELBOW BREADTH (in Inches)	HEIGHT WITHOUT SHOES (in Feet & Inches)	ELBOW BREADTH (in Inches)
5'1"–5'2"	2 1/2"–2 7/8"	4'9"–4'10"	2 1/4"–2 1/2"
5'3"–5'6"	2 5/8"–2 7/8"	4'11"–5'2"	2 1/4"–2 1/2"
5'7"–5'10"	2 3/4"–3"	5'3"–5'6"	2 3/8"–2 5/8"
5'11"–6'2"	2 3/4"–3 1/8"	5'7"–5'10"	2 3/8"–2 5/8"
6'3"	2 7/8"–3 1/4"	5'11"	2 1/2"–2 3/4"

(Derived from 1983 Metropolitan Height & Weight Tables: Stat Bull Metrop Life Found 64, No. 1: 5, 1983)

Techniques of Examination

Begin your observations from the first moment you see the patient. Does the patient hear you when called in the waiting room? rise with ease? walk easily or stiffly? If hospitalized when you first meet, what is the patient doing: sitting up and enjoying television? or lying in bed? What occupies the bedside table: a magazine? a flock of "get well" cards? a Bible or rosary? an emesis basin? or nothing at all? Each of these observations should raise one or more tentative hypotheses and guide your further assessments. Throughout the interview and examination, make note of the following:

STATE OF AWARENESS AND LEVEL OF CONSCIOUSNESS. Is the patient awake and alert? Does the patient seem to understand your questions and to respond appropriately and reasonably quickly, or to lose track of the topic, ramble, become silent, or even fall asleep?

Inattentiveness, drowsiness, stupor. See Table 3-1, Abnormalities of Consciousness (p. 109).

APPARENT STATE OF HEALTH. This judgment is an evaluative summary that should be supported by specific observations. Try to define the attributes that substantiate your conclusions. Thinness and weakness in an octogenarian with a tottering gait and a quavery voice suggest frailty, for example, while an ashen, sweaty face suggests an acute illness such as shock.

Acutely or chronically ill, frail, feeble

SIGNS OF DISTRESS. For example,

Cardiorespiratory distress

Labored breathing, wheezing, cough

Pain

Facial expression, sweating, protectiveness of a painful part

Anxiety

Anxious face, fidgety movements, cold moist palms

SKIN COLOR AND POSSIBLE LESIONS. See Chapter 6 for further details.

Pallor, cyanosis, jaundice, changes in pigmentation

STATURE AND HABITUS. If possible, measure the patient's height in stocking feet. Is the patient unusually short or tall? Is the build slender and lanky, muscular, or stocky? Is the body symmetrical? Note the general bodily proportions and look for any deformities.

Very short stature in Turner's syndrome and in achondroplastic, renal, and hypopituitary dwarfism; long limbs in proportion to the trunk in hypogonadism and Marfan's syndrome

SEXUAL DEVELOPMENT. Are the voice, facial hair, and breast size appropriate to the patient's age and gender?

Delayed or precocious puberty, hypogonadism, virilism

WEIGHT. Is the patient emaciated, slender, plump, obese, or somewhere in between? If obese, is the fat distributed rather evenly or does it concentrate in the trunk?

Generalized fat in simple obesity; truncal fat with relatively thin limbs in Cushing's syndrome

If possible, weigh the patient. Weight provides one index of caloric sufficiency, and changes over time give other valuable diagnostic data. Remember that weight may rise or fall with changes in body fluids as well as in fat or muscle.	Causes of weight loss include malignancy, diabetes mellitus, hyperthyroidism, chronic infection, depression, and successful dieting.
POSTURE, MOTOR ACTIVITY, AND GAIT. What is the patient's preferred posture?	Preference for sitting up in leftsided heart failure, and for leaning forward with arms braced in chronic obstructive pulmonary disease
Is the patient restless or quiet? How often does the patient move about? How fast are the movements?	Fast, frequent movements of hyperthyroidism; slumped posture and slowed activity of depression
Are there apparently involuntary motor activities, or are some bodily parts immobile?	Tremors or other involuntary movements; paralyses
Does the patient walk easily, with comfort, self-confidence, and good balance, or is there a limp, discomfort on walking, fear of falling, loss of balance, or abnormality in motor pattern?	See Table 17-3, Abnormalities of Gait and Posture (pp. 516–517).
DRESS, GROOMING, AND PERSONAL HYGIENE. How is the patient dressed? Is clothing appropriate to the temperature and weather? Is it clean, properly buttoned, and zipped? How does it compare with clothing worn by people of comparable age and social group?	Dress may reflect the cold intolerance of hypothyroidism, the embarrassment of a skin rash, or personal preferences in lifestyle.
Glance at the patient's shoes. Have holes been cut in them? Are the laces tied? Or is the patient wearing slippers?	Cut-out holes or slippers may indicate gout, bunions, or other painful foot conditions. Untied laces or slippers also suggest edema.
Is the patient wearing any unusual jewelry?	Copper bracelets are sometimes worn for arthritis.
Note the patient's hair and fingernails, together with any use of cosmetics.	Nail polish and hair coloring that have "grown out" suggest loss of interest in personal appearance and may even help you estimate its duration.
Do personal hygiene and grooming seem appropriate to the patient's age, lifestyle, occupation, and socioeconomic group? There are, of course, wide variations in norms.	Unkempt appearance may be seen in depression and chronic organic brain disease, but this appearance must be compared with the patient's probable norm.

Techniques of Examination	Examples of Abnormalities

ODORS OF BODY OR BREATH. Although odors may give important diagnostic clues, avoid one common mistake: never assume that alcohol on a patient's breath explains neurologic or mental status findings. Alcoholics may have other serious and potentially correctable problems such as hypoglycemia or a subdural hematoma, and an alcoholic breath does not necessarily mean alcoholism.

Breath odors of alcohol, acetone (diabetes), pulmonary infections, uremia, or liver failure

FACIAL EXPRESSION. Observe facial expression at rest, during conversation about specific topics, during the physical examination, and in interaction with others.

Anxiety, depression, embarrassment, anger, apathy; the stare of hyperthyroidism; the immobile face of parkinsonism

MANNER, AFFECT, AND RELATIONSHIP TO PERSONS AND THINGS. Note the patient's manner toward you and toward others such as family members, friends, or staff. Watch the face and gestures and listen to the words and voice of the patient for clues to affect and feelings.

Uncooperativeness, hostility, anger, resentment, depression, tearfulness, distrustfulness, suspiciousness, elation, relief, confidence, resignation, withdrawal, seductiveness

SPEECH. Listen for the pace of speech and its pitch, clarity, and spontaneity.

Fast speech of hyperthyroidism; slow, thick, hoarse voice of myxedema; lack of spontaneity in depression; aphasia; dysarthria

VITAL SIGNS. Note the pulse, blood pressure, respiratory rate, and temperature. You may choose to make these measurements at the beginning of the examination or to integrate them with your cardiovascular and thoracic assessments. If you do them now, count the radial pulse. Then, with your fingers still on the patient's wrist, count the respiratory rate without the patient's realizing it. (Breathing may change when a person becomes conscious that someone is watching.) Check the blood pressure; if it is high, repeat your measurement later in the examination.

See Table 9-15, Abnormalities of the Arterial Pulse (p. 297). See Table 8-1, Abnormalities in Rate and Rhythm of Breathing (p. 245).

Although measurement of temperature may be omitted in many ambulatory visits, take it if symptoms or signs suggest a possible abnormality. Oral thermometers are more convenient and more acceptable to patients than rectal ones, but oral glass thermometers should not be used when patients are unconscious, restless, or unable to close their mouths.

Hyperpyrexia refers to extreme elevation in body temperature, above 41.1° C (106° F). *Fever* or *pyrexia* refers to an elevated temperature, while *hypothermia* refers to an abnormally low temperature, below 35° C (95° F) rectally.

To take an *oral temperature* with a glass thermometer, shake the thermometer down to below 35.5° C (96° F), insert it under the tongue, instruct the patient to close both lips, and wait 3 to 5 minutes. Then read the thermometer, reinsert it for a minute, and read it again. If the temperature is still rising, repeat this procedure until the reading remains stable. It may take as long as 8 minutes to obtain an accurate oral temperature.

Causes of fever include infections, trauma (such as surgery or crushing injury), malignancies, infarctions, blood disorders (such as acute hemolytic anemia), and immune disorders (such as drug fevers and collagen diseases).

To take a *rectal temperature* select a rectal thermometer (with a stubby tip), lubricate it, and insert it about 3 cm to 4 cm (1½ inches) into the anal canal, in a direction pointing toward the umbilicus. Remove and read it after 3 minutes.

Electric thermometers with disposable probe covers are available for both rectal and oral temperatures. They shorten the time required to record an accurate temperature to about 10 seconds.

Whether an oral temperature is taken with a glass or an electric thermometer, drinking hot or cold liquids may alter it artifactually. Wait 10 to 15 minutes before measurement.

The chief cause of hypothermia is exposure to cold. Other predisposing causes include decreased muscular movement (as with paralysis), interference with vasoconstriction (as with alcohol and sepsis), starvation, hypothyroidism, and hypoglycemia. Elderly people are especially susceptible to hypothermia and are less likely to develop fever.

The average oral temperature, usually quoted at 37° C (98.6° F), fluctuates considerably and must be interpreted accordingly. In the early morning hours it may be as low as 35.8° C (96.4° F), in the late afternoon or evening as high as 37.3° C (99.1° F). Rectal temperatures average 0.4° to 0.5° C (0.7° to 0.9° F) higher than oral readings, but this difference varies considerably.

Rapid respiratory rates tend to increase the discrepancy between oral and rectal temperatures. Rectal measurements are then more reliable.

Chapter 6
The Skin

Anatomy and Physiology

The skin is composed of three layers: the epidermis, the dermis, and the subcutaneous tissues.

The most superficial layer, the *epidermis*, is thin, devoid of blood vessels, and itself divided into two layers: an outer horny layer of dead keratinized cells, and an inner cellular layer where both melanin and keratin are formed.

The epidermis depends on the underlying *dermis* for its nutrition. The dermis is well supplied with blood. It contains connective tissue, the sebaceous glands, and some of the hair follicles. It merges below with the *subcutaneous tissues* which contain fat, the sweat glands, and the remainder of the hair follicles.

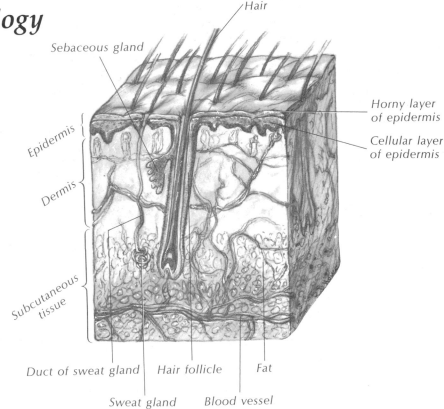

Hair, nails, and sebaceous and sweat glands are considered appendages of the skin. Adults have two types of hair: vellus and terminal. Vellus hair is short, fine, inconspicuous, and unpigmented, while terminal hair in contrast is coarser, thicker, more conspicuous, and usually pigmented. Scalp hair and eyebrows are examples of terminal hair.

Sebaceous glands secrete a protective fatty substance which gains access to the skin surface through the hair follicles. These glands are present on all skin surfaces except for the palms and soles. Sweat glands are of two types: eccrine and apocrine. The eccrine glands are widely distributed, open directly onto the skin surface, and by their sweat production help to control body temperature. In contrast, the apocrine glands are found chiefly in the axillary and genital regions, usually open into hair follicles, and are stimulated by emotional stress. Bacterial decomposition of apocrine sweat is responsible for adult body odor.

The color of normal skin depends primarily on four pigments: melanin, carotene, oxyhemoglobin, and deoxyhemoglobin. The amount of *melanin*, the brownish pigment of the skin, is genetically determined and is increased by sunlight. *Carotene* is a golden yellow pigment that exists in subcutaneous fat and in heavily keratinized areas such as the palms and soles.

Hemoglobin, which circulates in the red cells and carries most of the oxygen of the blood, exists in two forms. *Oxyhemoglobin*, a bright red pigment, predominates in the arteries and capillaries. An increase in blood flow through the arteries to the capillaries of the skin causes a reddening of the skin, while the opposite changes usually produce pallor. The skin of light-colored persons is normally redder on the palms, soles, face, neck, and upper chest.

As blood passes through the capillary bed, some of the oxyhemoglobin loses its oxygen to the tissues and thus changes to *deoxyhemoglobin*—a darker, less red, and somewhat bluer pigment. An increased concentration of deoxyhemoglobin in cutaneous blood vessels gives the skin a bluish cast known as *cyanosis*. Although cyanosis may signal serious disease, it may merely reflect a normal vascular response to various stimuli. When a person is anxious or exposed to a cold environment, for example, cutaneous blood flow decreases and slows, allowing the tissues to extract relatively more oxygen. The nailbeds then look bluish while the hands look pale and feel cool. When cyanosis results from increased tissue extraction of oxygen, it is called *peripheral* cyanosis. When it results from increased concentrations of deoxygenated hemoglobin in arterial blood, it is called *central* cyanosis.

In dark-skinned persons melanin may mask the other pigments, making it difficult to identify pallor, unusual redness, or cyanosis. The palms, soles, fingertips, and nailbeds of dark-skinned persons contain less melanin than other areas and may be helpful in this assessment.

Skin color is affected not only by pigments but also by the scattering of light as it is reflected back through the turbid superficial layers of the skin or vessel walls. This scattering makes the color look more blue and less red. The bluish color of a subcutaneous vein is due to this effect, for example; it is much bluer than the venous blood obtained on venipuncture.

CHANGES WITH AGE

During the pubertal years coarse, or terminal, hair appears in new places: the face in boys, and the axillae and pubic areas in both sexes. Hair on the trunk and limbs increases through and after puberty, more obviously in men. During puberty apocrine glands enlarge, axillary sweating increases, and the characteristic adult body odor appears.

As people age their skin wrinkles, becomes lax, and loses turgor. The vascularity of the dermis decreases and the skin of white persons tends to look paler and more opaque. Comedones (blackheads) often appear on the cheeks or around the eyes. Where skin has been exposed to the sun it looks weatherbeaten: thickened, yellowed, and deeply furrowed. Skin on the backs of the hands and forearms appears thin, fragile, loose, and transparent, and may show whitish, depigmented patches known as pseudoscars. Well demarcated, vividly purple macules or patches, termed senile purpura, may also appear in the same areas, fading after several weeks. These purpuric spots come from blood that has leaked through poorly supported capillaries and has spread within the dermis. Dry skin (asteatosis)—a common problem—is flaky, rough, and often itchy. It is frequently shiny, especially on the legs, where a network of shallow fissures often creates a mosaic of small polygons.

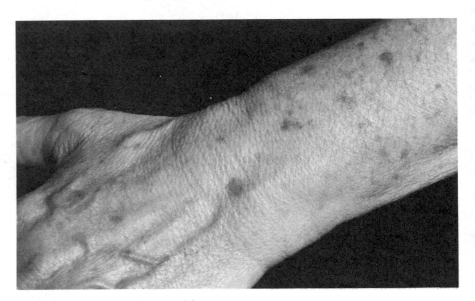

Senile lentigenes in a 58-year-old woman.

Brown macules known as liver spots, or senile lentigines, frequently appear on the backs of the hands and forearms or, less commonly, on the face. Unlike the familiar freckles, they do not fade spontaneously when protected from the sun. Also common are seborrheic keratoses—pigmented, raised, warty, and often slightly greasy lesions that develop most often on the trunk but also occur on the face and hands. (See Color Plate 3, Skin Tumors, p. 208.) Actinic (or senile) keratoses, which are less common, develop on exposed surfaces, first as small reddened areas and then as raised, rough, yellow to brown lesions (see p. 208). From middle life on, sebaceous hyperplasia may become evident on the face, especially on the forehead and nose. Hyperplastic sebaceous glands, which must be differentiated from basal cell epitheliomas, are yellowish, flattened papules with central depressions. They often look like diminutive doughnuts and range in size from 1 mm to 3 mm or more in diameter.

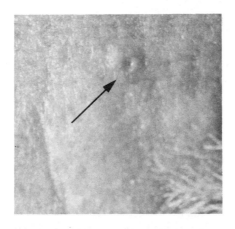

Sebaceous hyperplasia in a 53-year-old woman.

Cherry angiomas are very common, first appearing fairly early in adulthood (see p. 144). Most frequently found on the trunk, they have no significance.

While all these changes occur so frequently that they may be considered part of normal aging, two less common findings in older people are distinctly abnormal: squamous cell carcinoma, which sometimes develops in an actinic keratosis, and basal cell epithelioma. (See Color Plate 3, Skin Tumors, p. 208.)

Nails lose some of their luster with age and may yellow and thicken, especially on the toes.

Hair on the scalp loses its pigment, producing the well known graying. At as early as 20 years of age a man's hairline may start to recede at the temples; hair loss at the vertex follows. Many women show loss of hair in a similar pattern, but it is less severe. Balding in this distribution is genetically determined. In both sexes the number of scalp hairs decreases in a generalized, more subtle pattern, and the diameter of each hair diminishes.

Less familiar, but probably more important clinically, is the normal hair loss elsewhere on the body: the trunk, pubic areas, axillae, and limbs. These changes will be discussed, where relevant, in later chapters. Coarse facial hairs appear on the chin and upper lip of many women by the approximate age of 55, but do not increase further thereafter.

Many of the observations described here pertain to white persons and do not necessarily apply to other racial groups. For example, Native American men have relatively little facial and body hair compared to that of white men and should not be evaluated by white norms.

Techniques of Examination

Begin your observation of the skin and related structures during the general survey and continue it throughout the rest of your examination. The entire skin surface should be inspected in good light, preferably natural light or artificial light that resembles it. Correlate your findings with observations of the mucous membranes. Specific diseases may manifest themselves in both areas, and both are necessary for the assessment of skin color. Techniques of examining these membranes are described in later chapters.

Artificial light often distorts colors and masks jaundice.

SKIN. Inspect and palpate the skin. Note its:

Color. Patients may be more sensitive to a change in their own skin color than the clinician is. Ask about it. Look for increased pigmentation (brownness), loss of pigmentation, redness, pallor, cyanosis, and yellowing of the skin.

See Table 6-1, Variations in Skin Color (pp. 140–141).

The red color of oxyhemoglobin and the pallor due to a lack of it are best discerned where the horny layer of the epidermis is thinnest and causes the least scatter: the fingernails, the lips, and the mucous membranes, particularly those of the mouth and the palpebral conjunctivas. Inspect these areas in particular for pallor. In dark-skinned persons the palms and soles may also be useful.

Pallor due to decreased redness is seen in anemia and in decreased blood flow, as in fainting or arterial insufficiency.

The conjunctivas are not very helpful in assessing cyanosis, and the nailbeds are so frequently affected by peripheral factors that they are misleading. The lips, buccal mucosa, and tongue are usually best for the assessment of central cyanosis, although even the lips can become blue in the cold. Further, melanin pigment in the lips may give a false impression of cyanosis in some persons with dark complexions, especially those of Mediterranean heritage. The nails and the skin of the extremities are helpful in identifying peripheral cyanosis.

Causes of peripheral cyanosis include anxiety, cold exposure, and venous obstruction. Causes of central cyanosis include advanced lung disease, congenital heart disease, and abnormal hemoglobins. Cyanosis in congestive heart failure is usually peripheral, reflecting decreased blood flow, but in pulmonary edema it may also be central.

Look for the yellow color of excessive carotene in the palms, soles, and face. For the yellow color of jaundice, in contrast, look particularly in the bulbar conjunctivas against the background of the white scleras. Look for it also in the palpebral conjunctivas, the lips, and the hard palate, under the tongue, and in the skin itself. To see jaundice more easily in the lips, blanch out the red color by pressure with a glass slide.

Carotenemia

Jaundice suggests liver disease or excessive hemolysis of red blood cells.

Moisture. For example, dryness, sweating, oiliness

Dryness in hypothyroidism; oiliness in acne

Techniques of Examination	Examples of Abnormalities
Temperature. Use the backs of your fingers to make this assessment. In addition to identifying generalized warmth or coolness of the skin, note the temperature of any red areas.	Generalized warmth in fever, hyperthyroidism; coolness in hypothyroidism. Local warmth of inflammation.
Texture. For example, roughness, smoothness	Roughness in hypothyroidism
Mobility and Turgor. Lift a fold of skin and note the ease with which it is moved (mobility) and the speed with which it returns into place (turgor).	Decreased mobility in edema, scleroderma; decreased turgor in dehydration

Lesions. Observe any lesions of the skin.

1. First, identify the *anatomic location* of the lesions and their *distribution* over the entire surface of the body. Are they generalized or localized? Do they, for example, involve only the exposed surfaces, or the intertriginous (skin fold) areas, or areas exposed to specific contacts such as wrist bands or rings?

   Many skin diseases have characteristic distributions. For example, acne affects the face, upper chest, and back; psoriasis, the knees and elbows (among other areas); and Monilia infections, the intertiginous areas.

2. Then note the *grouping* or *arrangement* of the lesions. They may be, for example, linear, clustered, annular (in a ring), arciform (in an arc), or dermatomal (covering a skin band that corresponds to a sensory nerve root; see pp. 475–476).

   Vesicles in a unilateral dermatomal pattern are typical of herpes zoster.

3. Then try to identify the *type of skin lesions* (*e.g.*, macules, papules, vesicles). If possible, find representative and recent lesions that have not been traumatized by scratching or otherwise altered. Inspect them carefully and feel them.

   See Table 6-2, Basic Types of Skin Lesions (pp. 142–143).

   See Table 6-3, Vascular and Purpuric Lesions of the Skin (p. 144).

4. Note the *color* of the lesions.

   See Color Plate 3, Skin Tumors (p. 208).

NAILS. Inspect and palpate the fingernails and toenails. Note their color and shape, and any lesions. Longitudinal bands of pigment may be seen in the nails of normal black persons.

See Table 6-4, Abnormalities and Variations of the Nails (p. 145).

HAIR. Inspect and palpate the hair. Note its quantity, distribution, and texture.

The differential diagnosis of skin abnormalities is beyond the scope of this book. After familiarizing yourself with the basic types of lesions, you would do well to peruse a relatively brief but well illustrated textbook of dermatology. Whenever you see a skin lesion, make a consistent habit of looking it up in such a text. The type of lesions, their location, and their distribution, together with other information from the history and the examination, should equip you well for this search and, in time, for arriving at specific dermatologic diagnoses.

Table 6-1

Table 6-1 Variations in Skin Color

COLOR	PROCESS	SELECTED CAUSES	TYPICAL LOCALIZATION
BROWN	Deposition of melanin	Sunlight	Exposed area
		Pregnancy	Face (mask of pregnancy, or melasma), nipples, areolae, linea nigra, vulva
		Addison's disease and some pituitary tumors	Exposed areas, points of pressure and friction, nipples, genitalia, palmar creases (normally darker in black persons), recent scars; often generalized
GRAYISH TAN OR BRONZE	Deposition of melanin and hemosiderin	Hemochromatosis	Exposed areas, genitalia, scars; often generalized
BLUE (CYANOSIS)	Increased amount of deoxyhemoglobin secondary to hypoxia. This may be either—		
	Peripheral, or	Anxiety or cold environment	The nails, sometimes lips
	Central (arterial)	Heart or lung disease	Lips, buccal mucosa, tongue, nails
	Abnormal hemoglobin	Congenital or acquired methemoglobinemia; sulfhemoglobinemia	Lips, buccal mucosa, tongue, nails
REDDISH BLUE	Combination of increase in total amount of hemoglobin, increase in reduced hemoglobin, and capillary stasis	Polycythemia	Face, conjunctivas, mouth, hands, feet
RED	Increased visibility of normal oxyhemoglobin because of—		
	Dilatation or increased number of superficial blood vessels or increased blood flow	Fever, blushing, alcohol intake, local inflammation	Face and upper chest or local area of inflammation
	Decreased oxygen use in the skin	Cold exposure	The cold area (e.g., ears)

Table 6-1

	Process	Condition	Location/Distribution
YELLOW			
JAUNDICE	Increased bilirubin levels	Liver disease, red blood cell hemolysis	Conjunctivas, then other mucous membranes and generalized
CAROTENEMIA	Increased levels of carotene	Increased intake of carotene-containing vegetables and fruits; myxedema, hypopituitarism, diabetes mellitus, anorexia nervosa	Palms, soles, face; does not involve conjunctivas or other mucous membranes
CHRONIC UREMIA	Retention of urinary chromogens or other yellow pigments, superimposed on the pallor of anemia; increased melanin may also contribute	Chronic renal disease	Most evident in exposed areas, may be generalized; does not involve conjunctivas or other mucous membranes
DECREASED COLOR	Decreased melanin		
	Congenital inability to form melanin	Albinism	Generalized lack of pigment in skin, hair, eyes
	Acquired loss of melanin	Vitiligo	Patchy, symmetrical, often involving the exposed areas
		Tinea versicolor (a common fungus infection)	Chest, upper back, neck
	Decreased visibility of oxyhemoglobin		
	Decreased blood flow in superficial vessels	Syncope, shock, some normal variations	Most evident in face, conjunctivas, mouth, nails
	Decreased amount of oxyhemoglobin	Anemia	Most evident in face, conjunctivas, mouth, nails
	Edema. (Edema of the skin masks the colors of melanin and hemoglobin and prevents the appearance of jaundice.)	Nephrotic syndrome	The edematous areas

Table 6-2

Table 6-2 Basic Types of Skin Lesions

PRIMARY LESIONS (May Arise from Previously Normal Skin)

CIRCUMSCRIBED, FLAT, NONPALPABLE CHANGES IN SKIN COLOR

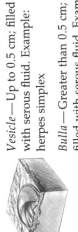

Macule—Small, up to 1 cm.* Example: freckle, petechia

Patch—Larger than 1 cm. Example: vitiligo

PALPABLE ELEVATED SOLID MASSES

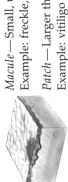

Papule—Up to 0.5 cm. Example: an elevated nevus

Plaque—A flat, elevated surface larger than 0.5 cm, often formed by the coalescence of papules

Nodule—0.5 cm to 1–2 cm; often deeper and firmer than a papule

Tumor—Larger than 1–2 cm

Wheal—A somewhat irregular, relatively transient, superficial area of localized skin edema. Example: mosquito bite, hive

CIRCUMSCRIBED SUPERFICIAL ELEVATIONS OF THE SKIN FORMED BY FREE FLUID IN A CAVITY WITHIN THE SKIN LAYERS

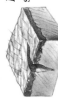

Vesicle—Up to 0.5 cm; filled with serous fluid. Example: herpes simplex

Bulla—Greater than 0.5 cm; filled with serous fluid. Example: 2nd degree burn

Pustule—Filled with pus. Examples: acne, impetigo

SECONDARY LESIONS (Result from Changes in Primary Lesions)

LOSS OF SKIN SURFACE

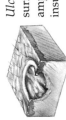

Erosion—Loss of the superficial epidermis; surface is moist but does not bleed. Example: moist area after the rupture of a vesicle, as in chickenpox

Ulcer—A deeper loss of skin surface; may bleed and scar. Examples: stasis ulcer of venous insufficiency, syphilitic chancre

Fissure—A linear crack in the skin. Example: athlete's foot

Table 6-2

MATERIAL ON THE SKIN SURFACE

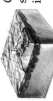

Crust—The dried residue of serum, pus, or blood. Example: impetigo

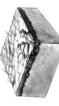

Scale—A thin flake of exfoliated epidermis. Examples: dandruff, dry skin, psoriasis

MISCELLANEOUS

Lichenification—Thickening and roughening of the skin with increased visibility of the normal skin furrows. Example: atopic dermatitis

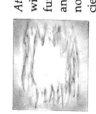

Atrophy—Thinning of the skin with loss of the normal skin furrows; the skin looks shinier and more translucent than normal. Example: arterial insufficiency

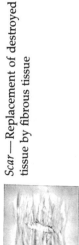

Scar—Replacement of destroyed tissue by fibrous tissue

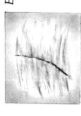

Keloid—A hypertrophied scar

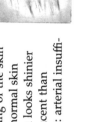

Excoriation—A scratch mark

Several additional terms, though technically neither primary nor secondary lesions, deserve mention. A *comedo* refers to the common blackhead and marks the plugged opening of a sebaceous gland. Comedones are one of the hallmarks of acne. *Telangiectasias* are dilated small vessels that look either red or bluish. They can appear by themselves or as parts of other lesions such as a basal cell carcinoma or radiodermatitis (skin injury from ionizing radiation). The common mole—a flat to slightly elevated, round, even pigmented lesion—is technically called a *nevus*, although there are additional kinds of nevi that look quite different.

* Authorities vary somewhat in their definitions of skin lesions by size. Dimensions given in this table should be considered approximate, not rigid.

Table 6-3

Table 6-3 Vascular and Purpuric Lesions of the Skin

	VASCULAR			PURPURIC	
	CHERRY ANGIOMA	SPIDER ANGIOMA	VENOUS STAR	PETECHIA	ECCHYMOSIS
COLOR	Bright or ruby red; may become brownish with age	Fiery red	Bluish	Deep red or reddish purple	Purple or purplish blue, fading to green, yellow, and brown with time
SIZE	1–3 mm	Very small up to 2 cm	Variable, from very small to several inches	Usually 1–3 mm	Variable, larger than petechiae
SHAPE	Round, flat or sometimes raised, may be surrounded by a pale halo	Central body, sometimes raised, surrounded by erythema and radiating legs	Variable. May resemble a spider or be linear, irregular, cascading	Round, flat	Round, oval, or irregular; may have a central subcutaneous flat nodule
PULSATILITY	Absent	Often demonstrable in the body of the spider, when pressure with a glass slide is applied	Absent	Absent	Absent
EFFECT OF PRESSURE	May show partial blanching, especially if pressure is applied with the edge of a pinpoint	Pressure on the body causes blanching of the spider.	Pressure over center does not cause blanching.	None	None
DISTRIBUTION	Trunk, also extremities	Face, neck, arms, and upper trunk; almost never below the waist	Most often on the legs, near veins; also anterior chest	Variable	Variable
SIGNIFICANCE	None; increase in size and numbers with aging	Liver disease, pregnancy, vitamin B deficiency, also occurs in some normal people	Often accompanies increased pressure in the superficial veins, as in varicose veins	Blood extravasated outside the vessels; may suggest increased bleeding tendency or emboli to skin	Blood extravasated outside the vessels; often secondary to trauma; also seen in bleeding disorders

Table 6-4

Table 6-4 Abnormalities and Variations of the Nails

CLUBBING OF THE NAILS

NORMAL

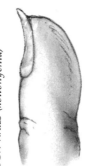

Normal angle 160°

The angle between the normal finger nail and nail base is about 160°. When palpated the nail base feels firm.

EARLY CLUBBING

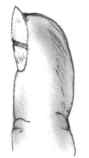

Straightened angle (180°) *Springy, floating*

In early clubbing the angle between nail and nail base straightens out. The nail base gives a springy or floating sensation when palpated. You can simulate this by squeezing your middle finger from each side between your thumb and ring finger of the same hand. Then palpate the nail base with the index finger of the opposite hand.

LATE CLUBBING

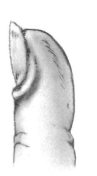

Angle greater than 180° *Swollen, springy, floating*

In late clubbing the base of the nail becomes visibly swollen and the angle between nail and nail base exceeds 180°.

Clubbing has many causes, including hypoxia and lung cancer.

CURVED NAILS

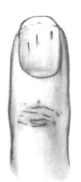

Curved nail *Normal angle*

Curved nails, a variant of normal, should not be confused with clubbing. Here, although the nails show a convex curve as they may in clubbing, the normal angle between nail and nail base is preserved.

SPOON NAILS *(koilonychia)*

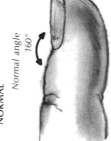

Spoon nails are characterized by concave curves. Spoon nails are sometimes seen in iron deficiency anemia, although they are not specific for this disorder.

BEAU'S LINES

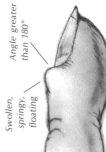

Beau's lines are transverse depressions in the nails associated with acute severe illness. Appearing some weeks later, they grow out with the nail gradually over several months.

PARONYCHIA

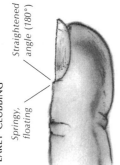

The term paronychia refers to inflammation of the skin around the nail. It is characterized by swelling and sometimes redness and tenderness.

SPLINTER HEMORRHAGES

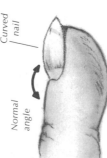

Splinter hemorrhages are red or brown linear streaks in the nail bed, parallel to the long axis of the fingers. Although traditionally associated with subacute bacterial endocarditis and trichinosis, they are non-specific, often occurring with minor trauma or without apparent cause. They have been described in from 10% to 20% of hospitalized adults.

Chapter 7
The Head and Neck

Anatomy and Physiology

THE HEAD

Regions of the head take their names from the underlying bones (*e.g.,* frontal area, occipital area). Familiarity with the anatomy of the skull is helpful, therefore, in localizing and describing physical findings.

Two salivary glands can be examined clinically: the parotid gland, which when enlarged is sometimes visible and palpable superficial to and behind the mandible, and the submaxillary (submandibular) gland, which is located deep to the mandible. Feel for the latter as you press your tongue against your upper incisors. Its lobular surface can often be felt against the tightened muscle. The openings of the parotid and submaxillary glands are visible within the oral cavity.

The superficial temporal artery passes upward just in front of the ear, where it is readily palpable. In many normal people, especially thin and elderly ones, its tortuous course can be traced across the forehead.

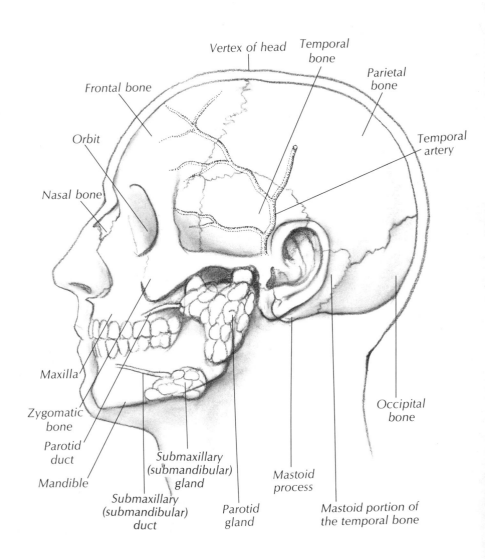

THE EYE

GROSS ANATOMY. Review the external anatomy of the eye, identifying the structures illustrated.

Note that the upper eyelid normally covers a portion of the iris but does not usually overlap the pupil. The opening between the eyelids is called the palpebral fissure. Peripherally the white sclera may look somewhat buff-colored—a color that should not be mistaken for the yellow of jaundice. Patches of normal brown pigment may occur in the scleras of black people.

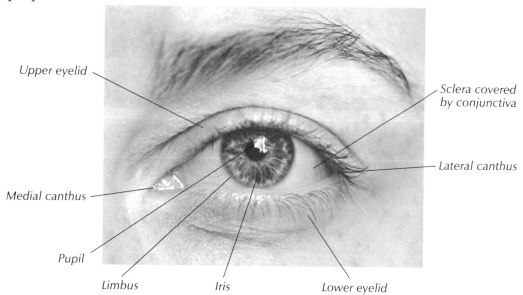

Upper eyelid

Sclera covered by conjunctiva

Medial canthus

Lateral canthus

Pupil

Limbus   Iris   Lower eyelid

Except for the cornea, the parts of the eyeball visible anteriorly are covered by the conjunctiva. At the margin of the cornea (limbus), the conjunctiva merges with the corneal epithelium. A portion of the conjunctiva with its vessels lies loosely on the surface of the sclera and is called the bulbar conjunctiva. Above and below, it forms a deep recess and then folds forward to join the tissues of the eyelids (palpebral conjunctiva). The eyelids themselves are given form and consistency by thin strips of connective tissue known as the tarsal plates. Within each tarsal plate lies a row of parallel meibomian glands which open near the posterior margin of the lid. By secreting sebaceous material they lubricate the lids. The levator palpebrae muscle, which raises the upper eyelid, has a dual innervation: from the oculo-

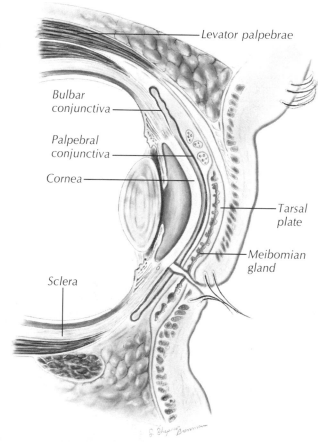

Levator palpebrae

Bulbar conjunctiva

Palpebral conjunctiva

Cornea

Tarsal plate

Meibomian gland

Sclera

SAGGITAL SECTION OF ANTERIOR EYE WITH LIDS CLOSED

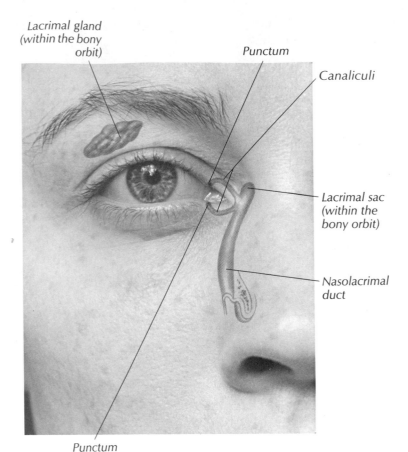

Lacrimal gland
(within the bony
orbit)

Punctum

Canaliculi

Lacrimal sac
(within the
bony orbit)

Nasolacrimal
duct

Punctum

motor nerve (3rd cranial nerve) and from the sympathetic system.

The conjunctiva and cornea are lubricated by secretions from the lacrimal gland and from the conjunctiva itself. The lacrimal gland lies mostly within the bony orbit, above and lateral to the eyeball. The tears spread across the eye and drain out of it medially through two tiny holes called lacrimal puncta. Each punctum can be found on a small elevation of the lid margin. The tears then pass through canaliculi into the lacrimal sac and on into the nose through the nasolacrimal duct. The lacrimal sac lies protected in a small bony depression inside the bony orbit. To press on it you must place your finger just inside the orbital rim.

The eyeball itself is a spherical structure designed to focus a controlled amount of light on the neurosensory elements within the retina. Muscles within the iris control pupillary size. Muscles of the ciliary body control the thickness of the lens, enabling the normal eye to focus in turn on objects near and far away. At the posterior pole of the eye the retinal surface shows a slight depression—the fovea centralis—which marks the point of central vision. The retina immediately around it is called the macula. The optic nerve with its retinal vessels joins the eye somewhat medial to this point. It is visible ophthalmoscopically as the optic disc. That portion of the eye posterior to the lens is termed the fundus of the eye. It includes most of the structures

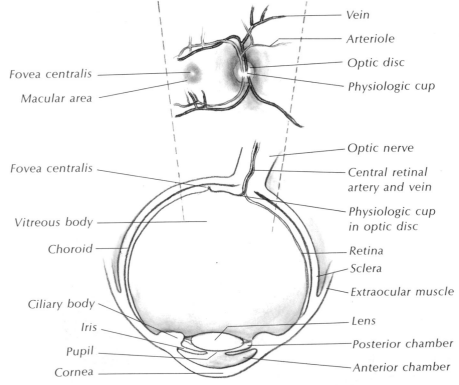

Fovea centralis

Macular area

Fovea centralis

Vitreous body

Choroid

Ciliary body

Iris

Pupil

Cornea

Vein

Arteriole

Optic disc

Physiologic cup

Optic nerve

Central retinal
artery and vein

Physiologic cup
in optic disc

Retina

Sclera

Extraocular muscle

Lens

Posterior chamber

Anterior chamber

**CROSS SECTION OF THE RIGHT EYE FROM ABOVE SHOWING A PORTION
OF THE FUNDUS COMMONLY SEEN WITH THE OPHTHALMOSCOPE**

normally inspected with the ophthalmoscope: retina, choroid, fovea, macula, optic disc, and retinal vessels. The most anterior parts of the retina and the ciliary body are visible only by special techniques.

A clear liquid called *aqueous humor* fills the anterior and posterior chambers of the eye. Aqueous humor is produced by the ciliary body, circulates from the posterior chamber through the pupil into the anterior chamber, and then drains out through the canal of Schlemm. Pressure within the eye depends primarily upon this circulatory system.

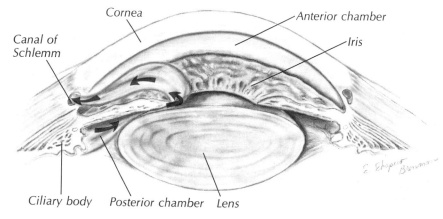

CIRCULATION OF AQUEOUS HUMOR

VISUAL PATHWAYS. For a clear visual image, reflected light from an object must pass through the cornea, aqueous humor, lens, and vitreous, and be focused on the retina. Images so formed are upside down and reversed right to left. An object in the upper temporal visual field, therefore, strikes the lower nasal quadrant of the retina.

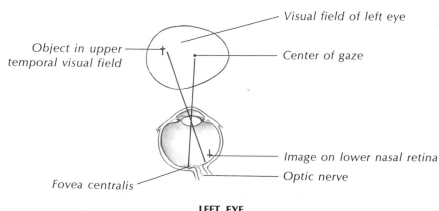

LEFT EYE

In response to this light stimulus, nerve impulses are conducted through the retina, the optic nerve, and the optic tract to the midbrain, and thence to the visual cortex of the occipital lobe. The spatial arrangements of nerve fibers in the retina are preserved in the optic nerves: temporal fibers run laterally in the nerve; nasal fibers run medially. At the optic chiasm, however, the nasal or medial fibers cross over so that the left optic tract contains fibers only from the left half of each retina and the right optic tract contains fibers only from the right half.

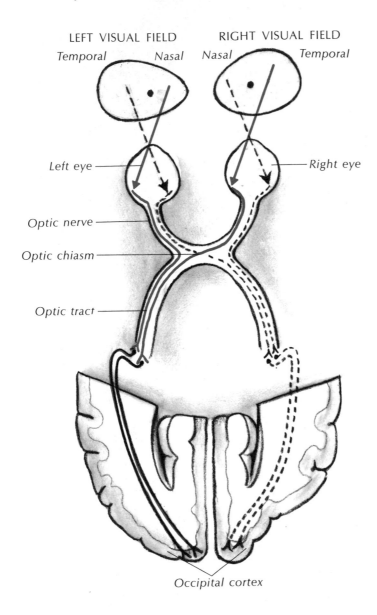

PUPILLARY REACTIONS.* Pupillary size changes in response to light and to the focus of gaze.

---

* Because of the complexity of these responses many authorities now prefer the term "reactions" to "reflexes."

The Light Reaction. A light beam shining onto the retina causes pupillary constriction in both that eye (the *direct reaction* to light) and the opposite eye (the *consensual reaction*).

The initial sensory pathways are similar to those described on page 150: retina, optic nerve, and optic tract. The pathways diverge, however, in the midbrain, and through a series of synapses impulses are transmitted through the oculomotor nerve (3rd cranial nerve) and thence to the constrictor muscles of the iris on each side.

The Near Reaction. When a person shifts gaze from a far object to a close one, the eyes respond in three ways: the pupils constrict (the near reaction), the eyes converge, and the lenses become more convex.

Pupillary constriction with near gaze, like that in response to light, is mediated by the oculomotor nerve. *Convergence* is also mediated by the oculomotor nerve, as described below under Extraocular Movements. The response of the lenses, called *accommodation*, is not visible. Their increased convexity is caused by contraction of the ciliary muscles and brings near objects into focus.

AUTONOMIC NERVE SUPPLY TO THE EYES. Fibers traveling in the oculomotor nerve and producing pupillary constriction as described above are part of the parasympathetic nervous system. The iris is also supplied by sympathetic fibers. When these are stimulated, pupillary dilata-

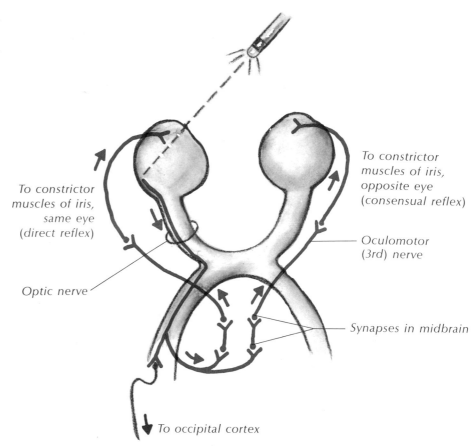

To constrictor muscles of iris, same eye (direct reflex)

To constrictor muscles of iris, opposite eye (consensual reflex)

Oculomotor (3rd) nerve

Optic nerve

Synapses in midbrain

To occipital cortex

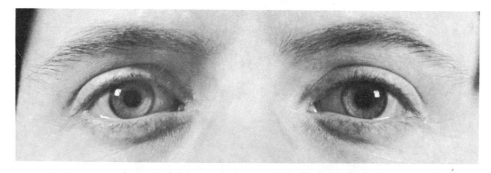

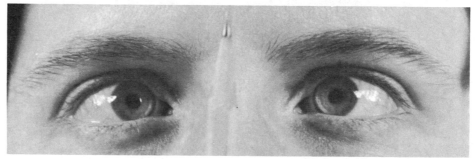

THE NEAR REACTION

tion and some elevation of the eyelid result. The sympathetic pathway starts in the hypothalamus, passes down through the brainstem and cervical cord, and continues out to the sympathetic trunk and ganglia of the neck. Sympathetic fibers then follow a nerve plexus around the carotid artery and its branches into the orbit.

EXTRAOCULAR MOVEMENTS. The movement of each eye is controlled by the coordinated action of six muscles, the four rectus and two oblique muscles. The function of each muscle, together with that of the nerve that supplies it, may be tested by asking the patient to move the eye in the direction predominantly controlled by that muscle. There are six such *cardinal directions.* When a person looks down and to the right, for example,

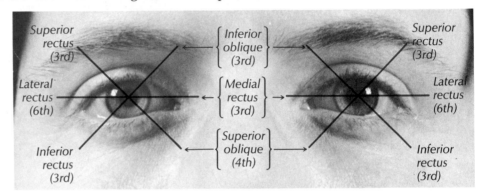

the right inferior rectus (3rd cranial nerve) is principally responsible for moving the right eye while the left superior oblique (4th cranial nerve) is principally responsible for moving the left. If one of these muscles is paralyzed, deviation of the eyes from their normal conjugate, or parallel, positions will be most obvious in this direction of gaze.

THE EAR

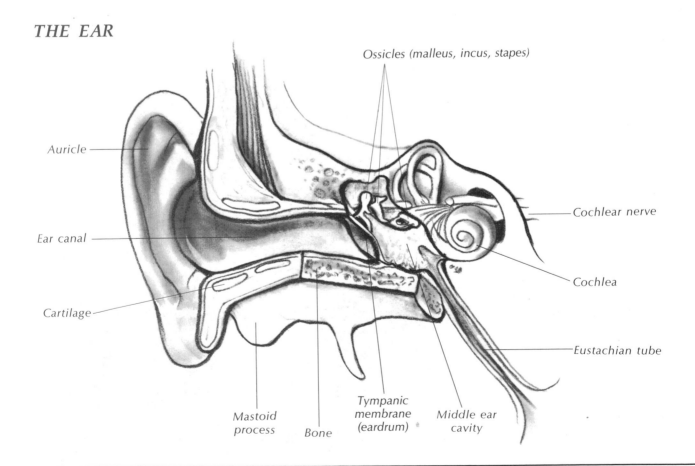

ANATOMY. The ear has three compartments: the external ear, the middle ear, and the inner ear.

The external ear comprises the auricle and ear canal. The auricle consists chiefly of cartilage covered by skin and has a firm, elastic consistency.

The ear canal opens behind the tragus and curves inward about 24 mm. Its outer portion is surrounded by cartilage. The skin in this outer portion is hairy and contains glands that produce cerumen (wax). The inner portion of the canal is surrounded by bone and lined by thin, hairless skin. Pressure on this latter area causes pain — a point to remember when you examine the ear.

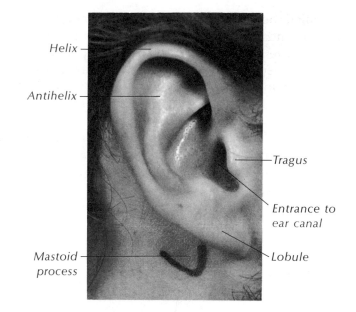

The bone behind and below the ear canal is the mastoid part of the temporal bone. The mastoid process is palpable behind the lobule.

At the end of the ear canal lies the tympanic membrane or eardrum, marking the lateral limits of the middle ear. The middle ear is an air-filled cavity across which sound is transmitted by way of three tiny bones, the ossicles. It is connected by the eustachian tube to the nasopharynx.

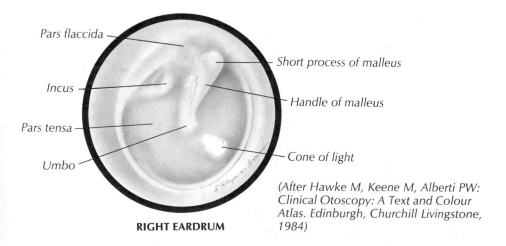

RIGHT EARDRUM

(After Hawke M, Keene M, Alberti PW: Clinical Otoscopy: A Text and Colour Atlas. Edinburgh, Churchill Livingstone, 1984)

The eardrum may be visualized as an oblique membrane pulled inward at its center by one of the ossicles, the malleus. Find the handle and the short process of the malleus — the two chief landmarks. From the umbo, where the eardrum meets the tip of the malleus, a light reflection called the cone of light fans downward and anteriorly. Above the short process lies a small portion of the eardrum called the pars flaccida. The remainder of the drum is the pars tensa. Anterior and posterior malleolar folds, which extend laterally and upward from the short process, separate the pars flaccida from the pars tensa but are usually invisible unless the eardrum is retracted. A second ossicle, the incus, can sometimes be seen through the drum.

Much of the middle ear and all of the inner ear are inaccessible to direct examination. Some inferences concerning their condition can be made, however, by testing auditory function.

PATHWAYS OF HEARING. Vibrations of sound pass through the air of the external ear and are transmitted through the eardrum and ossicles of the middle ear into the cochlea, a part of the inner ear.

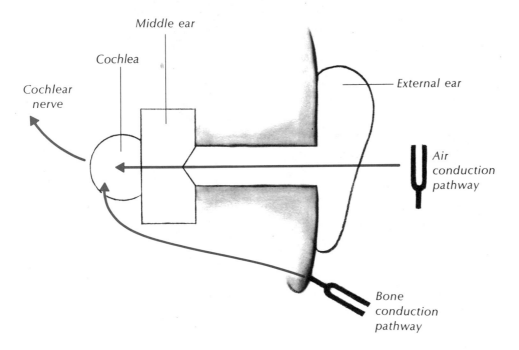

Here nerve impulses are initiated and sent to the brain by way of the cochlear nerve (a portion of the 8th cranial nerve). This pathway is the usual one in normal hearing. An alternate pathway used for testing purposes bypasses the external and middle ear by setting the bone of the skull into vibration and thereby stimulating the inner ear directly.

Hearing over the usual pathways, including the air-filled external and middle ear, is called air conduction. Hearing dependent upon sound transmitted through bone to the inner ear is called bone conduction. In the normal person, the usual pathway (*i.e.,* air conduction) is the more sensitive.

EQUILIBRIUM. The inner ear has an additional important function in controlling balance.

THE NOSE AND PARANASAL SINUSES

Review the terms used to describe the external anatomy of the nose.

Approximately the upper third of the nose is supported by bone, the lower two thirds by cartilage. Air enters the nasal cavity by way of the anterior naris on either side, then passes into a widened area known as the vestibule and on through the slitlike nasal passage to the nasopharynx. The medial wall of each nasal cavity is formed by the nasal septum which, like the external nose, is supported by both bone and cartilage. It is covered by a mucous membrane well supplied with blood. The vestibule, unlike the rest of the nasal cavity, is lined by hair-bearing skin, not mucosa.

Laterally the anatomy is more complex. Curving bony structures, the turbinates, covered by a highly vascular mucous membrane, protrude into the nasal cavity. Below each turbinate is a groove, or meatus, each named according to the turbinate above it. Into the inferior meatus drains the nasolacrimal duct; into the middle meatus drain most of the paranasal sinuses. Their openings are not usually visible.

The additional surface area provided by the turbinates and the mucosa covering them aids the nasal cavities in their principal functions: cleansing, humidification, and temperature control of inspired air.

Inspection of the nasal cavity through the anterior naris is usually limited to the vestibule, the anterior portion of the septum, and the

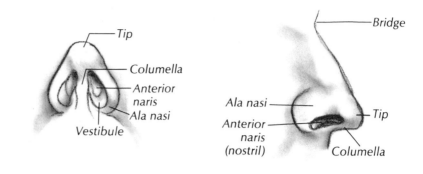

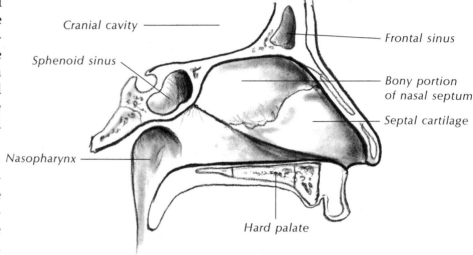

MEDIAL WALL—RIGHT NASAL CAVITY
(Mucous membrane removed to show the structure of the nasal septum)

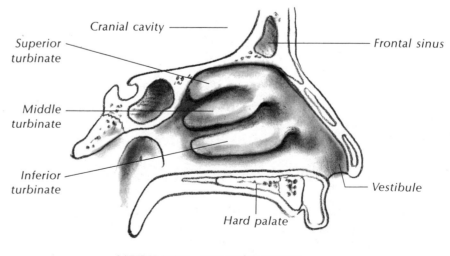

LATERAL WALL—LEFT NASAL CAVITY

lower and middle turbinates. Examination by means of a nasopharyngeal mirror is required for detection of posterior abnormalities. It is beyond the scope of this book.

The paranasal sinuses are air-filled cavities within the bones of the skull. Like the nasal cavities into which they drain, they are lined by mucous membrane. Their locations are diagrammed below. Only the frontal and maxillary sinuses are readily accessible to clinical examination.

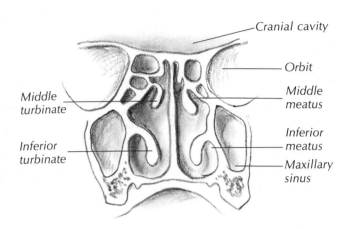

CROSS SECTION OF NASAL CAVITY—ANTERIOR VIEW

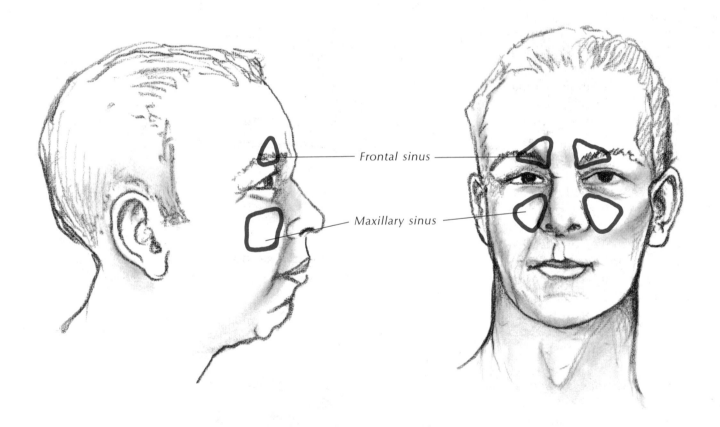

THE MOUTH AND THE PHARYNX

Structures in the mouth and pharynx are illustrated on page 157.

The dorsum of the tongue is covered by papillae, giving it a roughened surface. A thin white coating is frequent and normal. Often just visible toward the back of the tongue are the large vallate papillae. These should not be confused with tumor nodules.

Above and behind the tongue rises an arch formed by the anterior and posterior pillars, soft palate, and uvula. The tonsils can be seen in the fossae, or cavities, between the anterior and posterior pillars. In adults, however, the tonsils are often small or absent because of normal atrophy or surgical removal. The posterior pharynx may normally show small blood vessels and patches of lymphoid tissue on its surface.

The undersurface of the tongue is relatively smooth. At its base the ducts of the submaxillary gland (Wharton's ducts) pass forward to their openings near the midline. Each parotid duct (Stensen's duct) opens onto the buccal mucosa near the upper 2nd molar, where its location is frequently marked by a small papilla.

A full complement of 32 adult teeth (16 in each jaw) is identified here.

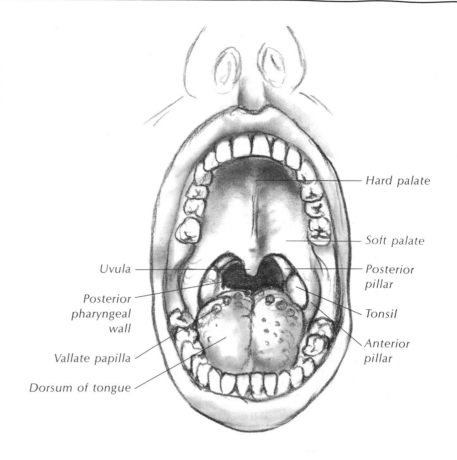

Hard palate

Soft palate

Uvula

Posterior pillar

Posterior pharyngeal wall

Tonsil

Anterior pillar

Vallate papilla

Dorsum of tongue

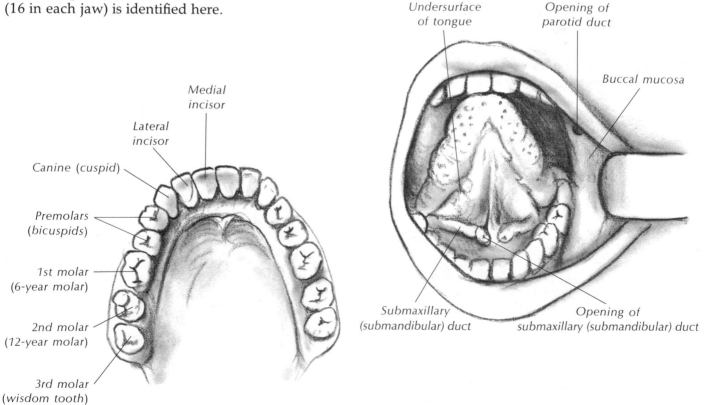

Medial incisor

Lateral incisor

Canine (cuspid)

Premolars (bicuspids)

1st molar (6-year molar)

2nd molar (12-year molar)

3rd molar (wisdom tooth)

Undersurface of tongue

Opening of parotid duct

Buccal mucosa

Submaxillary (submandibular) duct

Opening of submaxillary (submandibular) duct

THE NECK

For descriptive purposes each side of the neck is divided into two triangles by the sternomastoid muscle. The anterior triangle is bounded above by the mandible, laterally by the sternomastoid, and medially by the midline of the body. The posterior triangle extends from the sternomastoid to the trapezius and is bounded below by the clavicle. A portion of the omohyoid muscle crosses the lower portion of the posterior triangle and can be mistaken by the uninitiated for a lymph node or mass.

From above down identify the following midline structures: (1) the mobile hyoid bone just below the mandible, (2) the thyroid cartilage, readily identified by the notch on its superior edge, (3) the cricoid cartilage, (4) the tracheal rings, and (5) the softer thyroid isthmus which lies across the trachea below the cricoid. The lateral lobes of the thyroid curve posteriorly around the sides of the trachea and the esophagus. They are partially covered by the sternomastoid muscles. Women have larger and more easily palpable glands than do men.

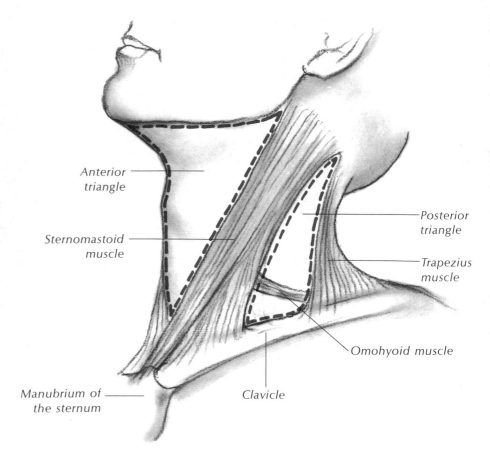

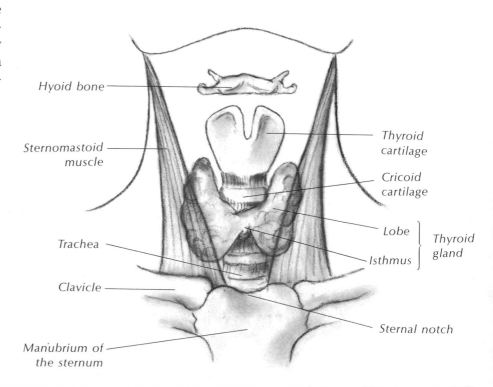

Deep to the sternomastoids run the great vessels of the neck: the carotid artery and internal jugular vein. The external jugular vein passes diagonally over the surface of the sternomastoid.

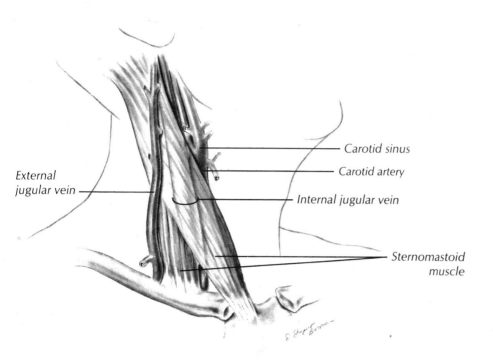

External jugular vein

Carotid sinus

Carotid artery

Internal jugular vein

Sternomastoid muscle

The lymph nodes of the head and neck have been classified in a variety of ways. One classification is shown here, together with the directions of lymphatic drainage. The deep cervical chain is largely obscured by the overlying sternomastoid muscle, but at its two extremes the tonsillar node and the supraclavicular nodes may be palpable. The submaxillary nodes lie superficial to the submaxillary gland, from which they should be differentiated. Nodes are normally round or ovoid, smooth, and smaller than the gland. The gland is larger and has a lobulated, slightly irregular surface.

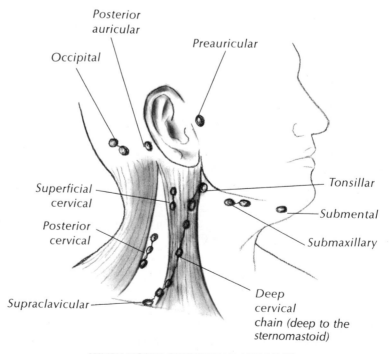

Posterior auricular

Preauricular

Occipital

Superficial cervical

Posterior cervical

Supraclavicular

Tonsillar

Submental

Submaxillary

Deep cervical chain (deep to the sternomastoid)

LYMPH NODES OF THE HEAD AND NECK

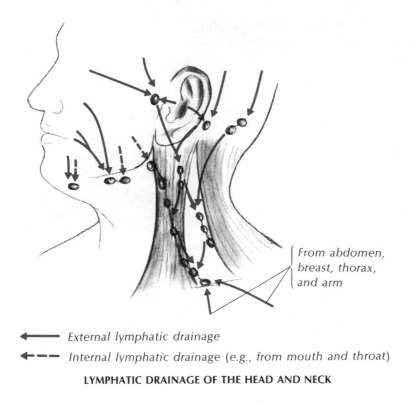

From abdomen, breast, thorax, and arm

⬅ *External lymphatic drainage*

⬅- - - *Internal lymphatic drainage (e.g., from mouth and throat)*

LYMPHATIC DRAINAGE OF THE HEAD AND NECK

Note that the tonsillar, submaxillary, and submental nodes drain portions of the mouth and throat as well as the more superficial tissues of the face. Knowledge of the lymphatic system is important to a sound clinical habit: whenever a malignant or inflammatory lesion is observed, look for involvement of the regional lymph nodes that drain it; whenever a node is enlarged or tender, look for a source in the area that it drains.

CHANGES WITH AGE

Several changes in the head and neck accompany adolescence. In boys the voice begins to deepen and the thyroid cartilage enlarges perceptibly during the adolescent growth spurt. Facial hair appears on the upper lip, then on the cheeks and the lower lip, and finally on the chin. The facial contours of both boys and girls change subtly as children turn into young adults. Lengthening of the eyeballs in their anteroposterior diameter may cause or accentuate myopia, or nearsightedness. The comedones (blackheads) and pustules of acne appear on the face so commonly that they are almost considered an adolescent norm. Lymphoid tissues, which grow rapidly in late childhood (see p. 525), are still relatively prominent in adolescents, and cervical lymph nodes are readily palpable in most teenagers. The frequency of palpable cervical nodes gradually diminishes with age and, according to one study, falls below 50% some time between the ages of 50 and 60. Tonsils, which are also composed of lymphoid tissue, become gradually smaller after the age of 5 years. In adulthood they become inconspicuous or invisible. In contrast to the lymph nodes, the submaxillary glands become easier to feel in older people.

The eyes, ears, and mouth bear the brunt of old age. Visual acuity remains fairly constant between the ages of 20 and 50 and then diminishes, gradually until about age 70 and more rapidly after that. Nevertheless most elderly people retain good to adequate vision — 20/20 to 20/70 as measured by standard charts. Near vision, however, begins to blur noticeably for virtually everyone. From childhood on, the lens gradually loses its elasticity and the eye grows progressively less able to focus on nearby objects. This loss of accommodative power, called presbyopia, usually becomes noticeable in one's 40s.

While aging alters function of the eyes it also alters structure. In some elderly people the fat that surrounds and cushions the eye within the bony orbit atrophies, allowing the eyeball to recede somewhat in the orbit. The skin of the eyelids becomes wrinkled, occasionally hanging in loose folds. Fat may push the fascia of the eyelids forward, creating soft bulges, especially in the lower lids and the inner third of the upper ones (p. 189). Combinations of a weakened levator palpebrae, relaxation of the skin, and increased weight of the upper eyelid may cause a senile ptosis. More important, the lower lid may fall outward away from the eyeball or turn inward onto it, resulting in ectropion and entropion respectively (p. 189). Because their eyes produce fewer lacrimal secretions, aging patients may complain of dryness of the eyes.

Corneal arcus, or arcus senilis, is common in elderly persons and in them has no clinical significance (p. 192). The corneas lose some of their luster. The pupils become smaller — a characteristic that makes it more difficult to examine the fundi of elderly people. The pupils may also become slightly irregular but should continue to respond to light and near effort. Except for possible impairment in upward gaze, extraocular movements should remain intact.

Lenses thicken and yellow with age, impairing the passage of light to the retinas, and elderly people need more light to read and do fine work. When the lens of an elderly person is examined with a flashlight it frequently looks gray, as if it were opaque, when in fact it permits good visual acuity and looks clear on ophthalmoscopic examination. Do not depend on your flashlight alone, therefore, to make a diagnosis of cataract — a true opacity of the lens (p. 192). Cataracts do become relatively common, however, affecting 1 out of 10 people in their 60s and 1 out of 3 in their 80s. Because the lens continues to grow over the years, it may push the iris forward, narrowing the angle between iris and cornea and increasing the risk of narrow-angle glaucoma (p. 169).

Ophthalmoscopic examination reveals fundi that have lost their youthful shine and light reflections. The arterioles look narrowed, paler, straighter, and less brilliant (p. 204). Drusen (colloid bodies) may be seen (p. 200). On a somewhat more anterior plane you may be able to see some vitreous floaters — degenerative changes that may cause annoying specks or webs in the field of vision. You may also find evidence of other more serious conditions that occur more often in elderly people than in younger ones: senile macular degeneration, glaucoma, retinal hemorrhages, or possibly retinal detachment.

Acuity of hearing, like that of vision, usually diminishes with age. Early losses, which start in young adulthood, involve primarily the high-pitched sounds beyond the range of human speech and have relatively little functional significance. Gradually, however, loss continues and begins to encroach on sounds in the middle and lower ranges. When a person fails to catch the upper tones of words while hearing the lower ones, words sound distorted and conversation is difficult to understand, especially in noisy environments. Hearing loss associated with aging, known as presbycusis, becomes increasingly evident after the approximate age of 50.

Diminished salivary secretions and a decreased sense of taste have been attributed to aging, but recent studies suggest that medications or various diseases probably account for most of these changes. Teeth may wear down or become abraded over time, or they may be lost to dental caries or other conditions (pp. 216–217). Periodontal disease is the chief cause of tooth loss in most adults (p. 216). If a person has no teeth the lower portion of the face looks small and sunken, with accentuated "purse-string" wrinkles radiating out from the mouth. Overclosure of the mouth may lead to maceration of the skin at the corners — angular stomatitis (p. 213). The bony ridges of the jaws that once surrounded the tooth sockets are gradually resorbed, especially in the lower jaw.

Techniques of Examination

THE HEAD

Because abnormalities covered by the hair are so easily missed, ask if the patient has noticed anything wrong with the scalp or hair. If a woman is wearing a wig, ask her to remove it.

Inspect and palpate:

THE HAIR. Note its quantity, distribution, pattern of loss if any, and texture. Identify nits (the eggs of lice) if present, differentiating them from dandruff.

Fine hair in hyperthyroidism; coarse hair in hypothyroidism. Tiny white ovoid nits adherent to hairs; loose white flakes of dandruff

THE SCALP. Part the hair in several places and look for scaliness, lumps, or other lesions.

Redness and scaling in seborrheic dermatitis, psoriasis

THE SKULL. Observe the general size and contour of the skull. Note any deformities, lumps, or tenderness. Familiarize yourself with the irregularities in a normal skull, such as those near the suture lines between the parietal and occipital bones.

Enlarged skull in hydrocephalus, Paget's disease of bone

THE FACE. Note the patient's facial expression and contours. Observe for asymmetry, involuntary movements, edema, and masses.

See Table 7-1, Selected Facies (p. 187).

THE SKIN. Observe the skin, noting its color, pigmentation, texture, thickness, hair distribution, and any lesions.

Acne in many adolescents. Hirsutism (excessive facial hair) in some women

THE EYES

TESTING VISION

Visual Acuity is a test of central vision. If possible use a Snellen eye chart and light it well. Position the patient 20 feet from the chart. Patients who use glasses other than reading glasses should wear them. Ask the patient to cover one eye with a card (to prevent peeking through the fingers) and to read the smallest line of print possible. Coaxing to attempt the next line may improve performance. A patient who cannot read the largest letter should be positioned closer to the chart and the distance from it noted. Determine the smallest line of print from which the patient can identify more than half the letters. Record the visual acuity designated at the side of this line, together with the use of glasses, if any. Visual acuity is expressed as a fraction (*e.g.,* 20/30), in which the numerator indicates the distance of the patient from the chart, the denominator the distance at which a normal eye can read the line of letters.

Vision of 20/200 means that the patient can read at 20 feet only very large letters, which a person with normal vision could read at 200 feet. The larger the denominator, the worse the vision. "20/40 corrected" means the patient could read the 40 line with glasses (a correction).

Testing near vision with a handheld card is especially useful with middle-aged and older people. Handheld cards also enable you to test visual acuity at the bedside. When the card is held at about 13 inches from the patient's eyes, the letters are equivalent in size to those on the larger 20-foot charts. You may, however, let patients choose their own distance. Patients who have reading glasses should wear them.

Presbyopia refers to the impaired near vision found in middle-aged and older people.

Both kinds of charts are available with numbers or with *E*s that face in different directions for people who cannot read letters.

If you have no charts, screen visual acuity with any available print. If patients cannot read even the largest letters, test their ability to count your upraised fingers and distinguish light (such as your flashlight) from dark.

Visual Fields by Confrontation is a rough clinical test of peripheral vision. This procedure is usually omitted in a routine examination but should be included whenever a neurologic problem is suspected. Because it is a rather crude method, it should be supplemented, if indicated, by special techniques such as perimetry or a tangent screen.

Poor peripheral vision can cause functional impairment even when visual acuity is normal.

Ask the patient to cover one eye, without pressing on it, and to look at your eye directly opposite. Close your other eye. Position yourself so that your face is directly in front of and level with the patient's.

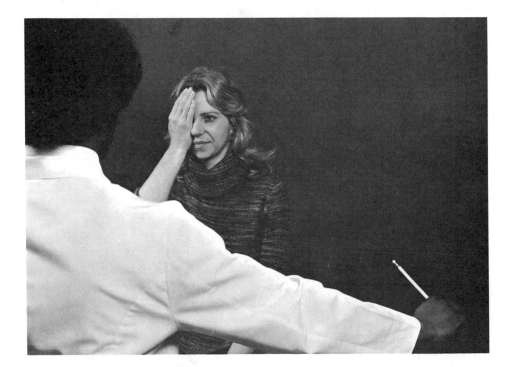

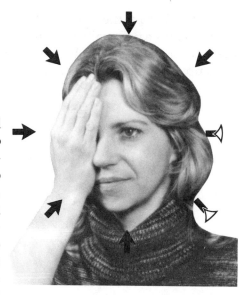

Slowly bring a pencil or other small test object from the periphery into the field of vision from the 8 directions shown, and ask the patient to say "now" as soon as it appears. During most of this examination keep the test object equidistant between your eye and the patient's so that you can compare the patient's visual field with your own. A normal person who is looking straight ahead, however, can see a moving object directly to one side (temporally) and also to the side and down (inferotemporally), even when the object is 90° or more from the line of vision. In order to assess peripheral vision in these two areas, therefore, you must first place your test object somewhat behind the patient, unavoidably within your own field.

Repeat with the other eye.

Visual fields are normally limited above by the brows, below by the cheeks, and medially by the nose. Variations in the prominence of these structures in relation to the eyes create minor variations in normal peripheral vision. These should be ignored. Visual fields are conventionally diagrammed from the patient's viewpoint.

Abnormalities detectable by confrontation may be diagrammed simply as follows:

Homonymous hemianopsia, a loss of vision on the same side of each field

A homonymous quadrantic defect

Bitemporal hemianopsia

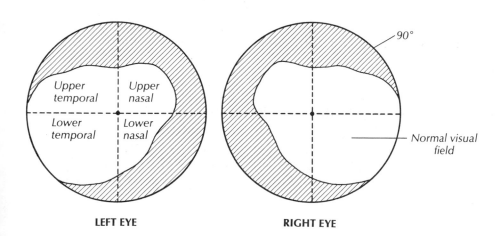

The central point of each circle indicates the focus of gaze; the circumference is 90° from this line of gaze as measured from the corneal surface.

See Table 7-2, Visual Field Defects Produced by Selected Lesions in the Visual Pathways (p. 188).

POSITION AND ALIGNMENT OF THE EYES. Survey the eyes for their position and alignment with each other. If you note unusually prominent eyes, especially on one side, inspect them from above. Stand behind the seated patient, draw the upper lids gently upward, and note the relationship of the corneas to the lower lids.

Exophthalmos refers to an abnormal protrusion of the eyeball. Bilateral exophthalmos suggests Graves' disease. Unilateral involvement suggests a tumor or inflammatory lesion of the orbit but may also be seen in Graves' disease.

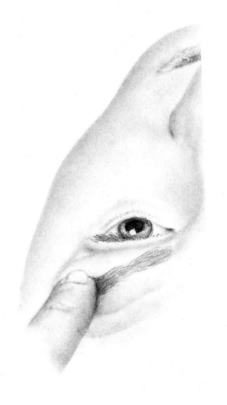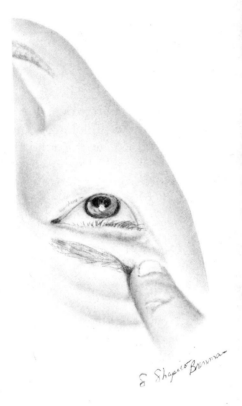

EYEBROWS. Inspect the eyebrows, noting their quantity and distribution and any scaliness of the underlying skin.

Scaliness in seborrheic dermatitis; loss of lateral 3rd in myxedema and in normal aging

EYELIDS. Note the position of the lids in relationship to the eyeballs. Inspect for:

Edema

Color (*e.g.,* redness)

Lesions

Condition and direction of the eyelashes

Adequacy with which the eyelids close. Look for this especially when the eyes are unusually prominent, when there is facial paralysis, or when the patient is unconscious.

See Table 7-3, Abnormalities of the Eyelids (p. 189). Blepharitis is an inflammation of the eyelids along the lid margins, often with crusting or scales.

Failure of the eyelids to close exposes the corneas to serious damage.

LACRIMAL APPARATUS. Briefly inspect the regions of the lacrimal gland and lacrimal sac for swelling.

See Table 7-4, Lumps and Swellings In and Around the Eyes (p. 190).

Look for excessive tearing or dryness of the eyes. The proper assessment of dryness may require special testing, as described in texts of ophthalmology.

Excessive tearing may be due to conjunctival or corneal inflammation, an ectropion, or obstruction of the drainage system.

Special Technique for Nasolacrimal Duct Obstruction. Ask the patient to look up. Press on the lower lid close to the medial canthus, just *inside* the rim of the bony orbit. You are thus compressing the lacrimal sac.

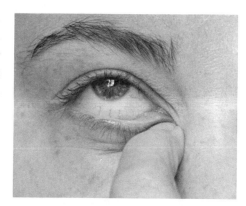

Look for fluid regurgitated out of the puncta into the eye. Avoid this test if the area is inflamed and tender.

Regurgitation of mucopurulent fluid from the puncta suggests an obstructed nasolacrimal duct.

CONJUNCTIVAS AND SCLERAS. Ask the patient to look up as you depress both lower lids with your thumbs, exposing the scleras and conjunctivas. Inspect the scleras and palpebral conjunctivas for color, and note the vascular pattern against the white scleral background. Look for any nodules or swelling.

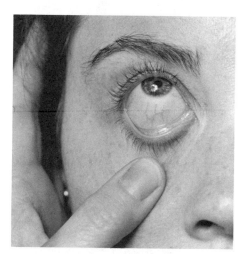

Apparently yellow scleras indicate jaundice. The pigment is actually in the overlying bulbar conjunctivas.

Pale palpebral conjunctivas of anemia

If you need a fuller view of the eye, rest your thumb and finger on the bones of the cheek and brow respectively and spread the lids.

Ask the patient to look to each side and down.

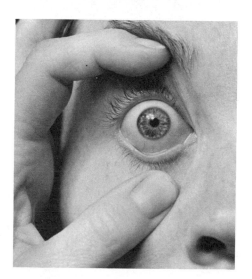

Increased number and size of visible vessels in inflammation and other disorders. See Table 7-5, Red Eyes (p. 191).

Special Technique for Inspection of the Upper Palpebral Conjunctiva. Adequate examination of the eye in search of a foreign body requires eversion of the upper eyelid. To do this:

1. Instruct the patient to look down.
2. Get the patient to relax the eyes—by reassurance and by gentle, assured, and deliberate movements.
3. Raise the upper eyelid slightly so that the eyelashes protrude, and then grasp the upper eyelashes and pull them gently down and forward.
4. Place a small stick such as an applicator or tongue blade at least 1 cm above the lid margin (and therefore at the upper border of the tarsal plate). Push down on the upper eyelid, thus everting it or turning it "inside out." Do not press on the eyeball itself.
5. Secure the upper lashes against the eyebrow with your fingers and inspect the palpebral conjunctiva.
6. After your inspection, grasp the upper eyelashes and pull them gently forward. Ask the patient to look up. The eyelid will return to its normal position.

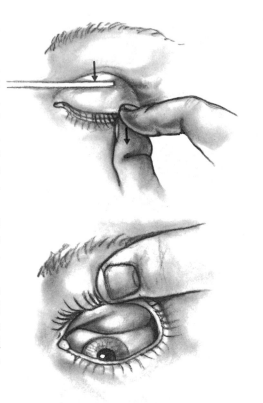

CORNEAS AND LENSES. With oblique lighting inspect the cornea of each eye for opacities and note any opacities in the lens that may be visible through the pupil.

See Table 7-6, Opacities of the Cornea and Lens (p. 192).

IRIDES. At the same time inspect the irides. The markings should be clearly defined. Now look for a crescentic shadow on the side away from your light. Since the iris normally forms a relatively open angle with the cornea, oblique lighting casts no shadow.

Occasionally the iris bows abnormally far forward, forming an unusually narrow angle with the cornea. The light then casts a crescentic shadow.

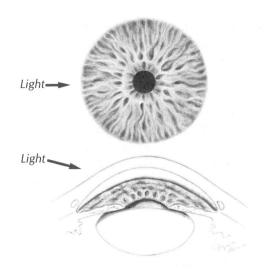

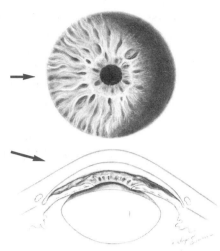

In the more common kind of glaucoma—open-angle glaucoma—the normal spatial relationship between iris and cornea is preserved and no shadow is cast.

This narrow angle increases the risk of acute narrow-angle (angle-closure) glaucoma—a sudden increase in intraocular pressure when drainage of aqueous humor is blocked.

PUPILS. Inspect the size, shape, and equality of the pupils. Slight inequality of the pupils (anisocoria) may be normal but must be carefully evaluated.

Miosis refers to constriction of the pupils, *mydriasis* to dilatation. See Table 7-7, Pupillary Abnormalities (pp. 193–194).

Test the *pupillary reaction to light.* Ask the patient to look into the distance, and shine a bright light obliquely into each pupil in turn. (Both the distant gaze and the oblique lighting help to prevent a near reaction.) Look for

1. The direct reaction (pupillary constriction in the same eye)
2. The consensual reaction (pupillary constriction in the opposite eye)

Always darken the room and use a bright light before deciding that a pupillary reaction is absent.

If the reaction to light is impaired or questionable, test the *near reaction.* Testing one eye at a time makes it easier to concentrate on pupillary responses, without the distraction of extraocular movement. Hold your finger or pencil about 10 cm from the patient's eye. Ask the patient to look alternately at it and into the distance directly behind it. Watch for pupillary constriction with near effort.

Testing the near reaction is helpful in diagnosing Argyll Robertson and tonic (Adie's) pupils. See p. 194.

EXTRAOCULAR MUSCLES. Look for weakness or imbalance of the extraocular muscles. From 2 or 3 feet directly in front of the patient shine a light onto the eyes and ask the patient to look at it. Observing from directly behind the light, inspect the reflections in the patient's corneas. They should be visible on or very slightly medial to the center of the pupils.

Asymmetry of the corneal reflections indicates a deviation from normal ocular alignment, which may be caused by muscle weakness. If you notice asym-

Then assess the extraocular movements. Ask the patient to follow your finger or pencil as you sweep through the six cardinal directions of gaze. Making a wide H in the air, lead the patient's gaze (1) to the patient's extreme right, (2) to the right and upward, and (3) down on the right; then (4) without pausing in the middle, to the extreme left, (5) to the left and upward, and (6) down on the left. Move your finger or pencil at a comfortable distance from the patient. Because middle-aged or older people may have difficulty focusing on near objects, it is helpful to make this distance greater for them than for young people. Pause during upward and lateral gaze to detect nystagmus. Some patients move their heads to follow your finger. If necessary, hold the head in the proper midline position.

metry or if a patient has complained of double vision or eyestrain, do a *cover test* (see p. 195). A cover test may bring out a latent muscle imbalance not otherwise seen.

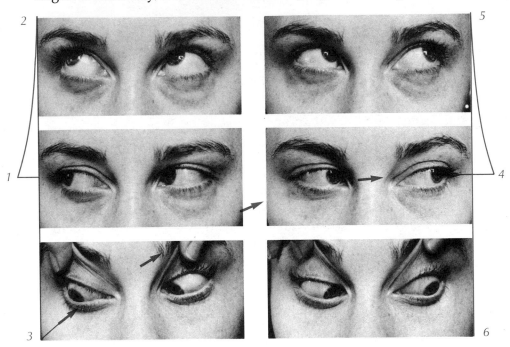

In paralysis of the left 6th nerve, illustrated below, the eyes are conjugate in right lateral gaze but not in left lateral gaze.

LOOKING RIGHT

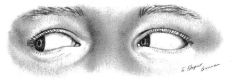

LOOKING LEFT

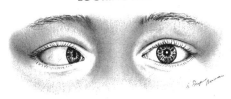

Inspect for

1. The normal conjugate, or parallel, movements of the eyes in each direction, or any deviation from normal

2. *Nystagmus*, a fine rhythmic oscillation of the eyes. A few beats of nystagmus on extreme lateral gaze are within normal limits. If you see it, bring your finger in to within the field of binocular vision and look again.

3. The relation of the upper eyelid to the globe as the eyes move from above downward. Normally the lid overlaps the iris slightly throughout this movement. If you suspect hyperthyroidism, ask the patient to follow your finger again as you move it slowly from up to down in the midline.

Finally, ask the patient to follow your finger or pencil as you move it in toward the bridge of the nose. Note convergence of the eyes. This is normally sustained to within 5 cm to 8 cm.

See Table 7-8, Deviations of the Eyes (p. 195).

Sustained nystagmus within the binocular field of gaze is seen in a variety of neurologic conditions. See Table 17-1, Nystagmus (pp. 512–513).

In the lid lag of hyperthyroidism a rim of sclera is seen between the upper lid and iris, and the lid appears to lag behind the globe.

Poor convergence in hyperthyroidism

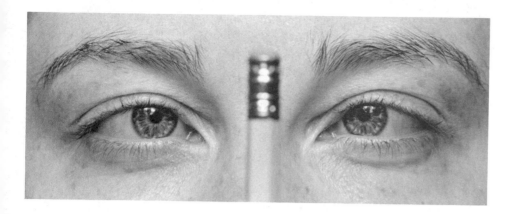

OPHTHALMOSCOPIC EXAMINATION. In general health care, you will usually examine your patients' eyes without dilating their pupils. Your view is therefore limited to the posterior structures illustrated on page 148. To see more peripheral structures, to evaluate the macula well, or to investigate unexplained visual loss, you will need to dilate the pupils unless there is a contraindication. Use an appropriate mydriatic drug such as tropicamide (Mydriacyl).

Contraindications for mydriatic drops include head injury and coma, where continuing observations of pupillary reactions are important, and any suspicion of narrow-angle glaucoma. Mydriatic drops cause temporary sensitivity to light and impairment of accommodation.

If you wear glasses for marked nearsightedness or severe astigmatism, leave them on. If patients have such refractive errors and you cannot focus clearly on their fundi, it may be easier to examine them with their glasses on. Patients with contact lenses may leave them in.

Darken the room. Switch on the ophthalmoscope light, and adjust it to the large round beam of white light.* Turn the lens disc to 0 diopters (a lens that neither converges nor diverges the light rays). Keep your index finger on the lens disc so that you can refocus the ophthalmoscope during the examination.

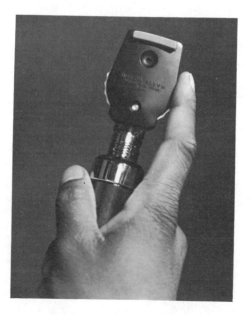

---

* Some clinicians like to use the large round beam for large pupils, the small round beam for small pupils. The other beams are rarely helpful. The slitlike beam is sometimes used to assess elevations or concavities in the retina, the green (or red-free) beam to detect small red lesions, and the grid to make measurements. Ignore the last three lights and practice with the large round white beam.

Use your *right hand* and *right eye* for the patient's *right eye*; your *left hand* and *left eye* for the patient's *left eye*. You thereby avoid facing your patient nose to nose, and your examination is closer, more mobile, and less intimate. Initially you will have difficulty using your nondominant eye, but persist. Hold your ophthalmoscope firmly braced up under the medial aspect of your bony orbit with its handle tilted laterally at about a 20° slant from the vertical. You should be able to see clearly through its aperture. Ask the patient to look slightly up and over your shoulder and gaze at a specific point on the wall.

From a position about 15 inches away from the patient and about 15° lateral to the patient's line of vision, shine the light beam on the pupil. Note the orange glow in the pupil—the *red reflex*. Also note any opacities interrupting the red reflex.

Absence of a red reflex suggests an opacity of the lens (cataract) or possibly of the vitreous. Less commonly, a detached retina may obscure this reflex. Do not be fooled by an artificial eye, which of course has no red reflex either.

Keeping the light beam focused on the red reflex, move in on the 15° line toward the pupil until your ophthalmoscope is very close to it, almost touching the patient's eyelashes. By placing the thumb of your other hand on the patient's eyebrow you gain extra proprioceptive guidance as you come closer to the patient, but this maneuver is not essential.

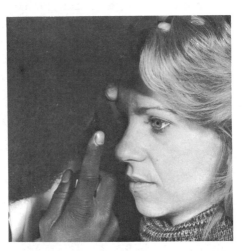

Try to keep both eyes open. Keep your eyes relaxed, as if gazing into the distance. You will thereby minimize the fluctuating blurriness caused by your automatic attempts to accommodate. Some patients find the light of modern ophthalmoscopes too bright. By lowering the light's intensity somewhat you can usually improve their comfort and cooperation without impairing your observations.

You should now be seeing the retina in the vicinity of the *optic disc*—a yellowish orange to creamy pink, oval or round structure. The disc will probably fill your field of gaze or even exceed it. If you do not see it, follow

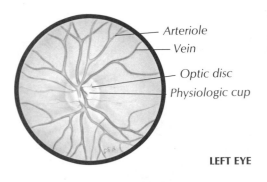

— Arteriole
— Vein
— Optic disc
Physiologic cup

LEFT EYE

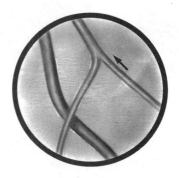

a blood vessel centrally until you do. You can tell which direction is central by noting the angles at which vessels branch and the progressive enlargement of vessel size at each junction as you approach the disc. Some trial and error may be necessary.

Now *bring the optic disc into sharp focus* by adjusting the lens disc. When examining a nearsighted (myopic) patient, whose eyeball is somewhat longer than normal, you will need to use a lens with a longer focus. To do this, rotate the lens disc counterclockwise to the lenses identified by the red numbers, indicating minus diopters.* When examining a farsighted patient or one whose own lens has been surgically removed, rotate the disc clockwise to the lenses of plus diopters, indicated by the black numbers. To illustrate these points:

When the lens has been surgically removed, its magnifying effect is lost. Retinal structures then look much smaller than usual, and you can see a much larger expanse of fundus.

When the patient's eye, as well as your own, is normal in size, you can usually focus clearly on the retina with a lens of 0 diopters (clear glass).

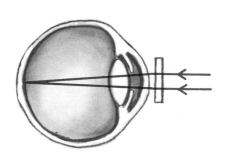

NORMAL EYE

When the patient is nearsighted, you will need a lens with a longer focus (minus diopters). When a nearsighted patient wears contact lenses, you do not need to make this adjustment.

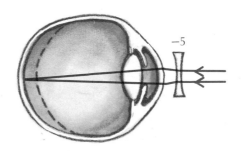

NEARSIGHTED EYE

In a nearsighted (myopic) eye, retinal structures are magnified more than usual. The disc exceeds the size of your view.

A lens with a shorter focus (*e.g.,* +1 or +2 diopters) is needed for farsighted eyes.

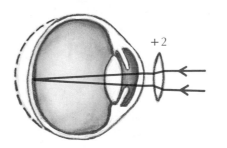

FARSIGHTED EYE

In a farsighted (hyperopic) eye, retinal structures look somewhat smaller than usual.

* A diopter is a unit which measures the power of a lens to converge or diverge light.

Note

1. The clarity of the disc outline. The nasal outline may normally be somewhat blurred.
2. The color of the disc, normally yellowish orange to creamy pink
3. The possible presence of normal white or pigmented rings or crescents around the disc
4. The size of the central physiologic cup, if present. This cup is normally yellowish white. Its horizontal diameter is usually less than half the horizontal diameter of the disc.

See Table 7-9, Normal Variations of the Optic Disc (p. 196).

See Table 7-10, Abnormalities of the Optic Disc (p. 197).

You may also see some pulsations of the veins as they cross the disc. Gentle pressure on the eye through the eyelid usually makes such pulsations evident even if you did not see them earlier. This maneuver is not, however, part of the routine examination.

The presence of venous pulsations at the disc gives some reassurance that cerebrospinal fluid pressure is normal, although exceptions occur.

Identify the *arterioles and veins.* They may be distinguished by the following features:

	ARTERIOLES	VEINS
COLOR	Light red	Dark red
SIZE	Smaller (⅔ to ⅘ the diameter of veins)	Larger
LIGHT REFLEX *(or reflection)*	Bright	Inconspicuous or absent

Follow the vessels peripherally in each of four directions, noting their relative sizes and the character of the arteriovenous crossings. Identify any lesions of the surrounding *retina* and note their size, shape, color, and distribution. As you search the retina, move your head and instrument as a unit, using the patient's pupil as an imaginary fulcrum. Until you gain experience, you may repeatedly lose your view of the retina because your light falls out of the pupil. You will improve with practice.

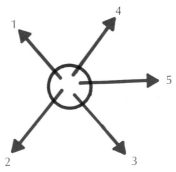

Sequence of inspection from disc to macula

LEFT EYE

See Table 7-11, Retinal Arterioles and Arteriovenous Crossings: Normal and Hypertensive (p. 198).

See Table 7-12, Red Spots and Streaks in the Fundi (p. 199).

See Table 7-13, Light-Colored Spots in the Fundi (pp. 200–201).

See Color Plate 1, Ocular Fundi (pp. 203–205).

Finally, by directing your light beam laterally or by asking the patient to look directly into the light, inspect the *macular area.* This is an avascular area somewhat larger than the disc but has no distinct margins. Except in older people the tiny bright reflection at its center — the fovea — helps to identify it. Shimmering light reflections in the macular area are common in young people.

The macular area is especially important because it is responsible for central vision. Senile macular degeneration is an important cause of impaired central vision in elderly people.

Visualizing the macula is unfortunately difficult. Unless you use a mydriatic, the patient's pupil constricts maximally; light reflections off the cornea may further obscure your view. Moving the ophthalmoscope slightly from side to side may help you get around the reflections.

It takes many forms, including hemorrhages, exudates, cysts, and "holes." A common form with altered pigmentation is illustrated here.

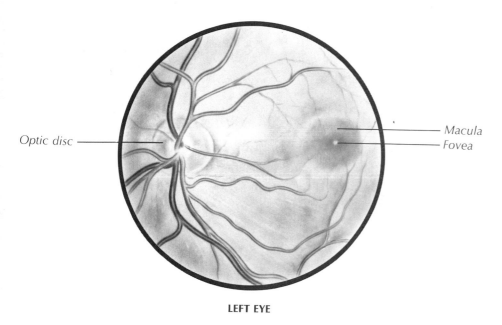

Optic disc

Macula
Fovea

LEFT EYE

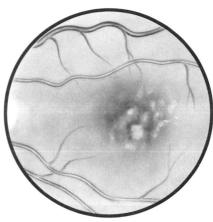

SENILE MACULAR DEGENERATION

If you suspect opacities in the *vitreous* or *lens,* inspect these normally transparent structures by rotating the lens disc progressively to diopters of around +10 or +12. This maneuver focuses on the anterior structures within the eyeball.

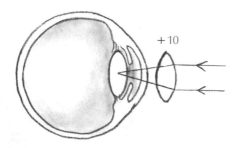

+10

ANTERIOR STRUCTURES

Vitreous floaters may be seen as dark specks or strands at levels between the fundus and the lens. Cataracts are more anterior and more homogeneous densities in the lens.

A NOTE ON MEASUREMENT WITHIN THE EYE. Lesions of the retina can be located in relationship to the optic disc and are measured in terms of "disc diameters" and diopters. For example, among the cotton wool patches illustrated on the right there is an irregular one between 1 and 2 o'clock, less than ½ disc diameter from the disc, and measuring about 1 × ½ disc diameters.

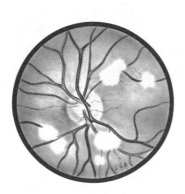

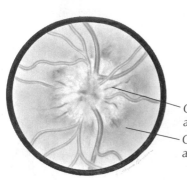

The elevated optic disc of papilledema can be measured by noting the differences in diopters of the two lenses used to focus clearly on the disc and on the uninvolved retina.

Clear focus here at +3 diopters
Clear focus here at −1 diopter

$+3 − (−1) = +4$, therefore a disc elevation of 4 diopters

FOR INTEREST. On ophthalmoscopic examination, the normal retina is magnified about 15 times, the normal iris about 4 times. The optic disc actually measures about 1.5 mm. At the retina, 3 diopters of elevation = 1 mm.

THE EARS

THE AURICLE. Inspect each auricle and surrounding tissues for deformities, lumps, or skin lesions.

See Table 7-14, Nodules In and Around the Ears (p. 209).

If ear pain, discharge, or inflammation is present, move the auricle up and down, press on the tragus, and press firmly just behind the ear.

Movement of the auricle and tragus is painful in acute otitis externa, but not in otitis media. Tenderness behind the ear may be present in otitis media.

EAR CANAL AND DRUM. For the otoscopic examination tip the patient's head to the opposite side. Grasp the auricle firmly but gently, while pulling it upward, back, and slightly out.

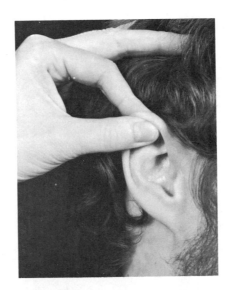

Insert into the canal, slightly down and forward, the largest ear speculum that the canal will accommodate. Two grips are illustrated. In the second, which is usually preferable, your hand is braced against the patient's head

Nontender nodular swellings covered by normal skin deep in the ear canals suggest osteomas.

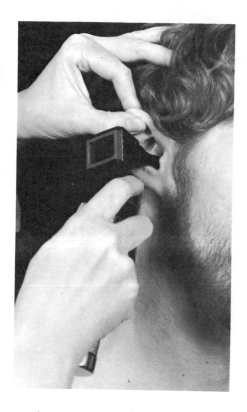

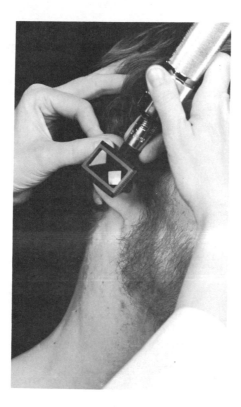

so that unexpected movements are less likely to injure the ear canal.

Identify any discharge or foreign bodies in the ear canal and note any redness or swelling. Cerumen, which varies in color and consistency from yellow and flaky to brown and sticky or even to dark and hard, may wholly or partly obscure your view.

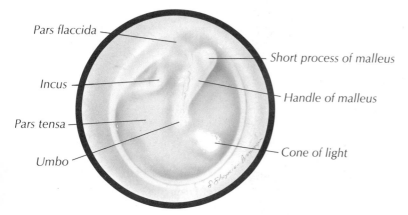

Pars flaccida

Short process of malleus

Incus

Handle of malleus

Pars tensa

Umbo

Cone of light

(*After Hawke M, Keene M, Alberti PW: Clinical Otoscopy: A Text and Colour Atlas. Edinburgh, Churchill Livingstone, 1984*)

Inspect the eardrum, noting its color and contour.

These are nonmalignant overgrowths, which may obscure the drum.

In acute otitis externa the canal is often swollen, narrowed, moist, pale, and tender, as shown below. It may be reddened.

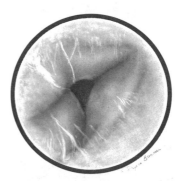

In chronic otitis externa the skin of the canal is often thickened, red, and itchy.

Red bulging drum of acute purulent otitis media, amber drum of a serous effusion

Identify the handle of the malleus, note its position, and inspect the short process. Find the cone of light.

Gently move the speculum so that you can see as much of the drum as possible, including the pars flaccida superiorly and the margins of the pars tensa. Look for any perforations. The anterior and inferior margins of the drum may not be visible.

Mobility of the eardrum can be evaluated with a pneumatic otoscope. See page 566.

AUDITORY ACUITY. To estimate hearing, test one ear at a time. Ask the patient to occlude one ear with a finger or, better still, occlude it yourself. When auditory acuity on the two sides is different, move your finger rapidly, but gently, in the patient's ear canal. The noise so produced will help to prevent the occluded ear from doing the work of the ear you wish to test. Then, standing 1 or 2 feet away, exhale fully (so as to minimize the intensity of your voice) and whisper softly toward the unoccluded ear. Choose numbers or other words with two equally accented syllables, such as "nine-four," or "baseball." If necessary, increase the intensity of your voice to a medium whisper, a loud whisper, and then a soft, medium, and loud voice. To make sure the patient does not read your lips, cover your mouth or obstruct the patient's vision.

If hearing is diminished, try to distinguish between conduction and sensorineural hearing loss. You need a quiet room and a tuning fork of 512 Hz, preferably, or possibly 1024 Hz. These frequencies fall within the range of human speech (300 Hz – 3000 Hz) — the functionally most important range. Forks with lower pitches may cause you to overestimate bone conduction and may also be felt as vibration in addition to being heard. Set the fork into *light* vibration by stroking it between thumb and index finger or by tapping it on your knuckles.

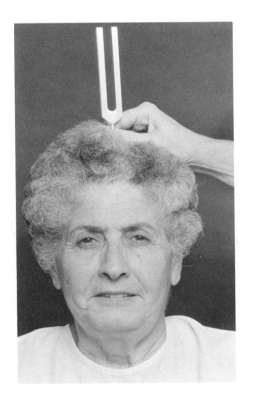

1. *Test for lateralization (Weber test).* Place the base of the lightly vibrating tuning fork firmly on top of the patient's head or on the midforehead. Ask where the patient hears it: on one or both sides. Normally the sound is heard in the midline or equally in both ears. If nothing is heard, try again, pressing the fork more firmly on the head.

An unusually prominent short process and a prominent handle that looks foreshortened suggest a retracted drum.

See Color Plate 2, Abnormalities of the Eardrum (pp. 206 – 207).

A serous effusion, a thickened drum, or purulent otitis media may decrease mobility.

In unilateral conduction hearing loss, sound is heard in, or lateralized to, the impaired ear. In unilateral sensorineural hearing loss, sound is heard in the good ear.

2. *Compare air (AC) and bone conduction (BC) (Rinne test).* Place the base of a lightly vibrating tuning fork on the mastoid bone, behind the ear and level with the canal. When the patient can no longer hear the sound, quickly place the fork close to the ear canal and ascertain whether the sound can be heard again. Here the "U" of the fork should face forward, thus maximizing its sound for the patient. Normally the sound is heard longer through air than through bone (AC > BC).

In conduction hearing loss, sound is heard through bone as long as or longer than it is through air (a negative Rinne test). In sensorineural hearing loss, sound is heard longer through air (the normal pattern and a positive Rinne test). See Table 7-15, Patterns of Hearing Loss (pp. 210–211).

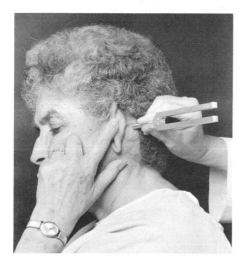
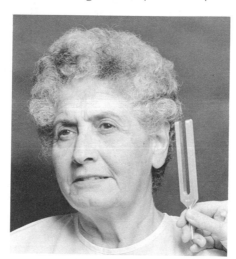

THE NOSE AND PARANASAL SINUSES

Inspect the external surface of the nose, noting any asymmetry, deformity, or inflammation.

To inspect the inside of the nose use an otoscope, preferably equipped with a short, wide nasal speculum and a magnifying lens. Tilt the patient's head back a bit and insert the speculum gently into the vestibule of each nostril, avoiding contact with the sensitive nasal septum. Hold the oto-

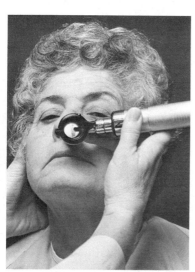
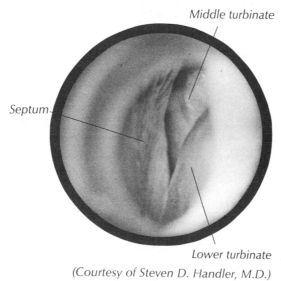

Middle turbinate

Septum

Lower turbinate

(Courtesy of Steven D. Handler, M.D.)

scope handle to one side to avoid the patient's chin and improve your mobility. By directing the speculum posteriorly, then somewhat upward, try to see both the lower and the upper portions of the nose. The passage itself is narrow and slitlike. Some asymmetry of the two sides is normal.

Inspect:

1. The nasal mucosa, including its color (normally somewhat redder than the oral mucosa). Look for swelling, exudate, and bleeding.

   Red swollen mucosa of acute rhinitis; pale mucosa of allergic rhinitis. See Table 7-16, Common Abnormalities of the Nose (p. 212).

2. The nasal septum, including evidence of bleeding, crusting, perforation, or deviation. Deviation of the nasal septum is common.

   The lower anterior portion of the septum (where the patient's finger can reach) is a common source of epistaxis (nosebleed).

3. The inferior and middle turbinates and the middle meatus between them for color, swelling, exudate, and polyps. Your view is limited to the anterior surfaces of these two turbinates.

   Causes of septal perforation include trauma, surgery, and the intranasal use of cocaine or amphetamines.

Make it a habit to place all nasal and ear specula outside your instrument case after using them. Then wash them thoroughly when you wash your hands after the physical examination. If a speculum (or other instrument) becomes contaminated with blood, it should be discarded, sterilized, or appropriately disinfected.

PALPATE THE SINUSES. Palpate for *frontal sinus tenderness* by pressing up from under the bony brow on each side. Avoid pressure on the eyes. Then press up on each *maxillary sinus*.

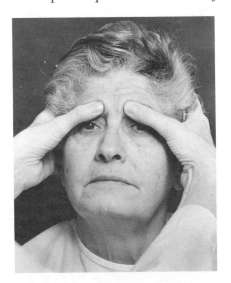 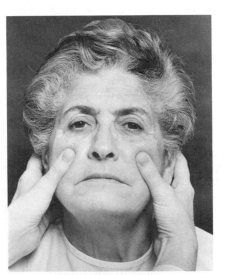

Local tenderness, together with symptoms such as pain, fever, and nasal discharge, suggests acute sinusitis involving the frontal or maxillary sinuses.

TRANSILLUMINATION OF THE SINUSES. Although transillumination is not routine, it is often helpful when sinus tenderness or other symptoms suggest sinusitis. The room should be thoroughly darkened. Using a

Absence of glow on one or both sides suggests a thickened mucosa or secretions in the

strong, narrow light source, place the light snugly deep under each brow, close to the nose. Shield the light with your hand. Look for a dim red glow as light is transmitted through the air-filled frontal sinus to the forehead.

frontal sinus, but it may also result from developmental absence of one or both sinuses.

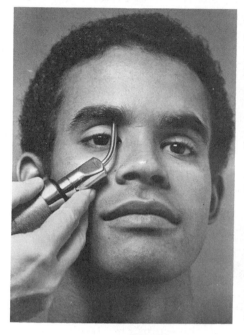
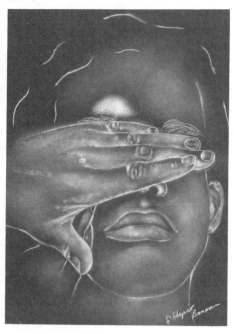

TRANSILLUMINATION OF FRONTAL SINUS

Ask the patient to open the mouth wide and tilt the head back. (An upper denture should first be removed.) Shine the light downward from just below the inner aspect of each eye. Look through the open mouth at the hard palate. A reddish glow indicates a normal air-filled maxillary sinus.

Absence of glow suggests thickened mucosa or secretions in the maxillary sinus. See page 570 for an alternative method of transilluminating the maxillary sinuses.

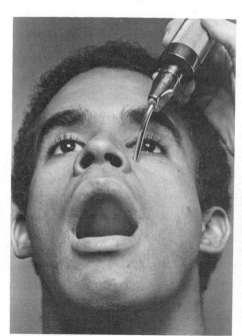
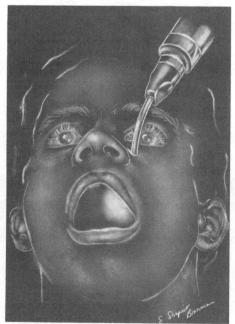

TRANSILLUMINATION OF MAXILLARY SINUS

THE MOUTH AND THE PHARYNX

If the patient wears dentures, offer a paper towel and ask the patient to remove them so that you can see the mucosa underneath. If suspicious ulcers or nodules are observed, put on a glove or finger cot and palpate the lesion, noting especially any thickening or infiltration of the tissues that might suggest malignancy.

Bright red edematous mucosa underneath a denture suggests denture sore mouth. There may be ulcers or papillary granulation tissue.

Inspect:

THE LIPS. Look for color, moisture, lumps, ulcers, or cracking.

Cyanosis, pallor. See Table 7-17, Abnormalities of the Lips (pp. 213–214).

THE BUCCAL MUCOSA. Ask the patient to open the mouth. With a good light and the help of a tongue blade inspect the buccal mucosa for color, pigmentation, ulcers, and nodules. Patchy pigmentation is normal in black people.

See Table 7-18, Abnormalities of the Buccal Mucosa and Hard Palate (p. 215).

THE GUMS AND TEETH. Look for

1. Inflammation, swelling, bleeding, retraction, or discoloration of the gums
2. Loose, missing, or carious teeth and any abnormalities in the position or shape of the teeth

See Table 7-19, Abnormalities of the Gums and Teeth (pp. 216–217).

THE ROOF OF THE MOUTH. Inspect the color and architecture of the hard palate.

Torus palatinus, a midline lump (see p. 215)

THE TONGUE. Inspect the dorsum of the tongue, including its color and papillae. Note any abnormal smoothness.

See Table 7-20, Abnormalities of the Tongue (p. 218).

Ask the patient to put out the tongue, and inspect it for symmetry—a test of the 12th (hypoglossal) cranial nerve. Note its size.

Asymmetrical protrusion in a 12th nerve lesion and in cancer of the tongue; enlargement in myxedema and acromegaly

Inspect the sides and the under surface of the tongue together with the floor of the mouth. These are the areas where malignancies are most likely to develop. Note any white or reddened areas, nodules, or ulcerations. Since cancer of the tongue is more common in men over age 50, especially in those who use tobacco and drink alcohol, a further maneuver is indicated for patients in this group. Explain what you plan to do and put on gloves. Ask the patient to protrude the tongue. With your right hand grasp the tip of the tongue with a square of gauze and gently pull it to the patient's left. Inspect the side of the tongue, and then palpate it with your gloved left hand, feeling for any induration. Reverse the procedure for the other side.

Cancer of the tongue is the second most common cancer of the mouth, second only to cancer of the lip. Any persistent nodule or ulcer, either red or white, must be suspect. Induration of the lesion further increases the possibility of malignancy. Cancer occurs most frequently on the side of the tongue, and next most often at its base.

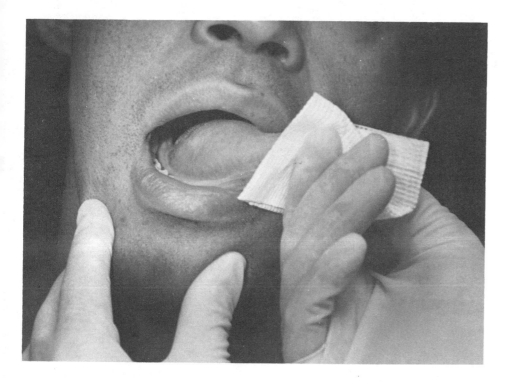

More common are tori mandibulares—innocuous bony nodules inside the lower jaw of some adults. At first small, tori may grow quite large, as shown below.

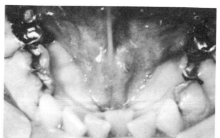

Palpate any other lesions you may have noticed in the mouth.

THE PHARYNX. Again ask the patient to open the mouth, this time without protruding the tongue. Press a tongue blade firmly down upon the midpoint of the arched tongue—far enough back to get good visualization of the pharynx but not so far that you cause gagging. Simultaneously ask the patient to say "ah" or to yawn. Note the rise of the soft palate—a test of the 10th cranial (vagus) nerve.

See Table 7-21, Abnormalities of the Pharynx (p. 219).

Inspect the soft palate, anterior and posterior pillars, uvula, tonsils, and posterior pharynx. Note their color and symmetry and any evidence of exudate, edema or ulceration, or tonsillar enlargement. If possible, palpate any suspicious area for induration or tenderness. Tonsils have crypts, or deep infoldings of squamous epithelium. Whitish spots of normal exfoliating epithelium may sometimes be seen in these crypts.

White patches of exudate associated with redness and swelling, however, suggest acute exudative pharyngitis.

Break or discard your tongue blade after use.

THE NECK

INSPECT THE NECK. Note symmetry, masses, and scars. Look for enlargement of the parotid or submaxillary glands, and note any visible lymph nodes.

A scar of past thyroid surgery may be the clue to unsuspected hypothyroidism.

LYMPH NODES. Palpate the lymph nodes. Using the pads of your index and middle fingers, move the skin over the underlying tissues in each area rather than moving your fingers over the skin. The patient should be relaxed, with the neck flexed slightly forward and, if needed, slightly toward the side of the examination. You can usually examine both sides at once. For the submental node, however, it is helpful to feel with one hand while bracing the top of the head with the other.

Feel in sequence for the following nodes:

1. Pre-auricular—in front of the ear
2. Posterior auricular — superficial to the mastoid process
3. Occipital—at the base of the skull posteriorly
4. Tonsillar—at the angle of the mandible
5. Submaxillary — midway between the angle and the tip of the mandible. These nodes are usually smaller and smoother than the lobulated submaxillary gland against which they lie.
6. Submental — in the midline behind the tip of the mandible
7. Superficial cervical—superficial to the sternomastoid
8. Posterior cervical chain — along the anterior edge of the trapezius
9. Deep cervical chain—deep to the sternomastoid and often inaccessible to examination. Hook your thumb and fingers around either side of the sternomastoid muscle to find them.
10. Supraclavicular—deep in the angle formed by the clavicle and the sternomastoid

A "tonsillar node" that pulsates is really the carotid artery.

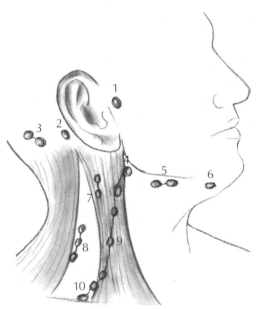

Enlargement of a supraclavicular node, especially on the left, suggests possible metastasis from a thoracic or abdominal malignancy.

Note their size, shape, delimitation (discrete or matted together), mobility, consistency, and any tenderness. Small, mobile, discrete, nontender nodes are frequently found in normal persons.

Tender nodes suggest inflammation; hard or fixed nodes suggest malignancy.

Enlarged or tender nodes, if unexplained, call for (1) reexamination of the regions they drain, and (2) careful assessment of lymph nodes elsewhere. Try to distinguish between regional and generalized lymphadenopathy.

Occasionally you may mistake a band of muscle or an artery for a lymph node. You should be able to roll a node in two directions: up and down, and side to side. Neither a muscle nor an artery will pass this test.

TRACHEA AND THYROID. Identify the thyroid and cricoid cartilages and the trachea below them. (The hyoid bone, high in the neck, should not be mistaken for a stony hard tumor.)

Inspect the trachea for any deviation from its usual midline position. Then feel for any deviation. Place your finger along one side of the trachea and note the space between it and the sternomastoid. Compare it with the other side. The spaces should be symmetrical.

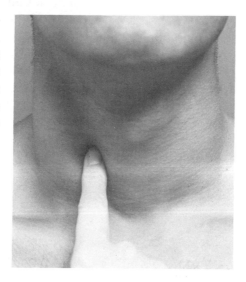

Masses in the neck or mediastinum may push the trachea to one side. Tracheal deviation may also signify important problems in the thorax, such as atelectasis or a large pneumothorax (see p. 252).

Inspect the neck for the thyroid gland. Ask the patient to bend the head back a bit. Inspect the region below the cricoid cartilage for the thyroid gland. Then ask the patient to take a sip from a glass of water, again extend the neck somewhat, and swallow. Watch for movement of the thyroid gland, noting its contour and symmetry.

An enlarged thyroid gland, and also many normal ones, may be visible even before swallowing. An enlarged thyroid gland is called a *goiter.*

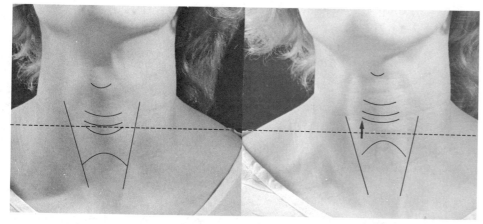

AT REST   SWALLOWING

The thyroid gland, the thyroid cartilage, and the cricoid cartilage all normally rise as the person swallows.

Now *palpate the thyroid gland.* Although there are many methods of performing this examination, palpation is probably best done from behind the patient. Because you cannot see what you are doing, you may initially find this position awkward. Orient yourself first to the patient's cricoid cartilage—the basic landmark for the examination. Feeling any visible thyroid tissue from in front of the patient first may also give you guidance.

From behind, place the fingers of both hands on the patient's neck so that the index fingers are just below the cricoid. The patient's neck should be extended, but not far enough to tighten the muscles. Adjust the degree of extension as you find necessary. As the patient swallows the thyroid isthmus should rise under your fingers. By rotating your fingers slightly downward and laterally, feel as much of the lateral lobes as possible, including their lower borders. During both maneuvers the patient should sip water as necessary to swallow as you repeat your palpation.

Although physical characteristics of the thyroid gland, such as size, shape, and consistency, are diagnostically important, they tell you little if anything about thyroid function. Assessment of thyroid function depends upon symptoms, signs elsewhere in the body, and laboratory tests. See Table 7-22, Thyroid Enlargement and Function (p. 220).

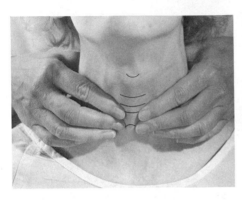

FEELING THE ISTHMUS

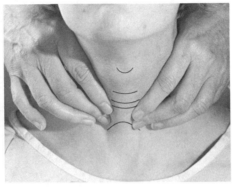

FEELING THE LATERAL LOBES

Note the size, shape, and consistency of the gland and identify any nodules or tenderness. The anterior surface of a lateral lobe is approximately the same size as the distal phalanx of the thumb; its consistency is somewhat rubbery.

The thyroid gland is usually easier to feel in a long slender neck than in a short stocky one. In the latter, further extension of the neck may help. In some persons, however, the thyroid gland is partially or wholly substernal.

If the thyroid gland is enlarged, listen over the lateral lobes with a stethoscope to detect a *bruit* (a sound similar to a cardiac murmur but of noncardiac origin).

A localized systolic or continuous bruit may be heard in hyperthyroidism.

THE CAROTID ARTERIES AND JUGULAR VEINS. You will probably wish to defer detailed examination of the great vessels of the neck until the patient lies down for the cardiovascular examination. Jugular venous distention, however, may be visible in the sitting position and should not be overlooked. You should also be alert to unusually prominent arterial pulsations. See Chapter 11 for further discussion.

Table 7-1

Table 7-1 Selected Facies

ACROMEGALY

The increased growth hormone of acromegaly produces enlargement of both bone and soft tissues. The head is elongated, with bony prominence of the forehead, nose, and lower jaw. Soft tissues of the nose, lips, and ears also enlarge. The facial features appear generally coarsened.

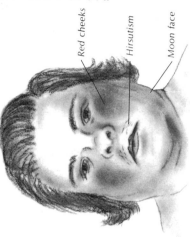

Brow prominent

Soft tissues of nose, ears, lips enlarged

Jaw prominent

CUSHING'S SYNDROME

The increased adrenal hormone production of Cushing's syndrome produces a round or "moon" face with red cheeks. Excessive hair growth may be present in the mustache and sideburn areas and on the chin.

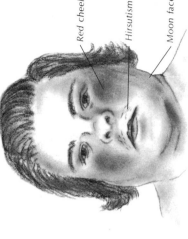

Red cheeks

Hirsutism

Moon face

MYXEDEMA

The patient with severe hypothyroidism, or myxedema, presents with a dull puffy facies. The edema, often particularly pronounced around the eyes, does not pit with pressure. The hair and eyebrows are dry, coarse, and thinned. The skin is dry.

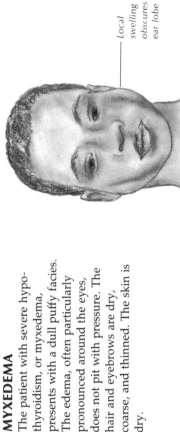

Hair dry, coarse, sparse

Lateral eyebrows thin

Periorbital edema

Puffy dull face with dry skin

PAROTID GLAND ENLARGEMENT

Chronic bilateral asymptomatic parotid gland enlargement may be associated with obesity, diabetes, cirrhosis, and other conditions. Note the swellings anterior to the ear lobes and above the angles of the jaw. Gradual unilateral enlargement suggests neoplasm. Acute enlargement is seen in mumps.

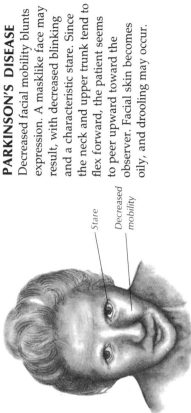

Local swelling obscures ear lobe

NEPHROTIC SYNDROME

The face is edematous and often pale. Swelling usually appears first around the eyes. The eyes may become slitlike when edema is severe.

Periorbital edema

Puffy pale face

Lips may be swollen

PARKINSON'S DISEASE

Decreased facial mobility blunts expression. A masklike face may result, with decreased blinking and a characteristic stare. Since the neck and upper trunk tend to flex forward, the patient seems to peer upward toward the observer. Facial skin becomes oily, and drooling may occur.

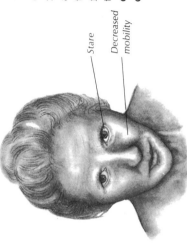

Stare

Decreased mobility

Table 7-2

Table 7-2 Visual Field Defects Produced by Selected Lesions in the Visual Pathways

BLACKENED FIELD INDICATES AREA OF NO VISION

VISUAL FIELDS

BLIND RIGHT EYE *(right optic nerve)*
A lesion of the optic nerve, and of course of the eye itself, produces unilateral blindness.

BITEMPORAL HEMIANOPSIA *(optic chiasm)*
A lesion at the optic chiasm may involve only the fibers that are crossing over to the opposite side. Since these fibers originate in the nasal half of each retina, visual loss involves the temporal half of each field.

LEFT HOMONYMOUS HEMIANOPSIA *(right optic tract)*
A lesion of the optic tract interrupts fibers originating on the same side of both eyes. Visual loss in the eyes is therefore similar (homonymous) and involves half of each field (hemianopsia).

HOMONYMOUS LEFT UPPER QUADRANTIC DEFECT *(optic radiation, partial)*
A partial lesion of the optic radiation may involve only a portion of the nerve fibers, producing, for example, a homonymous quadrantic defect.

LEFT HOMONYMOUS HEMIANOPSIA *(right optic radiation)*
A complete interruption of fibers in the optic radiation produces a visual defect similar to that produced by a lesion of the optic tract.

VISUAL PATHWAYS

LEFT VISUAL FIELD   RIGHT VISUAL FIELD

Temporal   Nasal   Temporal

Right eye

Left eye

Optic nerve

Optic tract

Optic radiation

RIGHT   LEFT

Table 7-3

Table 7-3   Abnormalities of the Eyelids

PTOSIS

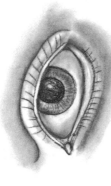

Ptosis refers to drooping of the upper eyelid. Causes include (1) muscular weakness, as in myasthenia gravis, (2) damage to the oculomotor nerve, which controls voluntary elevation of the eyelid, and (3) interference with the sympathetic nerves, which maintain smooth muscle tone of the lid (Horner's syndrome). A weakened muscle, relaxed tissues, and the weight of herniated fat may cause senile ptosis.

RETRACTION OR SPASM OF THE UPPER EYELID AND EXOPHTHALMOS

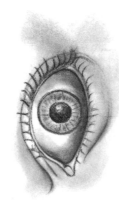

A retracted upper lid is identified by the rim of sclera between lid and iris. The eye has a stare, which is often accentuated by decreased blinking. Look for the associated lid lag when the eye moves slowly from upward to downward gaze. These signs suggest hyperthyroidism. They may simulate or accentuate exophthalmos — an actual forward protrusion of the eyeball (see p. 166).

ECTROPION

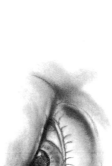

In ectropion the margin of the lid is turned outward, exposing the palpebral conjunctiva. When the punctum of the lower lid turns outward, the eye no longer drains satisfactorily and tearing occurs. Ectropion is more common in the elderly.

ENTROPION

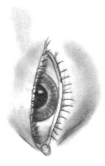

Entropion, also more common in the elderly, is an inward turning of the lid margin. The lower lashes, which are often invisible because they are turned inward, irritate the conjunctiva and lower cornea. Asking the patient to squeeze the lids together and then open them helps to demonstrate the problem when it is not obvious.

PERIORBITAL EDEMA

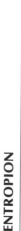

Since the skin of the eyelids is loosely attached to underlying tissues, edema tends to accumulate here more easily than elsewhere. Causes are many. Consider allergies, local inflammation, myxedema, fluid-retaining states such as the nephrotic syndrome, and finally, of course, recent crying.

HERNIATED FAT

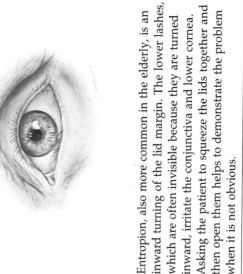

Puffy eyelids can be caused by fat as well as fluid. Fat pushes weakened fascia in the eyelids forward, producing bulges that involve the lower lids, the inner third of the upper ones, or both. Although these bulges appear more often in elderly people, they may also affect younger ones.

Table 7-4

Table 7-4   Lumps and Swellings In and Around the Eyes

PINGUECULA

A yellowish triangular nodule in the bulbar conjunctiva on either side of the iris, a pinguecula is harmless. Pingueculae appear almost uniformly with aging, first on the nasal and then on the temporal side.

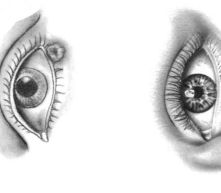

BASAL CELL EPITHELIOMA

A slowly progressive skin cancer, a basal cell epithelioma near the eye usually involves the lower lid. It appears as a papule with a pearly border and a depressed or ulcerated center.

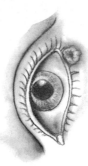

STY (Acute Hordeolum)

A painful, tender, red infection around a hair follicle of the eyelashes, a sty looks like a pimple or boil pointing on the lid margin.

INFLAMMATION OF THE LACRIMAL SAC (Dacryocystitis)

A swelling between the lower eyelid and nose suggests inflammation of the lacrimal sac. It may be acute or chronic. An *acute* inflammation is painful, red, and tender and may have a surrounding cellulitis. *Chronic* inflammation (illustrated) is associated with obstruction of the nasolacrimal duct. Tearing is prominent and pressure on the sac produces regurgitation of material through the puncta of the eyelids.

CHALAZION

A chalazion is a chronic inflammatory lesion involving a meibomian gland. A beady nodule in an otherwise normal lid, it is usually painless. Occasionally a chalazion becomes acutely inflamed but, unlike a sty, usually points inside the lid rather than on the lid margin.

ENLARGEMENT OF THE LACRIMAL GLAND

An enlarged lacrimal gland may displace the eyeball downward, nasally, and forward. A swelling is sometimes visible above the lateral third of the upper lid, giving the lid margin an S-shaped curve. Look for the enlarged gland by raising the temporal part of the upper eyelid as the patient looks down and medially. Causes of lacrimal gland enlargement include inflammation and tumors.

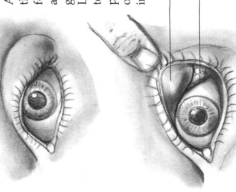

— Tarsal plate and conjunctiva

— Lacrimal gland

XANTHELASMA

Slightly raised, yellowish, well-circumscribed plaques in the skin, xanthelasmas appear along the nasal portions of one or both eyelids. They may accompany lipid disorders (*e.g.,* hypercholesterolemia), but may also occur in normal persons.

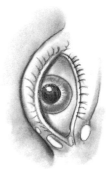
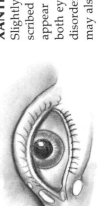
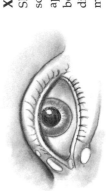

Table 7-5

Table 7-5 · Red Eyes

	CONJUNCTIVITIS	CORNEAL INJURY OR INFECTION	ACUTE IRITIS	ACUTE GLAUCOMA	SUBCONJUNCTIVAL HEMORRHAGE
PATTERN OF REDNESS	Conjunctival injection: diffuse dilatation of conjunctival vessels with redness that tends to be maximal peripherally	Ciliary injection: dilatation of deeper vessels that are visible as radiating vessels or a reddish violet flush around the limbus. Ciliary injection is an important sign of these three conditions but may not be apparent. The eye may be diffusely red instead. Other clues of these more serious disorders are pain, decreased vision, unequal pupils, and a less than perfectly clear cornea.			Leakage of blood outside of the vessels producing a homogeneous, sharply demarcated, red area that fades over days to yellow and then disappears
PAIN	Mild discomfort rather than pain	Moderate to severe, superficial	Moderate, aching, deep	Severe, aching, deep	Absent
VISION	Not affected except for temporary mild blurring due to discharge	Usually decreased	Decreased	Decreased	Not affected
OCULAR DISCHARGE	Watery, mucoid, or mucopurulent	Watery or purulent	Absent	Absent	Absent
PUPIL	Not affected	Not affected unless iritis develops	Small, and with time often irregular	Dilated	Not affected
CORNEA	Clear	Changes depending on cause	Clear or slightly clouded	Steamy, cloudy	Clear
SIGNIFICANCE	Bacterial, viral, and other infections; allergy; irritation	Abrasions and other injuries; viral and bacterial infections	Associated with many ocular and systemic disorders	Acute increase in intraocular pressure—an emergency	Often none. May result from trauma; bleeding disorders, or a sudden increase in venous pressure, as from cough.

Table 7-6

Table 7-6   Opacities of the Cornea and Lens

CORNEAL ARCUS

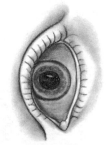

A corneal arcus is a thin grayish white arc or circle not quite at the edge of the cornea. It accompanies normal aging but may also be seen in younger people, especially blacks. In young people a corneal arcus suggests the possibility of hyperlipoproteinemia but does not prove it. Some surveys have revealed no relationship. An arcus does not interfere with vision.

CORNEAL SCAR

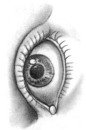

A corneal scar is a superficial grayish white opacity in the cornea, secondary to an old injury, for example, or to inflammation. Size and shape are variable. It should not be confused with the opaque lens of a cataract, visible on a deeper plane and only through the pupil.

PTERYGIUM

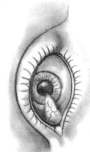

Not a true corneal opacity, a pterygium is a triangular thickening of the bulbar conjunctiva that grows slowly across the cornea, usually from the nasal side. Reddening may occur intermittently. A pterygium may interfere with vision as it encroaches upon the pupil.

CATARACTS

A cataract is an opacity of the lens and therefore can be viewed only through the pupil and on a deeper plane than corneal opacities. Cataracts are classified in many ways. When classification is by cause, old age leads the list—senile cataract. Cataracts may also be classified by location, as illustrated here in two forms—nuclear and peripheral cortical. Both are common in old age. In each of the illustrations the pupil has been widely dilated so that only a narrow rim of iris shows.

CROSS SECTION OF LENS

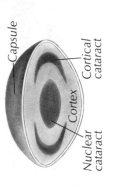

Capsule

Cortical cataract

Cortex

Nuclear cataract

NUCLEAR CATARACT

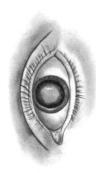

A nuclear cataract forms a central gray opacity, viewed here against a black background as you might see it with a flashlight. Through the ophthalmoscope it would appear black against the red reflex.

PERIPHERAL CORTICAL CATARACT

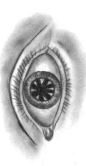

A peripheral cortical cataract produces spokelike shadows that point inward—gray against black as seen with a flashlight, or black against red with an ophthalmoscope.

Table 7-7

Table 7-7   *Pupillary Abnormalities*

BLIND EYE

Blind

Blind

When one eye is blind because of disease in the retina or optic nerve, sensory input for the light reaction is lost. A light shining into the blind eye produces no pupillary response in either eye. As long as the oculomotor nerve is intact, however, a light directed into the sound eye produces normal responses in both eyes. Unilateral blindness does not cause pupillary inequality.

Sympathetic nerve lesion (Horner's syndrome)

Oculomotor nerve paralysis

Argyll Robertson pupil

To occipital cortex

Retinal or optic nerve blindness

HORNER'S SYNDROME

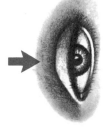

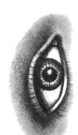

Horner's syndrome is caused by interruption of the sympathetic nerve supply, most often in the neck. The pupil is small and regular. It reacts normally to light and near effort. Involvement is unilateral. Ptosis of the eyelid is associated, often with loss of sweating on the forehead of the involved side. Because of the ptosis, the eye may look small.

BENIGN ANISOCORIA

Benign anisocoria refers to inequality of the pupils, usually slight, that has no demonstrable cause. Pupillary reactions are normal. Such inequality is relatively common but must be evaluated carefully. Compare it with the anisocoria of Horner's syndrome, oculomotor nerve paralysis, and tonic pupil.

Continued

Table 7-7

Table 7-7 (Cont'd.)

OCULOMOTOR NERVE PARALYSIS

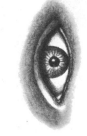 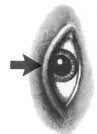

A dilated pupil that reacts neither to light nor with near effort may result from injury to the oculomotor nerve. Ptosis and deviation of the eye laterally may be associated.

ARGYLL ROBERTSON PUPILS

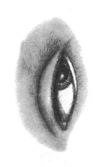

Argyll Robertson pupils are small, irregular, and bilateral. They do not react to light but do react with near effort. They are often, but not necessarily, related to central nervous system syphilis (tabes dorsalis).

DILATED FIXED PUPILS

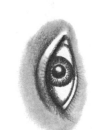 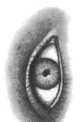

Bilaterally dilated and fixed pupils result from anticholinergic agents (e.g., atropine, mushrooms) and from glutethimide (Doriden) poisoning. Additional causes that should be considered in the comatose patient are severe brain damage and profound hypoxia.

TONIC (Adie's) PUPIL

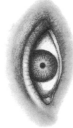 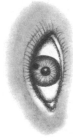

A tonic pupil is large, regular, and usually but not always unilateral. The reaction to light is diminished or absent while the near reaction, though slow and delayed, is present. Deep tendon reflexes are often decreased.

IRIDECTOMY

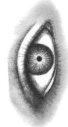 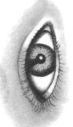

Peripheral

Complete

A common cause of pupillary irregularity in the elderly is iridectomy, a surgical incision in the iris. For cosmetic reasons it is made superiorly.

SMALL FIXED PUPILS

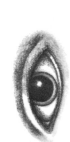 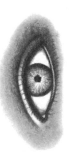

Bilaterally small, fixed, regular pupils result from morphine and related drugs, as well as from miotic drops given, for example, for glaucoma. In a comatose patient a pontine hemorrhage should also be considered.

Table 7-8

Table 7-8 Deviations of the Eyes

Deviation of the eyes from their normally conjugate position is termed *strabismus* or *squint*. Strabismus may be classified into two groups: (1) *nonparalytic*, in which the deviation is constant in all directions of gaze, and (2) *paralytic*, in which the deviation varies depending on the direction of gaze.

NONPARALYTIC STRABISMUS

Nonparalytic strabismus is caused by an imbalance in ocular muscle tone. It has many causes, may be hereditary, and often appears in childhood. Deviations are further classified according to direction:

CONVERGENT STRABISMUS
(*Esotropia*)

DIVERGENT STRABISMUS
(*Exotropia*)

COVER TEST

A cover test is helpful. Here is what you would see in the right monocular esotropia diagrammed in the last three steps on p. 561.

Corneal reflections are asymmetrical.

COVER

The right eye moves to fix on the light. (The left eye is not seen.)

UNCOVER

The left eye moves to fix on the light. The right eye deviates again.

PARALYTIC STRABISMUS

Paralytic strabismus is usually caused by weakness or paralysis of one or more extraocular muscles. Determine the direction of gaze that maximizes the deviation. For example:

A LEFT 6TH NERVE PARALYSIS

LOOKING TO THE RIGHT

Eyes are conjugate.

LOOKING STRAIGHT AHEAD

Esotropia appears.

LOOKING TO THE LEFT

Esotropia is maximum.

A LEFT 4TH NERVE PARALYSIS

LOOKING DOWN AND TO THE RIGHT

The left eye cannot look down when turned inward. Deviation is maximum.

A LEFT 3RD NERVE PARALYSIS

LOOKING STRAIGHT AHEAD

The eye is pulled outward by action of the 6th nerve. Upward, downward, and inward movements are impaired or lost. Ptosis and pupillary dilatation may be associated.

Table 7-9

Table 7-9 Normal Variations of the Optic Disc

PHYSIOLOGIC CUPPING	RINGS AND CRESCENTS	MEDULLATED NERVE FIBERS
Central cup *Temporal cup*		

The physiologic cup is a small whitish depression in the optic disc from which the retinal vessels appear to emerge. Although sometimes absent, the cup is usually visible either centrally or toward the temporal side of the disc. Grayish spots are often seen at its base.

Rings and crescents are often seen around the optic disc. These are developmental variations in which you can glimpse either white sclera, black retinal pigment, or both, especially along the temporal border of the disc. Rings and crescents are not part of the disc itself and should not be included in your estimates of disc diameters.

Medullated nerve fibers are a much less common but dramatic finding. Appearing as irregular white patches with feathered margins, they obscure the disc edge and retinal vessels. They have no pathologic significance.

Table 7-10

Table 7-10 Abnormalities of the Optic Disc

	NORMAL	OPTIC ATROPHY	PAPILLEDEMA	GLAUCOMATOUS CUPPING
PROCESS	Tiny disc vessels give normal color to the disc.	Death of optic nerve fibers leads to loss of the tiny disc vessels.	Venous stasis leads to engorgement and swelling.	Increased pressure within the eye leads to increased cupping (backward depression of the disc) and atrophy.
APPEARANCE	Color yellowish orange to creamy pink	Color white	Color pink, hyperemic	The base of the enlarged cup is pale.
	Disc vessels tiny	Disc vessels absent	Disc vessels more visible, more numerous, curve over the borders of the disc	
	Disc margins sharp (except perhaps nasally)		Disc swollen with margins blurred	
	The physiologic cup is located centrally or somewhat temporally. It may be conspicuous or absent. Its diameter from side to side is usually less than half that of the disc.		The physiologic cup is not visible.	The physiologic cup is enlarged, occupying more than half of the disc's diameter, at times extending to the edge of the disc. Retinal vessels sink in and under it, and may be displaced nasally.

Table 7-11

Table 7-11 Retinal Arterioles and Arteriovenous Crossings: Normal and Hypertensive

NORMAL RETINAL ARTERIOLE AND ARTERIOVENOUS (A–V) CROSSING

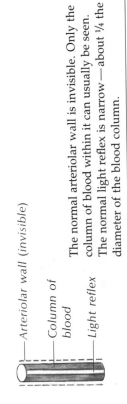

Arteriolar wall (invisible)

Column of blood

Light reflex

The normal arteriolar wall is invisible. Only the column of blood within it can usually be seen. The normal light reflex is narrow — about ¼ the diameter of the blood column.

Vein

Arteriolar wall

Arteriole

Since the arteriolar wall is transparent, a vein crossing beneath the arteriole can be seen right up to the column of blood on either side.

THE RETINAL ARTERIOLES IN HYPERTENSION

SPASM AND THICKENING OF ARTERIOLAR WALLS

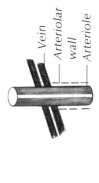

Narrowed column of blood

Narrowed light reflex

Focal narrowing

In hypertension the arterioles may show areas of focal or generalized spasm with narrowing of the column of blood. The light reflex is also narrowed. As the narrowing recurs or persists over many months or years, the arteriolar wall thickens and becomes less transparent.

COPPER WIRE ARTERIOLES

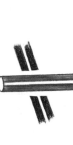

Sometimes the arterioles, especially those close to the disc, become full and somewhat tortuous and develop an increased light reflex with a bright metallic luster. Such a vessel is called a copper wire arteriole.

SILVER WIRE ARTERIOLES

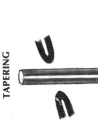

Occasionally a portion of a narrowed arteriole develops such an opaque wall that no blood is visible within it. This is a silver wire arteriole. This change typically occurs in the smaller branches.

ARTERIOVENOUS CROSSING

Thickening of the arteriolar walls is often associated with visible changes in the arteriovenous crossings. Decreased transparency of the retina probably also contributes to the first two of the following changes.

CONCEALMENT OR A–V NICKING

The vein appears to stop abruptly on either side of the arteriole.

TAPERING

The vein appears to taper down on either side of the arteriole.

BANKING

The vein is twisted on the distal side of the arteriole and forms a dark, wide knuckle.

Table 7-12

Table 7-12   Red Spots and Streaks in the Fundi

SUPERFICIAL RETINAL HEMORRHAGES

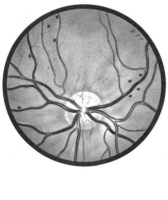

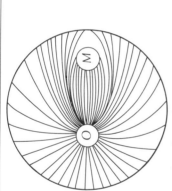

Superficial retinal hemorrhages are small, linear, flame-shaped, red streaks in the fundi. They are shaped by the superficial bundles of nerve fibers that radiate from the optic disc in the pattern illustrated (O = optic disc; M = macula). Sometimes the hemorrhages occur in clusters and then simulate a larger hemorrhage, but the linear streaking at the edges shows their true nature. Superficial hemorrhages are seen in severe hypertension, papilledema, and occlusion of the retinal vein, among other conditions.

An occasional superficial hemorrhage has a white center and may then be termed a *Roth spot*. It suggests the possibility of bacterial endocarditis or a blood disorder such as leukemia.

PRERETINAL (*Subhyaloid*) HEMORRHAGE

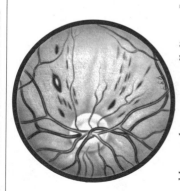

A preretinal (subhyaloid) hemorrhage develops when blood escapes into the potential space between retina and vitreous. This kind of hemorrhage is characteristically larger than retinal hemorrhages. Because it is anterior to the retina, it obscures any underlying retinal vessels. In an erect patient gravity may cause the red cells to settle, creating a horizontal line between plasma above and cells below. Causes include a sudden increase in intracranial pressure.

DEEP RETINAL HEMORRHAGES

Deep retinal hemorrhages are small, rounded, slightly irregular red spots that are sometimes called dot or blot hemorrhages. They occur in a deeper layer of the retina than flame-shaped hemorrhages. Diabetes mellitus is a common cause.

NEOVASCULARIZATION

Neovascularization refers to the formation of new blood vessels. They are more numerous, more tortuous, and narrower than other blood vessels in the area and form disorderly-looking red arcades. A common cause is the late, proliferative stage of diabetic retinopathy. The vessels may grow into the vitreous where bleeding may cause loss of vision.

MICROANEURYSMS

Microaneurysms are tiny, round, red spots seen commonly but not exclusively in and around the macular area. They are minute dilatations of very small retinal vessels, but the vascular connections are too small to be seen ophthalmoscopically. Microaneurysms are characteristic of diabetic retinopathy but not specific to it.

Table 7-13

Table 7-13   Light-Colored Spots in the Fundi

HARD EXUDATES

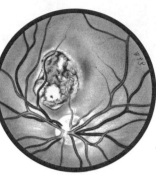

Hard exudates are creamy or yellowish, often bright lesions with well-defined (thus "hard") borders. They are small and round (as shown in the lower group of exudates) but may coalesce into larger irregular spots (as shown in the upper group). They often occur in clusters or in circular, linear, or star-shaped patterns. Causes include diabetes and hypertension.

HEALED CHORIORETINITIS

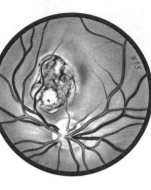

Here inflammation has destroyed the superficial tissues to reveal a well-defined, irregular patch of white sclera marked with dark pigment. Size varies from small to very large. Toxoplasmosis is illustrated. Multiple, small, somewhat similar-looking areas may be due to laser treatments.

COTTON WOOL PATCHES (Soft Exudates)

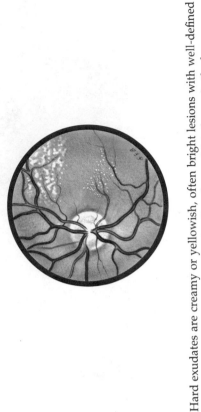

Cotton wool patches are white or grayish, ovoid lesions with irregular (thus "soft") borders. They are moderate in size but usually smaller than the disc. They are seen in hypertension and other conditions.

DRUSEN (Colloid Bodies)

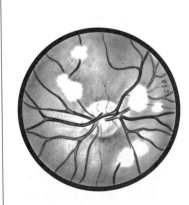

Drusen are yellowish round spots that vary from tiny to small. They are haphazardly distributed but may concentrate at the posterior pole. Drusen appear with normal aging.

Table 7-13

COLOBOMA

PROLIFERATIVE DIABETIC RETINOPATHY

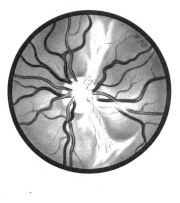

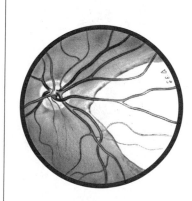

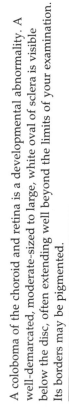

A coloboma of the choroid and retina is a developmental abnormality. A well-demarcated, moderate-sized to large, white oval of sclera is visible below the disc, often extending well beyond the limits of your examination. Its borders may be pigmented.

Bands or strands of white fibrous tissue develop in the late proliferative stage of diabetic retinopathy. They lie anterior to the retinal vessels and therefore obscure them. Neovascularization (p. 199) is typically associated.

Color Plate 1   Ocular Fundi

Out of a piece of paper, cut a circle about the size of an optic disc shown below. The circle simulates an ophthalmoscope's light beam. Lay it on each illustration, and inspect each fundus systematically.

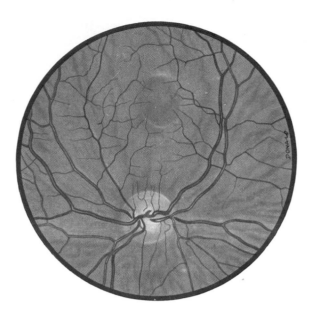

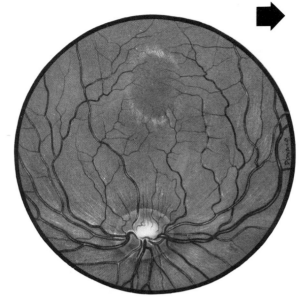

NORMAL FUNDUS OF A FAIR-SKINNED PERSON

Find and inspect the optic disc. Follow the major vessels in four directions, noting their relative sizes and the nature of the arteriovenous crossings—both normal here. Inspect the macula. The fovea is not visible in this subject. Look for any lesions in the retina. Note the striped, or tessellated, character of the fundus, especially in the lower field. This comes from normal choroidal vessels, unobscured by pigment.

NORMAL FUNDUS OF A BLACK PERSON

Again, inspect the disc, the vessels, the macula, and the retinal background. The ring around the macula is a normal light reflection. Compare the color of the fundus to that in the illustration above. It has a grayish brownish, almost purplish cast, which comes from pigment in the retina and the choroid. This pigment characteristically obscures the choroidal vessels, and no tessellation is visible. In contrast to either of these two figures, the fundus of a white person with brunette coloring is redder.

Continued

Color Plate 1 (Cont'd.)

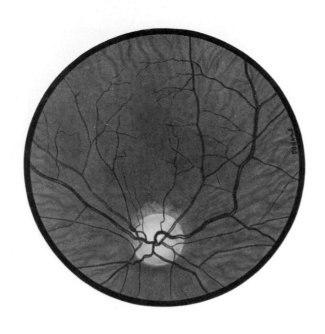

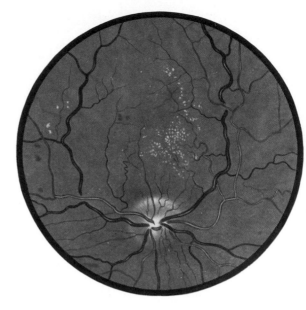

NORMAL FUNDUS OF AN AGED PERSON

Inspect the fundus as before. What differences do you observe? Two characteristics of the aging fundus can be seen in this example. The blood vessels are straighter and narrower than those in younger people, and the choroidal vessels can be seen easily. In this person the optic disc is less pink, and pigment may be seen temporal to the disc and in the macular area.

HYPERTENSIVE RETINOPATHY

Inspect the fundus as before. The nasal border of the optic disc is blurred. The light reflexes from the arterioles just above and below the disc are increased. Note the venous tapering—at the A–V crossing, about one disc diameter above the disc. Tapering and banking can be seen at 4:30 o'clock, two disc diameters from the disc. Punctate hard exudates and a few deep hemorrhages are readily visible.

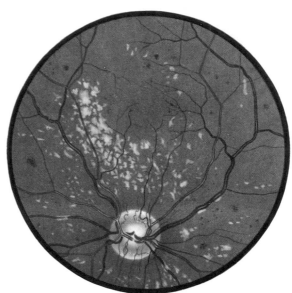

HYPERTENSIVE RETINOPATHY WITH MACULAR STAR

Punctate exudates are readily visible here. Some are scattered, while others radiate from the fovea to form a macular star. Note the two small, soft exudates about one disc diameter from the disc. A number of flame-shaped hemorrhages sweep toward 4 o'clock and 5 o'clock, and a few more may be seen toward 2 o'clock.

The changes shown in both this and the previous illustration of hypertensive retinopathy are typical of accelerated (malignant) hypertension. The other important abnormality that may accompany these changes is papilledema (p. 197).

DIABETIC RETINOPATHY

Punctate exudates have coalesced here into homogeneous, waxy-looking patches that are typical of diabetic retinopathy. What kinds of red spots can you find? Microaneurysms are most easily visible about one disc diameter below the disc. A few deep hemorrhages can also be seen, around 2 o'clock and 3 o'clock about three disc diameters from the disc.

This picture, with its combination of microaneurysms, deep hemorrhages, and hard exudates, is classified as background retinopathy. A later stage, known as proliferative retinopathy, includes neovascularization (p. 199), proliferating fibrous tissue (p. 201), and vitreous hemorrhages.

(Source of illustrations: Michaelson IC: Textbook of the Fundus of the Eye, 3rd ed, pp 52, 131, 141. Edinburgh, Churchill Livingstone, 1980)

Color Plate 2   Abnormalities of the Eardrum

NORMAL EARDRUM

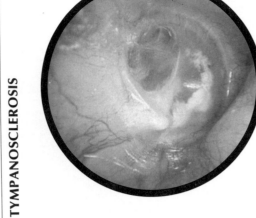

PERFORATION OF THE DRUM

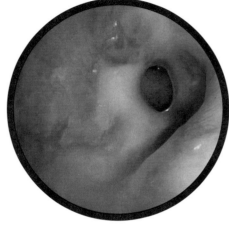

TYMPANOSCLEROSIS

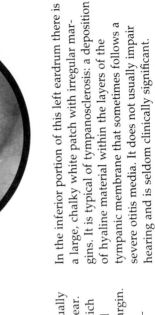

This normal right eardrum (tympanic membrane) is pinkish gray. The handle of the malleus lies in a somewhat oblique position behind the upper part of the drum. The short process of the malleus pushes the membrane laterally, creating a small white elevation. Above the short process lies a small portion of the eardrum called the pars flaccida. The remainder of the drum is the pars tensa. Anterior and posterior malleolar folds, which extend laterally and upward from the short process, separate the pars flaccida from the pars tensa, but they are often invisible unless the eardrum is retracted. From the umbo the bright cone of light fans anteriorly and downward. Other light reflections seen in this photo are artifactual. Posterior to the malleus, part of the incus is visible behind the drum. The small blood vessels that course along the handle of the malleus are within the range of normal and do not indicate inflammation. The ear canal, which surrounds the eardrum, looks flatter than it really is because of distortion inherent in the photographic technique.

Perforations are holes in the eardrum that usually result from purulent infections of the middle ear. They are classified as *central* perforations, which do not extend to the margin of the drum, and *marginal* perforations, which do involve the margin.

The more common central perforation is illustrated here. In this case a reddened ring of granulation tissue surrounds the perforation, indicating a chronic infectious process. The eardrum itself is scarred and no landmarks are discernible. Discharge from the infected middle ear may drain out through such a perforation, but none is visible here.

A perforation of the eardrum often closes in the healing process, as illustrated in the next photo. The membrane covering the hole may be exceedingly thin and transparent.

In the inferior portion of this left eardrum there is a large, chalky white patch with irregular margins. It is typical of tympanosclerosis: a deposition of hyaline material within the layers of the tympanic membrane that sometimes follows a severe otitis media. It does not usually impair hearing and is seldom clinically significant.

Other abnormalities in this eardrum include a *healed perforation* (the large oval area in the upper posterior drum) and signs of a *retracted drum*. A retracted drum is pulled medially, away from the examiner's eye, and the malleolar folds are tightened into sharp outlines. The short process often protrudes sharply, and the handle of the malleus, pulled inward at the umbo, looks foreshortened and more horizontal.

BULLOUS MYRINGITIS

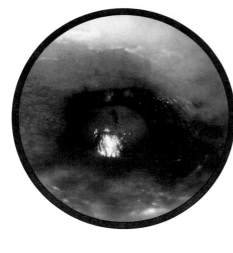

Bullous myringitis is a viral infection characterized by painful hemorrhagic vesicles that appear on the tympanic membrane, the ear canal, or both. Symptoms include earache, blood-tinged discharge from the ear, and hearing loss of the conduction type.

In this illustration a large vesicle on the posterior wall of the right ear canal contains serous fluid (as shown by its yellowish color) together with some dark red blood peripherally. The eardrum, not well seen here, would be likely to show similar lesions. The skin of the ear canal shows hemorrhagic patches.

Several different viruses may cause this condition.

ACUTE OTITIS MEDIA WITH PURULENT EFFUSION

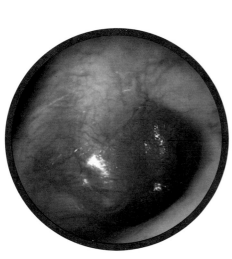

Acute otitis media with purulent effusion is caused by bacterial infection. Symptoms include earache, fever, and hearing loss. The eardrum reddens, loses its landmarks, and bulges laterally, toward the examiner's eye.

In this left ear the upper portion of the drum is reddened by dilated blood vessels and has begun to bulge. The short process and the handle of the malleus, though less distinct than normal, are still discernible. Later all landmarks are lost and the entire fiery red drum bulges laterally. Spontaneous rupture (perforation) of the drum may follow, with discharge of purulent material into the ear canal.

Moving the auricle and pressing on the tragus do not cause pain in otitis media as they usually do in acute otitis externa. Hearing loss is of the conduction type. Acute purulent otitis media is much more common in children than in adults.

SEROUS EFFUSIONS

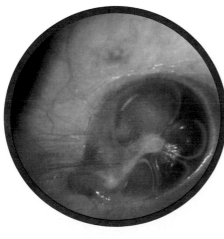

Serous effusions are usually caused by viral upper respiratory infections (*otitis media with serous effusion*) or by sudden changes in atmospheric pressure as from flying or diving (*otitic barotrauma*). The eustachian tube cannot equalize the air pressure in the middle ear with that of the outside air. Air is partly or completely absorbed from the middle ear into the bloodstream, and serous fluid accumulates there instead. Symptoms include fullness and popping sensations in the ear, mild conduction hearing loss, and perhaps some pain.

Amber fluid behind the eardrum is characteristic, as in this left drum of a patient with otitic barotrauma. A fluid level, a line between air above and amber fluid below, can be seen on either side of the short process. Air bubbles (not always present) can be seen here within the amber fluid.

(Sources of photos: *Normal Eardrum*—Hawke M, Keene M, Alberti PW: Clinical Otoscopy: A Text and Colour Atlas, p. 68. Edinburgh, Churchill Livingstone, 1984; *Eardrum abnormalities photos*—Courtesy of Michael Hawke, M.D., Toronto, Canada)

Color Plate 3   Skin Tumors

BASAL CELL EPITHELIOMA

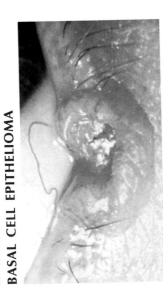

A basal cell epithelioma, though malignant, grows slowly and seldom metastasizes. It is most common in fair-skinned adults over 40, and usually appears on the face. An initial translucent nodule spreads, leaving a depressed center and a firm, elevated border. Telangiectatic vessels are often visible, as in this lesion on the eyelid.

SQUAMOUS CELL CARCINOMA

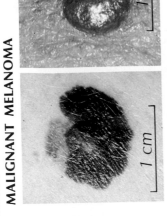

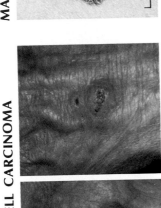

Squamous cell carcinoma usually appears on sun-exposed skin of fair-skinned adults over 60. It may develop in an actinic keratosis. It usually grows more quickly than a basal cell epithelioma, is firmer, and looks redder. The face and the back of the hand are often affected, as shown here.

MALIGNANT MELANOMA

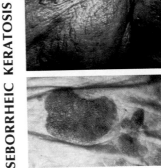

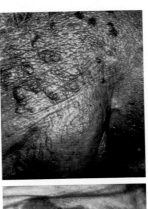

Noticeable growth or color change in a benign nevus (mole) warns of possible malignant melanoma, a highly malignant tumor most common in fair-skinned people. Suggestive signs are variation in color, an irregular perimeter, a raised and irregular surface, ulceration, and crusting. Two forms are illustrated: superficial spreading (left) and nodular (right).

KAPOSI'S SARCOMA IN AIDS

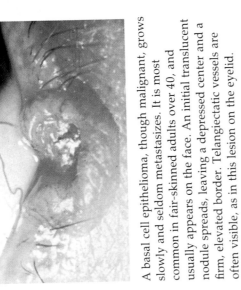

When Kaposi's sarcoma, a malignant tumor, accompanies AIDS, it may appear in many forms: macules, papules, plaques, or nodules almost anywhere in the body. Lesions are often multiple and may involve internal structures. On the left are ovoid, pinkish red plaques that typically lengthen along the skin lines. They may become pigmented. On the right is a purplish red nodule on the foot.

ACTINIC KERATOSIS

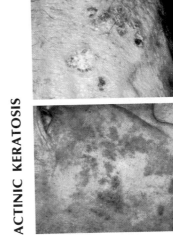

Actinic keratoses are superficial, flattened papules covered by a dry scale. Often multiple, they may be round or irregular, and are pink, tan or grayish. They appear on sun-exposed skin of older, fair-skinned persons. Though themselves benign, they may give rise to squamous cell carcinoma (suggested by rapid growth, induration, redness at the base, and ulceration). Keratoses on face and hand, typical locations, are shown.

SEBORRHEIC KERATOSIS

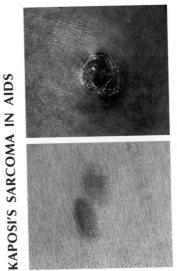

Seborrheic keratoses are common, benign, yellowish to brown, raised lesions that feel slightly greasy and velvety or warty. Typically multiple and symmetrically distributed on the trunk of older people, they may also appear on the face and elsewhere. In black people, often younger women, they may appear as small, deeply pigmented papules on the cheeks and temples (dermatosis papulosa nigra).

(Sources of photos: *Basal Cell Epithelioma, Squamous Cell Carcinoma, Actinic Keratosis,* and *Seborrheic Keratosis*—Sauer GC: Manual of Skin Diseases, 5th ed. Philadelphia, JB Lippincott, 1985; *Malignant Melanoma*— Balch CM, Milton GW [eds]: Cutaneous Melanoma. Philadelphia, JB Lippincott, 1985; *Kaposi's Sarcoma in AIDS*—DeVita VT Jr, Hellman S, Rosenberg SA [eds]: AIDS: Etiology, Diagnosis, Treatment, and Prevention. Philadelphia, JB Lippincott, 1985)

Table 7-14

Table 7-14 Nodules In and Around the Ears

LYMPH NODES	SEBACEOUS CYSTS	KELOID

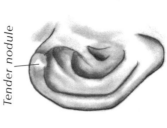

LYMPH NODES

Small lymph nodes just anterior to the tragus or overlying the mastoid process are quite common. Although sometimes visible, they are best detected by palpation.

SEBACEOUS CYSTS

Sebaceous cysts are common, especially behind the ear. They are characteristically *in* rather than beneath the skin and often show a central black dot or punctum which identifies the opening of the blocked sebaceous gland.

KELOID

A keloid, which is a nodular, hypertrophic mass of scar tissue, may develop in an earlobe pierced for earrings. Keloids are especially common in black people.

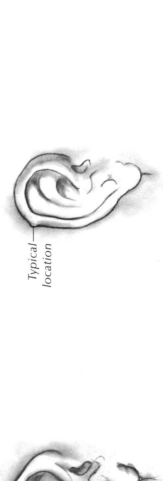

TOPHUS

Tophi are deposits of uric acid crystals characteristic of gout. They appear as hard nodules in the helix or antihelix. They occasionally discharge white chalky crystals.

DARWIN'S TUBERCLE

A small elevation in the rim of the ear, a Darwin's tubercle is a harmless congenital variation from normal—the equivalent of the tip of a mammalian ear. It should not be mistaken for a tophus.

CHONDRODERMATITIS HELICIS

This entity is characterized by a small, chronic, painful, tender nodule in the helix of the ear. It usually affects men, involving the right ear more often than the left. It may be confused with a tophus or skin cancer. Biopsy is important.

Table 7-15

Table 7-15   Patterns of Hearing Loss

Hearing loss is divided into two major types: (1) *conduction hearing loss*, in which a disorder of the external or middle ear impairs the conduction of sound to the inner ear, and (2) *sensorineural hearing loss*, in which a disorder of the inner ear, the cochlear nerve, or its central connections impairs the transmission of nerve impulses to the brain. A *mixed hearing loss* has both deficits.

	CONDUCTION LOSS	SENSORINEURAL LOSS
DISTORTION OF SOUNDS THAT IMPAIRS THE UNDERSTANDING OF WORDS	Relatively minor	Often present as the upper tones of words are disproportionately lost
EFFECT OF A NOISY ENVIRONMENT	Hearing may seem to improve: people talk more loudly.	Hearing typically worsens.
PATIENT'S OWN VOICE	Tends to be soft: the patient's voice is conducted through bone to a normal inner ear and cochlear nerve.	May be loud: the patient has trouble hearing his or her own voice.
USUAL AGE OF ONSET	Most often in childhood and young adulthood, up to age 40	Most often in the middle or later years
EAR CANAL AND DRUM	There is usually a visible abnormality, except in otosclerosis.	The problem is not visible.

Table 7-15

WEBER TEST (*in unilateral hearing loss*)

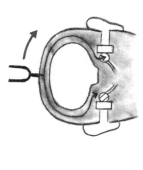

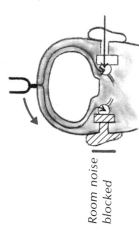

Room noise blocked

The sound lateralizes to the impaired ear. Because this ear is not distracted by room noise, it can detect vibrations better than normal. (Test yourself while occluding one ear with your finger.) This lateralization disappears in an absolutely quiet room.

The sound lateralizes to the good ear. The impaired inner ear or cochlear nerve is less able to transmit impulses no matter how the sound reaches the cochlea. The sound is therefore heard in the better ear.

RINNE TEST

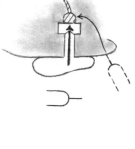

Bone conduction lasts longer than or is equal to air conduction (BC > AC or BC = AC, a negative Rinne). Pathways of normal conduction through the external or middle ear are blocked. Vibrations through bone bypass the obstruction to reach the cochlea.

Air conduction lasts longer than bone conduction (AC > BC, a positive Rinne). The inner ear or cochlear nerve is less able to transmit impulses regardless of how the vibrations reach the cochlea. The normal pattern prevails.

CAUSES INCLUDE:

Obstruction of the ear canal, otitis media, a perforated or relatively immobilized ear drum, and otosclerosis (a fixation of the ossicles by bony overgrowth)

Sustained exposure to loud noise, drugs, infections of the inner ear, trauma, tumors, congenital and hereditary disorders, and aging (presbycusis)

Further evaluation is done by audiometry and other specialized procedures.

Table 7-16

Table 7-16   Common Abnormalities of the Nose

FURUNCLE OF THE NOSE	ACUTE RHINITIS *(The Common Cold)*	ALLERGIC RHINITIS

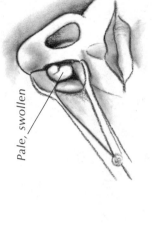

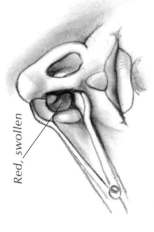

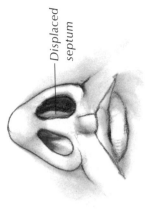

Pale, swollen

Red, swollen

White center

Red margin

Furuncles are quite common in the skin-lined vestibule. The area is tender and may be red and swollen; then a typical pustule forms. Examine it gently; manipulation may spread infection.

The nasal mucosa is red and swollen. Nasal discharge, which is at first watery and copious, becomes thick and mucopurulent.

The nasal mucosa is swollen, pale, boggy, and usually gray. A dull red or bluish color may also be seen. Similar findings are seen in some patients with nonallergic vasomotor rhinitis.

NASAL POLYPS

SEPTAL DEVIATION

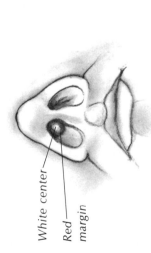

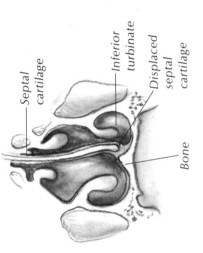

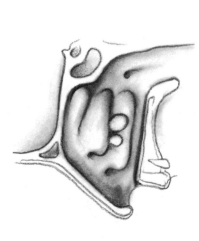

Displaced septum

Septal cartilage

Inferior turbinate

Displaced septal cartilage

Bone

CROSS SECTION VIEWED FROM THE FRONT

Nasal polyps may develop in patients with allergic rhinitis. They are usually found in the middle meatus, where they appear as gelatinous or soft, pale gray structures. Unlike the turbinates, for which they are sometimes mistaken, they are mobile.

Some degree of septal deviation is common in most adults. Illustrated here is one of the most frequent types—displacement of the septal cartilage in the anterior portion of the nose. Septal deviation may produce nasal obstruction but the turbinates often accommodate to the asymmetry. Most septal deviations are asymptomatic.

Table 7-17

Table 7-17   Abnormalities of the Lips

HERPES SIMPLEX
(Cold Sore, Fever Blister)

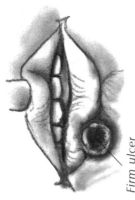

Blisters with crusting

The virus herpes simplex may produce recurrent vesicular eruptions of the lips and surrounding tissues. A small cluster of blisters develops. As these break, a crust is formed and healing ensues within 10 to 14 days.

CHANCRE

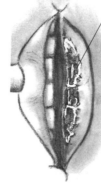

Firm ulcer

The primary lesion of syphilis may appear on the lip instead of in its more common location on the genitalia. It is a firm, buttonlike lesion which ulcerates and may become crusted. A chancre may resemble a carcinoma or a crusted cold sore. Use a glove for palpation. Dark field examination is necessary for diagnosis.

ANGULAR STOMATITIS
(Cheilosis)

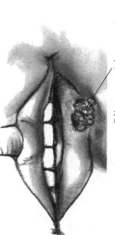

Softening, fissuring

Softening of the skin at the angles of the mouth, followed by fissuring or cracking, is called angular stomatitis or cheilosis. It may be secondary to riboflavin deficiency but it more commonly is caused by overclosure of the mouth (*e.g.*, in patients without teeth or with dentures that are too short in their vertical dimension). Saliva then wets and macerates the infolded skin, often leading to secondary infection from Monilia or bacteria. The mucous membrane remains uninvolved.

CHEILITIS

Fissures, scales and crusts

Painful fissuring with inflammation, scaling, and crust formation characterizes cheilitis. Involving chiefly the lower lip, cheilitis is often chronic. Its causes are several and may be obscure.

Continued

Table 7-17

Table 7-17 (Cont'd.)

MUCOUS RETENTION CYST
(*Mucocele*)

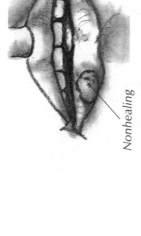

Round nodule

CARCINOMA OF THE LIP

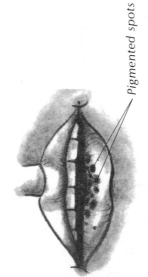

Nonhealing

A round, regular, partially translucent or bluish nodule in the lip is probably a mucous retention cyst or mucocele. This is a benign lesion, having chiefly cosmetic importance. Size varies from tiny up to 1–2 cm in diameter. The cysts may also occur inside the lower lip in the buccal mucosa.

Carcinoma of the lip usually involves the lower lip and may appear as a thickened plaque, ulcer, or warty growth. Much more frequent in men than in women, it is the most common form of oral cancer. Any sore or crusting lesion on the lip that does not heal must be considered suspicious.

PEUTZ–JEGHERS SYNDROME

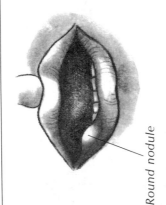

Pigmented spots

ANGIONEUROTIC EDEMA

Swollen

When pigmented spots on the lips are more prominent than freckling of the surrounding skin, suspect the Peutz–Jeghers syndrome. Look for abnormal pigment in the buccal mucosa to help confirm the diagnosis. Pigmented spots may also be found on the face, fingers, and hands. These findings are important because they are often associated with multiple intestinal polyps.

Angioneurotic edema is a diffuse, nonpitting, tense, subcutaneous swelling that may involve a number of structures, including the lips. It develops rather rapidly and usually disappears in a day or two. Although usually allergic in nature and sometimes associated with hives, it does not usually itch.

Table 7-18

Table 7-18 Abnormalities of the Buccal Mucosa and Hard Palate

APHTHOUS ULCER (*Canker Sore*)

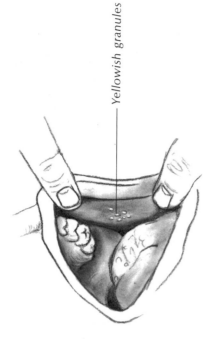

White ulcer surrounded by red

A small, round or oval, white ulcer surrounded by a halo of reddened mucosa characterizes the common aphthous ulcer. Such ulcers are painful, may be single or multiple, and are often recurrent. Any portion of the oral mucosa may be involved.

FORDYCE SPOTS (*Granules*)

Yellowish granules

Fordyce spots are small yellowish spots visible in the buccal mucosa of most adults. They may also involve the lips. They are sebaceous glands and should not be considered an abnormality. The patient who suddenly notices and worries about them may be reassured.

TORUS PALATINUS

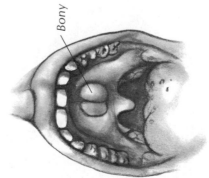

Bony

A torus palatinus is a fairly common midline bony outgrowth in the hard palate, usually developing in adult-hood. Its size and lobulation vary. Although alarming at first glance, it is of no clinical consequence except perhaps in the fitting of dentures. A nodule that is not in the midline is not a torus and should suggest a tumor.

MONILIASIS (*Candidiasis, Thrush*)

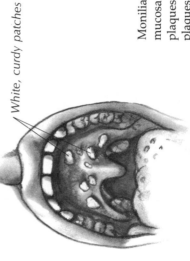

White, curdy patches

Moniliasis can involve the entire oral mucosa. It is characterized by white plaques resembling milk curds. The plaques are removable but not quite so easily as milk curds. The mucosa itself may be reddened or normal in color. Less commonly, moniliasis appears as shiny redness without the white patches. Definitive diagnosis depends on culture of the yeast.

Table 7-19

Table 7-19 Abnormalities of the Gums and Teeth

NORMAL GUMS

Pale red with normal stippling

Sharp interdental papilla

The gums (or gingivae) normally show a pale red stippled surface. Their margins about the teeth are sharp and the crevices between gums and teeth shallow (e.g., 1–2 mm). The teeth are seated firmly in their bony sockets.

GINGIVITIS

Marginal redness and swelling with bulbous interdental papillae

Redness and swelling of the margins of the gums characterize gingivitis, often the result of irritation by calculus formation. The normal stippling decreases or disappears. The gingivae between the teeth (interdental papillae) may become bulbous. The gums may bleed with light contact.

PERIODONTITIS (*Pyorrhea*)

Associated gingivitis

Gums recessed

If untreated, gingivitis may progress to periodontitis, an inflammation of the deeper tissues around the teeth. This is an extremely common cause of tooth loss in adults. The crevices between the gums and teeth enlarge, and pockets containing debris and purulent material develop in these areas. The gum margins recede, exposing the necks of the teeth. The teeth may become loose.

ACUTE NECROTIZING GINGIVITIS (*Trench Mouth, Vincent's Stomatitis*)

Grayish membrane over ulcerated gum margin

This is a painful gingivitis characterized by redness, swelling, and ulceration of the gingival tissues. The interdental papillae may be eroded by the ulcerative process. A grayish membrane forms over the inflamed and ulcerated gingival margins.

GINGIVAL ENLARGEMENT

Gums heaped up

Enlargement of the gums has a variety of causes including puberty, pregnancy, Dilantin therapy, and leukemia. The gingival tissues appear heaped up and partially cover the teeth.

EPULIS

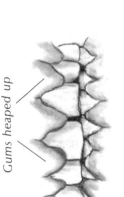

Local enlargement

Epulis is the term used to describe a localized gingival enlargement. Most are inflammatory, and some are neoplastic.

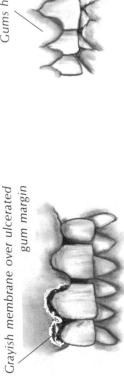

Table 7-19

LEAD OR BISMUTH LINE

Bluish black line

In chronic lead or bismuth poisoning a bluish black line may appear on the gums about 1 mm from the gum margin. It does not appear where teeth are absent. Distinguish it from the much more common melanin pigmentation.

MELANIN PIGMENTATION

Patchy brown pigment

A brownish melanin pigmentation of the gums is frequently observed. It is normal in blacks and other dark-skinned persons and may occasionally be seen even in light-skinned persons. A similar pigment pattern may be associated with Addison's disease.

DENTAL CARIES

Chalky white

Discolored, with cavitation

Dental caries is first visible as a chalky white deposit in the enamel surface of the tooth. This area may then discolor to brown or black, become soft, and cavitate. Special dental techniques including x-rays are necessary for early detection.

HUTCHINSON'S TEETH

Smaller teeth, more widely spaced

Sides taper   *Central notches*

Hutchinson's teeth are notched on their biting surfaces, smaller than normal, and more widely spaced. Their sides taper in. The upper central incisors are most often affected; the permanent, rather than deciduous, teeth are involved. They are a sign of congenital syphilis.

ABRASION OF TEETH WITH NOTCHING

Notches

Sides normal, do not taper

The biting surface of the teeth may become abraded or notched by recurrent trauma (*e.g.*, from opening bobby pins with one's teeth, or holding nails between the teeth). Unlike Hutchinson's teeth, the sides of these teeth show their normal contours; size and spacing are unaffected.

ATTRITION OF TEETH

Exposed dentin

The teeth of many elderly people have been worn down by repetitive chewing. This flattening of the biting surfaces is called attrition. The enamel may be worn away, exposing the underlying dentin. The latter often takes on a yellow or brownish stain.

Table 7-20

Table 7-20 Abnormalities of the Tongue

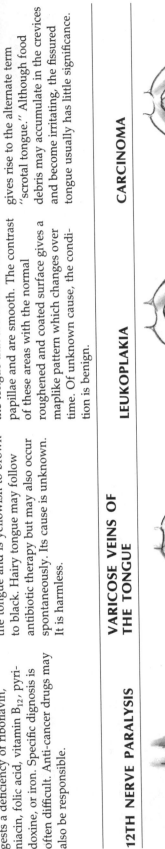
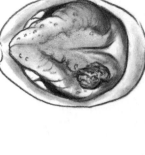
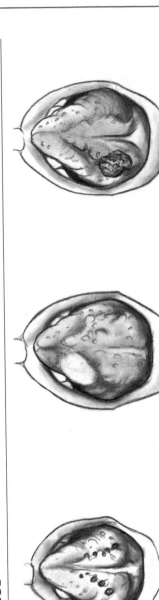

SMOOTH TONGUE

A smooth, slick, and often sore tongue that has lost its papillae suggests a deficiency of riboflavin, niacin, folic acid, vitamin B₁₂, pyridoxine, or iron. Specific dignosis is often difficult. Anti-cancer drugs may also be responsible.

HAIRY TONGUE

The "hair" of hairy tongue consists of elongated papillae on the dorsum of the tongue and is yellowish to brown to black. Hairy tongue may follow antibiotic therapy but may also occur spontaneously. Its cause is unknown. It is harmless.

GEOGRAPHIC TONGUE

Geographic tongue is characterized by scattered red areas on the dorsum of the tongue that are denuded of their papillae and are smooth. The contrast of these areas with the normal roughened and coated surface gives a maplike pattern which changes over time. Of unknown cause, the condition is benign.

FISSURED TONGUE

Fissures may appear in the tongue with increasing age and at times become numerous. Their appearance gives rise to the alternate term "scrotal tongue." Although food debris may accumulate in the crevices and become irritating, the fissured tongue usually has little significance.

12TH NERVE PARALYSIS

Paralysis of the 12th cranial (hypoglossal) nerve produces atrophy and fasciculations of the involved half of the tongue. Deviation toward the paralyzed side occurs when the tongue is protruded.

VARICOSE VEINS OF THE TONGUE

Small purplish or blue black round swellings may appear under the tongue with age and have aptly been called "caviar lesions." They have no significance. As with several other tongue findings, familiarity with them pays dividends when the patient or the examiner first notices them. Reassurance is in order.

LEUKOPLAKIA

Leukoplakia is a term applied to a thickened white patch adherent to the mucous membrane. Its appearance has been likened to dried white paint. Although tongue involvement is illustrated here, leukoplakia may involve any part of the oral mucosa. Its primary significance lies in the fact that it may be premalignant.

CARCINOMA

Carcinoma of the tongue is uncommon on the dorsum of the tongue where it might be most readily noticed. Look for it at the base or edges of the tongue. Any ulcer or nodule which fails to heal in 2 to 3 weeks must be considered suspicious.

Table 7-21

Table 7-21 Abnormalities of the Pharynx

VIRAL PHARYNGITIS	STREPTOCOCCAL PHARYNGITIS	DIPHTHERIA

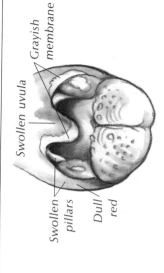

Swollen uvula

Grayish membrane

Swollen pillars

Dull red

Red

Enlarged tonsils with white patches

Swollen uvula

Slight redness

Prominent lymphoid patches

Viral pharyngitis may show few if any signs. Mild redness, slight swelling of the pillars, and prominent lymphoid patches on the posterior pharynx are frequent. Signs that suggest infectious mononucleosis as the cause of sore throat are petechiae on the palate and enlargement or tenderness of the posterior auricular, inguinal, and (if marked) axillary lymph nodes.

Classically streptococcal infection produces redness and swelling of the tonsils, pillars, and uvula, with white or yellow patches of exudate on the tonsils. Accurate clinical diagnosis is frequently impossible, however, since streptococcal pharyngitis may occur without exudate, and some viral illnesses, including infectious mononucleosis, may produce an exudative pharyngitis.

Now rare, diphtheria is included here because without prompt diagnosis and treatment it may prove fatal. The throat is dull red and swollen. A thick exudate forms on the tonsils and, unlike a streptococcal exudate, may spread over the soft palate and uvula. The throat is less painful than might be expected from the severity of the patient's illness.

TONSILLAR HYPERTROPHY | PARALYSIS OF THE 10TH CRANIAL (VAGUS) NERVE | PERITONSILLAR ABSCESS *(Quinsy Sore Throat)*

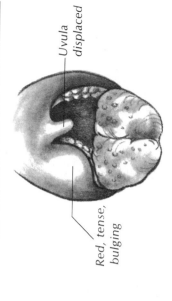

Uvula displaced

Red, tense, bulging

Deviated to left

Failure to rise

Enlarged tonsils

The tonsils may be enlarged without being infected. They may protrude medially beyond the edges of the pillars even to the midline when the tongue is protruded. The size of the tonsils is not in itself an indicator of disease.

When the patient says "ah" the soft palate on the paralyzed side fails to rise. The uvula deviates to the uninvolved side.

Peritonsillar abscess occasionally complicates acute tonsillitis. Usually caused by streptococci or staphylococci, the infection spreads from tonsil to adjacent soft tissue, producing a very painful, usually unilateral, red bulge that may extend beyond the midline. Painful swallowing may cause drooling.

Table 7-22

Table 7-22 Thyroid Enlargement and Function

Evaluation of the thyroid gland includes a description of the gland and a functional assessment.

DIFFUSE ENLARGEMENT	MULTINODULAR GOITER	SINGLE NODULE

A diffusely enlarged gland, or goiter, includes the isthmus and the lateral lobes, but there are no discretely palpable nodules. Causes include Graves' disease, Hashimoto's thyroiditis, and endemic goiter (related to iodine deficiency, now uncommon in the United States). Sporadic goiter refers to an enlarged gland with no apparent cause.

This term refers to an enlarged thyroid gland that contains two or more identifiable nodules. Multiple nodules suggest a metabolic rather than a neoplastic process, but irradiation during childhood, a positive family history, enlarged cervical nodes, or continuing enlargement of one of the nodules raises the suspicion of malignancy.

A clinically single nodule may be a cyst, a benign tumor, or one nodule within a multinodular gland, but it also raises the question of a malignancy. Prior irradiation, hardness, rapid growth, fixation to surrounding tissues, enlarged cervical nodes, and occurrence in males increase the probability of malignancy.

SYMPTOMS OF THYROID DYSFUNCTION

HYPERTHYROIDISM	HYPOTHYROIDISM
Nervousness	Fatigue, lethargy
Weight loss despite an increased appetite	Modest weight gain with anorexia
Excessive sweating and heat intolerance	Dry coarse skin and cold intolerance
Palpitations	Swelling of face, hands, and legs
Frequent bowel movements	Constipation
Muscular weakness of the proximal type and tremor	Weakness, muscle cramps, arthralgias, paresthesias, impaired memory and hearing

SIGNS OF THYROID DYSFUNCTION

HYPERTHYROIDISM	HYPOTHYROIDISM
Tachycardia or atrial fibrillation	Bradycardia and, in late stages, hypothermia
Increased systolic and decreased diastolic blood pressures	Decreased systolic and increased diastolic blood pressures
Hyperdynamic cardiac pulsations with an accentuated S_1	Intensity of heart sounds sometimes decreased
Warm, smooth, moist skin	Dry, coarse, cool skin, sometimes yellowish from carotene, with nonpitting edema and loss of hair
Tremor and proximal muscle weakness	Impaired memory, mixed hearing loss, somnolence, peripheral neuropathy, carpal tunnel syndrome
With Graves' disease, eye signs such as stare, lid lag, and exophthalmos	Periorbital puffiness

Chapter 8
The Thorax and Lungs

Anatomy and Physiology

Review the *anatomy of the chest wall,* identifying the structures illustrated.

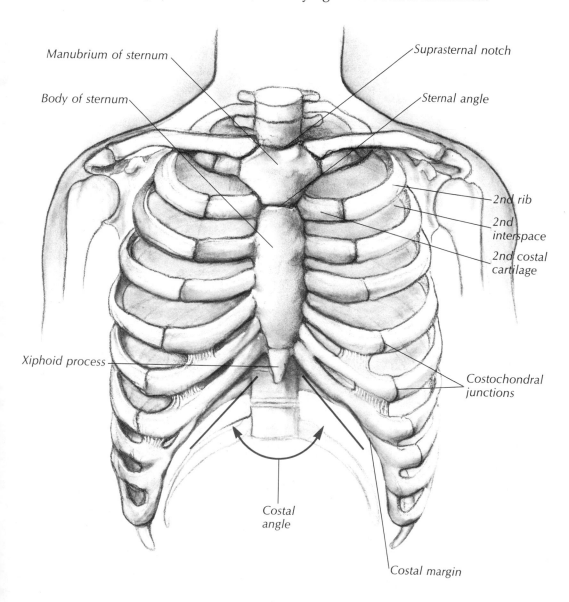

Manubrium of sternum

Body of sternum

Suprasternal notch

Sternal angle

2nd rib

2nd interspace

2nd costal cartilage

Xiphoid process

Costochondral junctions

Costal angle

Costal margin

To localize and describe a finding in relation to the chest wall you must be able to number the ribs and the interspaces between them accurately. The sternal angle (or angle of Louis) is the best guide. To find it, first identify the suprasternal notch, then move your finger down about 5 cm or a little more to find the horizontal bony ridge that joins the manubrium to the body of the sternum. Then move your finger laterally and find the adjacent 2nd rib and costal cartilage. The interspace immediately below is the 2nd interspace. From here, using two fingers, you can "walk down the interspaces," one space at a time, on an oblique line illustrated by the red numbers below. Do not try to count interspaces along the lower edge of the sternum because the ribs there are too close together. To find the interspaces in a woman with large breasts, either displace the breast laterally or palpate a little more medially than illustrated. Avoid pressing too hard on tender breast tissue.

Note that the costal cartilages of only the first seven ribs articulate with the sternum. Those of the 8th, 9th, and 10th ribs articulate with the costal cartilages just above. The 11th and 12th ribs, the so-called floating ribs, have free anterior tips. The cartilaginous tip of the 11th rib can usually be felt laterally, and the 12th may be felt posteriorly. Costal cartilages are not distinguishable from ribs by palpation.

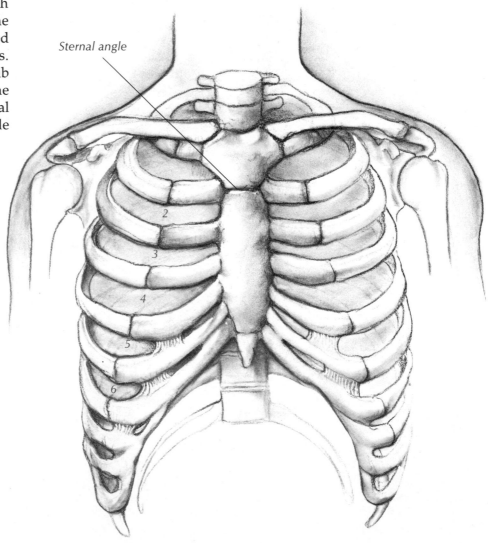

Sternal angle

Posteriorly the 11th and 12th ribs give you another possible starting point for counting ribs and interspaces. This is especially helpful in localizing findings in the lower posterior chest, but is also useful occasionally when the anterior approach is unsatisfactory. First, with the fingers of one hand, press inward and up against the lower border of the rib cage, roughly in the area indicated by the red arrow. Identify the 12th rib. Then "walk" upward in the interspaces on the red numbers or, alternatively, obliquely upward and around to the front of the chest.

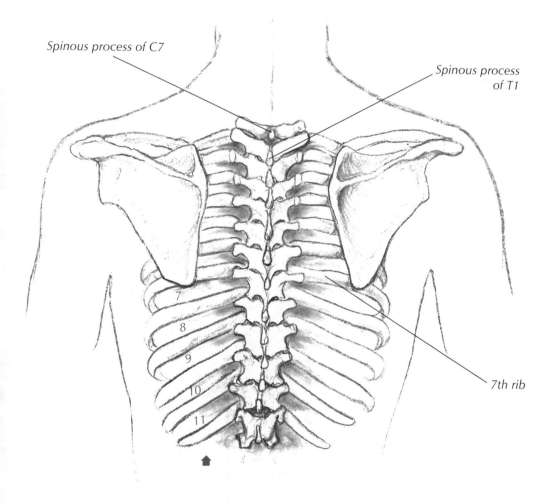

Spinous process of C7

Spinous process of T1

7th rib

7
8
9
10
11

Other bony landmarks and relationships are sometimes useful. The inferior angle of the scapula lies approximately at the level of the 7th rib or interspace. Findings may also be localized according to their relationship to the spinous processes of the vertebrae. When a person flexes the neck forward, the most prominent process (the vertebra prominens) is usually that of the 7th cervical. When two processes appear equally prominent, they are the 7th cervical and 1st thoracic. The processes below them can often be felt and counted, especially when the spine is flexed.

Localization of findings depends upon their relationship not only to ribs and vertebrae but also to imaginary lines drawn on the chest. Become familiar with the lines illustrated. Estimation of the midclavicular line requires the accurate identification of the lateral end of the clavicle. For this refer to p. 430.

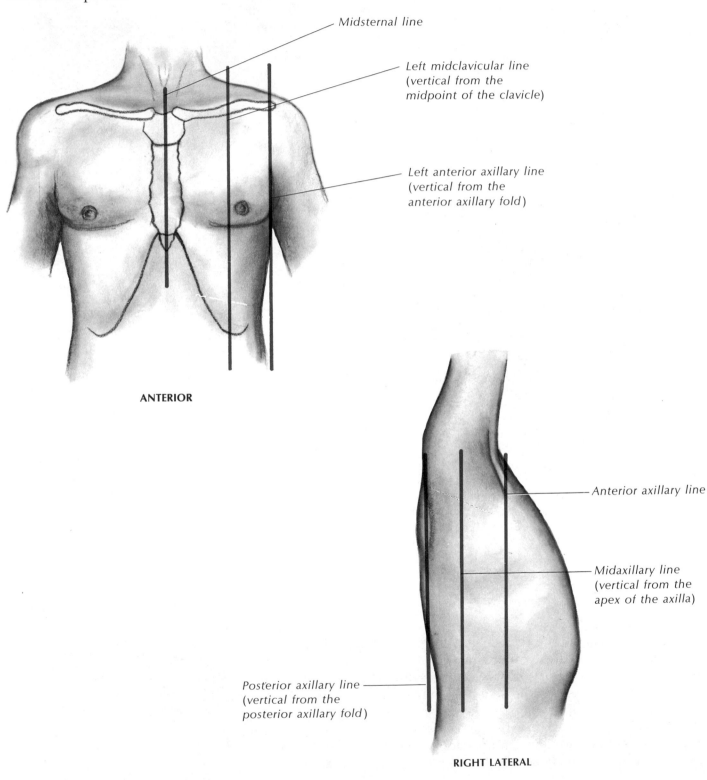

Midsternal line

Left midclavicular line
(vertical from the
midpoint of the clavicle)

Left anterior axillary line
(vertical from the
anterior axillary fold)

ANTERIOR

Anterior axillary line

Midaxillary line
(vertical from the
apex of the axilla)

Posterior axillary line
(vertical from the
posterior axillary fold)

RIGHT LATERAL

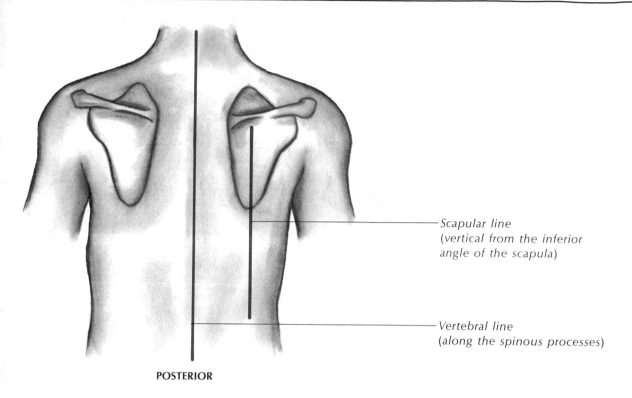

Scapular line
(*vertical from the inferior
angle of the scapula*)

Vertebral line
(*along the spinous processes*)

POSTERIOR

More general terms are also helpful: supraclavicular (above the clavicle), infraclavicular (below the clavicle), interscapular (between the scapulae), and infrascapular (below the scapula).

While examining the chest, keep in mind the probable location of the underlying lungs and their lobes. These locations can be mentally projected onto the chest wall. Key points in these surface projections include the following:

*The apex of each lung
rises about 2–4 cm
above the inner
third of the clavicle.*

*The inferior border
crosses the 6th rib at
the midclavicular line,
and the 8th rib at
the midaxillary line.*

ANTERIOR

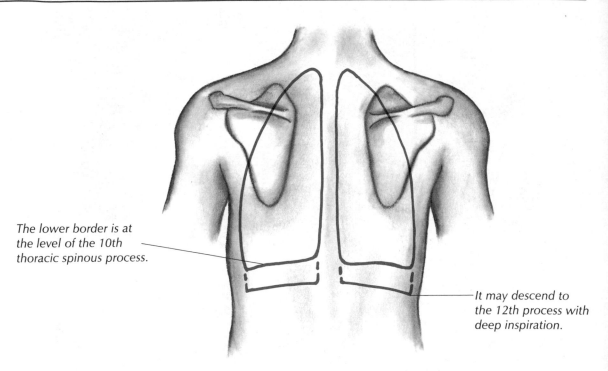

The lower border is at the level of the 10th thoracic spinous process.

It may descend to the 12th process with deep inspiration.

POSTERIOR

Each lung is divided approximately in half by an oblique or major fissure. Posteriorly the locations of the oblique fissures are approximated by lines drawn from the 3rd thoracic spinous process obliquely down and laterally. These lines are close to the vertebral borders of the scapulae when a person's hands are placed on top of the head. They divide upper from lower lobes.

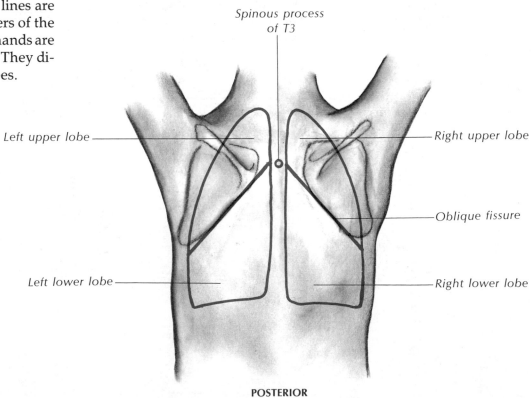

Spinous process of T3

Left upper lobe

Right upper lobe

Oblique fissure

Left lower lobe

Right lower lobe

POSTERIOR

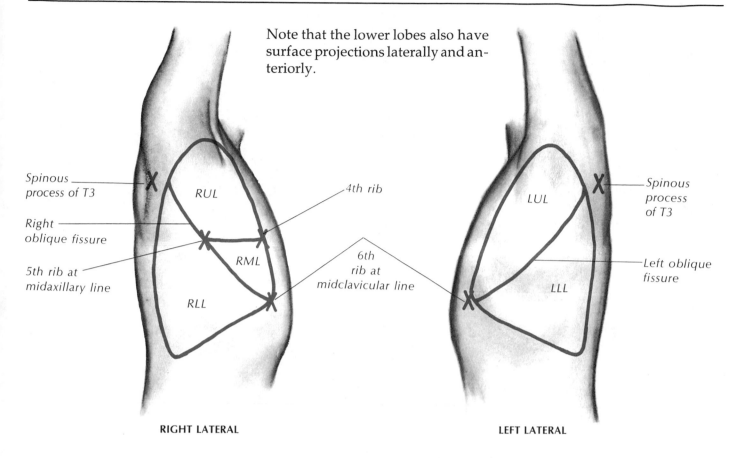

Note that the lower lobes also have surface projections laterally and anteriorly.

Spinous process of T3

Right oblique fissure

5th rib at midaxillary line

RUL

RML

RLL

4th rib

6th rib at midclavicular line

LUL

LLL

Spinous process of T3

Left oblique fissure

RIGHT LATERAL

LEFT LATERAL

The right lung is further divided by the horizontal (or minor) fissure into the right upper and right middle lobes. This fissure runs from the right midaxillary line at the level of the 5th rib across anteriorly at the level of the 4th rib.

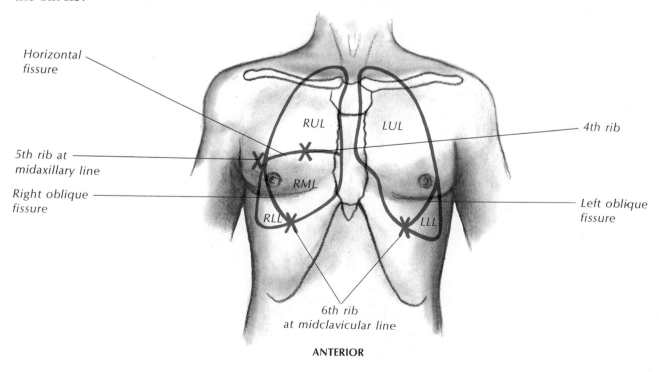

Horizontal fissure

5th rib at midaxillary line

Right oblique fissure

RUL

LUL

RML

RLL

LLL

4th rib

Left oblique fissure

6th rib at midclavicular line

ANTERIOR

Although you should be mindful of the probable location of lung lobes when examining a patient's chest and when making correlations with radiologic findings, you should usually describe your physical findings in terms that are less explicit anatomically: upper, middle, and lower lung fields, for example, or the bases (lowermost portions) of the lungs. You may then infer what lobes are involved. Signs in the right upper lung field, for example, probably originate in the right upper lobe, while those at the left base almost certainly come from the left lower lobe. Signs in the right middle lung field laterally, however, could come from any of three different lobes.

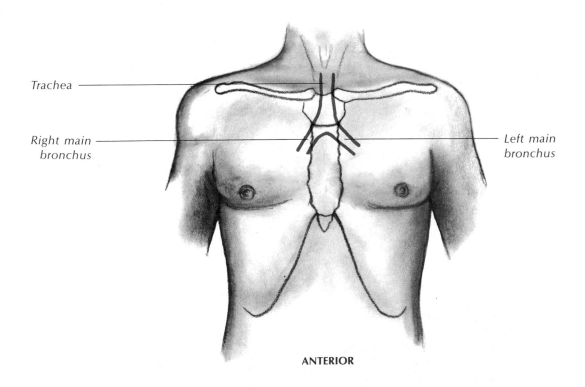

Trachea

Right main bronchus

Left main bronchus

ANTERIOR

Since certain physical findings in the chest are influenced by the closeness of the chest wall to the trachea and large bronchi, the location of these structures should also be familiar. Note that the trachea bifurcates at about the level of the sternal angle anteriorly and of the 4th thoracic spinous process posteriorly.

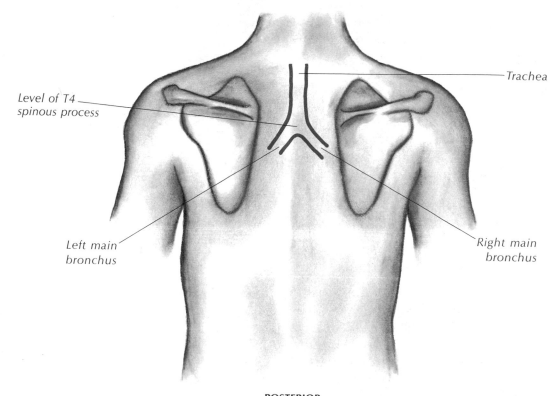

Trachea

Level of T4
spinous process

Left main
bronchus

Right main
bronchus

POSTERIOR

Breathing is largely an automatic act, controlled in the brain stem and mediated by the muscles of respiration. During inspiration the diaphragm and intercostal muscles contract, enlarging the thorax and expanding the lungs in the pleural cavities. The chest wall moves upward, anteriorly, and laterally while the diaphragm descends. As inspiratory effort stops, the lungs recoil, the diaphragm rises passively, and the chest wall relaxes into its resting position. When breathing is labored because of exercise or disease, additional muscles come into play: the trapezii, sternomastoids, and scalenus muscles in the neck during inspiration and the abdominal muscles during expiration. Watch the muscles in your own neck in a mirror as you inhale as deeply as possible.

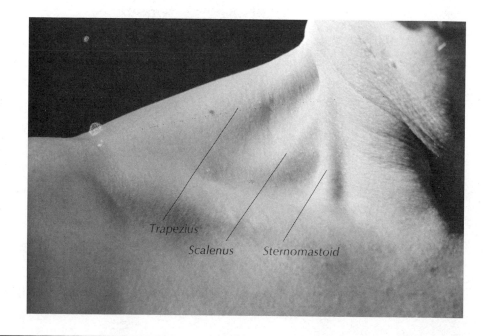

Trapezius

Scalenus   Sternomastoid

Normal breathing is quiet—barely audible near the open mouth as a faint whish. This sound has no definite pitch because it has components over a wide range of frequencies. Sound of this kind is called white noise.

Respiratory sounds originate in the larger airways and are transmitted through lung tissue to the chest wall, where you can hear them with a stethoscope. The tissues through which they pass, however, filter out their higher-pitched components. What you hear over most of the lungs are soft, relatively low-pitched sounds that last through inspiration and fade out of your range of hearing relatively early in expiration. Such sounds have been termed *vesicular breath sounds.* Listen for them on yourself or a colleague in the lower portion of the lung—in the midaxillary line, for example, or more posteriorly. Although the expiratory component of vesicular breath sounds *seems* short to the human ear, expiration in fact continues, lasting longer than normal inspiration.

When you listen near the trachea—over the manubrium or between the scapulae, for example—your stethoscope is close enough to the source of the breath sounds so that little filtration occurs. Here the breath sounds are louder and higher in pitch. This difference is most noticeable during expiration, and you can hear relatively high-pitched breath sounds throughout expiration. These expiratory sounds last as long as the inspiratory ones or even longer. Sounds similar to these when heard at greater distances from the large airways are abnormal and are called *bronchial breath sounds.*

The characteristics of these two kinds of sounds are summarized in the table below. Note the *basic qualities for the analysis of any sound: duration, pitch, and intensity.*

Characteristics of Breath Sounds

BREATH SOUNDS	DURATION OF INSPIRATION AND EXPIRATION	RELATIVE PITCH OF EXPIRATION	RELATIVE INTENSITY OF EXPIRATION	NORMAL LOCATIONS
VESICULAR	Inspiratory sounds last longer than expiratory sounds.	Low	Soft	Most of the lungs, away from the trachea and large bronchi
BRONCHIAL	Expiratory sounds are equal to or longer than inspiratory sounds.	High	Loud	Near the large airways (*i.e.,* near the manubrium and between the scapulae, especially on the right)

Just as breath sounds are transmitted through the lung and chest wall to the surface, so are the sounds of the voice. You can feel their vibrations with your hand as *fremitus* or hear them through a stethoscope as *voice sounds*. As with breath sounds, the higher-pitched components of these voice sounds are filtered out and much attenuated as they pass through normal tissues to the surface. Normal speech is heard as a relatively low-pitched, indistinct mumble; whispered words, which lack low-pitched components, are scarcely heard at all. Abnormalities of the lungs may change both breath sounds and voice sounds and are described in Table 8-3, Alterations in Breath and Voice Sounds (p. 247).

CHANGES WITH AGE

Throughout adult life a person's vital capacity (the maximal volume of air that can be expired after a full inspiration) declines slowly. So does the maximal rate of expiration. These functional changes (and others as well) result partly from the aging process, partly from disease. Skeletal changes associated with aging often accentuate the dorsal curve of the thoracic spine, producing kyphosis and an increased anteroposterior diameter of the chest. The resulting "barrel chest," however, does not by itself impair function.

Techniques of Examination

GENERAL APPROACH

1. The patient should be undressed to the waist and examined with good lighting.
2. Proceed in an orderly fashion:
   a. Inspect, palpate, percuss, and auscultate.
   b. Compare one side with the other. Variations between patients are great; to some extent at least, comparison of one side with the other allows a patient to serve as his or her own control.
   c. Develop a pattern that assures relatively complete coverage, such as from apices to the lung bases.
3. Throughout your examination, try to visualize the underlying tissues, including the lobes of the lungs.
4. Examine the posterior thorax and lungs while the patient is still in the sitting position. The patient's arms should be folded across the chest with the hands resting, if possible, on the opposite shoulders. This position moves the scapulae partly out of the way and increases your access to the lung fields.
5. Then ask the patient to lie down while you examine the anterior thorax and lungs. This supine position makes the examination of women easier because the breasts are less likely to interfere. (Many clinicians, however, prefer to examine both the back and the front of the chest with the patient sitting. Either technique is satisfactory.)

When the patient cannot sit up without aid, try to get help so that you can examine the posterior chest in the sitting position. If this is impossible, roll the patient to one side and then the other. Percuss the upper lung and auscultate both lungs in each position. Because ventilation is relatively greater in the dependent lung, your chances of hearing wheezes or crackles are greater on the dependent side.

EXAMINATION OF THE POSTERIOR CHEST

Inspection

Observe the *rate, rhythm, depth,* and *effort* of breathing. A normal resting adult breathes quietly and regularly about 8 to 16 times a minute. An occasional sigh is normal.

See Table 8-1, Abnormalities in Rate and Rhythm of Breathing (p. 245).

From a midline position behind the patient note the *shape of the chest and the way in which it moves,* including:

Deformities or asymmetry of the thorax

See Table 8-2, Deformities of the Thorax (p. 246).

Abnormal retraction of the interspaces during inspiration. Retraction is most apparent in the lower interspaces.

Severe asthma, chronic obstructive pulmonary disease, tracheal or laryngeal obstruction

Asymmetry in respiratory movement or a unilateral lag (or delay) in that movement

Unilateral impairment or lagging of respiratory movement suggests disease of the underlying lung or pleura.

Palpation

Palpation of the chest has four potential uses:

1. *Identification of tender areas.* Carefully palpate any area where pain has been reported or where lesions are evident.
2. *Assessment of observed abnormalities* such as masses or sinus tracts (blind, inflammatory, tubelike structures opening onto the skin)
3. *Further assessment of respiratory expansion.* Place your thumbs about at the level of and parallel to the 10th ribs, your hands grasping the lateral rib cage. As you position your hands, slide them medially a bit in order to raise loose skin folds between thumbs and spine. Ask the patient to inhale deeply.

Intercostal tenderness of an inflamed pleura
Although rare, sinus tracts usually indicate infection of the underlying pleura and lung (*e.g.*, tuberculosis, actinomycosis).

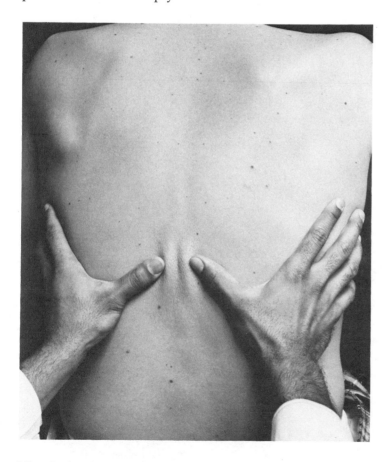

Watch the divergence of your thumbs during inspiration and feel for the range and symmetry of respiratory movement.

4. *Assessment of tactile fremitus.* Fremitus refers to the palpable vibrations transmitted through the bronchopulmonary system to the chest wall when the patient speaks. Ask the patient to repeat the words

Causes of unilateral diminution or delay in chest expansion include chronic fibrotic disease of the underlying lung or pleura, pleural effusion, the pulmonary consolidation of lobar pneumonia, pleural pain with associated splinting, and unilateral bronchial obstruction. Fremitus is decreased or absent when the voice is soft or when the transmission of vibrations

"ninety-nine" or "one-one-one." If fremitus is faint, ask the patient to speak more loudly or in a lower voice.

Palpate and compare symmetrical areas of the lungs, using either the ball of your hand (the bony part of the palm at the base of the fingers) or the ulnar surface of your hand. In either case you are using the vibratory sensitivity of the bones in your hand to pick up fremitus. Use one hand until you become thoroughly familiar with the feel of fremitus. Some clinicians find this technique more accurate. The simultaneous use of both hands to compare sides, however, increases speed.

from the larynx to the surface of the chest is impeded. Causes include an obstructed bronchus; chronic obstructive pulmonary disease; separation of the pleural surfaces by fluid (pleural effusion), fibrosis (pleural thickening), air (pneumothorax), or an infiltrating tumor; and also a very thick chest wall.

Fremitus is increased when transmission is increased, as through the consolidated lung of lobar pneumonia.

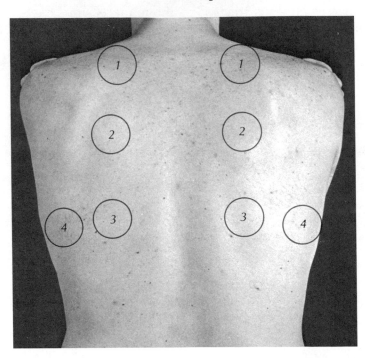

Identify, describe, and localize any areas of increased or decreased fremitus. Fremitus is typically more prominent in the interscapular area than in the lower lung fields and is often more prominent on the right side than on the left. It disappears below the diaphragm.

Tactile fremitus is a relatively rough tool, but as a scouting maneuver it directs your attention to possible abnormalities. Later in the examination you will check any hypotheses that it raises by listening for breath sounds, voice sounds, and whispered voice sounds. All these attributes tend to increase or decrease together.

Percussion

Percussion of the chest sets the chest wall and underlying tissues into motion, producing audible sounds and palpable vibrations. Percussion helps to determine whether the underlying tissues are air-filled, fluid-filled, or solid. It penetrates only about 5 cm to 7 cm into the chest, however, and will therefore not help you to detect deep-seated lesions.

The *technique of percussion* can be practiced on any surface. The key points, as described for a right-handed person, are:

Hyperextend the middle finger of your left hand (the pleximeter finger). Press its distal interphalangeal joint *firmly* on the surface to be percussed. Avoid contact by any other part of the hand, since this would damp the vibrations.

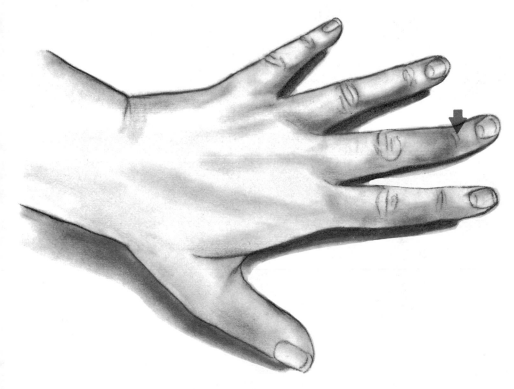

Position your right forearm quite close to the surface with the hand cocked upward. The right middle finger should be partially flexed, relaxed, and poised to strike.

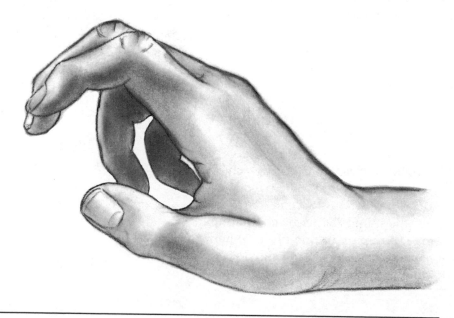

With a quick, sharp, but relaxed wrist motion, strike the pleximeter finger with the right middle finger (the plexor). Aim at your distal interphalangeal joint. You are trying to transmit vibrations through the bones of this joint to the underlying chest wall.

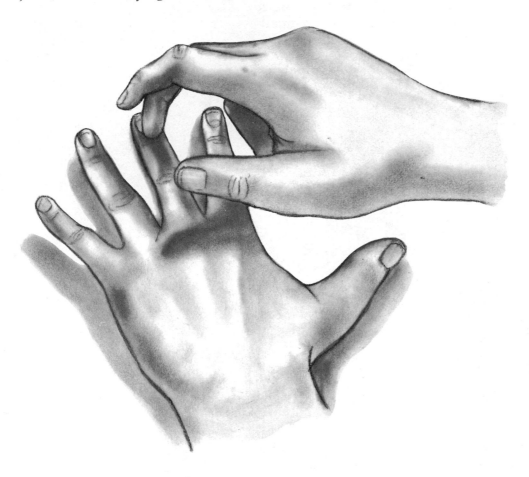

Use the tip of your plexor finger, not the finger pad. Your striking finger should be almost at right angles with the pleximeter. (A very short fingernail is required to avoid self-mutilation!)

Withdraw your striking finger quickly to avoid damping the vibrations that you have created.

In summary, the movement is at the wrist. It is direct, brisk yet relaxed, and a bit bouncy.

Use the lightest percussion that will produce a clear note. A thick chest wall requires heavier percussion than a thin one. In comparing two areas, however, keep your technique constant. Thump about twice in one location and then move on. You will perceive the sounds better by comparing one area with another than by repetitive thumping in one place. When percussing the lower posterior chest, stand somewhat to the side rather than directly behind the patient. Your hand position will feel more natural, and you will produce a clearer note.

Learn to identify five percussion notes, four of which you can reproduce on yourself. These notes can usually be distinguished by differences in their basic qualities of sound: intensity, pitch, and duration. Train your ear to detect these differences by concentrating on one quality at a time as you percuss first in one location, then in another.

Percussion Notes and Their Characteristics			
	RELATIVE INTENSITY	**RELATIVE PITCH**	**RELATIVE DURATION**	**EXAMPLE LOCATION**
FLATNESS	Soft	High	Short	Thigh
DULLNESS	Medium	Medium	Medium	Liver
RESONANCE	Loud	Low	Long	Normal lung
HYPERRESONANCE	Very loud	Lower	Longer	Emphysematous lung
TYMPANY	Loud	High*	*	Gastric air bubble or puffed-out cheek

* Distinguished mainly by its musical timbre

While the patient keeps both arms crossed in front of the chest, percuss the thorax in symmetrical locations from the apices to the lung bases. Compare one side with the other.

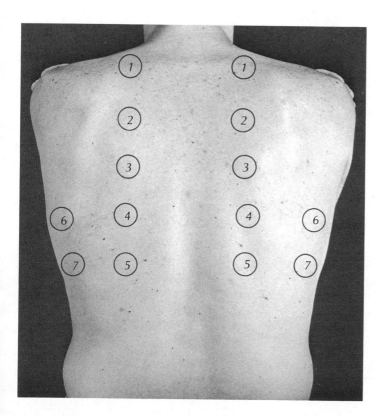

Dullness replaces resonance when fluid or solid tissue replaces air-containing lung or occupies the pleural space deep to your percussing fingers. Examples include: lobar pneumonia, in which the alveoli of the lungs are consolidated by blood cells, and pleural accumulations of serous fluid (pleural effusion), blood (hemothorax), pus (empyema), fibrous tissue, or tumor.

Generalized hyperresonance may be heard over the hyperinflated lungs of emphysema or asthma, but it is not a reliable sign. Unilateral hyperresonance suggests a large pneumothorax or possibly a large air-filled bulla in the lung.

Omit the scapular areas, since the thickness of musculoskeletal structures usually precludes worthwhile percussion there.

Identify, describe, and localize any area of abnormal percussion note.

With the pleximeter finger held parallel to the expected border of diaphragmatic dullness, percuss in progressive steps downward. Identify the level of diaphragmatic dullness on each side during quiet respiration. Check the level laterally as well as medially. As you percuss toward diaphragmatic dullness, you may first perceive a slight impairment of resonance. Continue on to frank dullness.

An abnormally high level suggests pleural effusion or a high diaphragm, as from atelectasis or diaphragmatic paralysis.

A typical left pleural effusion of moderate size is represented below.

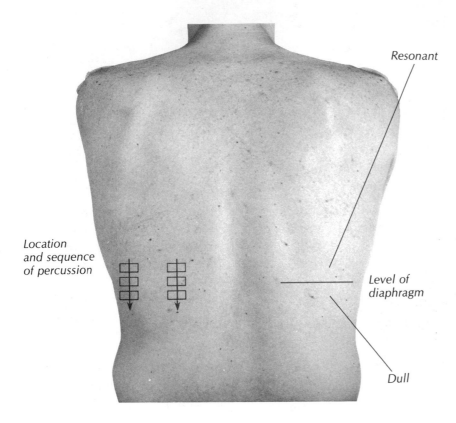

Resonant

Location and sequence of percussion

Level of diaphragm

Dull

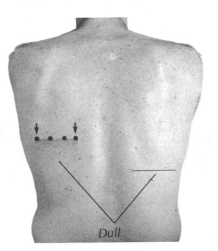

Dull

Diaphragmatic excursion may be estimated by noting the distance between the levels of dullness on full expiration and full inspiration, normally around 5 cm or 6 cm. This estimate, however, does not correlate well with radiologic assessment of diaphragmatic movement.

Note that, on each of the patient's sides, you are percussing the boundary between resonant lung tissue above and dullness below. If this boundary lies at a normal level, you infer that it reflects the normal diaphragmatic boundary between lung and solid subdiaphragmatic tissue. You cannot find the diaphragm itself by percussion, or determine where it is within a dull area like that on this patient's left.

Auscultation

Auscultation of the lungs is useful in estimating air flow through the tracheobronchial tree, detecting obstruction, and assessing the condition of the surrounding lungs and pleural space. Some clinicians prefer to use the diaphragm of the stethoscope; others, the bell.

With your stethoscope listen to the lungs as the patient breathes somewhat more deeply than normal through an open mouth. Using locations similar to those recommended for percussion, compare symmetrical areas of the lungs, from above down. Listen to at least one full breath in each location. Be alert for patient discomfort secondary to hyperventilation (*e.g.,* light-headedness, faintness), and allow the patient to rest as needed. Listen for:

Sounds from bedclothes, paper gowns, and the chest itself can generate confusion in auscultation. Hair on the chest may cause crackling sounds. Either press harder or wet the hair. If the patient is cold or tense, you may hear muscle contraction sounds—muffled, low-pitched rumbling or roaring noises. A change in position often helps.

1. The *breath sounds.* Note their intensity. Breath sounds may be decreased when the patient fails to breathe deeply enough or has a very thick chest wall, as in obesity.

   Listen for the pitch, intensity, and duration of the expiratory and inspiratory sounds. In normal vesicular breathing, the expiratory sound is relatively low-pitched, soft, and shorter than the inspiratory sound. Is this kind of sound normally distributed over the patient's chest wall? Or are there bronchial breath sounds in unexpected places?

Breath sounds may be decreased when air flow is decreased (as by obstructive lung disease or muscular weakness), or when pleural fluid or air blocks the transmission of sound (as in pleural effusion or pneumothorax).

See Table 8-3, Alterations in Breath and Voice Sounds (p. 247).

2. Any *added (adventitious) sounds* such as crackles, wheezes, or rubs. Note what kinds of sounds you hear, where in the respiratory cycle you hear them, and where on the chest wall they are located.

See Table 8-4, Added Lung Sounds: Crackles, Wheezes, and Rubs (pp. 248–249).

If breath sounds are diminished, or if you suspect but cannot hear signs of obstructive breathing, ask the patient to breathe hard and fast with mouth open. The diminished breath sounds associated with obesity may become readily audible; wheezes that were previously inaudible may appear. At the very end of a forced hard expiration, however, many normal people have a brief expiratory polyphonic wheeze.

Breath sounds remain decreased in emphysema. Wheezes may appear in asthma or bronchitis.

If you have discovered abnormalities in tactile fremitus, percussion, or auscultation, continue on to check *spoken and whispered voice sounds.*

See Table 8-3, Alterations in Breath and Voice Sounds (p. 247).

1. Ask the patient to say "ninety-nine" or "eee." Listen in symmetrical areas of the lungs, noting the intensity and clarity of the sounds. Normally the sounds are muffled. Listen also for the quality of the "ee" sound. It should be discernible as an "ee."

A change from "ee" to "ay" indicates egophony (p. 247).

See Table 8-5, Physical Signs in Selected Abnormalities of Bronchi and Lungs (pp. 250–252).

2. Ask the patient to whisper "ninety-nine" or "one, two, three." Normally the whispered voice is heard only faintly and indistinctly.

EXAMINATION OF THE ANTERIOR CHEST

The patient, when examined in the supine position, should lie comfortably with arms somewhat abducted. An orthopneic patient should be examined in the sitting position or with the bed elevated to a comfortable level.

Persons with severe chronic obstructive lung disease often prefer to sit leaning forward, with lips pursed during exhalation and arms supported on knees or table.

Inspection

Observe the *rate, rhythm, depth,* and *effort* of breathing. A normal resting patient can lie supine without respiratory difficulty and does not use the accessory muscles of respiration. If breathing seems labored and wheezy, note whether inspiration or expiration is noisier and more difficult.

The sternomastoids, scaleni, and trapezii may contract visibly when breathing is labored. Stridor is a loud, harsh musical breathing sound that unlike the wheezes of bronchial origin is chiefly inspiratory. It suggests partial obstruction of the larynx or trachea.

At the same time *listen to the patient's breathing.* In the normal resting person inspiratory breath sounds are not audible at a distance of more than a few centimeters from the mouth.

In asthma and chronic bronchitis the white noise of inspiratory breath sounds increases in intensity and may be audible even across the room.

Observe the *shape of the patient's chest* and *the way in which it moves.* Note:

Deformities or asymmetry of the thorax

See Table 8-2, Deformities of the Thorax (p. 246).

Abnormal retraction of the interspaces and supraclavicular fossae during inspiration

Severe asthma, chronic obstructive pulmonary disease, tracheal or laryngeal obstruction

Local lag or impairment in respiratory movement

Underlying disease of lung or pleura

Palpation

Palpation has four potential uses:

1. *Identification of tender areas*

2. *Assessment of observed abnormalities*

3. *Further assessment of respiratory expansion.* Place your thumbs along each costal margin, your hands along the lateral rib cage. As you position your hands, slide them medially a bit to raise a loose skin fold

Tender pectoral muscles or costal cartilages tend to corroborate, but do not prove, a musculoskeletal origin of chest pain.

between the thumbs. Ask the patient to inhale deeply. Watch for divergence of your thumbs as the thorax expands, and feel for the range and symmetry of respiratory movement.

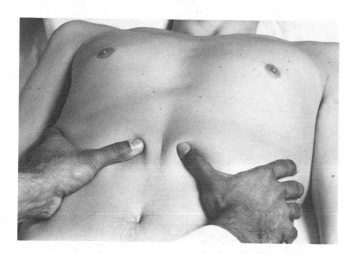

4. *Assessment of tactile fremitus.* Compare both sides of the chest, using the ball or ulnar surface of your hand. Fremitus is usually decreased or absent over the precordium. When examining a woman, gently displace the breasts as necessary.

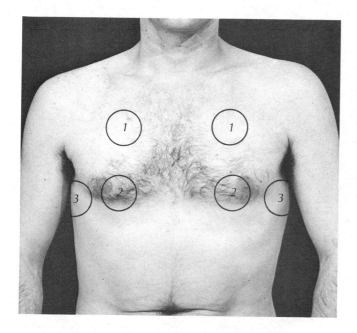

Percussion

Percuss the anterior and lateral chest, again comparing both sides. The heart normally produces an area of dullness to the left of the sternum from the 3rd to the 5th interspaces. Percuss the left lung lateral to it.

Dullness replaces resonance when fluid or solid tissue replaces air-containing lung or

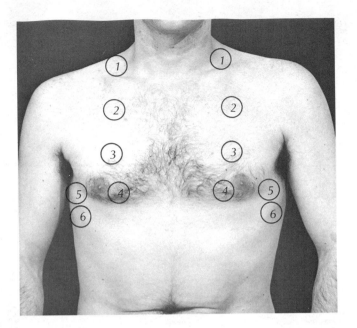

occupies the pleural space. Since pleural fluid usually sinks to the lowest part of the pleural space (posteriorly in a supine patient), only a very large effusion can be detected anteriorly.

The hyperresonance of emphysema may totally replace cardiac dullness.

When a woman's breast interferes with percussion, gently displace it with your left hand while percussing with the right.

The dullness of right middle lobe pneumonia typically occurs behind the right breast. Unless you displace the breast, you may miss the abnormal percussion note.

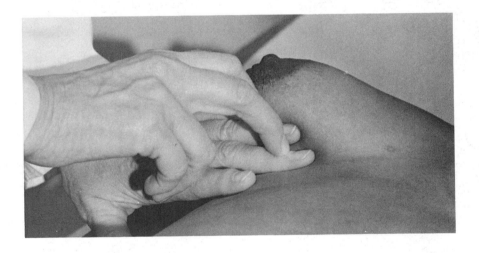

Alternatively you may ask the patient to move her breast for you.

Identify, describe, and localize any area of abnormal percussion note.

With your pleximeter finger parallel to the expected upper border of liver dullness, percuss in progressive steps downward in the right midclavicular line. Identify the upper border of liver dullness. Later, during the abdominal examination, you will use this method to estimate the size of the liver. As you percuss down the chest on the left, the resonance of normal lung usually changes to the tympany of the gastric air bubble.

An emphysematous lung often displaces this border downward. It also lowers the level of diaphragmatic dullness posteriorly.

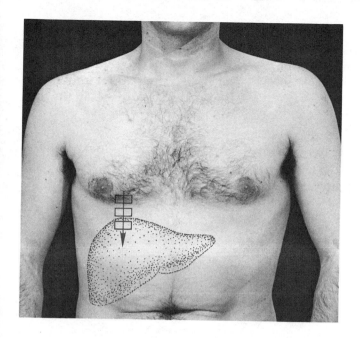

Auscultation

Listen to the chest, anteriorly and laterally, as the patient breathes through the mouth somewhat more deeply than normal. Compare symmetrical areas of the lungs, using the pattern suggested for percussion.

1. Listen to the *breath sounds*, noting their intensity and identifying any variations from normal vesicular breathing. Bronchial breathing may be heard over the large airways, especially on the right.

2. Identify any *added sounds*, time them in the respiratory cycle, and locate them on the chest wall.

See Table 8-4, Added Lung Sounds: Crackles, Wheezes, and Rubs (pp. 248–249).

If breath sounds are diminished, or if you suspect but cannot hear signs of obstructive breathing, ask the patient to breathe hard and fast with mouth open.

If indicated, proceed to *spoken and whispered voice sounds.*

SPECIAL MANEUVERS

CLINICAL ASSESSMENT OF PULMONARY FUNCTION. An informative but frequently overlooked way to assess the complaint of breathlessness in an ambulatory patient is to walk with the patient down the hall or climb one flight of stairs.

Obstructive pulmonary disease is characterized by a slowed expiratory phase. This can be clinically quantitated by measuring the forced expiratory time. Ask the patient to take a deep breath in and then breathe out as quickly and completely as possible, with mouth open. Listen over the trachea with the bell of a stethoscope and time the audible expiration. It should last less than 5 seconds. Try to get three consistent readings, allowing a short rest between efforts if necessary.

IDENTIFICATION OF A FRACTURED RIB. Local pain and tenderness of one or more ribs raise the question of fracture. By anteroposterior compression of the chest you can help to distinguish a fracture from soft tissue injury. With one hand on the sternum and the other on the thoracic spine, compress the chest. Is this painful, and where?

A forced expiration time longer than 6 seconds strongly suggests obstructive pulmonary disease if the patient understands and cooperates in the test.

An increase in the local pain (distant from your hands) favors rib fracture over soft tissue injury.

Table 8-1

Table 8-1   Abnormalities in Rate and Rhythm of Breathing

When observing respiratory patterns think in terms of *rate, depth,* and *regularity* of the patient's breathing. Describe what you see in these terms. Traditional terms, such as tachypnea, are given below so that you will understand them, but simple descriptions are recommended for use.

NORMAL

Inspiration   Expiration

— *Time* —

Volume of air

The respiratory rate is about 8–16 per min in adults and up to 44 per min in infants.

RAPID SHALLOW BREATHING (*Tachypnea*)

Rapid shallow breathing has a number of causes, including restrictive lung disease, pleuritic chest pain, and an elevated diaphragm.

RAPID, DEEP BREATHING (*Hyperpnea, Hyperventilation*)

Rapid deep breathing also has a number of causes, including exercise, anxiety, and metabolic acidosis. In the comatose patient, infarction, hypoxia, or hypoglycemia affecting the midbrain or pons should be considered. *Kussmaul breathing* is deep breathing associated with metabolic acidosis. It may be fast, normal in rate, or slow.

SLOW BREATHING (*Bradypnea*)

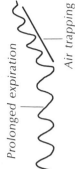

Slow breathing may be secondary to such causes as diabetic coma, drug-induced respiratory depression, and increased intracranial pressure.

CHEYNE–STOKES BREATHING

Hyperpnea   Apnea

Respiration waxes and wanes cyclically so that periods of deep breathing alternate with periods of apnea (no breathing). Children and aging people may normally show this pattern in sleep. Other causes include heart failure, uremia, drug-induced respiratory depression, and brain damage (typically on both sides of the cerebral hemispheres or diencephalon).

ATAXIC BREATHING (*Biot's Breathing*)

Ataxic breathing is characterized by unpredictable irregularity. Breaths may be shallow or deep and stop for short periods. Causes include respiratory depression and brain damage, typically at the medullary level.

SIGHING RESPIRATION

Sighs

Breathing punctuated by frequent sighs should alert you to the possibility of hyperventilation syndrome — a common cause of dyspnea and dizziness.

Occasional sighs are normal.

OBSTRUCTIVE BREATHING

Prolonged expiration

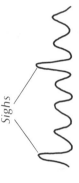

Air trapping

In obstructive lung disease expiration is prolonged because of increased airway resistance. If the respiratory rate increases, the patient lacks sufficient time for full expiration. The chest overexpands (air trapping) and breathing becomes more shallow.

Table 8-2

Table 8-2 Deformities of the Thorax

NORMAL INFANT

CROSS SECTION OF THORAX	CLINICAL APPEARANCE

The chest of the normal infant is approximately round or barrel-shaped in cross section.

NORMAL ADULT

CLINICAL APPEARANCE	CROSS SECTION OF THORAX

As a child grows to adulthood, the thorax enlarges laterally more than it does anteroposteriorly. Some increase in its anteroposterior diameter often accompanies aging.

BARREL CHEST

CROSS SECTION OF THORAX	CLINICAL APPEARANCE

A barrel chest has an increased anteroposterior diameter. It may occur with the kyphosis of aging or the hyperinflation of pulmonary emphysema.

FUNNEL CHEST (*Pectus Excavatum*)

CROSS SECTION OF THORAX	CLINICAL APPEARANCE

A funnel chest is characterized by a depression in the lower portion of the sternum. Compression of the heart and great vessels may cause murmurs.

PIGEON CHEST (*Pectus Carinatum*)

CROSS SECTION OF THORAX	CLINICAL APPEARANCE

Groove

Anteriorly displaced sternum

In a pigeon chest the sternum is displaced anteriorly, increasing the anteroposterior diameter. Grooves in the chest wall accentuate the deformity.

THORACIC KYPHOSCOLIOSIS

CROSS SECTION OF THORAX	CLINICAL APPEARANCE

High shoulder
High scapula
Thoracic convexity to right
Interspaces flared

In thoracic kyphoscoliosis the spine is curved and the thorax shows corresponding deformities. Distortion of the underlying lungs may make interpretation of lung findings very difficult.

Table 8-3

Table 8-3   Alterations in Breath and Voice Sounds

When normally air-filled lung tissue becomes airless or solid, the sounds transmitted to the chest wall through an open bronchial tree undergo much less attenuation than normal. Higher-pitched components of the sounds, which are normally filtered out, come through more readily. Characteristic alterations in breath and voice sounds occur in areas superficial to the abnormal tissue. These changes have been known as bronchial breath sounds, bronchophony, egophony, and whispered pectoriloquy, although some authorities recommend simple descriptions such as "increased clarity of whispered and spoken voice." Changes such as these are found in lobar pneumonia and near the upper border of a large pleural effusion.

BRONCHIAL BREATH SOUNDS	The expiratory sound is higher-pitched and louder than in vesicular breath sounds. It is equal to or lasts longer than the inspiratory component. Sounds like these are normal over the trachea and large bronchi but not in the more peripheral parts of the lung.
EGOPHONY	Altered filtration of sound may give a nasal bleating quality to voice sounds and change the patient's "ee" to what sounds like "ay."
BRONCHOPHONY	Voice sounds are louder and clearer than usual because their higher-pitched components are better transmitted through an open bronchial tree that is surrounded by airless lung tissue.
WHISPERED PECTORILOQUY	Like the voice sounds in bronchophony, whispered sounds in whispered pectoriloquy are louder and heard more clearly than normal. Their higher-pitched components are better transmitted through an open bronchial tree that is surrounded by airless lung tissue.

Table 8-4

Table 8-4   Added Lung Sounds: Crackles, Wheezes, and Rubs

Added (adventitious) sounds in the lungs are of two basic kinds: (1) discrete, noncontinuous sounds, called *crackles*, and (2) continuous musical sounds of greater duration, called *wheezes*. Pleural rubs are technically categorized as crackling sounds. The terminology of lung sounds, confused for over a century, is changing, and common usages vary. Rales and crepitations, for example, are older terms for crackles, and many American clinicians like to distinguish two types: the soft, very short, and high-pitched *fine crackles* and the louder, slightly longer, and lower-pitched *coarse crackles*. Moreover, a distinction may be made between two continuous sounds: the sonorous, low-pitched *rhonchus* and the sibilant, higher-pitched *wheeze*. Presented here is a simple classification that is currently gaining acceptance.

CRACKLES

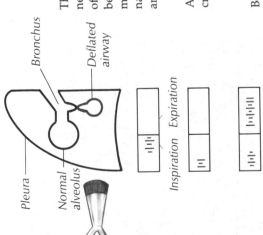

Pleura
Bronchus
Deflated airway
Normal alveolus

Inspiration   Expiration

The discrete, noncontinuous sounds termed crackles may be simulated by rolling a lock of hair between your fingers near your ear. Crackles that are heard relatively late in inspiration, as illustrated on the left, are attributed to a series of tiny explosions produced when previously deflated airways are reinflated during inspiration and air pressures between the two previously separated air-containing compartments are suddenly equalized. These conditions are met in pneumonia, and in the dependent portions of patients' lungs in congestive heart failure and diffuse pulmonary fibrosis. Crackles may also be present at the lung bases of elderly, bedridden, and some other normal people, and clear with deep breathing. These latter crackles have no pathologic significance.

A few crackles may be heard in obstructive chronic bronchitis. In contrast to the previous group of late inspiratory crackles, these tend to occur early in inspiration and are audible at the mouth.

Both early inspiratory and expiratory crackles have been described in bronchiectasis.

Loud gurgling and bubbling sounds during both inspiration and expiration may be produced by secretions in the trachea and large bronchi. Such sounds may be heard in pulmonary edema and in moribund or other patients who cannot cough up their secretions.

WHEEZES

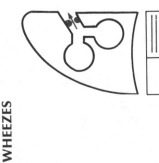

Wheezes are musical sounds produced by the rapid passage of air through a bronchus that is narrowed to the point of closure. The walls of the bronchus oscillate between closed and barely open positions, and generate audible sound.

Wheezes are characteristic of obstructive lung disease. They are typically expiratory but may occur in both inspiration and expiration. Although wheezes vary in pitch, no inferences can be made from the pitch as to the size of the airways involved. Wheezes may be subdivided according to their timing and complexity.

Expiratory polyphonic wheezes of simultaneous onset have several musical components, each with a different pitch, all starting and stopping at the same time. When these occur during quiet breathing, they indicate widespread airflow obstruction.

Table 8-4

Monophonic, random-onset wheezes also have several components with differing pitches, but the components start and stop at different times. These wheezes, which may be both inspiratory and expiratory, are often heard in bronchial asthma.

Occasionally patients with severe obstructive lung disease worsen to the point that they are no longer able to force enough air through the narrowed bronchi to produce wheezing. The disappearance of wheezing in such patients should signal concern and not be mistaken for improvement.

A persistent single, monophonic wheeze may indicate partial obstruction of a bronchus by tumor, scarring, or a foreign body. It may be inspiratory, expiratory, or both.

PLEURAL RUBS

Normal pleural surfaces move smoothly and noiselessly against each other during respiration. When pleural surfaces become inflamed, however, they move jerkily as they are momentarily and repeatedly delayed by increased friction. These movements, with their associated vibrations, produce creaking, grating sounds known as a pleural rub. The sounds are usually confined to a relatively small area of the chest wall. They are often both inspiratory and expiratory but are sometimes confined to inspiration. A friction rub is often heard only during the first day or two of a pleurisy. When inflamed pleural surfaces are separated by fluid, they no longer produce a rub.

Pleural rubs resemble crackles acoustically, although they are produced by quite different pathologic processes. Rubs, especially when confined to inspiration, may therefore be difficult to distinguish from pulmonary crackles.

The crackling sounds of a rub may be discrete, but sometimes they are so numerous that they merge into a continuous sound.

MEDIASTINAL CRUNCH
(Hamman's sign)

A mediastinal crunch is a series of precordial crackles synchronous with the heart beat, not with respiration. Best heard in the left lateral position, it is due to mediastinal emphysema.

Table 8-5

Table 8-5   Physical Signs in Selected Abnormalities of Bronchi and Lungs

CONDITION	DESCRIPTION	PERCUSSION NOTE	TACTILE FREMITUS VOICE SOUNDS, WHISPERED VOICE SOUNDS	BREATH SOUNDS	ADDED SOUNDS
NORMAL *Bronchus* *Pleura* *Alveoli*	The tracheobronchial tree and alveoli are clear; the pleurae are thin and close together; the mobility of the chest wall is unimpaired.	Resonant	Normal	Vesicular, except perhaps for bronchial breath sounds near the large bronchi	None, except perhaps for a few transient, inspiratory crackles at the bases after recumbency or sleep
LEFT-SIDED HEART FAILURE *Swollen mucosa (sometimes)* *Deflated airway*	In left-sided heart failure, some airways in the dependent portions of the lungs are deflated abnormally during expiration. The bronchial mucosa may be swollen. A pleural effusion may occur in left-sided heart failure but is not included in this section.	Resonant	Normal	Normal, or sometimes prolonged expiration	Crackles at lung bases; sometimes wheezes
PLEURAL FLUID OR THICKENING *Pleural fluid or thickening*	Pleural fluid (such as serous effusion, blood, or pus) and pleural thickening (due to scar tissue) muffle all sounds.	Dull to flat	Decreased to absent; however, bronchophony, egophony, and whispered pectoriloquy may appear near the top of a large effusion	Decreased vesicular or absent; however, a bronchial quality may appear near the top of a large effusion	None unless there is underlying disease

Table 8-5

		Percussion	Fremitus/Voice	Breath Sounds	Adventitious Sounds
PULMONARY CONSOLIDATION (e.g., lobar pneumonia) 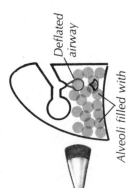 *Deflated airway* *Alveoli filled with fluid, red and white cells*	A consolidated lung is dull to percussion but, as long as the large airways are clear, fremitus and breath and voice sounds are transmitted as if they came directly from the larynx and trachea. Abnormally deflated portions of the lungs produce crackles.	Dull	Increased, with bronchophony, egophony, whispered pectoriloquy	Bronchial	Crackles
BRONCHITIS *Bronchial constriction* *Deflated airway*	In bronchitis, there may be partial bronchial obstruction from secretions or constrictions. Abnormally deflated portions of lung may produce crackles.	Resonant	Normal	May be normal but expiration is often prolonged	Vary from none to crackles or expiratory, simultaneous-onset, polyphonic wheezes
EMPHYSEMA 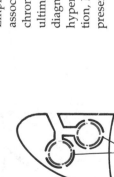 *Overinflated alveoli with destruction of walls*	Emphysema is often inextricably associated with manifestations of chronic bronchitis and is ultimately a pathological diagnosis. Persisting signs of hyperinflation and poor ventilation, however, suggest its presence.	Ranges from normal to hyper-resonant, obscuring cardiac dullness and lowering diaphragmatic dullness	Decreased	Decreased vesicular, often with prolonged expiration	None, or signs of bronchitis

Continued

Table 8-5

Table 8-5 (Cont'd.)

CONDITION	DESCRIPTION	PERCUSSION NOTE	TACTILE FREMITUS VOICE SOUNDS, WHISPERED VOICE SOUNDS	BREATH SOUNDS	ADDED SOUNDS
PNEUMOTHORAX 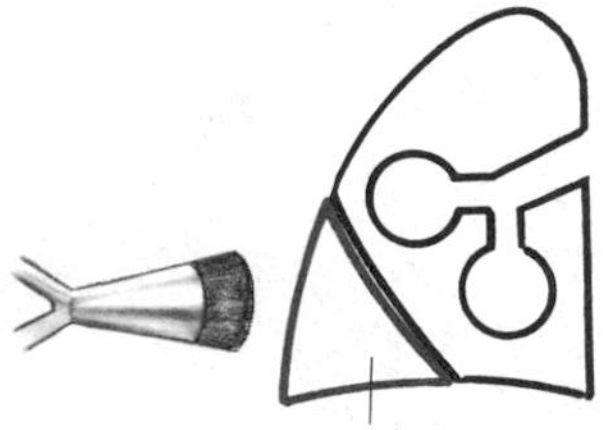 *Pleural air*	The free pleural air of pneumothorax may mimic obstructive lung disease but is usually unilateral and may shift the trachea to the opposite side. The air-filled pleural space, when big enough, gives a hyperresonant percussion note but muffles voice and breath sounds.	Normal to hyperresonant	Decreased to absent	Decreased to absent	None
ATELECTASIS 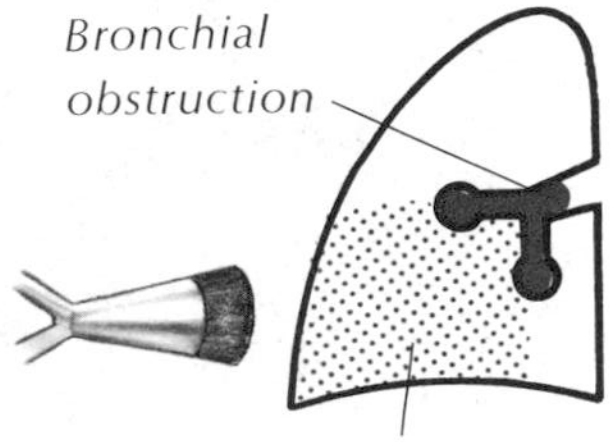 *Bronchial obstruction* *Collapsed portion of lung*	A collapsed or atelectatic lung is dull to percussion. Bronchial obstruction (shown here but not always present) prevents transmission of breath and voice sounds. The trachea may shift to the same side.	Dull	Decreased to absent	Decreased vesicular or absent	None

The changes described in this table vary importantly with the extent, severity, and nature of the disorder. A small pneumothorax may produce no abnormal signs, for example, and small areas of atelectasis are usually undetectable by clinical methods. Deep-seated abnormalities usually produce fewer signs than superficial ones and are often clinically silent. Many kinds of pneumonia, such as Mycoplasma and viral pneumonias, moreover, do not ordinarily produce extensive consolidation of lung tissue and do not, therefore, cause changes in the percussion note, breath sounds, or voice sounds. Crackles are often present, but are admittedly nonspecific.

Chapter 9
The Cardiovascular System

Anatomy and Physiology

SURFACE PROJECTIONS OF THE HEART AND GREAT VESSELS

The heart is assessed chiefly by examination through the anterior chest wall. Most of the anterior cardiac surface is made up of right ventricle. This chamber and the pulmonary artery may be visualized roughly as a wedge lying behind and to the left of the sternum.

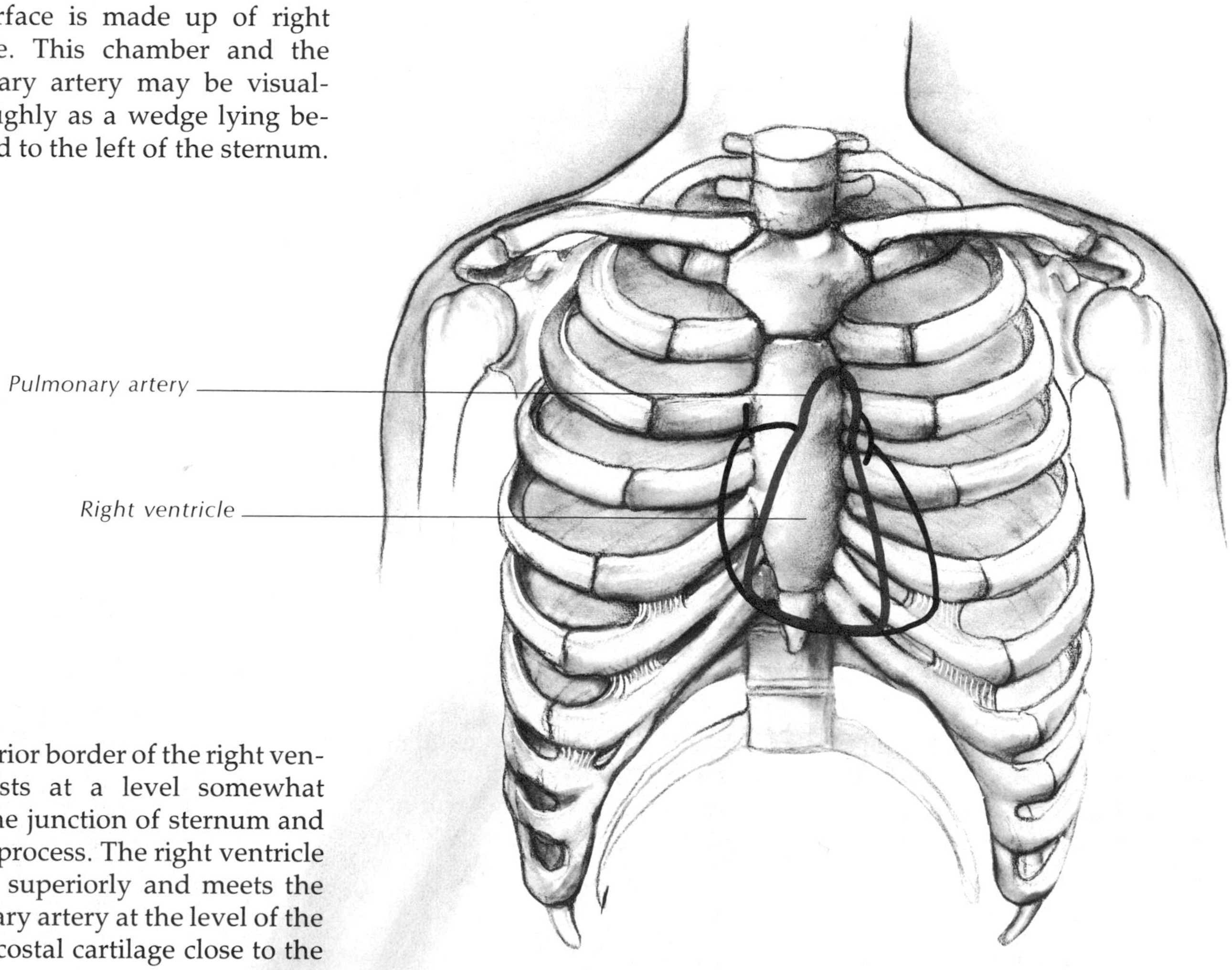

Pulmonary artery —————————

Right ventricle —————————

The inferior border of the right ventricle rests at a level somewhat below the junction of sternum and xiphoid process. The right ventricle narrows superiorly and meets the pulmonary artery at the level of the 3rd left costal cartilage close to the sternum.

The left ventricle, lying to the left and behind the right ventricle, makes up only a small portion of the anterior cardiac surface. It is clinically important, however, forming the left border of the heart and producing the apical impulse.* This impulse is a brief systolic beat usually found in the 5th interspace, 7 cm to 9 cm from the midsternal line.

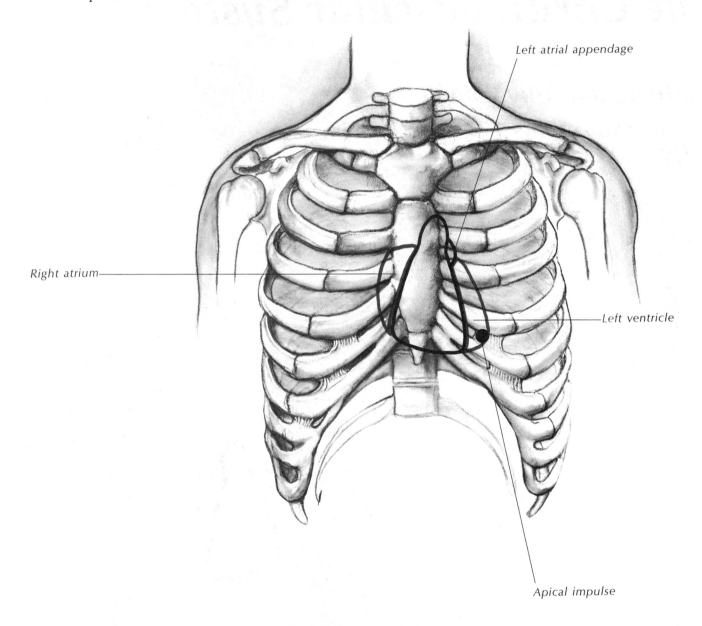

Left atrial appendage

Right atrium

Left ventricle

Apical impulse

The right border of the heart is formed by the right atrium, a chamber not usually identifiable on physical examination. The left atrium is mostly posterior and cannot be examined directly, although its small atrial appendage may make up a segment of the left cardiac border between pulmonary artery and left ventricle.

* The apical impulse is sometimes called the point of maximum impulse, or P.M.I. Since in some conditions the most prominent cardiac impulse may not be apical, this term is not recommended.

Above the heart lie the great vessels. The pulmonary artery, already mentioned, bifurcates quickly into its left and right branches. The aorta curves upward from the left ventricle to the level of the sternal angle, where it arches backward and then down. On the right the superior vena cava empties into the right atrium.

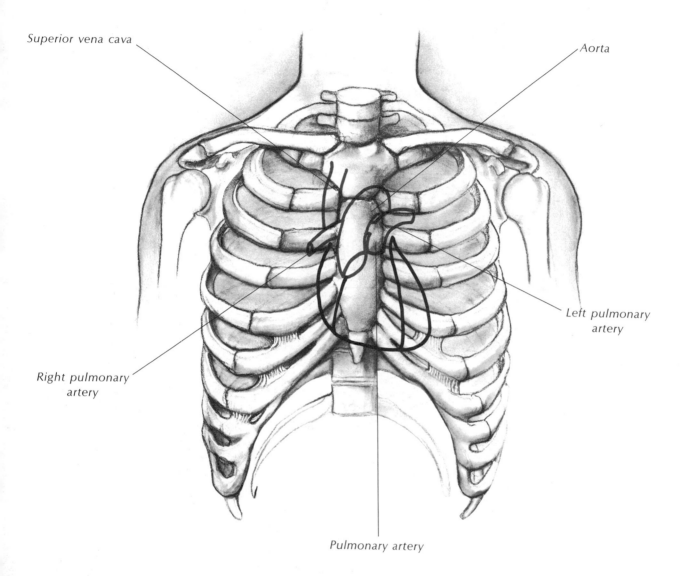

Superior vena cava

Aorta

Left pulmonary artery

Right pulmonary artery

Pulmonary artery

Although not illustrated above, the inferior vena cava also empties into the right atrium. The superior and inferior venae cavae carry venous blood from the upper and lower portions of the body respectively.

CARDIAC CHAMBERS, VALVES, AND CIRCULATION

Circulation through the heart is illustrated in the following diagram, which identifies the cardiac chambers, valves, and direction of blood flow. Because of their positions, the tricuspid and mitral valves are often called

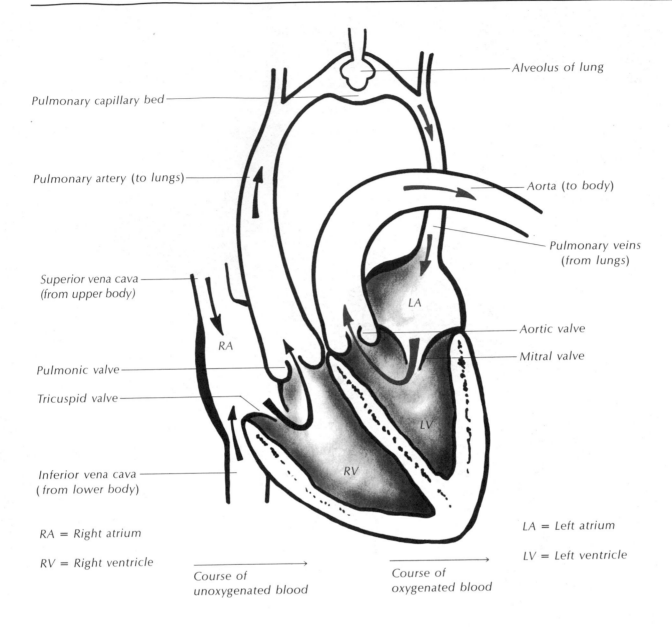

Pulmonary capillary bed

Alveolus of lung

Pulmonary artery (to lungs)

Aorta (to body)

Pulmonary veins
(from lungs)

Superior vena cava
(from upper body)

LA

Aortic valve

Mitral valve

RA

Pulmonic valve

Tricuspid valve

LV

Inferior vena cava
(from lower body)

RV

RA = Right atrium

LA = Left atrium

RV = Right ventricle

LV = Left ventricle

Course of
unoxygenated blood

Course of
oxygenated blood

atrioventricular valves. The aortic and pulmonic valves are called semi-lunar valves because their leaflets have a half-moon configuration.

Although this diagram shows all valves in an open position, they are not all open at the same time in the living heart. Closure of the valves is responsible for normal heart sounds. The positions and movements of the valves must be understood in relation to events in the cardiac cycle.

EVENTS IN THE CARDIAC CYCLE

If one were to measure the pressure in the left ventricle throughout the cardiac cycle, one would find a pressure curve like the following:

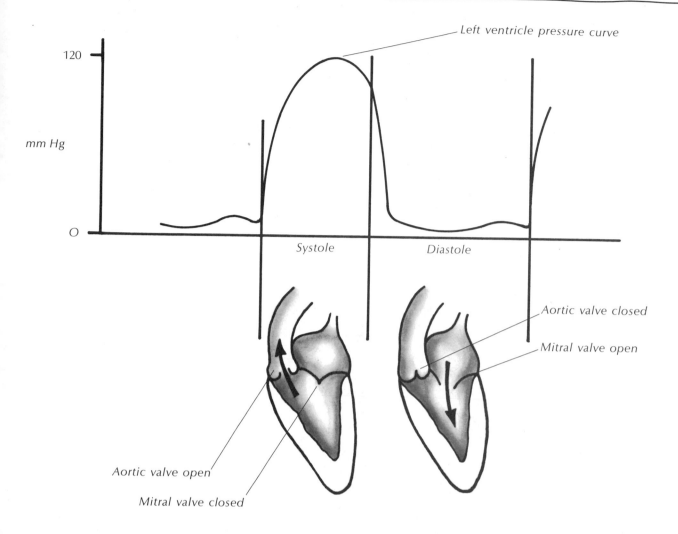

During systole the ventricle contracts, producing a rapid rise in pressure followed by a rounding off as its blood is ejected. As the ventricle relaxes in diastole, pressure falls almost to 0. Late in diastole there is a small rise in pressure because of the extra volume of blood sent into the ventricle by atrial contraction.

Note that during systole the aortic valve is open, allowing ejection of blood from the left ventricle into the aorta. The mitral valve is closed, preventing blood from regurgitating back into the left atrium. In contrast, during diastole the aortic valve is closed, preventing regurgitation of blood from the aorta back into the left ventricle. The mitral valve is open, allowing blood to flow from the left atrium into the relaxed left ventricle.

The interrelationships of the pressures in these three chambers—left atrium, left ventricle, and aorta—together with the position and movement of the valves are fundamental to the understanding of heart sounds. Events on the right side of the heart also contribute, of course, but for the sake of clarity will be discussed later.

During diastole, pressure in the blood-filled left atrium slightly exceeds that in the relaxed left ventricle, and blood flows from left atrium to left ventricle across the open mitral valve. Just before the onset of ventricular systole, atrial contraction produces a slight pressure rise in both chambers.

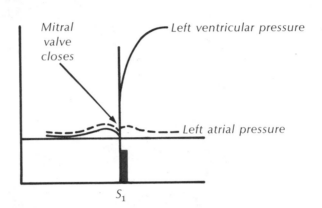

As the ventricle starts to contract, pressure within it rapidly exceeds left atrial pressure, thus shutting the mitral valve. Closure of the mitral valve produces the first heart sound (S_1).*

As the ventricular pressure continues to rise, it exceeds the diastolic pressure in the aorta and forces the aortic valve open. Opening of the aortic valve is not usually heard, but in some pathologic conditions is accompanied by an early systolic ejection sound (Ej).

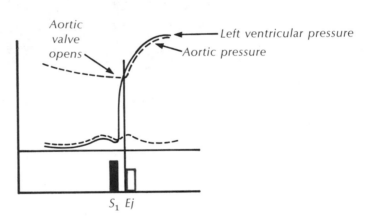

As the ventricle ejects most of its blood, its pressure begins to fall. When left ventricular pressure drops below the aortic pressure, the aortic valve shuts. Aortic valve closure causes the second heart sound (S_2).

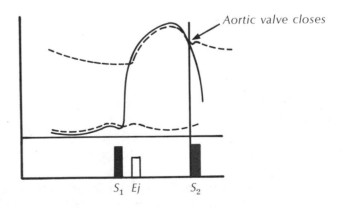

* An extensive literature deals with the exact causes of heart sounds (*e.g.*, actual closure of valve leaflets, tensing of related structures, and the impact of columns of blood). The explanations given here are oversimplified but retain clinical usefulness.

As the left ventricular pressure continues to drop during ventricular relaxation, it falls below left atrial pressure. The mitral valve opens. This is usually a silent event but may be audible as an opening snap (O.S.) in mitral stenosis.

Next occurs a period of rapid ventricular filling as blood flows early in diastole from left atrium to left ventricle. In children and young adults this period may be marked by a third heart sound (S_3).

Finally, although not often heard in normal adults, a fourth heart sound (S_4) marks atrial contraction. It immediately precedes S_1 of the next beat.

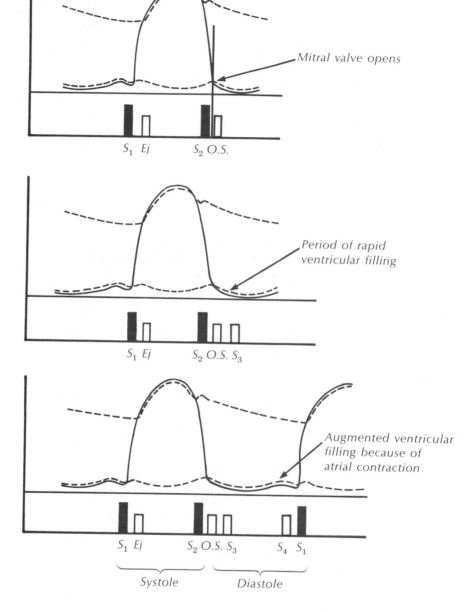

Mitral valve opens

S_1 Ej S_2 O.S.

Period of rapid ventricular filling

S_1 Ej S_2 O.S. S_3

Augmented ventricular filling because of atrial contraction

S_1 Ej S_2 O.S. S_3 S_4 S_1

Systole   Diastole

THE SPLITTING OF HEART SOUNDS

While these events are occurring on the left side of the heart, similar changes are occurring on the right, involving the right atrium, right ventricle, tricuspid valve, pulmonic valve, and pulmonary artery. Right ventricular and pulmonary arterial pressures are significantly lower than corresponding levels on the left side. Furthermore, right-sided events usually occur slightly later than those on the left. Instead of a single heart sound, therefore, you may hear two discernible components, the first from left-sided valvular closure, the second from right-sided closure.

Consider the second heart sound and its two components, A_2 and P_2, which come from closure of the aortic and pulmonic valves respectively. During expiration these two components are fused into a single sound, S_2. During inspiration, however, A_2 and P_2 separate slightly, and S_2 splits into its two audible components.

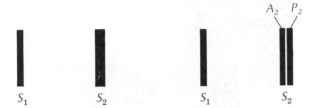

Explanations for this change are a bit complicated. Inspiration makes intrathoracic pressure more negative, draws more blood into the right heart from the systemic venous system, increases right ventricular stroke volume, prolongs right ventricular systole, and thus delays closure of the pulmonic valve. At the same time inspiration has opposite effects on the left side of the heart. The capacity of the pulmonary vascular tree is increased during inspiration, venous return to the left side of the heart decreases, left ventricular systole shortens slightly, and aortic closure occurs earlier.

Of the two components of the second heart sound A_2 is normally the louder, reflecting the high pressure in the aorta. It is heard throughout the precordium. P_2, in contrast, is relatively soft, reflecting the lower pressure in the pulmonary artery. It can usually be heard only in its own area— chiefly the 2nd and 3rd left interspaces close to the sternum. It is here that you will search for splitting of the second heart sound.

The first heart sound also has two components, an earlier mitral and a later tricuspid sound. The mitral sound, its principal component, is much louder, again reflecting the high pressures on the left side of the heart. It can be heard throughout the precordium and (like S_1 itself) is loudest at the cardiac apex. The softer tricuspid component is usually limited to the lower left sternal border, and it is here, therefore, that you should listen for a split S_1. The earlier, louder mitral component may mask the tricuspid sound, however, and splitting is not always detectable. Splitting of the first heart sound does not vary with respiration.

HEART MURMURS

Heart murmurs are distinguishable from heart sounds by their longer duration. Heart murmurs, which are generally attributable to turbulent blood flow or to vibrations of the heart valves, may be physiologic or pathologic. In the absence of heart disease, for example, blood flowing across a normal pulmonic valve may sometimes cause an audible murmur that is physiologic. Because blood is normally ejected through the pulmonic valve during systole, such a murmur is systolic in timing. If the pulmonic valve is narrowed (or stenotic), a pathologic systolic murmur is heard. If the valve is competent, *i.e.,* if it closes tightly as it should throughout diastole, no blood flows through the pulmonic valve during diastole, and diastole is silent. In contrast, if the valve is incompetent and fails to close completely during diastole, it allows blood to regurgitate back into the right ventricle, and a diastolic murmur is heard.

Knowledge of the cardiac cycle and what is happening to the chambers, valves, and blood flow during systole and diastole is essential to your understanding of the cardiac examination. Further description of murmurs is given in Tables 9-11 through 9-15.

RELATION OF AUSCULTATORY FINDINGS TO THE CHEST WALL

The locations on the chest wall where you hear heart sounds and murmurs give you important information as to their likely origins. Sounds and murmurs that originate in the mitral valve are usually best heard at and around the cardiac apex. Those that originate in the tricuspid valve are best

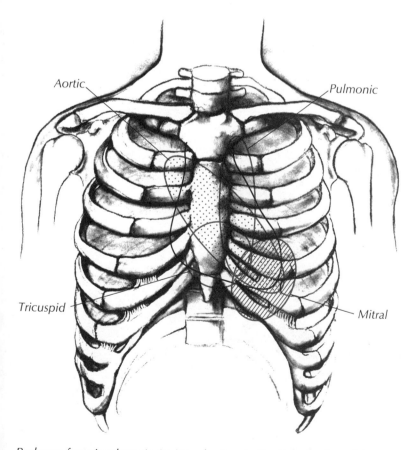

Redrawn from Leatham A: An Introduction to the Examination of the Cardiovascular System, 2nd ed, p 20. Oxford: Oxford University Press, 1979

heard at or near the lower left sternal border. Those originating in the pulmonic valve are usually best heard in the 2nd and 3rd left interspaces close to the sternum, but at times they may also be heard at higher or lower levels. And those originating in the aortic valve may be heard anywhere from the right 2nd interspace to the apex. Unfortunately these areas overlap, as illustrated on page 261, and clinicians must often infer the origin of any single finding from other data.

THE CONDUCTION SYSTEM

An electrical conduction system stimulates and coordinates the contraction of cardiac muscle.

Each normal impulse is initiated in a group of cardiac cells known as the sinus node. Located in the right atrium, the sinus node acts as cardiac pacemaker and automatically discharges an impulse about 60 to 100 times a minute. This impulse travels through both atria to the atrioventricular (or AV) node, a specialized group of cells located low in the atrial septum. Here the impulse is delayed somewhat before its passage down the bundle of His and its branches and thence to the ventricular myocardium. Muscular contraction follows: first the atria, then the ventricles. The normal conduction pathway is diagrammed in simplified form at the right.

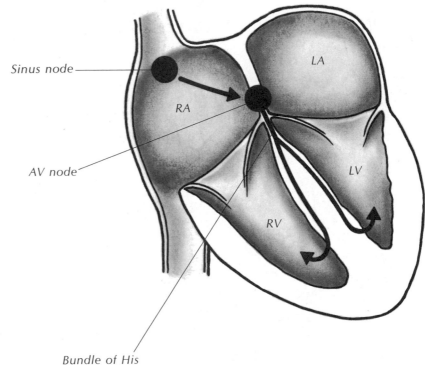

The electrocardiogram records these events. Each normal impulse produces a series of waves:

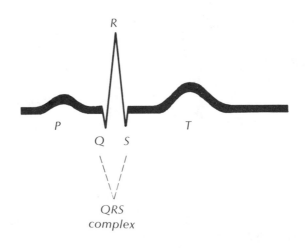

A *small P wave* of atrial depolarization (electrical activation)

A *larger QRS complex* of ventricular depolarization. Each consists of one or more of the following:

A *Q wave,* formed whenever the initial deflection is downward

An *R wave*, the upward deflection

An *S wave*, a downward deflection following an R wave

A *T wave* of ventricular repolarization (or recovery)

The electrical impulse slightly precedes the myocardial contraction that it stimulates. The relation of electrocardiographic waves to the cardiac cycle is shown below.

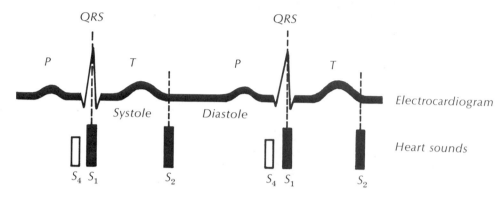

THE HEART AS A PUMP

The left and right ventricles pump blood into the systemic and pulmonary arterial trees respectively. *Cardiac output,* the volume of blood ejected from each ventricle during one minute, is the product of *heart rate* and *stroke volume.* Stroke volume (the volume of blood ejected with each heartbeat) depends in turn on preload, myocardial contractility, and afterload.

Preload refers to the load that stretches the cardiac muscle prior to contraction. The volume of blood in the right ventricle at the end of diastole, then, constitutes its preload for the next beat. Right ventricular preload is increased by increasing venous return to the right heart. Physiologic causes include inspiration and the increased volume of blood that flows from exercising muscles. The increased volume of blood in a dilated ventricle of congestive heart failure also increases preload. Causes of decreased right ventricular preload include exhalation, decreased left ventricular output, and pooling of blood in the capillary bed or venous system.

Myocardial contractility refers to the ability of the cardiac muscle, when given a load, to shorten. Contractility is increased by action of the sympathetic nervous system and decreases when the myocardium is damaged.

Afterload refers to the resistance against which the ventricle must contract. Sources of resistance to left ventricular contraction include the walls of the aorta and large arteries, the peripheral vascular tree (primarily the small arteries and arterioles), the volume of blood already in the aorta, and the viscosity of the blood.

Pathologic increases in preload and afterload, called *volume overload* and *pressure overload* respectively, produce different kinds of changes in the affected ventricles. These changes may be detectable by palpable differences in the ventricular impulses, by alterations in the heart sounds, and by the appearance of pathologic heart sounds and heart murmurs.

ARTERIAL PULSES AND BLOOD PRESSURE

With each contraction the left ventricle ejects a volume of blood into the aorta and thence on into the arterial tree. A pressure wave moves rapidly through the arterial system where it can be felt as the *arterial pulse.* Although the pressure wave travels quickly—many times faster than the blood itself—a palpable delay between ventricular contraction and peripheral pulses makes the pulses in the arms and legs unsuitable for timing cardiac events.

Blood pressure in the arterial system varies with the cardiac cycle, reaching a systolic peak and a diastolic trough, the levels of which are measured by sphygmomanometry. The difference between systolic and diastolic pressures is known as the pulse pressure.

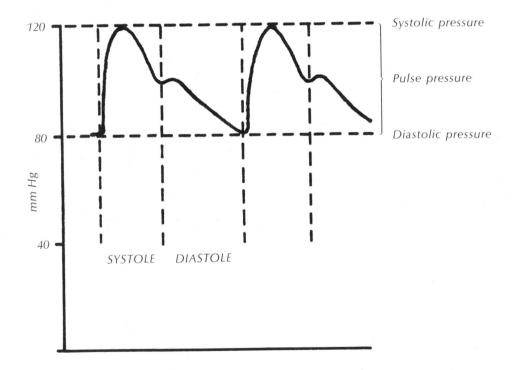

Several factors influence arterial pressure:

1. Left ventricular stroke volume
2. The distensibility of the aorta and large arteries
3. The peripheral vascular resistance, principally at the arteriolar level. This is controlled by the autonomic nerve system.
4. The volume of blood in the arterial system
5. The viscosity of the blood

Changes in any of these five factors alter systolic pressure, diastolic pressure, or both. Blood pressure levels fluctuate strikingly through any 24-hour period, varying, for example, with physical activity, emotional state, pain, noise, environmental temperature, the use of coffee, tobacco, and other drugs, and even with the time of day.

JUGULAR VENOUS PRESSURE AND PULSES

Systemic venous pressure is much lower than the arterial pressure. It is ultimately dependent upon left ventricular contraction, but much of this force is dissipated as the blood passes through the arterial tree and capillary bed. Other important determinants of systemic venous pressure include blood volume and the capacity of the right heart to receive blood and to eject it onward into the pulmonary arterial system. When any of these variables is altered pathologically, abnormalities in venous pressure result. For example, the venous pressure falls when left ventricular output or blood volume is significantly reduced; it rises when the right heart fails or when increased pressure in the pericardial sac impedes the return of blood to the right atrium.

In the laboratory, venous pressure is measured from a zero point in the right atrium. Since it is difficult to establish this point reliably during physical examination, a stable and reproducible landmark is substituted —the sternal angle. In most positions, whether a patient is upright or supine, the sternal angle is roughly 5 cm above the right atrium.

Although it is possible to measure venous pressure elsewhere in the venous system, the best estimate of right atrial pressure, and therefore of right heart function, is made from the internal jugular veins. If these are impossible to see the external jugular veins can be used, but they are less reliable. The level of venous pressure is determined by finding the highest point of oscillation in the internal jugular veins or, if necessary, the point above which the external jugular veins appear collapsed. The vertical distance in centimeters between either of these points and the sternal angle is recorded as the venous pressure. The zero point (*i.e.*, the sternal

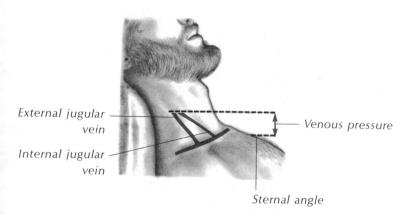

External jugular vein

Internal jugular vein

Venous pressure

Sternal angle

angle) should also be stated. A jugular venous pressure 2 cm above the sternal angle is roughly equivalent to a central venous pressure of 7 cm.

In order to see the venous pressure level, it may be necessary to alter the patient's position. In the illustration on page 265, for example, consider an internal jugular venous pressure of 0—just level with the sternal angle. The venous pulsations would be visible scarcely, if at all, just above the clavicle. By lowering the head of the patient's bed you should see them more satisfactorily higher in the patient's neck. Conversely, if the patient's pressure were extremely high—up to the ear lobe, for example—you could not be sure of its top. If you sat the patient upright, however, the top of the oscillating column would probably drop into view.

Pressures more than 3 cm or 4 cm above the sternal angle are considered elevated.

The oscillations that you see in the internal jugular veins (and sometimes in the externals as well) do not arise in the venous system itself. They reflect instead changing pressures within the right atrium. Of all the visible veins, the right internal jugular has the most direct channel to the right atrium and usually, therefore, reflects these pressure changes most satisfactorily.

Careful observation reveals that the undulating pulsations of the internal jugular veins (and sometimes the externals as well) are composed of two quick elevations and two troughs.

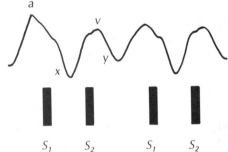

The first elevation, the *a wave*, reflects the slight rise in atrial pressure that accompanies atrial contraction. It occurs just before the first heart sound and before the carotid pulse. The following trough, the *x descent*, starts with atrial relaxation. It continues as the right ventricle, contracting during systole, pulls the floor of the atrium downward. During ventricular systole blood continues to flow into the right atrium from the venae cavae. The tricuspid valve is closed, the chamber begins to fill, and right atrial pressure begins to rise again, creating the second elevation, the *v wave*. When the tricuspid valve opens early in diastole, blood in the right atrium flows passively into the right ventricle, and right atrial pressure falls again, creating the second trough or *y descent*. To remember these four oscillations in a somewhat oversimplified way, think of the following sequence: atrial contraction, atrial relaxation, atrial filling, and atrial emptying.

To the naked eye the two descents are the most obvious events in the normal jugular pulse. Of the two, the sudden collapse of the *x* descent late in systole is the more prominent, occurring just before the second heart sound. The *y* descent follows the second heart sound early in diastole.

CHANGES WITH AGE

Cardiovascular findings vary importantly with age. The apical impulse, which is usually felt easily in children and young adults, may get harder to find with age as the chest deepens in its anteroposterior diameter. For the same reason, splitting of the second heart sound may be harder to hear in older people as its pulmonic component becomes less audible. A physiologic third heart sound, commonly heard in children and young adults, may persist as late as the age of 40, especially in women. After the approximate age of 40, however, an S_3 strongly suggests either ventricular failure or volume overloading of the ventricle caused by valvular heart disease such as mitral regurgitation. In contrast, an S_4 is seldom heard in young adults. It may be heard in apparently healthy older people, but is also frequently associated with heart disease. (See Table 9-9, Extra Heart Sounds in Diastole, p. 302.) Unlike the general population, most trained athletes have an audible S_3 and many have an S_4.

At some time over the life span almost everyone has cardiovascular murmurs. Most of these murmurs are benign in that they occur without other evidence of cardiovascular abnormality and may therefore be considered normal variants. The nature of these common murmurs varies importantly with age, and familiarity with their patterns helps you to distinguish normal from abnormal.

Children, adolescents, and young adults frequently have soft *pulmonic systolic murmurs* (see p. 306).

Many women late in pregnancy and during lactation have a so-called mammary souffle* secondary to increased blood flow in their breasts. Although this murmur may be noted anywhere in the breasts, it is often most easily heard in the 2nd or 3rd interspace on either side of the sternum. A mammary souffle is typically both systolic and diastolic, but sometimes only the louder systolic component is audible.

Many middle-aged and older adults have *aortic systolic murmurs.* These have been heard in about a third of people near the age of 60, and in well over half of those reaching 85. Aging thickens the bases of the aortic cusps with fibrous tissue, calcification follows, and audible vibrations result. Turbulence produced by blood flow into a dilated aorta may contribute to this murmur. In most people this valvular fibrosis and calcification—known as aortic sclerosis—do not impede blood flow. In some, however, the valve cusps become progressively calcified and immobile, and true aortic stenosis, or obstruction of flow, develops. The aortic systolic murmur then loses its benignity. Clinical differentiation between benign aortic sclerosis and the pathologic aortic stenosis may be extremely difficult.

---

* Souffle is pronounced soó-fl, not like cheese soufflé. Both words come from a French word meaning puff.

A similar aging process affects the mitral valve, usually about a decade later than aortic sclerosis. Here degenerative changes with calcification impair the ability of the mitral valve to close normally during systole, and cause the *systolic murmur of mitral regurgitation*. Although these changes are fairly common, a murmur of mitral regurgitation cannot be considered benign.

Murmurs may originate in large blood vessels as well as in the heart. The *jugular venous hum*, which is very common in children and may still be heard through young adulthood, illustrates this point (see p. 310). A second, more important example is the *cervical systolic murmur* or *bruit*. In older people systolic bruits heard in the middle or upper portions of the carotid arteries suggest, but do not prove, a partial arterial obstruction secondary to atherosclerosis. In contrast, cervical bruits in younger people are usually innocent. In children and young adults systolic murmurs (or bruits) are frequently heard just above the clavicle. One study has shown that, while cervical bruits can be heard in almost 9 out of 10 children under the age of 5, their prevalence falls steadily to about 1 out of 3 in adolescence and young adulthood and to less than 1 out of 10 in middle age. For further information on cardiovascular murmurs, see Tables 9-11 through 9-15, pages 304 to 310.

The aorta and large arteries stiffen with age as they become arteriosclerotic. As the aorta becomes less distensible, a given stroke volume causes a greater rise in systolic blood pressure; *systolic hypertension* with a *widened pulse pressure* may ensue. Peripheral arteries tend to lengthen, become tortuous, and feel harder and less resilient. These changes do not necessarily indicate atherosclerosis, however, and you can make no inferences from them as to disease in the coronary or cerebral vessels. Lengthening and tortuosity of the aorta and its branches occasionally result in kinking or buckling of the carotid artery low in the neck, especially on the right. The resulting pulsatile mass, which occurs chiefly in hypertensive women, may be mistaken for a carotid aneurysm. A tortuous aorta occasionally raises the pressure in the jugular veins on the left side of the neck by impairing their drainage in the chest.

In western societies systolic blood pressure tends to rise from childhood through old age. Diastolic blood pressure stops rising, however, roughly around the sixth decade. On the other extreme, some elderly people develop an increased tendency toward *postural* (or *orthostatic*) *hypotension* —a sudden drop in blood pressure when they rise to a sitting or standing position. This is an important problem with multiple, often correctable causes, and should not be missed.

Techniques of Examination

The cardiovascular examination usually starts with the heart rate and blood pressure, although both may be taken along with other vital signs at the beginning of the physical examination. The clinician then examines the arterial pulsations, the jugular venous pulsations, and finally the heart itself. Position yourself on the patient's right side.

THE ARTERIAL PULSE

By examining arterial pulses you can count the rate of the heart, determine its rhythm, assess the amplitude and contour of the pulse wave, and sometimes detect obstructions to blood flow.

HEART RATE. The radial pulse is conveniently used to assess the heart rate. With the pads of your index and middle fingers, compress the radial artery until a maximal pulsation is detected. If the rhythm is regular and the rate seems normal, count the rate for 15 seconds and multiply by 4. If the rate is unusually fast or slow, however, count it for 60 seconds.

When the rhythm is irregular, the rate should be evaluated by cardiac auscultation because beats that occur earlier than others may not be detected peripherally and the pulse rate can thus be seriously underestimated.

Irregular rhythms of this kind include atrial fibrillation and frequent premature contractions.

RHYTHM. Initial assessment of rhythm is also made at the radial pulse. Abnormalities are best assessed, however, during cardiac auscultation. In either case, the questions are the same. Is the rhythm regular or irregular? If irregular, try to identify a pattern: (1) Do early beats appear on a basically regular rhythm? (2) Does the irregularity vary consistently with respiration? Or (3), is the rhythm totally irregular?

See Tables 9-1 to 9-3, Differentiation of Selected Heart Rates and Rhythms (pp. 293–296).

AMPLITUDE AND CONTOUR. These are best assessed in the carotid or brachial arteries. The carotid reflects the aortic pulsation most accurately, but in patients with carotid obstruction, kinking, or thrills, it is unsuitable. Although either of these arteries can be felt with the fingers, the thumb is convenient and can be positioned more comfortably.

When feeling the carotid artery, first inspect the neck for pulsations. Carotid pulsations may be visible just medial to the sternomastoid muscles. Then place your left thumb on the right carotid artery in the lower third of the neck, press posteriorly, and feel for the pulsations.

A tortuous and kinked carotid artery produces a unilateral pulsatile bulge.

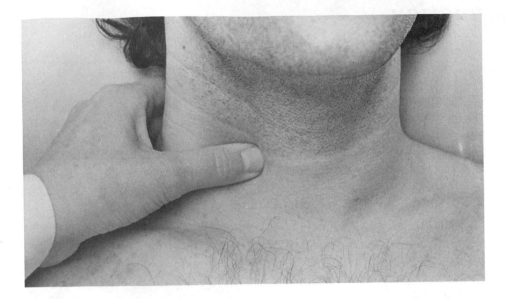

Decreased pulsations may be caused by decreased stroke volume, but may also be due to local factors in the artery such as atherosclerotic narrowing or occlusion.

Your thumb should press just inside the medial border of a well relaxed sternomastoid muscle, roughly at the level of the cricoid cartilage. Avoid pressing on the carotid sinus, which lies at the level of the top of the thyroid cartilage. For the left carotid, use your right thumb. Do not press on both carotids at the same time because you might thereby decrease the blood supply to the brain in some patients.

Pressure on the carotid sinus may cause a reflex drop in pulse rate or blood pressure.

When feeling the brachial artery, use the thumb of your opposite hand. Cup your hand under the patient's elbow and feel for the pulse just medial to the biceps tendon. The patient's arm should rest with the elbow extended, palm up. With your free hand you may need to flex the elbow to a varying degree to get optimal muscular relaxation.

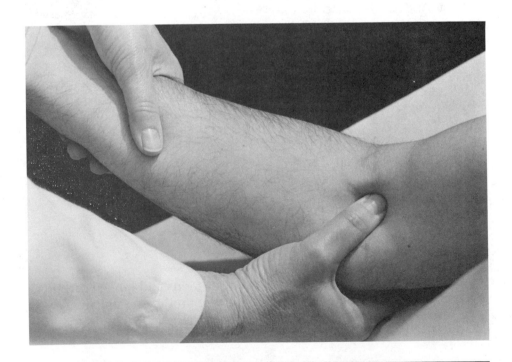

Whichever artery you use, slowly increase the pressure of your thumb until you feel a maximal pulsation, and then slowly release it. Try to assess

1. The amplitude of the pulse. This correlates reasonably well with the pulse pressure.
2. The contour of the pulse wave (*i.e.*, the speed of its upstroke, the duration of its summit, and the speed of its downstroke). The normal upstroke is smooth and rapid and follows the first heart sound almost immediately. The summit is smooth, rounded, and roughly midsystolic. The downstroke is less abrupt than the upstroke.
3. Any variations in amplitude
   a. From beat to beat

   b. With respiration

BRUITS AND THRILLS. During palpation of the carotid artery you may detect humming vibrations that feel like the throat of a purring cat. These are termed a *thrill.* If you feel them, listen over the area with the bell of a stethoscope for a *bruit,* a murmurlike sound of vascular rather than cardiac origin.

You should also listen over the carotid arteries if the patient is middle-aged or elderly or if you suspect cerebrovascular disease. Ask the patient to stop breathing for a moment so that breath sounds do not obscure the vascular sound. Heart sounds alone do not constitute a bruit.

Further examination of arterial pulses is described in Chapter 15, The Peripheral Vascular System.

BLOOD PRESSURE

CHOICE OF SPHYGMOMANOMETER. Blood pressure may be measured satisfactorily with a sphygmomanometer of either the aneroid or the mer-

See Table 9-4, Abnormalities of the Arterial Pulse (p. 297).

Small, weak pulses and large, bounding pulses (see p. 297)

Pulsus alternans, bigeminal pulse (see p. 297)
Paradoxical pulse (see p. 297)

A carotid bruit with or without a thrill in a middle-aged or older person suggests but does not prove arterial narrowing. An aortic murmur may radiate to the carotid artery and simulate a bruit.

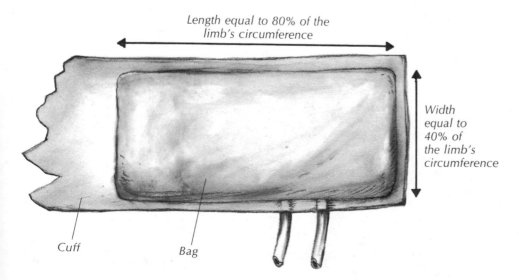

Length equal to 80% of the limb's circumference

Width equal to 40% of the limb's circumference

Cuff   Bag

cury type. Since an aneroid instrument often becomes inaccurate with repeated use, it should be recalibrated periodically. Select a cuff with an inflatable bag of appropriate size. Proper size depends on the circumference of the limb on which the cuff is to be used. The width of the bag should be about 40% of this circumference—12 cm to 14 cm in an average adult. The length of the bag should be about 80% of this circumference (range 60% to 100%)—almost long enough to encircle the arm.

TECHNIQUE. The patient should be as comfortable and relaxed as possible, the arm free of clothing. Center the inflatable bag over the brachial artery on the inside of the arm. The lower border should be about 2.5 cm above the antecubital crease. Secure the cuff snugly. Position the patient's arm so that it is slightly flexed at the elbow. Support it yourself or rest it on a pillow, table, or other steady surface, making sure that the cuff lies at heart level. Find the brachial artery—usually just medial to the biceps tendon.

Cuffs that are too short or narrow may give falsely high readings. Using a regular cuff on an obese arm may lead to a false diagnosis of hypertension. For an obese arm, select a cuff with a larger than standard bag.

A loose cuff or a bag that balloons outside the cuff leads to falsely high readings. If the patient supports the arm, the sustained muscular contraction may raise the diastolic pressure as much as 10%.

If the brachial artery is much below heart level the blood pressure will appear falsely high. Conversely, if the artery is much above heart level blood pressure will appear falsely low. A 13.6 cm difference between arterial and cardiac levels produces a blood pressure error of 10 mm Hg.

An occasional patient has an auscultatory gap—a silent interval part way between systolic and diastolic pressures. If this is not recognized, it may lead to serious underestimation of systolic pressure (*e.g.*, 150/98 in the example below) or overestimation of diastolic pressure.

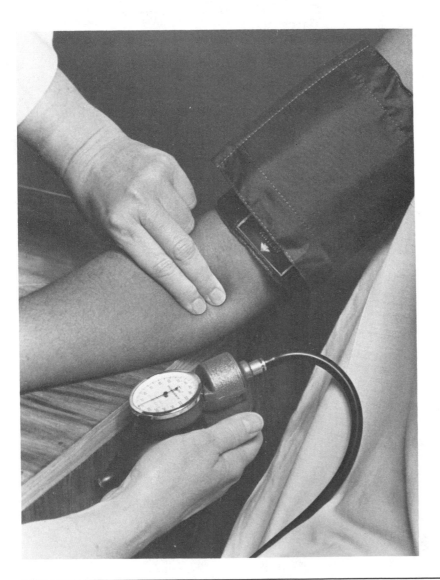

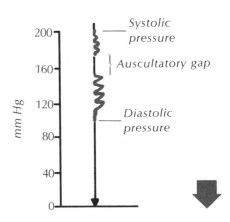

With the thumb or fingers of one hand resting on the brachial artery, rapidly inflate the cuff to about 30 mm Hg above the level at which the pulsations disappear. Deflate the cuff slowly until you again feel the pulse. This is the palpatory systolic pressure and helps you avoid being misled by an auscultatory gap. Deflate the cuff completely.

Now place the bell of a stethoscope lightly over the brachial artery. Since the sounds to be heard (often called Korotkov sounds) are relatively low in pitch, they can be heard better with a bell. The diaphragm, however, is often easier to hold in place on the arm.

If you find an auscultatory gap, record your findings completely (*e.g.,* 200/98 with an auscultatory gap from 170 to 150).

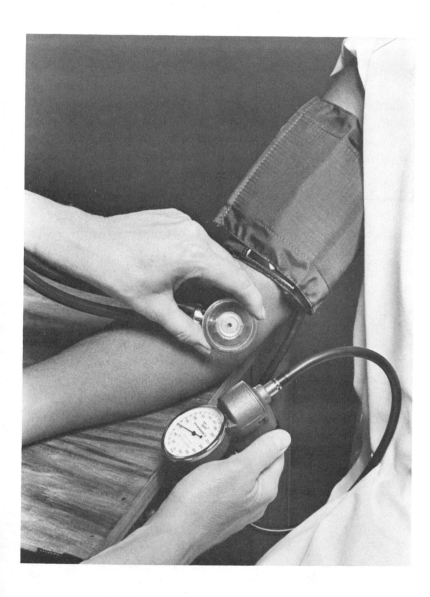

Inflate the cuff again, to about 30 mm Hg above the palpatory systolic pressure. Then deflate the cuff slowly, allowing the pressure to drop at a rate of about 2 to 3 mm Hg per second. Note the level at which you hear the sounds of at least two consecutive beats. This is the systolic pressure.

Rapid deflation will lead to underestimation of the systolic and overestimation of the diastolic pressure.

Continue to lower the pressure slowly until the sounds become muffled and then disappear. Then deflate the cuff rapidly to zero. The disappearance point, which is usually only a few mm Hg below the muffling point, marks the generally accepted diastolic pressure.

Read both the systolic and the diastolic levels to the nearest 2 mm Hg.

In some people the muffling point and the disappearance point are farther apart. Occasionally, as in aortic regurgitation, the sounds never disappear. If there is more than 10 mm Hg difference, record both figures (*e.g.*, 154/80/68).

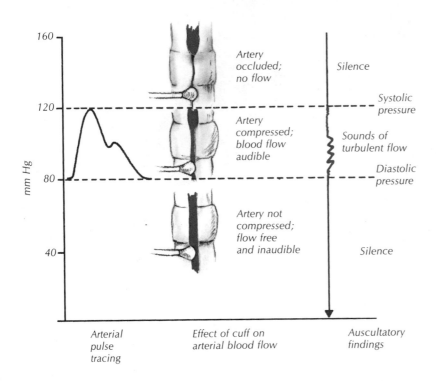

Arterial
pulse
tracing

Effect of cuff on
arterial blood flow

Auscultatory
findings

When using a mercury sphygmomanometer, keep the manometer vertical (unless you are using a tilted floor model) and make all readings at eye level with the meniscus. When using an aneroid instrument, hold the dial so that it faces you directly. Avoid slow or repetitive inflations of the cuff, because the resulting venous congestion can cause false readings. If you need to repeat your measurements, wait a minute or two after the cuff has deflated completely.

By making the sounds less audible, venous congestion may produce artifactually low systolic and high diastolic pressures.

Blood pressure should be taken in both arms at least once. You should do this too when evaluating a patient with symptoms of cerebrovascular insufficiency. Normally there may be a difference in pressure of 5 mm Hg, and sometimes up to 10 mm Hg. Subsequent readings should be made on the arm with the higher pressure.

Pressure difference of more than 10–15 mm Hg suggests arterial compression or obstruction on the side with the lower pressure. With cerebrovascular symptoms, consider the subclavian steal syndrome.

When the patient is taking antihypertensive medications, when there is a history of fainting or postural dizziness, or when you suspect depletion of blood volume, take the blood pressure in three positions — supine, sitting, and standing (unless, of course, these positions are contraindicated). Normally, as the patient rises from the horizontal to a standing position sys-

A substantial fall in systolic pressure (20 mm Hg or more), especially when accompanied by symptoms, indicates orthostatic (postural) hypotension.

tolic pressure drops slightly or remains unchanged while diastolic pressure rises slightly.

The diastolic pressure may also fall. Causes include drugs, depletion of blood volume, prolonged bedrest, and diseases of the peripheral autonomic nervous system.

Upper limits of normal adult blood pressure are unavoidably arbitrary points on a continuum. In 1984 the Joint National Committee on Detection, Evaluation, and Treatment of High Blood Pressure recommended that the diagnosis of hypertension be considered confirmed in adults (aged 18 or over) when on at least two subsequent visits two or more diastolic pressures average 90 mm Hg or higher, or when the systolic pressures on two or more subsequent visits are consistently greater than 140 mm Hg. Hypertension is further classified according to its diastolic level: mild from 90 to 104, moderate from 105 to 114, and severe at or greater than 115. Diastolic pressures from 85 to 89 are considered high normal.

Assessment of hypertension also includes the effects on its target organs—the eyes, the heart, the brain, and the kidneys. Look for evidence of hypertensive retinopathy, left ventricular hypertrophy, and neurologic deficits suggesting a stroke. (Renal assessment requires urinalysis and blood tests.)

When the systolic pressure is at or greater than 160, but the diastolic is less than 90, isolated systolic hypertension is said to be present. A systolic pressure between 140 and 159 with a diastolic pressure less than 90 is called borderline isolated systolic hypertension.

Lower limits of normal blood pressure, sometimes estimated at 90/60 in adults, should always be interpreted in the light of past readings and the patient's present clinical state.

A pressure of 110/70 might well be normal, for example, but could also indicate significant hypotension in a patient whose past pressures have been high.

SPECIAL PROBLEMS

The Apprehensive Patient. Anxiety is a frequent cause of high blood pressure, especially on a first visit. Try to get the patient relaxed. Repeat your measurements later during the encounter and on subsequent visits before concluding that the patient has persistent hypertension.

The Obese Arm. If you have difficulty fitting the cuff to an obese arm, you may apply a standard cuff to the forearm and listen over the radial artery.

Leg Pulses and Pressures. In order to rule out coarctation of the aorta, two observations should be made at least once with every hypertensive patient:

1. Compare the volume and timing of the radial and femoral pulses.
2. Compare blood pressures in the arm and leg.

A diminished, delayed femoral pulse in relation to the radial pulse suggests coarctation of the aorta or occlusive aortic disease. Blood pressure lower in the legs than in the arms is confirmatory.

To determine blood pressure in the leg, use a wide long cuff on the lower third of the thigh. Center the bag over the posterior surface, wrap it securely, and listen over the popliteal artery. If possible the patient should be prone. Alternatively, ask the supine patient to flex one leg slightly, with the heel resting on the bed. By sphygmomanometry, systolic pressure in the legs is usually found to be substantially higher than in the brachial artery. This does not reflect a true difference in intra-arterial pressures. A systolic pressure lower in the legs than the arms is abnormal.

Weak or Inaudible Korotkov Sounds. Consider the following possibilities and act accordingly:

1. Erroneous placement of your stethoscope. Search again for the brachial artery.

2. Venous engorgement of the arm from repeated inflation of the cuff. With the cuff deflated, raise the patient's arm overhead and ask the patient to open and close the hand rapidly 5 to 10 times. Try again, inflating the cuff rapidly.

3. Shock. Try to get the systolic pressure by palpation. It may be impossible to measure the blood pressure of a patient in shock without direct arterial puncture.

Arrhythmias. Irregular rhythms produce variations in pressure and therefore unreliable measurements. Ignore the effects of an occasional premature contraction. With frequent premature contractions and in atrial fibrillation, take an average of several observations and note that your measurements are approximate.

JUGULAR VENOUS PRESSURE AND PULSES

Examination of the jugular veins and their pulsations allows quite accurate estimation of the central venous pressure, and therefore gives important information about cardiac compensation. The internal jugular pulsations, although somewhat harder to see than the external jugulars, give a more accurate reading. In children under 12 years of age, however, the jugular veins and pulses are difficult to see and are therefore of little use in evaluating the cardiovascular system in this age group.

Position the patient so as to promote comfort, with the head slightly elevated on a pillow and the sternomastoid muscles relaxed. Start with the head of the bed or table elevated about 30°; then adjust it so as to maximize the jugular venous pulsations and make them visible in the lower half of the neck.

Use tangential (oblique) lighting and *examine both sides of the neck.* Unilateral distention, especially of an external jugular vein, may be deceptive: it can be caused by local factors in the neck.

Identify the external jugular vein on each side. Then *find the pulsations of the internal jugular vein.* Since this vein lies deep to muscle, you will not see the vein itself. Watch instead for the pulsations transmitted through the sur-

When the patient's venous pressure is increased, an elevation up to 60° or even 90° may be required. A hypovolemic patient, in contrast, may have to lie flat before you can see the veins. In all these positions the sternal angle remains roughly 5 cm bove the right atrium, although individual variations do occur.

rounding soft tissues. Look for them in the suprasternal notch, between the attachments of the sternomastoid on the sternum and clavicle, or just posterior to the sternomastoid. Distinguish these pulsations from those of the adjacent carotid artery by the following points:

INTERNAL JUGULAR PULSATIONS	CAROTID PULSATIONS
Rarely palpable	Palpable
Soft undulating quality, usually with two elevations and two troughs	A more vigorous thrust with a single outward component
Pulsations eliminated by light pressure on the vein(s) just above the sternal end of the clavicle	Pulsation not eliminated by this pressure
Level of the pulsations usually descends with inspiration	Level of the pulsation not affected by inspiration
Level of the pulsations changes with position, dropping as patient becomes more upright	Level of the pulsation unchanged by position

Identify the highest point at which pulsations of the internal jugular vein can be seen. With a centimeter ruler measure the vertical distance between this point and the sternal angle. Establishing true vertical and horizontal lines is difficult—much like the problem of hanging a picture straight when you are close to it. Place your ruler on the sternal angle and line it up with something in the room that you know to be vertical. Any long rectangle, such as a packaged tongue blade, makes a good horizontal line. If its short edge is parallel to the vertical ruler, its long edge should be truly horizontal. A second observer at some distance from you can often see a slanting line better than you can and help you to correct it.

Increased pressure suggests right-sided heart failure or, less commonly, constrictive pericarditis, tricuspid stenosis, or superior vena cava obstruction. In patients with obstructive lung disease, venous pressure may appear elevated on expiration only; the veins collapse on inspiration. This finding does not indicate congestive heart failure.

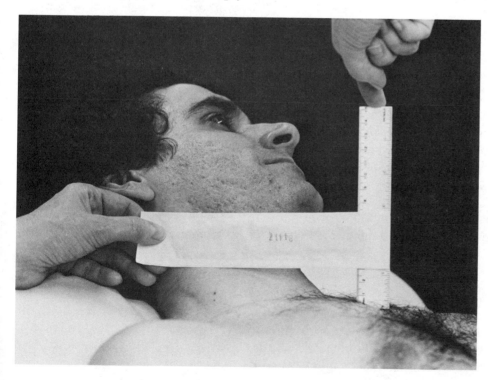

The highest point of venous pulsations may lie below the level of the sternal angle. Under these circumstances venous pressure is not elevated and seldom needs to be measured.

If you are unable to visualize pulsations in the internal jugular veins, look for them in the external jugulars, although they are not usually visible here. If you see none, identify *the point above which the external jugular veins appear to be collapsed.* Make this observation on each side of the neck. Measure the vertical distance of this point from the sternal angle.

Unilateral distention of the external jugular vein is usually due to local kinking or obstruction. Occasionally even bilateral distention has a local cause.

By either technique round your measurement off to the nearest centimeter and record it. The angle at which the patient was lying should also be included because of its possible effects on the measurement. Thus, "The internal jugular venous pulse is 6 cm above the sternal angle, with the head of the bed elevated to 45°." Venous pressure greater than 3 cm or 4 cm above the sternal angle is considered elevated.

If congestive heart failure is suspected, whether or not the jugular venous pressure appears elevated, *check for an abdominojugular (hepatojugular) reflux.* Adjust the position of the patient so that the highest level of pulsation is readily identifiable in the lower half of the neck. Place the palm of your hand on the center of the abdomen and slowly press it inward, exerting firm and sustained pressure for 30 to 60 seconds. Your hand must be warm, and the patient should remain relaxed and breathing easily. If your hand is pressing on a tender area, move it elsewhere on the abdomen. Watch for an increase in the jugular venous pressure. A transient rise is normal.

Rapid pressure, a cold hand, and producing pain may provoke a Valsalva response, thus raising the venous pressure in a normal person.

A sustained rise in pressure otherwise suggests right ventricular failure but may also be seen in obstructive pulmonary disease.

Observe the amplitude and timing of the jugular venous pulsations. In order to time these pulsations, feel the left carotid artery with your right thumb or listen to the heart simultaneously. The *a* wave just precedes S_1 and the carotid pulse, the *x* descent can be seen as a systolic collapse, the *v* wave almost coincides with S_2, and the *y* descent follows early in diastole. Look for absent or unusually prominent waves.

The *a* waves disappear in atrial fibrillation.

Giant *a* waves are seen in tricuspid stenosis and severe cor pulmonale.

Considerable practice and experience are required to master jugular venous pulsations. A beginner is probably well advised to concentrate primarily on jugular venous pressure.

Large *v* waves characterize tricuspid regurgitation.

THE HEART

For most of the cardiac examination the patient should be supine with the upper body raised by elevating the head of the bed or table to about 30°. When examining a woman with large breasts, gently displace the left breast upward or laterally as necessary. Alternatively, ask her to do this for you. The room must be quiet.

Abnormalities should be described in terms of

1. Their timing in relation to the cardiac cycle
2. Their location on the chest wall as defined by interspaces and their distance from the midsternal, midclavicular, or axillary lines. Although the midsternal line offers the most reliable zero point for measurement, the midclavicular line gives a reference point that varies appropriately with the size of the patient.
3. The effects of special maneuvers such as changing the patient's position or having the patient breathe in particular ways

Inspection and Palpation

By inspecting the anterior chest you can often see cardiovascular pulsations. You may even be able to see ventricular movements such as those associated with S_3 and S_4 without being able to feel them. Further, visible pulsations help you to place your palpating fingers correctly. Tangential lighting is necessary to see these movements. Use a good, steady penlight or a gooseneck lamp. Observing the chest surface tangentially is also useful, allowing you to see the pulsations at their maximal amplitude.

Palpation yields further information. In addition to feeling S_3 and S_4 you may be able to detect relatively high-pitched and invisible heart sounds such as an accentuated S_2. When feeling for impulses that accompany heart sounds, use the undersurfaces of your fingertips. Use light pressure when feeling for the low-pitched S_3 and S_4, and firmer pressure when feeling for the relatively high-pitched S_1 and S_2.

You may also be able to feel the thrills that accompany loud heart murmurs. Thrills, like tactile fremitus, are usually best felt through bone — the ball of your hand pressed firmly on the chest surface. Apical thrills are best felt with the patient lying on the left side and holding the breath out. Aortic and pulmonic thrills are best felt during held expiration but with the patient supine or leaning forward.

Thrills most often accompany loud harsh or rumbling murmurs such as those of aortic stenosis, patent ductus arteriosus, ventricular septal defect, and mitral stenosis.

The term "thrill," which patients can easily misinterpret, should be explained to them whenever it is used.

In order to time what you observe in relation to the cardiac cycle, you can use two methods:

1. Listen simultaneously to the heart with a stethoscope. When listening at the apex you can watch the movements of the stethoscope as they reflect left ventricular contraction and can note their relation to the first and second heart sounds. You can also listen at the apex while watching or feeling impulses elsewhere on the chest.

At normal and slow rates, S_1 is the first of the paired heart sounds, following the longer diastolic period and preceding the shorter systole. The first sound at the apex is usually, but not always, louder than the second.

If S_1 is softer than usual and indistinguishable from S_2 because of a rapid heart rate, try listening at the base of the heart, where S_2 is usually louder.

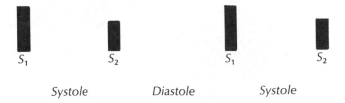

S_1 S_2 S_1 S_2

Systole   *Diastole*   *Systole*

2. Feel the carotid impulse in the neck with your left thumb as you inspect or palpate the chest. The carotid impulse is systolic.

As you start your observations walk to the foot of the bed or table briefly and inspect the chest from this position, noting any asymmetry of the thorax.

A left precordial bulge suggests cardiac enlargement that developed before puberty. It is occasionally seen in cardiomegaly of adult onset.

Return to the patient's right side and carefully inspect the entire anterior chest for pulsations, paying special attention to the five areas illustrated here:

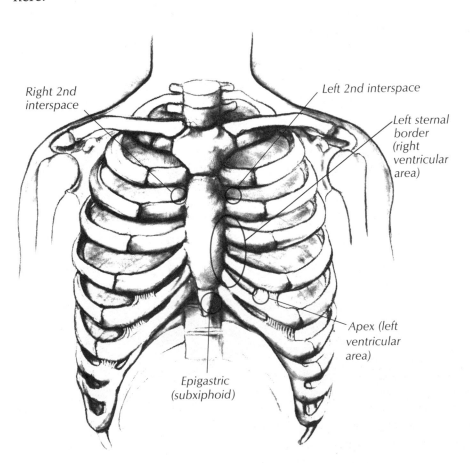

Right 2nd interspace

Left 2nd interspace

Left sternal border (right ventricular area)

Apex (left ventricular area)

Epigastric (subxiphoid)

THE CARDIAC APEX (LEFT VENTRICULAR AREA). This is normally at or medial to the midclavicular line in the 5th or possibly the 4th interspace. Here you can often see the apical impulse, the brief early systolic pulsation of the left ventricle as it rotates to the right and upward and touches the chest wall.

The apical impulse may not be visible in the supine patient and is typically best felt in the partial left lateral decubitus position. Ask the patient to roll partly onto the left side and look again. Then feel for the impulse. If inspection does not reveal its location, search for it first with the palmar surfaces of several fingers.

Cardiac impulses lateral to the midclavicular line suggest cardiac enlargement or displacement.

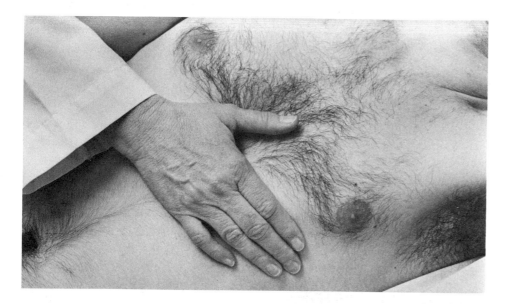

An occasional patient has dextrocardia—a heart situated on the right side. The apical impulse will then be found on the right. If you cannot find an apical impulse, percuss for the dullness of heart and liver and for the tympany of the stomach. In situs inversus, all three of these structures are on opposite sides from normal. A right-sided heart (dextrocardia) with a normally placed liver and stomach is usually associated with congenital heart disease.

If you cannot find it, ask the patient to exhale fully and stop breathing for a few seconds. Once you have found the apical impulse, make finer assessments with your fingertips, and then with one finger.

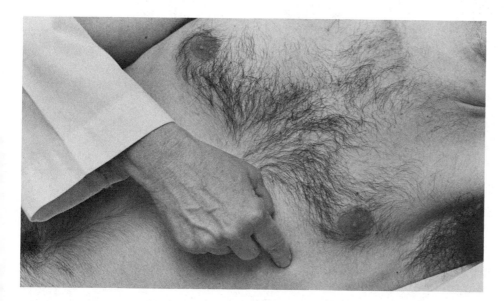

Obesity, a very muscular chest wall, and pulmonary emphysema may make the apical impulse undetectable.

Assess the location, diameter, amplitude, and duration of the apical impulse. Having the patient breathe out and briefly stop breathing is helpful in this assessment.

Location. The left lateral decubitus position displaces the apical impulse to the left and makes the assessment of location more difficult. If it is at or inside the midclavicular line, however, the location is normal. Otherwise try to assess it again later when the patient is in the supine position. Note the interspace(s) that the impulse occupies and its distance from the midsternal or midclavicular line.

Diameter. The diameter of the normal apical impulse is about 1 cm to 2 cm.

Amplitude. The usual apical impulse is small in amplitude and feels like a gentle tap. An increased amplitude, referred to as a hyperkinetic impulse, may be felt in some young, thin persons, especially with excitement or after exercise. Duration of the impulse, however, is normal.

Duration. To assess duration listen to the heart sounds while you are feeling the apical impulse, or watch the movement of your stethoscope as you listen at the apex. Estimate the proportion of systole occupied by the apical impulse. The normal impulse may be sustained during the first two thirds of systole, often less, but does not continue to the second heart sound.

By inspection and palpation you may also be able to detect the ventricular movements that are synchronous with pathologic third and fourth heart sounds. For the left ventricular impulses, feel the apical beat gently with one finger. The patient should lie partly on the left side, breathe out, and briefly stop breathing. A brief mid-diastolic impulse indicates an S_3; an impulse just before the systolic apical beat itself indicates an S_4. By inking an X on the apex you may be able to see these movements.

THE LEFT STERNAL BORDER IN THE 3RD, 4TH, AND 5TH INTERSPACES (RIGHT VENTRICULAR AREA). The patient should rest supine at 30°. Place the tips of your curved fingers in the 3rd, 4th, and 5th interspaces

---

Examples of Abnormalities

See Table 9-5, Variations and Abnormalities of the Ventricular Impulses (p. 298).

The apical impulse may be displaced upward and to the left by pregnancy or a high left diaphragm. It may also be displaced by deformities of the thorax, by a mediastinal shift, or by enlargement of the heart.

An area greater than 2 × 2 cm suggests left ventricular enlargement.

Amplitude is increased in hyperkinetic states (*e.g.,* hyperthyroidism, severe anemia), in pressure overload of the left ventricle (*e.g.,* aortic stenosis), and in volume overload of the left ventricle (*e.g.,* mitral regurgitation).

Sustained contraction that approaches the second heart sound indicates left ventricular enlargement. A sustained impulse without displacement suggests pressure overload as the cause. A sustained but hypokinetic impulse (decreased amplitude) is noted in the dilated heart of cardiomyopathy.

For the significance of these movements and their associated sounds, see Table 9-9, Extra Heart Sounds in Diastole (p. 302).

and try to feel the systolic impulse of the right ventricle. Again, asking the patient to breathe out and hold the breath out improves your observation.

A marked increase in amplitude with little or no change in duration occurs in chronic volume overload of the right ventricle, as from an atrial septal defect.

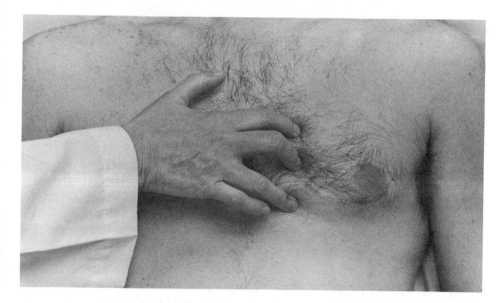

If an impulse is palpable, assess it according to location, amplitude, and duration. A brief systolic tap of low or slightly increased amplitude is sometimes felt in thin or shallow-chested persons, especially when stroke volume is increased, as by anxiety.

An impulse with increased amplitude and duration occurs with pressure overload of the right ventricle, as in pulmonic stenosis or pulmonary hypertension.

The diastolic movements of right-sided third and fourth heart sounds may also be felt. Feel for them in the 4th and 5th left interspaces. Time them by auscultation or carotid palpation.

See Table 9-9, Extra Heart Sounds in Diastole (p. 302).

THE EPIGASTRIC (SUBXIPHOID) AREA, where the right ventricle may also be felt. With your hand flattened, press your index finger just under the rib

In pulmonary emphysema, hyperinflated lung may prevent palpation of an enlarged right ventricle in the left parasternal area. The impulse is easily felt, however, high in the epigastrium. In such patients heart sounds are often heard best here also.

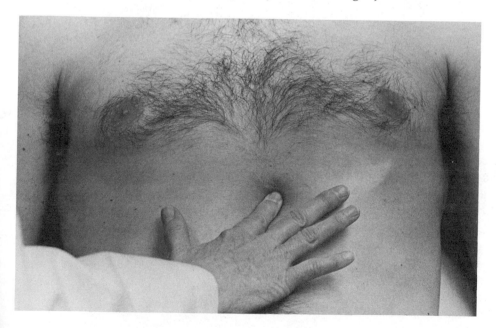

cage and up toward the left shoulder and try to feel right ventricular pulsations.

Asking the patient to inhale and hold the breath is helpful here. The inspiratory position moves your hand well away from the pulsations of the abdominal aorta, which might otherwise be confusing.

The diastolic movements of S_3 and S_4 may also be felt in this location.

THE LEFT 2ND INTERSPACE, which overlies the *pulmonary artery*. During held expiration, look and feel for an impulse and feel for possible heart sounds. Firmer pressure is needed for the heart sounds. In thin or shallow-chested people the pulsation of a pulmonary artery may sometimes be felt here, especially after exercise or with excitement.

A prominent pulsation here often accompanies dilatation or increased flow in the pulmonary artery. A palpable second heart sound suggests increased pressure in the pulmonary artery (pulmonary hypertension).

THE RIGHT 2ND INTERSPACE. You are again searching for pulsations and palpable heart sounds by the techniques just described.

A palpable second heart sound suggests systemic hypertension.

Percussion

In most cases palpation has replaced percussion in the estimation of cardiac size. When you cannot feel the apical impulse, however, percussion may suggest where to search for it. Occasionally percussion may be your only tool. Under these circumstances cardiac dullness often occupies a large area. Starting well to the left on the chest, percuss from resonance toward cardiac dullness in the 3rd, 4th, 5th, and possibly the 6th interspaces.

A markedly dilated failing heart may have a hypokinetic apical impulse that is displaced far to the left. A large pericardial effusion may make the impulse undetectable.

Auscultation

LOCATIONS. You should listen to the heart with your stethoscope in the right 2nd interspace close to the sternum, along the left sternal border in each interspace from the 2nd through the 5th, and at the apex.

In the past most of these areas have had auscultatory names (shown in parentheses on p. 285 because they are still commonly used). Because murmurs of more than one origin may occur in a given area these names may be misleading, and some authorities now discourage their use.

The areas designated on page 285 should not limit your auscultation. If the heart is enlarged or displaced, you should alter your pattern accordingly. You should also listen in any area where you have observed an abnormality, and you should listen in areas adjacent to murmurs in order to determine where they are loudest and to trace their radiation.

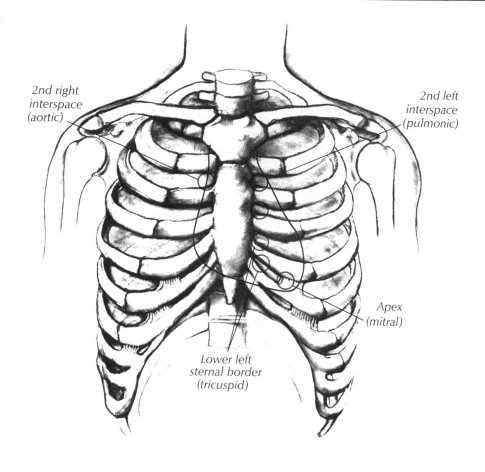

*2nd right
interspace
(aortic)*

*2nd left
interspace
(pulmonic)*

*Apex
(mitral)*

*Lower left
sternal border
(tricuspid)*

Heart sounds and murmurs that originate in the four valves are illustrated in the diagram below. Pulmonary sounds are usually best heard in the 2nd and 3rd left interspaces but may extend further.

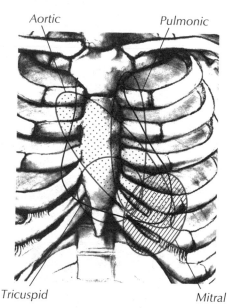

Aortic   *Pulmonic*

Tricuspid   *Mitral*

(*Redrawn from Leatham A: Introduction to the Examination of the Cardiovascular System, 2nd ed, p 20. Oxford: Oxford University Press, 1979*)

SEQUENCE. Clinicians vary in their sequence of auscultation, some preferring to start at the base, others preferring to start at the apex. Either pattern is satisfactory.

USE OF THE STETHOSCOPE. You should listen throughout the precordium with the diaphragm of your stethoscope, pressing it firmly on the chest. The diaphragm is better for picking up relatively high-pitched sounds such as S_1, S_2, the murmurs of aortic and mitral regurgitation, and pericardial friction rubs. The bell is more sensitive to low-pitched sounds such as S_3, S_4, and the murmur of mitral stenosis. Use the bell at the apex and more medially along the lower sternal border. Apply it lightly, with just enough pressure to produce an air seal with its full rim.

PATIENT POSITIONS. Listen to the entire precordium with the patient supine, as previously described, but use two other positions in addition:

1. Ask the patient to *roll partly onto the left side,* thus bringing the left ventricle closer to the chest wall. Place the bell of your stethoscope lightly on the apical impulse.

This position accentuates or brings out a left-sided S₃ and S₄ and mitral murmurs, especially the murmur of mitral stenosis. You may otherwise miss these important findings.

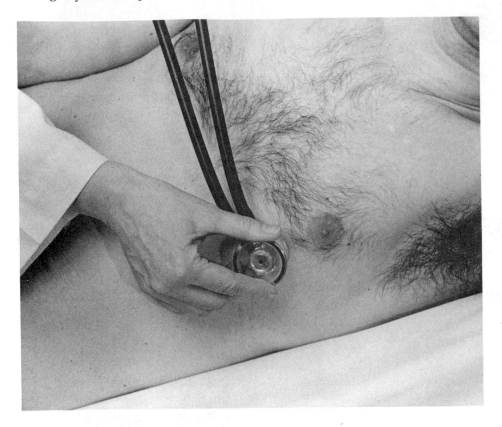

2. Ask the patient to *sit up, lean forward, exhale completely,* and *stop breathing* in expiration. With the diaphragm of your stethoscope pressed on the chest, listen along the left sternal border and at the apex, pausing periodically so the patient may breathe.

This position accentuates or brings out aortic murmurs. You may easily miss the murmur of aortic regurgitation unless you use this position.

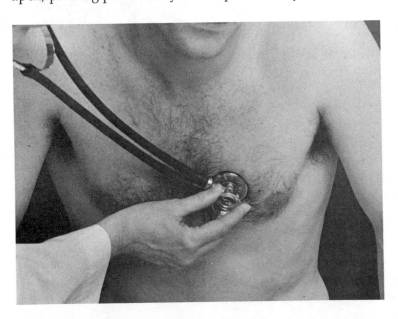

Asking the patient to sit up from a lying position may also be useful. Do this when evaluating a split S_2 that fails to disappear when the patient is supine. Expiratory splitting should disappear when the patient sits up. Moreover, innocent pulmonic murmurs often disappear when the patient is in the sitting position.

WHAT TO LISTEN FOR. Throughout your examination take your time at each auscultatory area, concentrating in turn on each of the six following points:

1. Listen carefully to the first heart sound. Note its intensity and any apparent splitting. Normal splitting is often detectable along the lower left sternal border.

See Table 9-6, Variations in the First Heart Sound (p. 299).

2. Listen to the second heart sound. Note its intensity. In the left 2nd and 3rd interspaces pay special attention to splitting of this sound. Ask the patient to breathe quietly, then slightly more deeply than normal. Does S_2 split? When? How wide is the split? Does the split decrease or disappear, as it should, during expiration?

See Table 9-7, Variations in the Second Heart Sound (p. 300).

If splitting persists in expiration, two maneuvers may fuse it, thus suggesting its normality: (a) listen with the patient sitting up, and (b) ask the patient to strain down (a Valsalva maneuver).

Causes of persistent splitting include delayed closure of the pulmonic valve (as in right bundle branch block, pulmonic stenosis, atrial septal defect, and right ventricular failure) and early closure of the aortic valve (as in mitral regurgitation).

A thick chest wall or an increased anteroposterior diameter of the chest, as in aging, may make the pulmonic component of S_2 inaudible. In some patients deeper breathing may bring out the splitting.

3. Listen for extra sounds in systole such as ejection sounds or systolic clicks. Note their location, timing, intensity, pitch, and the effects of respiration on the sounds.

The systolic click of mitral valve prolapse is the most common of these sounds. See Table 9-8, Extra Heart Sounds in Systole (p. 301).

4. Listen for extra sounds in diastole such as S_3, S_4, or an opening snap. Note their location, timing, intensity, pitch, and the effects of respiration on the sounds.

See Table 9-9, Extra Heart Sounds in Diastole (p. 302).

See Table 9-10, Causes of an Apparently Split First Heart Sound (p. 303).

5. Listen for systolic murmurs. Murmurs are differentiated from heart sounds by their longer duration.

See Table 9-11, Mechanisms of Heart Murmurs (p. 304).

6. Listen for diastolic murmurs.

If a murmur is present, describe it in terms of its timing, shape, intensity, pitch, quality, location of maximal intensity, and radiation.

TIMING. You must first be sure whether you are hearing a *systolic murmur,* which occurs somewhere between S_1 and S_2, or a *diastolic murmur,* which occurs somewhere between S_2 and S_1.

Diastolic murmurs usually indicate heart disease. Systolic murmurs may indicate heart disease but often occur when the heart is entirely normal.

An occasional murmur, such as that caused by a patent ductus arteriosus, starts in systole and continues without pause through S_2 into but not necessarily throughout diastole. It is then called a *continuous* murmur.

The combination of two murmurs—one systolic and the other diastolic, each with its own characteristics—is not a continuous murmur although it might have similar timing.

Systolic murmurs are further divided into two principal categories:

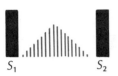 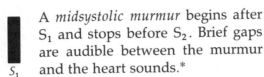

A *midsystolic murmur* begins after S_1 and stops before S_2. Brief gaps are audible between the murmur and the heart sounds.*

Midsystolic murmurs most often are related to blood flow across the semilunar valves. See Table 9-12, Midsystolic Murmurs (pp. 305–306).

 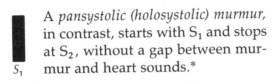

A *pansystolic (holosystolic) murmur,* in contrast, starts with S_1 and stops at S_2, without a gap between murmur and heart sounds.*

Pansystolic murmurs often occur with regurgitant (backward) flow across the atrioventricular valves. See Table 9-13, Pansystolic Murmurs (p. 307).

Diastolic murmurs are divided into 3 categories:

An *early diastolic* murmur starts immediately after S_2, without a discernible gap, and then usually fades into silence before the next S_1.*

Early diastolic murmurs typically accompany regurgitant flow across incompetent semilunar valves.

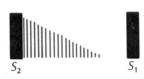

A *middiastolic murmur* starts a short time after S_2. It may fade away, as illustrated, or merge into a late diastolic murmur.

Middiastolic and presystolic murmurs are related to turbulent flow across the atrioventricular valves. See Table 9-14, Diastolic Murmurs (pp. 308–309).

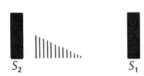

A *late diastolic (presystolic)* murmur starts late in diastole and typically continues up to S_1.

Some murmurs and other cardiovascular sounds, such as pericardial friction rubs or venous hums, have *both systolic and diastolic components*. Observe and describe these sounds according to the same characteristics used for systolic and diastolic murmurs.

See Table 9-15, Differentiation of Cardiovascular Sounds With Both Systolic and Diastolic Components (p. 310).

SHAPE. The shape or configuration of a murmur is determined by its intensity over time.

* To be more precise, systolic and early diastolic murmurs should be timed in relation to A_2 or P_2, depending on whether the murmur is aortic or pulmonic respectively. This subtle difference, however, is difficult to discern, especially for beginning students.

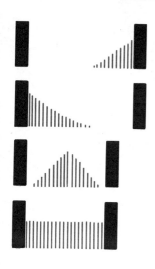

A *crescendo murmur* grows louder.

The presystolic murmur of mitral stenosis in normal sinus rhythm

A *decrescendo murmur* grows softer.

The early diastolic murmur of aortic regurgitation

A *crescendo–decrescendo murmur* first rises in intensity and then falls.

The midsystolic murmur of aortic stenosis

A *plateau murmur* has the same intensity throughout.

The pansystolic murmur of mitral regurgitation

LOCATION OF MAXIMAL INTENSITY. This is determined by the site where the murmur originates. Find the location by exploring the area in which you can hear the murmur, and describe where you hear it best in terms of the interspace and its relation to the sternum, the apex, the midsternal, the midclavicular, or one of the axillary lines.

For example, a murmur best heard in the 2nd right interspace usually originates at or near the aortic valve.

RADIATION OR TRANSMISSION FROM THE POINT OF MAXIMAL INTENSITY. This is determined not only by the site of origin but also by the intensity of the murmur and the direction of blood flow. Explore the area around a murmur and determine where else you can hear it.

A loud murmur of aortic stenosis often radiates into the neck (in the direction of arterial flow).

INTENSITY. This is usually graded on a 6-point scale and expressed as a fraction. The numerator describes the intensity of the murmur wherever it is loudest, and the denominator indicates the scale you are using. (There is also a 4-point scale.)

The *6 categories* are defined as follows:

Grade 1—very faint, heard only after the listener has "tuned in"; may not be heard in all positions

Grade 2—quiet but heard immediately upon placing the stethoscope on the chest

Grade 3—moderately loud

Grade 4—loud

Grade 5—very loud, may be heard with a stethoscope partly off the chest

Grade 6—may be heard with the stethoscope entirely off the chest

Intensity is influenced by the thickness of the chest wall and the presence of intervening tissue. For example, an identical degree of turbulence would cause a louder murmur in a thin person than in a very muscular or obese one. Emphysematous lungs may diminish the intensity of murmurs.

PITCH. This is categorized as high, medium, and low.

QUALITY. This is described in terms such as blowing, harsh, rumbling, and musical.

For a final example, a harsh, medium-pitched, grade 3/6, midsystolic crescendo–decrescendo murmur, best heard in the 2nd right interspace, with radiation to the neck

Other useful characteristics of murmurs—and heart sounds too—include their variations, if any, with respiration, with the position of the patient, or with other special maneuvers.

Murmurs originating in the right side of the heart tend to change more with respiration than do left-sided murmurs.

A Note on Cardiovascular Assessment

A good cardiovascular examination requires more than observation. You need to think about the possible meanings of your individual observations, fit them together in a logical pattern, and correlate your cardiac findings with the patient's blood pressure, arterial pulses, venous pulsations, and venous pressure, and with the remainder of your history and physical examination.

Evaluating the common systolic murmur illustrates this point. In examining an asymptomatic teenager, for example, you might hear a Grade 2 midsystolic murmur localized in the 2nd and 3rd left interspaces. Since this suggests a murmur of pulmonic origin, you should pay special attention to the size of the right ventricle by carefully palpating the left parasternal area. Because pulmonic stenosis and atrial septal defects can occasionally cause such murmurs, listen carefully to the splitting of the second heart sound and try to hear any ejection sounds. Listen to the murmur after the patient sits up. Look for evidence of anemia, hyperthyroidism, or pregnancy that could produce such a murmur by increasing the flow across the pulmonic valve. If all your findings are normal, your patient probably has an *innocent murmur*—one with no pathologic significance.

In contrast, in examining a 60-year-old person with anginal pains, you might hear a Grade 3 harsh midsystolic murmur maximal in the right 2nd interspace and radiating to the neck vessels. You cannot feel a thrill. These findings suggest aortic stenosis, but could be related to a sclerotic valve without stenosis, to a dilated aorta, or to increased flow across a normal valve. Evaluate the apical impulse for evidence of left ventricular enlargement. Listen for the murmur of aortic regurgitation as the patient leans forward and exhales. Assess the carotid pulse contour and the blood pressure for evidence of aortic stenosis. Put all this information together and make a tentative hypothesis as to the nature of the murmur.

Special Maneuvers

AUSCULTATORY AIDS. Elsewhere in this chapter you have already read how to improve your auscultation of the heart by positioning the patient in different ways. Two additional maneuvers extend these methods.

Squatting. When a person squats, venous return to the heart increases and so does peripheral vascular resistance. Arterial blood pressure, stroke

The transient increase in left ventricular volume decreases

volume, and the volume of blood in the left ventricle all rise. On standing, changes occur in opposite directions. These changes help (1) to identify a prolapsed mitral valve, and (2) to distinguish hypertrophic cardiomyopathy from aortic stenosis.

the prolapse of a mitral valve, delays the click and murmur, and may decrease the intensity of the murmur. Standing reverses these changes.

Secure the patient's gown so that it will not interfere with your examination, and ready yourself for prompt auscultation. Instruct the patient in how to squat next to the examining table and how to hold on to it for balance. Listen to the heart with the patient in the squatting position and again in the standing position.

The increased stroke volume increases the intensity of the murmur of aortic stenosis. In contrast, the increase in left ventricular volume decreases the outflow obstruction in hypertrophic cardiomyopathy and decreases the intensity of its murmur. Standing reverses both changes.

Valsalva Maneuver. When a person strains down against a closed glottis, venous return to the right heart is decreased, and after a few seconds left ventricular volume and arterial blood pressure both fall. Release of the effort has the opposite effects. These changes, like those of squatting, help to identify prolapse of the mitral valve and hypertrophic cardiomyopathy.

The decreased left ventricular volume increases the tendency of the mitral valve to prolapse, moves the click earlier in systole, and lengthens the murmur.

The patient should be lying down. Place one hand on the midabdomen and instruct the patient to strain against it. By adjusting your pressure you can alter the patient's effort to the desired level. Use your other hand to place your stethoscope on the patient's chest.

The decreased left ventricular volume increases the obstruction of hypertrophic cardiomyopathy and usually increases the intensity of the murmur. The murmur of aortic stenosis, in contrast, decreases.

PULSUS ALTERNANS. If you suspect left-sided heart failure, feel the pulse specifically for alternating amplitudes. These are usually best felt in the radial or femoral arteries. A blood pressure cuff gives you a more sensitive method. After raising the cuff pressure, lower it slowly to the systolic level and then below it. While you do this, the patient should breathe quietly or stop breathing in the respiratory midposition. If dyspnea prevents this, help the patient sit up, with legs dangling over the side of the bed.

Alternately loud and soft Korotkov sounds or a sudden doubling of the apparent heart rate as the cuff pressure declines indicates a pulsus alternans (see p. 297).

The upright position may accentuate the alternation.

PARADOXICAL PULSE. If you have noted that the pulse varies in amplitude with respiration or if you suspect pericardial tamponade (because of increased jugular venous pressure, a rapid and diminished pulse, and dyspnea, for example), look for a paradoxical pulse with a blood pressure cuff. As the patient breathes, quietly if possible, lower the cuff pressure

A paradoxical pulse varies more widely with respiration than normal. The level identified by first hearing Korotkov sounds is the highest systolic pressure

slowly to the systolic level. Note the pressure level at which the first sounds can be heard. Then drop the pressure very slowly until sounds can be heard throughout the respiratory cycle. Again note the pressure level. The difference between these two levels is normally no greater than 3 or 4 mm Hg.

during the respiratory cycle. The level identified by hearing sounds throughout the cycle is the lowest systolic pressure. A difference between these levels of more than 10 mm Hg suggests pericardial tamponade, possibly constrictive pericarditis, but, most commonly, obstructive airway disease. (See p. 297.)

Table 9-1

Table 9-1 Approach to the Differentiation of Selected Heart Rates and Rhythms

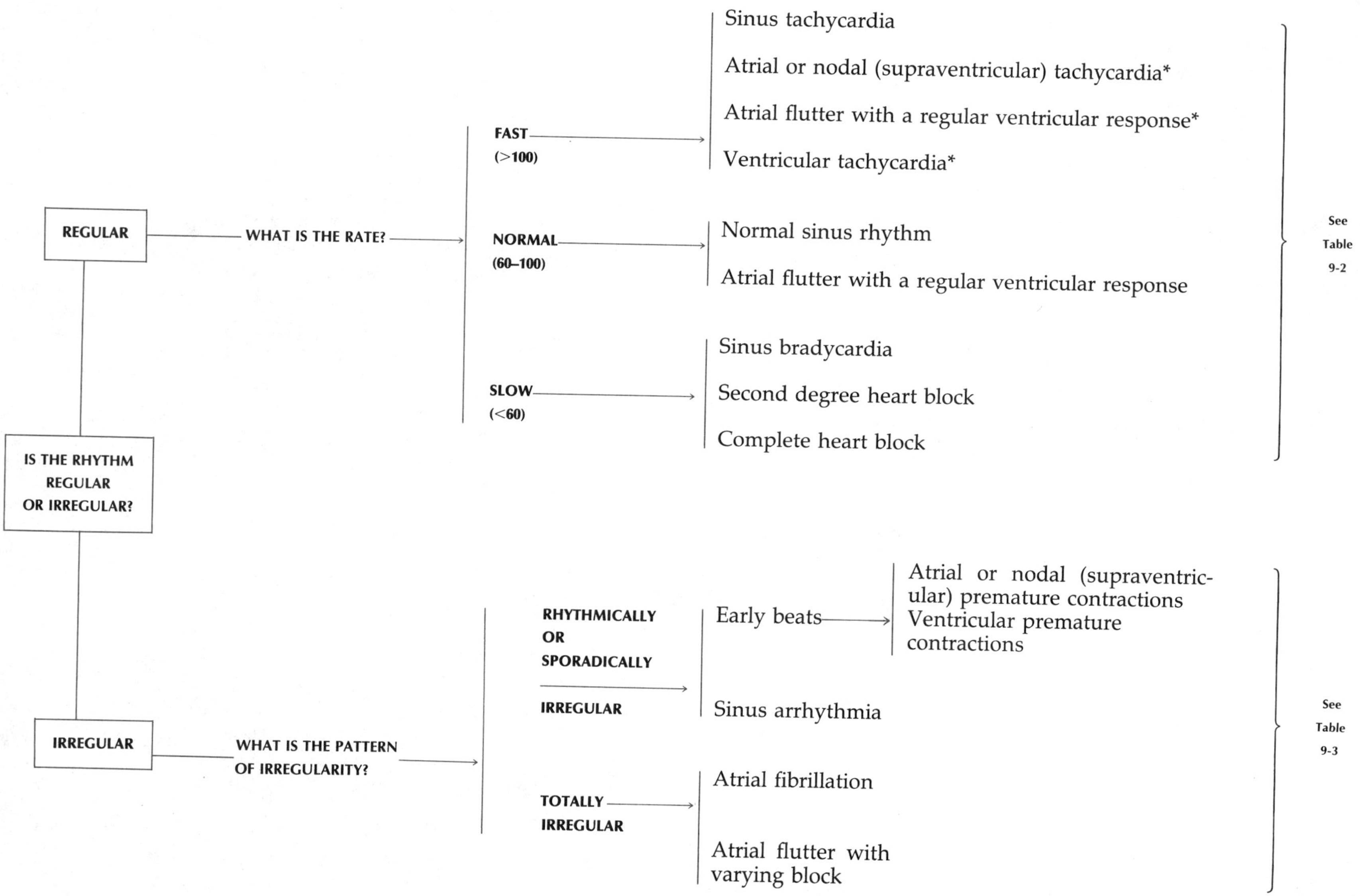

IS THE RHYTHM REGULAR OR IRREGULAR?

REGULAR → **WHAT IS THE RATE?**

- **FAST (>100)**
  - Sinus tachycardia
  - Atrial or nodal (supraventricular) tachycardia*
  - Atrial flutter with a regular ventricular response*
  - Ventricular tachycardia*

  (See Table 9-2)

- **NORMAL (60–100)**
  - Normal sinus rhythm
  - Atrial flutter with a regular ventricular response

- **SLOW (<60)**
  - Sinus bradycardia
  - Second degree heart block
  - Complete heart block

IRREGULAR → **WHAT IS THE PATTERN OF IRREGULARITY?**

- **RHYTHMICALLY OR SPORADICALLY IRREGULAR**
  - Early beats →
    - Atrial or nodal (supraventricular) premature contractions
    - Ventricular premature contractions
  - Sinus arrhythmia

  (See Table 9-3)

- **TOTALLY IRREGULAR**
  - Atrial fibrillation
  - Atrial flutter with varying block

* Less commonly these arrhythmias may also occur with slower ventricular rates.

Table 9-2

Table 9-2 Differentiation of Selected Regular Rhythms

DESCRIPTION	CLINICAL MANIFESTATIONS			FIRST AND SECOND HEART SOUNDS
	VENTRICULAR RATE			
	USUAL RESTING RATE	RESPONSE TO EXERCISE	RESPONSE TO VAGAL STIMULATION*	

RHYTHMS WITH FAST VENTRICULAR RATES

DESCRIPTION	USUAL RESTING RATE	RESPONSE TO EXERCISE	RESPONSE TO VAGAL STIMULATION*	FIRST AND SECOND HEART SOUNDS
SINUS TACHYCARDIA — A fast rhythm originating normally in the sinus node and conducted over normal pathways through the heart. Causes include exercise, anxiety, fever, hyperthyroidism, and blood loss.	100–150		Smooth slowing	Normal
ATRIAL OR NODAL (*Supraventricular*) TACHYCARDIA — A fast rhythm typically occurring in episodes or paroxysms. Young adults with no other evidence of heart disease are often affected. Conduction within the atria is abnormal, but the ventricles usually respond to each impulse.	160–200		Abrupt slowing or no change	Normal
ATRIAL FLUTTER WITH A REGULAR VENTRICULAR RESPONSE — A very fast atrial rhythm, often around 300–320 per min. There is usually a partial conduction block at the AV node. In a 2:1 block, for example, every second atrial beat is followed by a ventricular response.	150–160		Abrupt slowing or no change	Normal
VENTRICULAR TACHYCARDIA — A fast rhythm originating in the ventricles. This is an ominous arrhythmia, usually associated with organic heart disease, and may herald ventricular fibrillation and sudden death.	150–200		No change	Split S_1, S_2; varying intensity of S_1

Table 9-2

		Ventricular Rate (per minute)	Effect of Exercise	Effect of Carotid Sinus Massage*	Heart Sounds
RHYTHMS WITH NORMAL VENTRICULAR RATES					
NORMAL SINUS RHYTHM	A rhythm of normal origin and conduction through the heart. Note, however, that a regular rhythm with a normal rate is not necessarily a normal sinus rhythm.	60–100	Smooth increase	Smooth slowing	Normal
ATRIAL FLUTTER WITH A REGULAR VENTRICULAR RESPONSE	A very fast atrial rhythm, as described above, but with a greater degree of AV block, *e.g.*, a 4:1 block, in which every fourth atrial impulse is followed by a ventricular response.	60–100	Abrupt increase or no change	Abrupt slowing or no change	Normal
RHYTHMS WITH SLOW VENTRICULAR RATES					
SINUS BRADYCARDIA	A slow rhythm with normal sinus origin and normal conduction. A very common rhythm. Other causes include excellent physical fitness, hypothyroidism, hypothermia, acute myocardial infarction, the sick sinus syndrome, and drugs such as digitalis and propranolol.	50–60, may be down to 40	Smooth increase		Normal
SECOND DEGREE HEART BLOCK	A slow rhythm produced by impaired conduction through the AV node or the bundle of His. Some of the atrial impulses fail to get through to the ventricles. Causes include heart disease and drugs such as digitalis.	35–60	Smooth increase		Normal S_1, S_2; atrial sounds may also be heard
COMPLETE HEART BLOCK	A very slow rhythm produced by a complete block of conduction through the AV node or the bundle of His or its branches. Ventricular beats originate in the ventricles themselves. The most common cause is an acute myocardial infarction.	25–45, may be up to 60	No change		Varying intensity of S_1

*Vagal stimulation may be produced by holding a deep breath, by the induction of gagging or retching, and by carotid sinus massage. Careful monitoring is required.

Table 9-3 Differentiation of Selected Irregular Rhythms

TYPE OF RHYTHM	DIAGRAMMATIC REPRESENTATION	RHYTHM	HEART SOUNDS
ATRIAL OR NODAL (*Supraventricular*) PREMATURE CONTRACTIONS	QRS, Normal QRS and T, Aberrant P wave, P, T, S_1 S_2, S_1 S_2, Early beat, Pause	A beat of atrial or nodal origin comes earlier than the next expected normal beat. A pause follows and then the rhythm resumes.	S_1 may differ in intensity from the S_1 of normal beats, and S_2 may be decreased. Both sounds are otherwise similar to normal beats.
VENTRICULAR PREMATURE CONTRACTIONS	No P wave, Aberrant QRS and T, S_1 S_2, Early beat with split sounds, Pause	A beat of ventricular origin comes earlier than the expected normal beat. A pause follows and the rhythm resumes.	S_1 may differ in intensity from the S_1 of the normal beats, and S_2 may be decreased. Both sounds are likely to be split.
SINUS ARRHYTHMIA	S_1 S_2 S_1 S_2 S_1 S_2 S_1 S_2, INSPIRATION, EXPIRATION	The heart varies cyclically, usually speeding up with inspiration and slowing down with expiration.	Normal, although S_1 may vary with the heart rate.
ATRIAL FIBRILLATION AND ATRIAL FLUTTER WITH VARYING AV BLOCK	No P waves, Fibrillation waves, S_1 S_2 S_1 S_2 S_1 S_2 S_1 S_2 S_1 S_2 S_1 S_2	The ventricular rhythm is totally irregular, although short runs may seem regular.	S_1 varies in intensity.

Table 9-4

Table 9-4   Abnormalities of the Arterial Pulse

NORMAL (mm Hg)	The pulse pressure is about 30–40 mm Hg. The pulse contour is smooth and rounded. (The notch on the descending slope of the pulse wave is not palpable.)
SMALL, WEAK PULSES	The pulse pressure is diminished, and the pulse feels weak and small. The upstroke may feel slowed, the peak prolonged. Causes include (1) decreased stroke volume as in heart failure, hypovolemia, and severe aortic stenosis; and (2) increased peripheral resistance, as in exposure to cold and severe congestive heart failure.
LARGE, BOUNDING PULSES	The pulse pressure is increased and the pulse feels strong and bounding. The rise and fall may feel rapid, the peak brief. Causes include (1) an increased stroke volume, a decreased peripheral resistance, or both, as in fever, anemia, hyperthyroidism, aortic regurgitation, arteriovenous fistulas, and patent ductus arteriosus; (2) an increased stroke volume due to slow heart rates, as in bradycardia and complete heart block; and (3) decreased compliance (increased stiffness) of the aortic walls, as in aging or atherosclerosis.
BISFERIENS PULSE	A bisferiens pulse is an increased arterial pulse with a double systolic peak. Causes include pure aortic regurgitation, combined aortic stenosis and regurgitation, and, though less commonly palpable, hypertrophic cardiomyopathy.
PULSUS ALTERNANS	The pulse alternates in amplitude from beat to beat even though the rhythm is basically regular (and must be for you to make this judgment). When the difference between stronger and weaker beats is slight it can be detected only by sphygmomanometry. Pulsus alternans indicates left ventricular failure and is usually accompanied by a left-sided S_3.
BIGEMINAL PULSE (*Premature contractions*)	This is a disorder of rhythm that may masquerade as pulsus alternans. A bigeminal pulse is caused by a normal beat alternating with a premature contraction. The stroke volume of the premature beat is diminished in relation to the normal beats, and the pulse varies in amplitude accordingly.
PARADOXICAL PULSE (*Expiration — Inspiration*)	A paradoxical pulse may be detected by a palpable decrease in the pulse's amplitude on quiet inspiration. If the sign is less pronounced, a blood pressure cuff is needed. Systolic pressure decreases by more than 10 mm Hg. A paradoxical pulse is found in pericardial tamponade, constrictive pericarditis (though less commonly), and obstructive lung disease.

Table 9-5

Table 9-5 Variations and Abnormalities of the Ventricular Impulses

When a ventricle works under conditions of chronic pressure overload (increased afterload), its walls thicken. Volume overload (increased preload), in contrast, produces dilatation of the ventricle as well as thickening of its walls. A hyperkinetic impulse results from an increased stroke volume. An impulse may feel hyperkinetic when the chest wall is unusually thin.

CHARACTERISTICS OF THE IMPULSE	LEFT VENTRICLE				RIGHT VENTRICLE			
	NORMAL	HYPERKINETIC	PRESSURE OVERLOAD	VOLUME OVERLOAD	NORMAL	HYPERKINETIC	PRESSURE OVERLOAD	VOLUME OVERLOAD
LOCATION	5th or possibly 4th interspace, medial to the midclavicular line	Normal	Normal	Displaced to the left and downward	Indeterminate	3rd, 4th, or 5th interspaces	3rd, 4th or 5th interspaces, also subxiphoid	Left sternal border, extending toward the left cardiac border, also subxiphoid
DIAMETER	Not more than 1–2 cm in adults (1 cm in children)	Normal, though increased amplitude may make it seem larger	Increased	Increased	Indeterminate	Not useful	Not useful	Not useful
AMPLITUDE	Small, gentle	Increased	Increased	Increased	Not palpable beyond infancy	Slightly increased	Increased	Slightly to markedly increased
DURATION	Usually less than two thirds of systole; the impulse stops before S_2	Normal	Prolonged, may be sustained up to S_2	Often slightly prolonged	Indeterminate	Normal	Prolonged	Normal to prolonged
EXAMPLES OF CAUSES		Anxiety, hyperthyroidism, severe anemia	Aortic stenosis, systemic hypertension	Aortic or mitral regurgitation		Anxiety, hyperthyroidism, severe anemia	Pulmonic stenosis, pulmonary hypertension	Atrial septal defect

Table 9-6

Table 9-6 Variations in the First Heart Sound

NORMAL VARIATIONS

S_1 is softer than S_2 at the *base* (right and left 2nd interspaces).

S_1 is often but not always louder than S_2 at the *apex*.

ACCENTUATED S_1

S_1 is accentuated (1) by tachycardia and by high cardiac output states (*e.g.*, exercise, anemia, hyperthyroidism), and (2) in mitral stenosis. In both situations the mitral valve is still open wide at the onset of ventricular systole. The valve then slams shut.

DIMINISHED S_1

S_1 is diminished in first degree heart block (delayed conduction from atria to ventricles). Here the mitral valve has had time after atrial contraction to float back into an almost closed position before ventricular contraction shuts it. It closes less loudly. S_1 is also diminished when the mitral valve is calcified and relatively immobile, as in mitral regurgitation.

VARYING S_1

S_1 varies in intensity (1) in complete heart block, where atria and ventricles are beating independently of each other, and (2) in any totally irregular rhythm (*e.g.*, atrial fibrillation). In these situations the mitral valve is in varying positions before being shut by ventricular contraction. Its closure sound, therefore, varies in loudness.

SPLIT S_1

S_1 may be split normally along the lower left sternal border where the tricuspid component, often too faint to be heard, becomes audible. When S_1 seems to be split at the apex, you are usually hearing two sounds: S_1, together with an S_4, an early systolic ejection sound, or an early systolic click (see Table 9-10, p. 303). Abnormal splitting of both heart sounds may be heard in right bundle branch block and in beats of ventricular origin such as premature ventricular contractions.

Table 9-7

Table 9-7   Variations in the Second Heart Sound

	EXPIRATION	INSPIRATION	
PHYSIOLOGIC SPLITTING	S_1 S_2	S_1 A_2 P_2 S_2	*Physiologic splitting* of the second heart sound can usually be detected in the 2nd or 3rd left interspace. The pulmonic component of S_2 is usually too faint to be heard at the apex or aortic area where S_2 is single and derived from aortic valve closure alone. In Normal splitting is accentuated by inspiration and usually disappears on expiration. In some patients, however, especially younger ones, S_2 may not become completely single on expiration. It may do so when the patient sits up.
PATHOLOGIC SPLITTING *(All of these suggest heart disease.)*	S_1 S_2	S_1 S_2	*Wide splitting* of S_2 refers to an increase in the usual splitting that persists throughout the respiratory cycle. Wide splitting can be caused by delayed closure of the pulmonic valve (*e.g.*, by pulmonic stenosis or right bundle branch block). As illustrated here, right bundle branch block also causes splitting of S_1 into its mitral and tricuspid components. Wide splitting can also be caused by early closure of the aortic valve, as in mitral regurgitation.
	S_1 S_2	S_1 S_2	*Fixed splitting* refers to wide splitting that does not vary with respiration. It occurs in atrial septal defect and right ventricular failure.
	S_1 P_2 A_2 S_2	S_1 S_2	*Paradoxical or reversed splitting* refers to splitting that appears on expiration and disappears on inspiration. Closure of the aortic valve is abnormally delayed so that A_2 follows P_2 in expiration. Normal inspiratory delay of P_2 makes the split disappear. The most common cause of paradoxical splitting is left bundle branch block.

INCREASED INTENSITY OF S_2 IN THE RIGHT SECOND INTERSPACE (where only A_2 can usually be heard) occurs in systemic hypertension because of the increased pressure. It also occurs when the aortic root is dilated, probably because the aortic valve is then closer to the chest wall.

A DECREASED OR ABSENT S_2 IN THE RIGHT SECOND INTERSPACE is noted in calcific aortic stenosis because of immobility of the valve. If A_2 is inaudible, no splitting is heard.

INCREASED INTENSITY OF THE PULMONIC COMPONENT OF S_2. When P_2 is equal to or louder than A_2, pulmonary hypertension may be suspected. Other causes include a dilated pulmonary artery and an atrial septal defect. Splitting of the second heart sound that is heard widely, even at the apex and right base, indicates an accentuated P_2.

A DECREASED OR ABSENT P_2 is most commonly due to the increased anteroposterior diameter of the chest associated with aging. It can also result from pulmonic stenosis. If P_2 is inaudible, no splitting is heard.

Table 9-8

Table 9-8 Extra Heart Sounds in Systole

Extra heart sounds in systole are of two kinds: (1) early ejection sounds, and (2) clicks, most commonly heard in mid- and late systole.

EARLY SYSTOLIC EJECTION SOUNDS

S_1 E_j S_2

Early systolic ejection sounds occur shortly after the first heart sound, coincident with the opening of the aortic and pulmonic valves. They are relatively high in pitch, have a sharp, clicking quality, and are heard better with the diaphragm of the stethoscope.

An *aortic ejection sound* is heard at both base and apex and may be louder at the apex. It does not usually vary with respiration. An aortic ejection sound may accompany a dilated aorta or aortic valve disease.

A *pulmonic ejection sound* is best heard in the 2nd and 3rd left interspaces. When the first heart sound, usually relatively soft in this area, appears to be loud, you may instead be hearing a pulmonic ejection sound. Decreased intensity of the sound during inspiration gives another clue. Causes include dilatation of the pulmonary artery, pulmonary hypertension, and pulmonic stenosis.

SYSTOLIC CLICKS

S_1 S_2

Systolic clicks are usually due to *mitral valve prolapse*—an abnormal systolic ballooning of part of the mitral valve into the left atrium. The clicks are usually mid- or late systolic, but occasionally they are early systolic. Prolapse of the mitral valve is a common cardiac abnormality, affecting about 5% of young adults. It is more common in women. The click is usually single, but more than one are sometimes heard. A click is best heard at or medial to the apex but may also be heard at the lower left sternal border. It is high-pitched and clicking in quality and is heard better with the diaphragm. The click is often followed by an apical systolic murmur (see p. 307). Findings often vary from time to time: a click only, a click and a murmur, or only a late systolic murmur. Findings also vary with the patient's body position, and several positions are recommended for detection of mitral prolapse: supine, seated, standing, and squatting.

Table 9-9

Table 9-9   Extra Heart Sounds in Diastole

OPENING SNAP	S_1 S_2 *O.S.*	The *opening snap* is a very early diastolic sound usually produced by the opening of a stenotic mitral valve. It is best heard just medial to the apex and along the lower left sternal border. When it is loud an opening snap radiates to the apex and to the pulmonic area, where it may be mistaken for the pulmonic component of a split S_2. Its high pitch and snapping quality help distinguish it from an S_3. It is heard better with the diaphragm.
S_3	S_1 S_2 S_3	A *physiologic third heart sound* is frequently heard in children. It may persist in young adults to the approximate age of 35 or 40. It is common during the last trimester of pregnancy. Occurring early in diastole during rapid ventricular filling, it is later than an opening snap, dull and low-pitched, and best heard at the apex in the left lateral decubitus position. The bell of the stethoscope should be used with very light pressure. A *pathologic S_3 or ventricular gallop* sounds just like a physiologic S_3. An S_3 in a person over 40 (possibly a little older in women) is almost certainly pathologic. Causes include myocardial failure and, less commonly, volume overloading of a ventricle, as from aortic, mitral, or tricuspid regurgitation. A left-sided S_3 is typically heard at the apex in the left lateral position. A right-sided S_3 is usually heard along the lower left sternal border or below the xiphoid with the patient supine. It is louder on inspiration. The term *gallop* comes from the cadence of three heart sounds, especially at rapid heart rates.
S_4	S_1 S_2 S_4 S_1	An S_4 (*atrial sound* or *atrial gallop*) occurs just before S_1. It is low-pitched, dull, and better heard with the bell. An S_4 is occasionally heard in an apparently normal person, especially in trained athletes and also in older age groups. More commonly it is due to increased resistance to ventricular filling following atrial contraction. This increased resistance is related to decreased compliance (increased stiffness) of the ventricular myocardium. Causes of a left-sided S_4 include hypertensive heart disease, coronary artery disease, aortic stenosis, and cardiomyopathy. A left-sided S_4 is best heard at the apex in the left lateral position. The less common right-sided S_4 is heard along the lower left sternal border or below the xiphoid. It often increases with inspiration. Causes of a right-sided S_4 include pulmonary hypertension and pulmonic stenosis. An S_4 may also be associated with delayed conduction between atria and ventricles. This delay separates the normally faint atrial sound from the louder S_1, and makes it audible. An S_4 is never heard in the absence of atrial contraction, as in atrial fibrillation. An occasional patient has both an S_3 and an S_4, producing a *quadruple rhythm* of four heart sounds. At rapid heart rates the S_3 and S_4 may merge into one loud extra heart sound called a *summation gallop*.

Table 9-10 Causes of An Apparently Split First Heart Sound

Normal splitting of the first heart sound occurs when the soft second tricuspid component is audible. Additional causes of an apparently split S_1 are compared below. A pulmonic ejection sound is not included in this table because its location in the 2nd and 3rd left interspaces should alone make the differentiation. An early systolic click has the same significance as a midsystolic or late systolic click—mitral valve prolapse.

	LEFT-SIDED S_4	RIGHT-SIDED S_4	SPLIT S_1	AORTIC EJECTION SOUND	EARLY SYSTOLIC CLICK
LOCATION OF MAXIMAL INTENSITY	Apex	Lower left sternal border or subxiphoid	Lower left sternal border	Aortic area, apex, or both	Apex, medial to it, or at the lower left sternal border
PITCH AND QUALITY	Low-pitched, dull	Low-pitched, dull	High-pitched; both components of similar quality	High-pitched, clicking	High-pitched, clicking
BETTER HEARD WITH	Bell	Bell	Diaphragm	Diaphragm	Diaphragm
PALPABLE SPLIT	Often, as a double impulse at the apex	May be present as a double impulse at the left sternal border or in the subxiphoid area	Absent	Absent	Absent
SPECIAL AUSCULTATORY AIDS	The left lateral decubitus position accentuates this S_4.	Inspiration often accentuates this S_4.	None	None	The squatting position delays the click and widens the split.

Table 9-11

Table 9-11   *Mechanisms of Heart Murmurs*

Heart murmurs are of longer duration than heart sounds. They originate within the heart itself or in its great vessels and are usually caused by one of the following mechanisms:

1. Flow across a partial obstruction (*e.g.*, aortic stenosis)

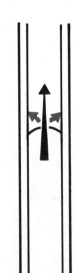

2. Flow across a valvular or intravascular irregularity without obstruction (*e.g.*, a bicuspid aortic valve without true stenosis)

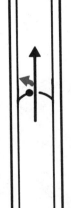

3. Increased flow through normal structures (*e.g.*, aortic systolic murmur associated with anemia)

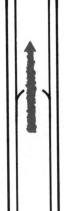

4. Flow into a dilated chamber (*e.g.*, aortic systolic murmur associated with aneurysmal dilatation of the ascending aorta)

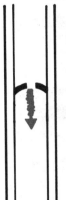

5. Backward or regurgitant flow across an incompetent valve or defect (*e.g.*, mitral regurgitation)

6. Shunting of blood out of a high pressure chamber or artery through an abnormal passage (*e.g.*, ventricular septal defect, patent ductus arteriosus)

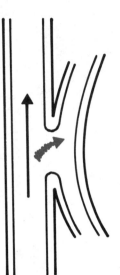

Table 9-12

Table 9-12 Midsystolic Murmurs

Midsystolic (ejection) murmurs constitute the most common kind of heart murmur. They may be (1) *organic* (*i.e.,* secondary to structural cardiovascular abnormality): (2) *functional* (*i.e.,* secondary to a physiologic alteration with or without heart disease); or (3) *innocent* (*i.e.,* not associated with any functional or structural abnormality). Systolic ejection murmurs are relatively easy to identify but often hard to interpret. The entire cardiovascular examination, in fact a thorough evaluation of the whole patient, is frequently necessary.

Midsystolic ejection murmurs are associated with forward flow through the semilunar valves or outflow tracts. Constriction, structural irregularity, an increased rate of flow, or flow into a dilated great vessel produces the systolic noise. The murmur has a crescendo–decrescendo (or diamond-shaped) pattern and is usually separated from the first and second heart sounds.

Organic causes of midsystolic ejection murmurs include aortic and pulmonic stenosis (*i.e.,* failure of the aortic and pulmonic valves, respectively, to open as fully as they should during systole). Occasionally the constriction of flow occurs above or below the valve instead of in the valve itself. The murmurs of aortic and pulmonic valvular stenosis are contrasted below. Other causes of these murmurs are discussed on the next page.

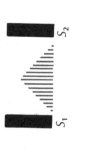

S_1 S_2

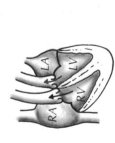

AORTIC STENOSIS

Systole

LOCATION	2nd right interspace
RADIATION	Into the neck, down the left sternal border, and sometimes to the apex. Note that an apical ejection murmur, despite its location, often originates in the aortic valve.
INTENSITY	Variable. If loud, a thrill may be felt in the aortic area and neck.
PITCH	Medium
QUALITY	Often harsh, more musical when heard at the apex
ASSOCIATED SIGNS MAY INCLUDE	1. A diminished S_2 2. An early aortic ejection sound, a left-sided S_4 3. A thrusting, sustained apical impulse of left ventricular hypertrophy 4. A slowly rising carotid pulse contour 5. A narrow pulse pressure

PULMONIC STENOSIS

Systole

LOCATION	2nd or 3rd left interspace
RADIATION	Toward the left shoulder and upward toward the neck vessels, especially on the left
INTENSITY	Variable. If loud, a thrill may be felt in the pulmonic area.
PITCH	Medium
QUALITY	Often harsh
ASSOCIATED SIGNS MAY INCLUDE	1. A widely split S_2 and diminished to absent P_2. (If P_2 is absent, there can be no splitting.) 2. An early pulmonic ejection sound, a right-sided S_4 3. A right ventricular impulse that is increased in amplitude and prolonged in duration

Continued

Table 9-12

Table 9-12 (Cont'd.)

OTHER CAUSES OF AORTIC SYSTOLIC MURMURS	OTHER CAUSES OF PULMONIC SYSTOLIC MURMURS
Structural abnormality of the aortic valve without true stenosis may cause a midsystolic or early systolic ejection murmur indistinguishable from mild aortic stenosis. Two common examples are a congenitally *bicuspid but nonstenotic aortic valve* and the *sclerotic aortic valve associated with aging.* The lack of associated signs may help you to make these diagnoses, but prolonged followup is often necessary.	*Increased blood flow* across the pulmonic valve may produce a murmur that sounds like that of pulmonic stenosis. It is this mechanism, not flow through the defect, that produces the systolic murmur of *atrial septal defect.* Wide splitting of S_2 may accompany both atrial septal defect and pulmonic stenosis.
Flow into an aorta dilated by syphilitic aortitis or by atherosclerosis may also cause this kind of systolic murmur.	Increased blood flow from causes such as anemia, pregnancy, fever, or hyperthyroidism can also cause a pulmonic flow murmur.
Functional murmurs associated with increased blood flow across the aortic valve must also be considered in the differential diagnosis. Anemia, pregnancy, fever, and hyperthyroidism, for example, may cause such murmurs. If so, the murmur will disappear when the underlying condition is corrected. Aortic regurgitation increases left ventricular volume and thus augments systolic flow across the aortic valve. By this mechanism aortic regurgitation may produce an early or midsystolic murmur (in addition to its own diastolic murmur) in the absence of true valvular stenosis.	Distinguishing the pulmonic murmurs of organic heart disease from the much more common *innocent murmurs* of children and young adults is a frequent and important problem. Innocent murmurs are usually (but not always) soft, grade 1 or 2, short, midsystolic, and best heard in the left 2nd and 3rd interspaces. Splitting of the second sound is normal, no ejection sound is heard, and palpation of the right ventricle is normal. There should be no diastolic murmurs. The character of an innocent murmur frequently changes with change in position, phase of respiration, and heart rate. Chest x-ray, electrocardiogram, and other tests may be needed to make sure of this diagnosis.
Hypertrophic cardiomyopathy is yet another cause of a midsystolic murmur. Markedly hypertrophied and stiffened heart muscle impairs left ventricular filling and often obstructs left ventricular outflow. This obstruction creates a harsh crescendo–decrescendo murmur best heard at the left sternal border and apex. Unlike aortic stenosis, this murmur is not well heard in the 2nd right interspace and does not radiate to the neck. The murmur may merge with an associated murmur of mitral regurgitation at the apex. An S_4 is prominent, and the initial upstroke of the carotid artery is brisk. Squatting and the Valsalva maneuver are also useful in identifying this condition (see pp. 290–291).	

Table 9-13

Table 9-13 *Pansystolic (Holosystolic) Murmurs*

Pansystolic (holosystolic) murmurs are heard when blood flows from a chamber of high pressure to one of lower pressure through a valve or other structure that should be closed. These murmurs are sometimes called "regurgitant," referring to the backward flow across the atrioventricular valves. Causes of pansystolic murmurs include mitral regurgitation (LV → LA), tricuspid regurgitation (RV → RA), and ventricular septal defect (LV → RV). The murmur begins immediately with the first heart sound and continues up to the second heart sound.

Three types of pansystolic murmurs are contrasted below.

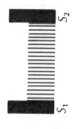

	MITRAL REGURGITATION	TRICUSPID REGURGITATION	VENTRICULAR SEPTAL DEFECT
	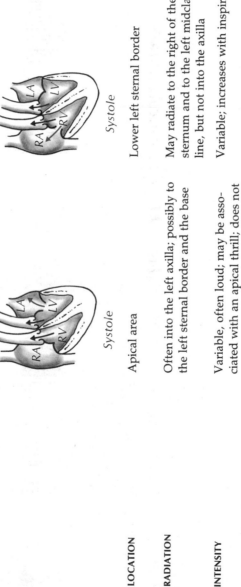 *Systole*	*Systole*	*Systole*
LOCATION	Apical area	Lower left sternal border	Left sternal border in the 3rd, 4th, and 5th interspaces
RADIATION	Often into the left axilla; possibly to the left sternal border and the base	May radiate to the right of the sternum and to the left midclavicular line, but not into the axilla	May radiate over the precordium but not into the axilla
INTENSITY	Variable, often loud; may be associated with an apical thrill; does not increase with inspiration	Variable; increases with inspiration	Often very loud and accompanied by a thrill
PITCH	High	High	High
QUALITY	Blowing	Blowing	Often harsh
ASSOCIATED SIGNS MAY INCLUDE	Decreased S₁ An S₃ An enlarged and sustained apical impulse of increased amplitude, displaced to the left and downward	A right ventricular impulse that is increased in amplitude and may be prolonged Systolic pulsations in the jugular venous pulse and sometimes in the liver	Signs vary with severity of defect and with associated lesions.

Another form of mitral regurgitation occurs with a *prolapsed mitral valve.* Here the murmur associated with regurgitant flow is usually late systolic and often follows a mid- or late systolic click. In about 10% of cases the murmur is pansystolic. For further discussion see Systolic Clicks, p. 301.

Table 9-14

Table 9-14   Diastolic Murmurs

Unlike systolic murmurs, diastolic murmurs are almost always indicative of heart disease. Two general types may be distinguished: (1) the diastolic rumble originating in the atrioventricular valves, and (2) the early diastolic murmurs of semilunar valve incompetence.

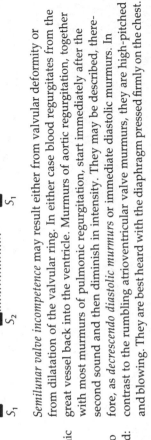

Diastolic rumbling murmurs are caused by (1) flow across distorted or stenotic mitral or tricuspid valves, or (2) increased blood flow across normal mitral or tricuspid valves. Because these valves open only after the aortic and pulmonic valves close, a short period of silence separates S₂ from the beginning of diastolic rumbles. These murmurs are low in pitch, rumbling in quality, and heard best with the bell of the stethoscope in light skin contact. They tend to be loudest in the two phases of diastole when ventricular filling is most rapid: early in diastole immediately after valvular opening, and again during atrial contraction (presystole). When the atria do not contract, as in atrial fibrillation, the presystolic component is often lacking, and only a middiastolic rumble remains.

Semilunar valve incompetence may result either from valvular deformity or from dilatation of the valvular ring. In either case blood regurgitates from the great vessel back into the ventricle. Murmurs of aortic regurgitation, together with most murmurs of pulmonic regurgitation, start immediately after the second sound and then diminish in intensity. They may be described, therefore, as *decrescendo diastolic murmurs* or immediate diastolic murmurs. In contrast to the rumbling atrioventricular valve murmurs, they are high-pitched and blowing. They are best heard with the diaphragm pressed firmly on the chest.

The most common examples of these two types of diastolic murmurs are those of mitral stenosis and aortic regurgitation. They are contrasted on the next page.

Table 9-14

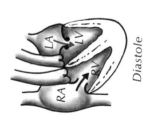

Diastole

Diastole

MITRAL STENOSIS

LOCATION	Apical area
RADIATION	Very little
INTENSITY	Variable; may be brought out or accentuated in the left lateral decubitus position and by exercise
PITCH	Low (heard better with a bell)
QUALITY	Rumbling
ASSOCIATED SIGNS MAY INCLUDE	Increased S_1 in the apical area
	Opening snap
	Increased P_2 and increased amplitude and duration of the right ventricular impulse if pulmonary hypertension has developed

AORTIC REGURGITATION

Usually the mid-left sternal border

Toward the right 2nd interspace and down the left sternal border to the apex; possibly also along the right sternal border

Variable, often faint; may be brought out by asking the patient to sit leaning forward with breath exhaled

High (heard better with a diaphragm)

Blowing

Aortic systolic murmur from increased flow. A relatively large volume of blood regurgitates back into the left ventricle with each diastole and adds importantly to the volume of blood ejected across the aortic valve in the next systole.

A low rumbling apical diastolic murmur resembling the murmur of mitral stenosis. This is called an *Austin Flint murmur* and is caused by a regurgitant stream of blood that impinges on the anterior leaflet of the mitral valve during diastole.

S_3

A thrusting apical impulse displaced downward and laterally (left ventricular enlargement)

Wide pulse pressure, large bounding pulses

Table 9-15

Table 9-15 Differentiation of Cardiovascular Sounds With Both Systolic and Diastolic Components

Some cardiovascular sounds are not confined to one portion of the cardiac cycle. Three examples are (1) a pericardial friction rub, produced by inflammation of the pericardial sac; (2) patent ductus arteriosus, a congenital abnormality in which an open channel persists between aorta and pulmonary artery; and (3) a venous hum, a benign sound produced by turbulence of blood in the jugular veins (common in children). Their characteristics are contrasted below. The term "continuous murmur" is defined as one that begins in systole and continues through the second sound into all or part of diastole. It need not continue through diastole. The murmur of patent ductus arteriosus, therefore, may be classified as continuous.

	PERICARDIAL FRICTION RUB	PATENT DUCTUS ARTERIOSUS	VENOUS HUM
TIMING	May have three short components, each associated with cardiac movement: (1) atrial systole, (2) ventricular systole, and (3) ventricular diastole. Usually the first two components are present; all three make diagnosis easy; only one (which is usually the systolic) invites confusion with a murmur.	Continuous murmur in both systole and diastole, often with a silent interval late in diastole. Is loudest in late systole, obscures S_2, and fades in diastole	Continuous murmur without a silent interval. Loudest in diastole
LOCATION	Variable but usually best heard in the 3rd interspace to the left of the sternum	Left 2nd interspace	Above the medial third of the clavicles, especially on the right
RADIATION	Little	Toward the left clavicle	1st and 2nd interspaces
INTENSITY	Variable. May increase when the patient leans forward and exhales	Usually loud, sometimes associated with a thrill	Soft to moderate. Can be obliterated by pressure on the jugular veins
QUALITY	Scratchy, scraping	Harsh, machinerylike	Humming, roaring
PITCH	High (heard better with a diaphragm)	Medium	Low (heard better with a bell)

Chapter 10
The Breasts and Axillae

Anatomy and Physiology

The female breast lies between the 2nd and 6th ribs, between the sternal edge and midaxillary line. About two thirds of it is superficial to the pectoralis major, about one third to the serratus anterior. The nipple and the areola that surrounds it are somewhat lateral to the center of the breast. Sebaceous glands on the areola (glands of Montgomery) appear as small round elevations.

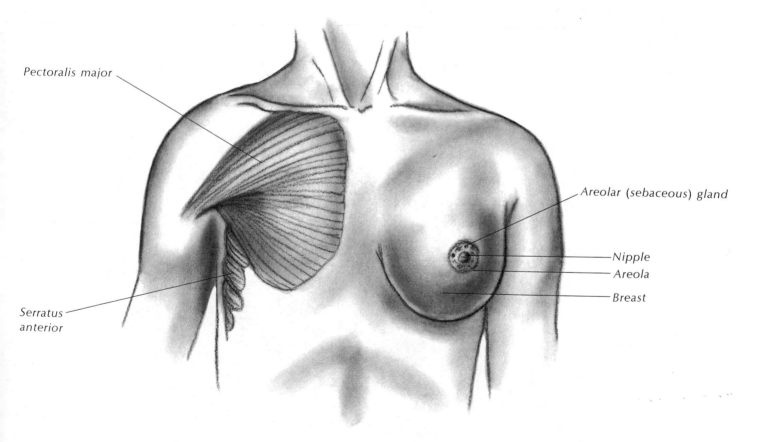

Pectoralis major

Serratus anterior

Areolar (sebaceous) gland

Nipple

Areola

Breast

For purposes of description, the breast may be divided into four quadrants by horizontal and vertical lines crossing at the nipple. In addition a tail of breast tissue frequently extends toward or into the axilla. An alternative method of localizing findings visualizes the breast as the face of a clock. A lesion may be located by the ''time'' (*e.g.*, 4 o'clock) and by the distance in centimeters from the nipple.

Breast tissue has three principal components. (1) The *glandular tissue* is organized into 12 to 20 lobes, each of which terminates in a duct that opens on the surface of the nipple. (2) This glandular tissue is supported by *fibrous tissue*, including suspensory ligaments that are connected both to the skin and to fascia underlying the breast. (3) *Fat* surrounds the breast and predominates both superficially and peripherally. The proportions of these components vary with age, the general state of nutrition, pregnancy, and other factors.

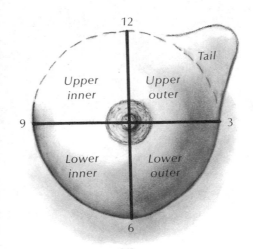

LEFT BREAST

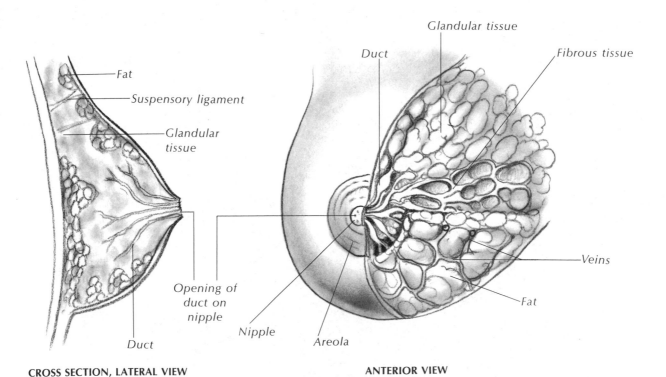

CROSS SECTION, LATERAL VIEW

ANTERIOR VIEW

The male breast consists chiefly of a small nipple and areola. These overlie a thin disc of undeveloped breast tissue that may not be distinguishable clinically from the surrounding tissues.

CHANGES WITH AGE

Development of a woman's breasts begins during puberty. The preadolescent breast consists of a small elevated nipple with no elevation of underlying breast tissue. Between the ages of 8 and 13 (average around 11) secondary sex characteristics become apparent. Breast buds appear, and further enlargement of breasts and areolae follows. The five stages of breast development as defined by Tanner's sex maturity ratings (SMR) are shown below.

Sex Maturity Ratings in Girls: Breasts

STAGE 1

Preadolescent. Elevation of nipple only

STAGE 2	**STAGE 3**
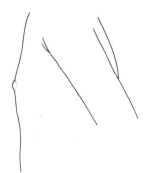	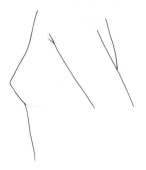
Breast bud stage. Elevation of breast and nipple as a small mound; enlargement of areolar diameter	Further enlargement and elevation of breast and areola, with no separation of their contours

STAGE 4	**STAGE 5**
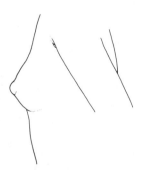	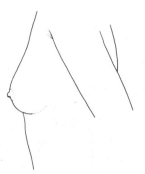
Projection of areola and nipple to form a secondary mound above the level of breast	Mature stage; projection of nipple only. Areola has receded to general contour of the breast (although in some normal individuals the areola continues to form a secondary mound)

(Illustrations through the courtesy of W.A. Daniel, Jr, Division of Adolescent Medicine, University of Alabama, Birmingham)

Concomitantly, pubic hair appears and spreads, as illustrated on page 375. These two developmental changes—in breasts and pubic hair—are useful in assessing growth and maturation, although they do not necessarily proceed synchronously in any given person. The sequence from SMR 2 to SMR 5 takes about 3 years on the average, with a range of 1.5 to 6 years. Axillary hair usually appears about 2 years after pubic hair.

Menarche ordinarily occurs when a girl is in breast stage 3 or 4. By the time of menarche a girl has characteristically reached the peak of her adolescent growth spurt. Although she may continue to grow somewhat, her rate of growth has begun to taper off. The relationships of menarche to breast development and to the growth spurt are useful in counselling a girl who is worried that she may grow too tall or that her menarche is too late. The usual sequence of these changes is summarized in the diagram below.

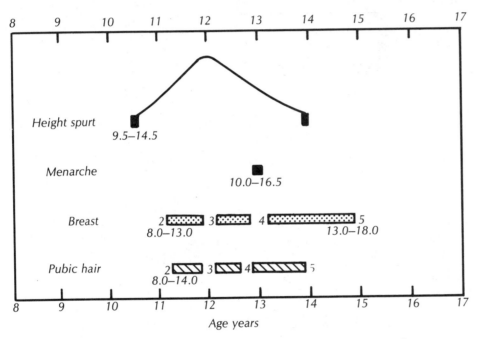

Numbers below the bars indicate the ranges in age within which certain changes occur. (Redrawn from Marshall WA, Tanner JM: Variations in the pattern of pubertal changes in boys. Arch Dis Child 45:22, 1970)

Tanner's figures are based on studies of white English girls. An American survey indicates that black girls tend to be more advanced in their secondary sex characteristics than are whites of the same age. Black girls, too, develop axillary hair earlier than their white counterparts, sometimes before their pubic hair appears. These differences, together with the relatively fine, sparse pubic hair described in Oriental women, illustrate the caution required in applying group norms.

Breasts vary normally in several ways. In about 1 out of 12 girls breasts develop at different rates, and considerable asymmetry may result. This is usually a temporary phenomenon and, unless the difference is unusually marked, reassurance is indicated.

In many girls and premenopausal women the breasts enlarge and become tender and possibly painful during the premenstrual period. At the same time the texture of the breast becomes increasingly lumpy, irregular, or nodular. This condition has in the past been termed fibrocystic disease, but it is so common that it may simply represent a physiologic response. The alternate term "physiologic nodularity" has been proposed. Until the issue is further clarified, the term "fibrocystic disease" deserves at least mental quotation marks.

Pregnancy brings further changes to the breasts. Starting in the second month the breasts enlarge progressively and become somewhat nodular as glandular and ductal tissue increases. The nipples enlarge and become darker and more erectile. Later the areolae also darken and the venous pattern over the breasts becomes accentuated. Colostrum, a thick, yellowish fluid, can often be expressed from the nipple by gentle massage during the latter part of pregnancy.

The breasts of an aging woman tend to diminish in size as glandular tissue atrophies and is replaced by fat. Although the proportion of fat increases, its total amount may also decrease. The breasts often get flabby and hang lower on the chest, as shown on page 127. The ducts surrounding the nipple may become more easily palpable as firm stringy strands. Axillary hair diminishes.

Although adult male breasts are usually relatively small, approximately 2 out of 3 adolescent boys develop temporary breast enlargement, or gynecomastia, on one or both sides. Usually this is a slight change consisting only of a firm plaque of breast tissue deep to the areola. Occasionally, however, more obvious enlargement develops and may cause considerable embarrassment (see p. 328). Pubertal gynecomastia usually resolves spontaneously.

Recent studies indicate that palpable breast tissue may persist in adult men much more frequently than clinicians have recognized it. One report demonstrates a direct correlation with body mass. Aging itself appears to have relatively little if any relationship.

LYMPHATICS

Since the lymphatics of much of the breast drain toward the axilla, an understanding of the axillary lymph nodes will help you in assessing the breasts. Of these, the central axillary nodes are most frequently palpable. They are located high in the axilla, close to the ribs and serratus anterior. Into them drain channels from three other groups of lymph nodes:

1. The pectoral (or anterior) group of nodes is located along the lower border of the pectoralis major inside the anterior axillary fold. These nodes drain the anterior chest wall and most of the breast.

2. The subscapular (or posterior) group is located along the lateral border of the scapula and is felt deep in the posterior axillary fold. These nodes drain the posterior chest wall and a portion of the arm.

3. The lateral group is felt along the upper humerus. These nodes drain most of the arm.

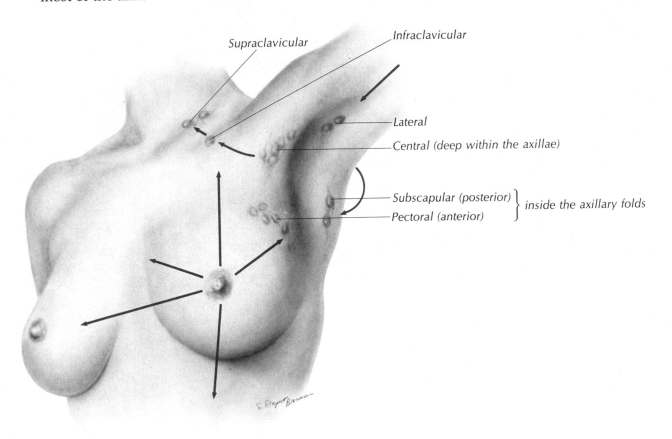

Arrows indicate direction of lymph flow

Lymph drains from the central axillary nodes to the infraclavicular and supraclavicular nodes.

Note that the lymphatics of the breast do not all drain into the axilla. Depending upon the location of a lesion in the breast, spread may occur directly to the infraclavicular nodes, into deep channels within the chest or abdomen, and even to the opposite breast.

Techniques of Examination

THE FEMALE BREAST

General Approach

Many student examiners, especially men, initially find it embarrassing to examine a woman's breasts. These feelings are normal. Women patients, too, may be embarrassed or dislike the exposure involved. With practice you can learn to do a competent examination yet remain sensitive to the patient's feelings.

Tell the patient that you are going to examine her breasts. This may be a good time to ask if she has noted any lumps or other problems or whether she does monthly self-examinations. An adequate inspection requires full exposure of the chest, but later in the examination you may find it helpful to cover one breast while you are palpating the other. Gentleness, courtesy, and a matter-of-fact approach all help the patient to relax.

If the patient is unfamiliar with self-examination, you have a good opportunity to explain what you are doing and help her to repeat maneuvers after you. Self-examination should probably start around the age of 25 to 30, when the incidence of breast cancer rises. An earlier start may be indicated when the family history is strongly positive.

Inspection

With the patient in the sitting position, disrobed to the waist and with her arms at her sides —

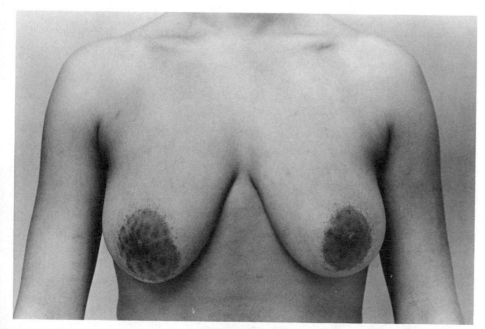

ARMS AT SIDES

Inspect the breasts. Note:

1. Their size and symmetry. Some difference in the size of the breasts, including the areolae, is common and is usually normal, as shown in the photograph on page 317.

2. Their contour, with special reference to masses, dimpling, or flattening

    See Table 10-1, Visible Signs of Breast Cancer (p. 325).

3. The appearance of the skin, including

    Color

    Redness in infection or inflammatory carcinoma

    Thickening or edema

    Edema or increased venous prominence in carcinoma

    Venous pattern

Inspect the nipples. Note:

See Table 10-2, Abnormalities of Nipple and Areola (p. 326).

1. Their size and shape. Simple inversion of long standing is common and usually normal.

    Recent or fixed inversion of the nipple and asymmetry in the directions in which the nipples point suggest cancer.

2. The direction in which they point

3. Rashes or ulcerations

    Paget's disease of the breast (see p. 326)

4. Discharge

When examining an adolescent girl, assess her breast development according to Tanner's sex maturity ratings (SMR) described on page 313. Because an adolescent girl is often concerned about her breasts, it may be helpful to tell her that she is developing normally (if she is) and, using the diagrams, to review with her the usual developmental sequence. You will rate pubic hair development separately, later in the examination.

In order to bring out dimpling or retraction that may otherwise be overlooked, ask the patient (1) to raise her arms over her head, and (2) to press her hands against her hips. Again inspect the breast contour carefully.

Dimpling or retraction of the breasts with either of these maneuvers suggests an underlying cancer. Occasionally these signs may be associated with benign lesions such as post-traumatic fat necrosis, but they must always be evaluated with great care.

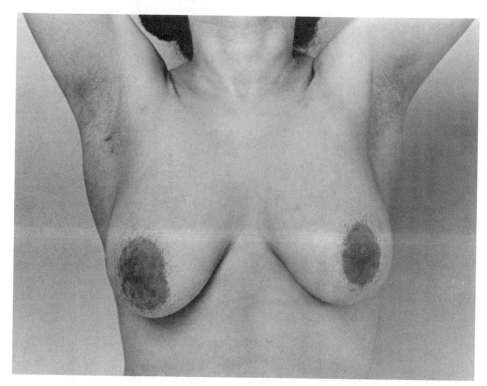

ARMS OVER HEAD

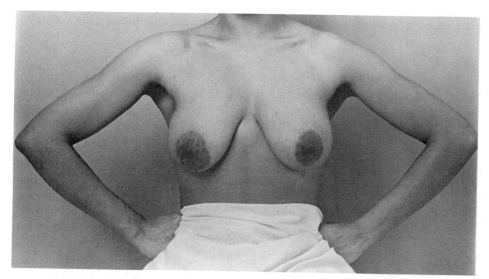

HANDS PRESSED AGAINST HIPS

Contraction of the pectoral muscles produced by pressing the hands against the hips may cause dimpling or retraction that is not visible when the arms are in a resting position.

Occasionally, other maneuvers may be useful:

If the breasts are large or pendulous, ask the patient to stand and lean forward, supported by the back of a chair or the examiner's hands.

This position may reveal an asymmetry of the breast or nipple not otherwise visible and may thus help you to identify a cancer.

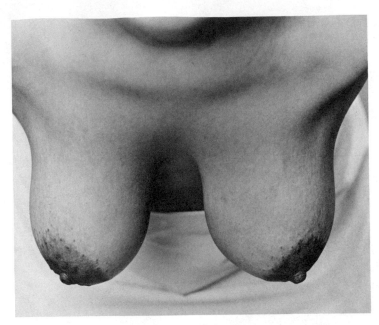

LEANING FORWARD

If you suspect a mass, gently move or compress the breast and watch for dimpling.

Dimpling suggests an underlying cancer.

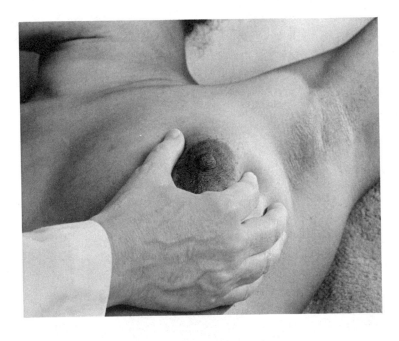

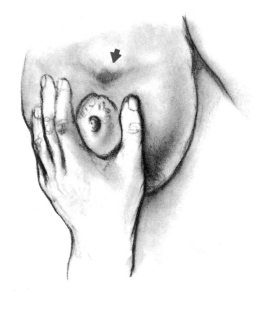

Palpation

Ask the patient to lie down. Unless the breasts are small, place a small pillow under the patient's shoulder on the side you are examining and ask her to rest her arm over her head. These maneuvers help to spread the breast more evenly across the chest and make it easier to find nodules.

Use the pads of your three fingers in a rotary motion to compress the breast tissue gently against the chest wall. Proceed systematically, examining the entire breast including the periphery, tail, and areola.

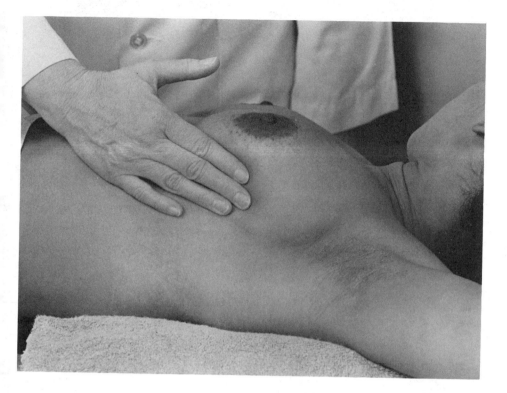

Use a uniform pattern of palpation to assure that you examine the entire breast from the clavicle to the inframammary fold, from the midsternal line to the posterior axillary line, and well into the axilla for the tail of the breast. Patterns include a spiral and a series of parallel lines that move from the sternum and from the posterior axillary line toward the nipple line.

The term "dominant mass" refers to a lump that is larger or qualitatively different from the rest of the breast tissue. It suggests a pathologic rather than a physiologic change.

Note:

The *consistency of the tissues.* Normal variations include the firm elasticity of the young breast, the lobular feel of glandular tissue, and the somewhat stringy feel of some older breasts. Premenstrual fullness, nodularity, and tenderness are common. Especially in large breasts a firm transverse ridge of compressed tissue may be present along the lower edge of the breast. This is the normal inframammary ridge and should not be confused with a tumor.

Tenderness

Tenderness suggests premenstrual fullness, fibrocystic disease, or inflammation, but cancers may also be tender.

Nodules. If any are present, describe the following:

1. Their location, by quadrant or the clock method, with centimeters from the nipple
2. The size in centimeters
3. Shape (*e.g.,* round or discoid, regular or irregular)
4. Consistency (*e.g.,* soft, firm, or hard)
5. Delimitation in relationship to surrounding tissues (*e.g.,* well circumscribed or not)
6. Tenderness
7. Mobility, with special reference to the skin, the pectoral fascia, and the underlying chest wall. Try to move the skin over the mass. Next try to move the mass itself while the patient relaxes her arm and then while she presses her hand against her hip.

See Table 10-3, Differentiation of Common Breast Nodules (p. 327).

Hard, irregular, poorly circumscribed nodules, fixed to the skin or underlying tissues, strongly suggest cancer.

If a mobile mass becomes fixed when the patient presses her hand against her hip, the mass is attached to the pectoral fascia. If it is immobile with the patient relaxed, it is attached to the ribs and intercostal muscles.

Palpate each nipple, noting its elasticity. Compress the nipple and adjacent areola gently between your thumb and index finger, trying to strip them of any discharge.

Loss of nipple elasticity in cancer

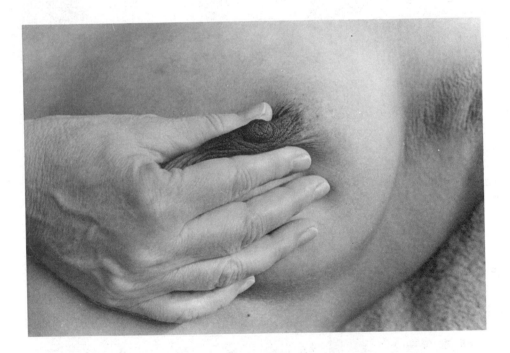

If you see any discharge, or if there is a history of nipple discharge, try to determine its origin by compressing the areola with your index finger placed in radial positions around the nipple. Watch for discharge appearing through one of the duct openings on the nipple's surface. Small amounts of milky discharge may occasionally persist for long periods after lactation.

Bloody discharge may accompany an intraductal papilloma. A milky discharge, not due to a prior pregnancy and usually bilateral, suggests galactorrhea. A unilateral discharge from one

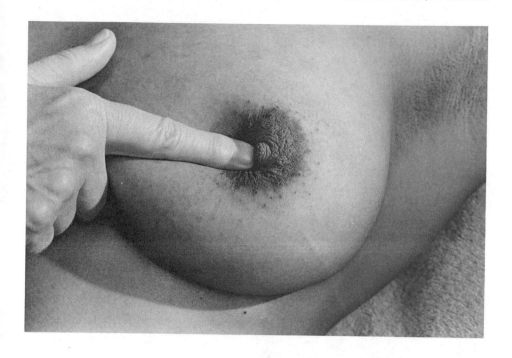

or two ducts suggests a local lesion such as fibrocystic disease, intraductal papilloma, or possibly cancer.

The tactile stimulation of examination may produce temporary erection of the nipple and wrinkling or puckering of the areola. These normal phenomena should not be confused with signs of cancer.

Inversion, flattening, or retraction of the nipple and edema of the areola suggest cancer.

THE MALE BREAST

Examination of the male breast may be brief but should not be omitted.

Inspect the nipple and areola for nodules, swelling, or ulceration.

See Table 10-4, Abnormalities of the Male Breast (p. 328).

Palpate the areola for nodules. If the breast appears enlarged, distinguish between the soft fatty enlargement that may accompany obesity and the firm disc of glandular enlargement.

A firm disc of glandular enlargement in a male is called *gynecomastia.*

THE AXILLAE

Although the axillae may be examined with the patient lying down, a sitting position is preferable.

Inspection

Inspect the skin of each axilla, noting evidence of:

Rash

Infection

Deodorant and other rashes

Sweat gland infections (hidradenitis suppurativa)

Unusual pigmentation

Deeply pigmented, velvety axillary skin suggests the rare acanthosis nigricans, one form of which is associated with internal malignancy.

Palpation

To examine the left axilla, ask the patient to relax with the left arm down. Help by supporting the left wrist or hand with your left hand. Cup together the fingers of your right hand and reach as high as you can toward the apex of the axilla. Your fingers should lie directly behind the pectoral muscles, pointing toward the midclavicle. Now press your fingers in toward the chest wall and slide them downward, trying to feel the central nodes against the chest wall. Of the axillary nodes these are the most often palpable. One or more soft, small, nontender nodes are frequently felt.

Enlarged axillary nodes are most commonly due to infection of the hand or arm, but a search for them is an important part of the evaluation for breast cancer.

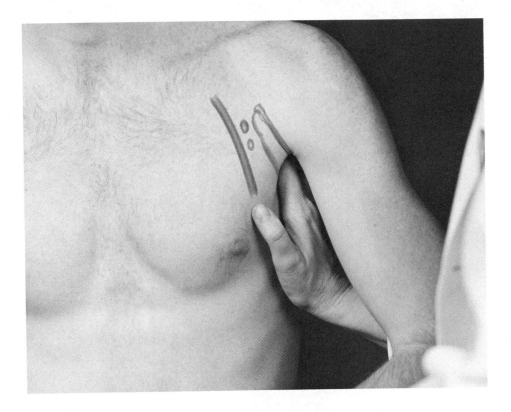

Feel inside the anterior and posterior axillary folds and against the humerus for the pectoral, subscapular, and lateral axillary nodes respectively. The subscapular and lateral nodes may be more easily identified by standing behind the patient.

Now, using your left hand, reverse the procedure to examine the right axilla.

If you detect enlarged or tender nodes, feel for infraclavicular nodes and reexamine the supraclavicular nodes.

Table 10-1

Table 10-1 Visible Signs of Breast Cancer

RETRACTION SIGNS

A breast cancer frequently causes fibrosis, or scar tissue formation. Contraction of this fibrotic tissue produces *retraction signs*, including dimpling of the skin, alteration in breast contours, and flattening or deviation of the nipple.

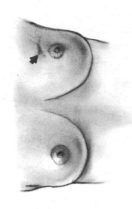

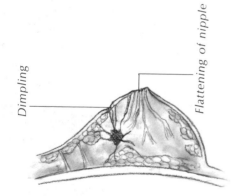

Dimpling

Flattening of nipple

SKIN DIMPLING

Dimpling of the skin suggests an underlying malignancy. Look for this sign when arms are at rest, during special positioning, and on moving or compressing the breasts.

Dimpling and retraction may also be due to benign lesions such as fat necrosis.

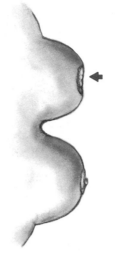

ABNORMAL CONTOURS

ARMS OVER HEAD

Alterations in contour are identified by careful inspection of the normally convex surfaces of the breasts and by comparison of one breast with the other. Changing the patient's position (*e.g.,* by elevation of her arms) also helps.

LEANING FORWARD

Here an abnormal contour and nipple retraction appear when the patient leans forward.

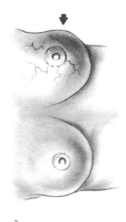

In addition, vascular signs may be noted. These include:

EDEMA OF THE SKIN

Edema of the skin is produced by lymphatic blockade. This is manifested by thickened skin with enlarged pores — the so-called pig skin or orange peel (peau d'orange) appearance.

VENOUS PROMINENCE

Prominence of the venous pattern, especially when unilateral, raises suspicion of underlying disease.

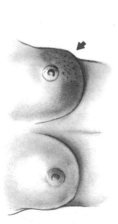

Table 10-2

Table 10-2   Abnormalities of Nipple and Areola

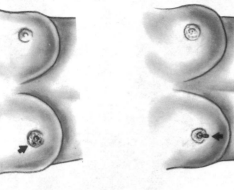

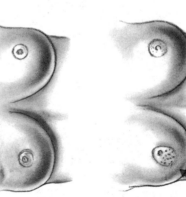

NIPPLE INVERSION

Simple nipple inversion is a common variant of normal and is usually of long standing. It may be unilateral or bilateral. The nipple can usually be pulled out of the sulcus in which it lies. Flattening, broadening, and true retraction are absent. The recent development of inversion in a previously erect nipple, however, is highly suggestive of malignancy.

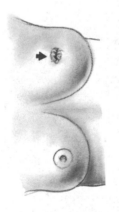

NIPPLE FLATTENING OR RETRACTION

The fibrosis associated with a cancer behind the nipple pulls the nipple inward and may broaden and flatten it.

NIPPLE DEVIATION OR POINTING

The fibrosis associated with cancer may deviate the axis in which the nipple points. The nipple deviates toward the cancer.

EDEMA OF NIPPLE AND AREOLA

The pig skin or orange peel appearance produced by lymphatic blockade often affects the areola first. It strongly suggests cancer.

PAGET'S DISEASE OF THE BREAST

A form of breast cancer, Paget's disease progresses slowly from a smooth redness to rough thickening to erosion or ulceration of the nipple and areola. In any persisting dermatitis of nipple and areola, cancer must be suspected.

NIPPLE DISCHARGE

There are many causes of nipple discharge, most of them nonmalignant. Note the color of the discharge and if possible identify its source.

SUPERNUMERARY BREASTS

One or more extra breasts may be located along the "milk line," most commonly in the axillae or below the normal breasts. A supernumerary breast usually consists of a small nipple and areola and may be mistaken for a mole. Less commonly glandular tissue is present.

Table 10-3

Table 10-3   Differentiation of Common Breast Nodules

The three most common kinds of breast nodules are the cysts of fibrocystic disease (physiologic nodularity), fibroadenoma (a benign tumor), and breast cancer. The classic characteristics of these three conditions, as listed below, are not, however, always predictive of the condition. Definitive diagnosis usually depends on aspiration of cysts or surgical biopsy.

	CYSTS	FIBROADENOMA	CANCER
FINDINGS BY PALPATION (The illustrations do not imply visibility to inspection.)			
USUAL AGE	30–55, regresses after menopause	Puberty and young adulthood, up to age 55	30–90, most common in middle-aged and elderly women
NUMBER	Single or multiple	Usually single, may be multiple	Usually single, although may coexist with other nodular lesions
SHAPE	Round	Round, discoid, or lobular	Irregular or stellate
CONSISTENCY	Soft to firm, usually elastic	May be soft, usually firm	Firm or hard
DELIMITATION	Well delineated	Well delineated	Not clearly delineated from surrounding tissues
MOBILITY	Mobile	Very mobile	May be fixed to skin or underlying tissues
TENDERNESS	Often tender	Usually nontender	Usually nontender
RETRACTION SIGNS	Absent	Absent	Often present

Table 10-4

Table 10-4 Abnormalities of the Male Breast

GYNECOMASTIA

A smooth, firm, mobile, often tender disc of breast tissue centrally located behind the male areola indicates gynecomastia. It may be unilateral or bilateral, mild or severe. Temporary gynecomastia frequently accompanies normal puberty, usually between the ages of 14 and 15.6. Although it usually resolves spontaneously, it may cause considerable psychological distress.

Until recently gynecomastia in adult men has been attributed to decreased androgenic effects, increased estrogenic effects, or both, and various diseases and drugs have been implicated in causing it. The importance of these factors needs to be reevaluated in light of the reportedly high prevalence of palpable breast tissue.

CANCER

Breast cancer is uncommon among men, with only one case occurring for roughly 100 cases among women.

A hard, irregular nodule in the areola of a man's breast suggests this diagnosis. The nodule is usually eccentrically placed. Frequently fixed to both nipple and underlying tissue, it tends to distort the nipple and areola.

Check the axillae for evidence of metastases.

Chapter 11
The Abdomen

Anatomy and Physiology

Review the anatomy of the abdominal wall, identifying the landmarks illustrated. The rectus abdominis muscles can be identified when a person raises head and shoulders from the supine position.

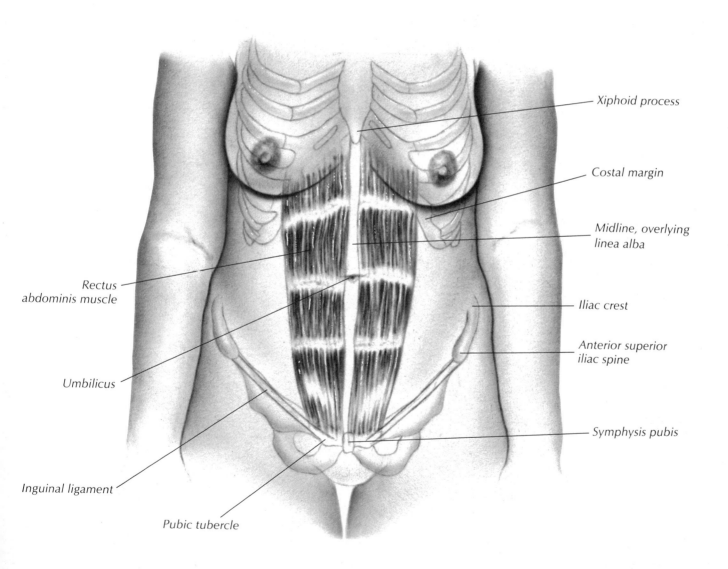

Xiphoid process

Costal margin

Midline, overlying linea alba

Iliac crest

Anterior superior iliac spine

Symphysis pubis

Rectus abdominis muscle

Umbilicus

Inguinal ligament

Pubic tubercle

For descriptive purposes the abdomen is generally divided into four quadrants by imaginary lines crossing at the umbilicus: right upper, right lower, left upper, and left lower quadrants. Another system divides the abdomen into nine sections. Terms for three of them are commonly used: epigastric, umbilical, and hypogastric or suprapubic.

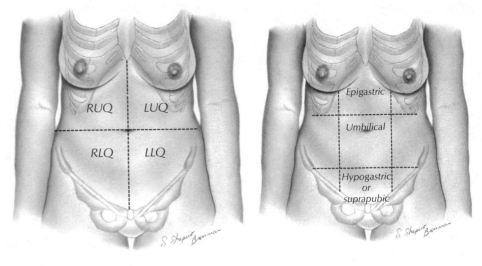

When examining the abdomen you may be able to feel several normal structures. The sigmoid colon is frequently palpable as a firm, narrow tube in the left lower quadrant while the cecum and part of the ascending colon form a softer, wider tube in the right lower quadrant. Portions of the transverse and descending colon may also be palpable. None of these structures should be mistaken for a tumor. Although the normal liver often extends down just below the right costal margin, its soft consistency makes it difficult to feel through the abdominal wall. Occasionally, however, it may be palpable. Also in the right upper quadrant, but usually on a deeper level, lies the lower pole of the right kidney. It may be palpable, especially in thin women with relaxed abdominal walls. Pulsations of the abdominal aorta are frequently visible and usually palpable in the upper abdomen, while the pulsations of the iliac arteries may sometimes be felt in the lower quadrants.

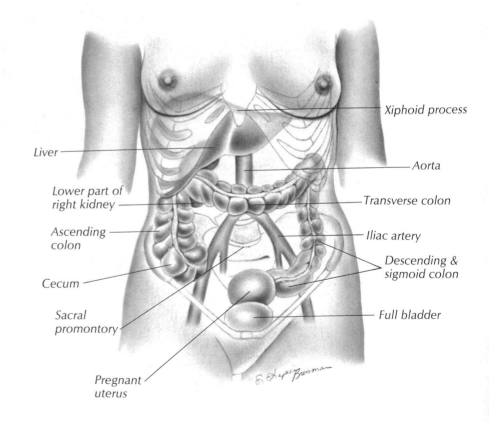

A distended bladder and a pregnant uterus each may rise above the symphysis pubis. With deep palpation several centimeters below the umbilicus in thin relaxed persons you can sometimes feel the sacral promontory, the anterior edge of the first sacral vertebra. Until you are familiar with this normal structure, you may mistake its stony hard outlines for a tumor. Another stony hard lump that can sometimes mislead you, and also alarms an occasional patient who discovers it first, is a normal xiphoid process.

The abdominal cavity extends up under the rib cage to the dome of the diaphragm. In this protected location, beyond the reach of the palpating hand, are much of the liver and stomach and all of the normal spleen. Percussion may help you to assess these organs. Most of the normal gallbladder lies deep to the liver, from which it cannot be clinically distinguished. The duodenum and pancreas lie deep in the upper abdomen where they are not normally palpable.

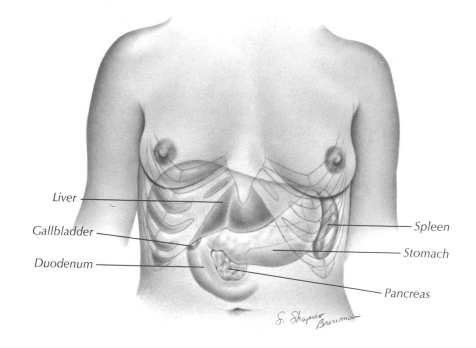

The kidneys are posterior organs, the upper portions of which are protected by the ribs. The costovertebral angle—the angle formed by the lower border of the 12th rib and the transverse processes of the upper lumbar vertebrae—defines the region to assess for kidney tenderness.

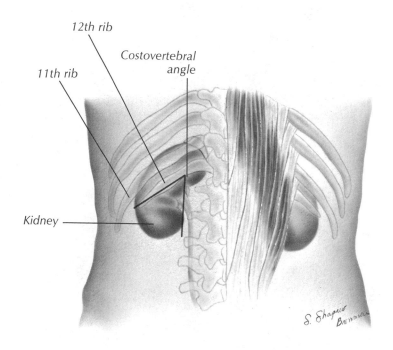

CHANGES WITH AGE

During the middle and later years fat tends to accumulate in the lower abdomen and near the hips, even when total body weight is stable. This accumulation, together with weakening of the abdominal muscles, often produces a potbelly. An occasional person, noting this change with concern or alarm, may interpret it as fluid or evidence of disease.

Techniques of Examination

General Approach

Essential conditions for a good abdominal examination include (1) good light, (2) a relaxed patient, and (3) full exposure of the abdomen from above the xiphoid process to the symphysis pubis. The groins should be visible although the genitalia should be kept draped. To encourage relaxation:

1. The patient should *not* have a full bladder.

2. Make the patient comfortable in a supine position with a pillow for the head and perhaps another under the knees. You can ascertain whether or not the patient is relaxed flat on the table by trying to insert your hand underneath the low back.

An arched back thrusts the abdomen forward, thus tightening the abdominal muscles.

3. The patient should keep arms at the sides or folded across the chest. Although patients commonly put their arms over their heads, this move should be discouraged because it stretches and tightens the abdominal wall and makes palpation difficult.

4. Have warm hands, a warm stethoscope, and short fingernails. Rubbing your hands together or running hot water over them may help to warm them. Anxious examiners, unfortunately, often have cold hands. This problem decreases over time.

5. Ask the patient to point to any areas of pain, and examine tender areas last.

6. Approach slowly and avoid quick, unexpected movements.

7. Distract the patient if necessary with conversation or questions.

8. If the patient is very frightened or very ticklish, begin palpation with his or her own hand beneath yours. In a few moments you can slip your hand underneath to palpate directly.

9. Monitor your examination by watching the patient's face.

Make a habit of visualizing each organ in the region you are examining. From the patient's right side proceed in an orderly fashion: inspection, auscultation, percussion, palpation.

Inspection

Starting from your usual standing position at the right side of the bed, inspect the abdomen. When looking at the contour of the abdomen and watching for peristalsis, it is helpful to sit or bend down so that you can view the abdomen tangentially.

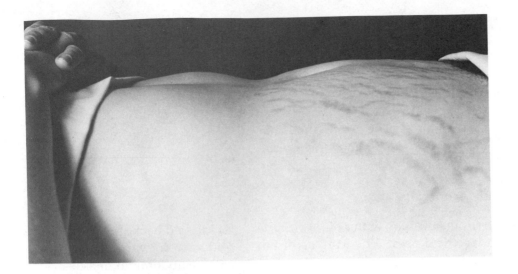

Note:

1. *The skin,* including:

   Scars. Describe their location.

   Striae. Old silver striae or stretch marks, as illustrated above, are normal.

   Dilated veins. A few small veins may be visible normally.

   Rashes and lesions

2. *The umbilicus*—its contour and location, and any signs of inflammation or hernia

3. *The contour of the abdomen.* Is it flat, rounded, protuberant, or scaphoid (markedly concave or hollowed)? Do the flanks bulge or are there any local bulges? Include in this survey the inguinal and femoral areas.

4. *Symmetry*

5. *Enlarged organs.* As the patient breathes, watch for an enlarged liver or spleen to descend below the rib cage.

6. *Masses*

7. *Peristalsis.* Observe for several minutes if you suspect intestinal obstruction. Peristalsis may be visible normally in very thin people.

8. *Pulsations.* The normal aortic pulsation is frequently visible in the epigastrium.

Pink purple striae of Cushing's syndrome

Dilated veins of hepatic cirrhosis or of inferior vena cava obstruction

See Table 11-1, Abdominal Hernias and Bulges (p. 351).

See Table 11-2, Protuberant Abdomens (p. 352).

Bulging flanks of ascites

Suprapubic bulge of distended bladder or pregnant uterus

Asymmetry of an enlarged organ or mass

Lower abdominal mass of an ovarian or uterine tumor

Increased peristaltic waves of intestinal obstruction

Increased pulsation of aortic aneurysm or of increased pulse pressure

Auscultation

Auscultation of the abdomen is useful in assessing bowel motility and abdominal complaints, in searching for renal artery stenosis as a cause of hypertension, and in exploring for other vascular obstructions. You should practice the technique until you become thoroughly familiar with normal variations and can listen intelligently when you need to. In most other situations, however, auscultation may safely be omitted.

Listen to the abdomen before percussing and feeling it, because the latter maneuvers may alter the frequency of bowel sounds. Place the diaphragm of your stethoscope gently on the abdomen.

Listen for *bowel sounds* and note their frequency and character. Normal sounds consist of clicks and gurgles, the frequency of which has been estimated at from 5 to 34 per minute. Occasionally you may hear borborygmi—loud prolonged gurgles of hyperperistalsis—the familiar "stomach growling." Since bowel sounds are widely transmitted through the abdomen, listening in one spot, such as the right lower quadrant, is generally enough.

Bowel sounds may be altered in diarrhea, intestinal obstruction, paralytic ileus, and peritonitis. See Table 11-3, Sounds in the Abdomen (p. 353).

If the patient has high blood pressure, listen in the epigastrium and in each upper quadrant for *bruits*—vascular sounds resembling heart murmurs. Later in the examination, when the patient sits up, listen also in the costovertebral angles. Epigastric bruits confined to systole may be heard in normal persons.

In a hypertensive patient an epigastric bruit with systolic and diastolic components strongly suggests renal artery stenosis.

If you suspect arterial insufficiency in the legs, listen for bruits over the aorta, the iliac arteries, and the femoral arteries. Bruits confined to systole are relatively common, however, and do not necessarily signify occlusive disease.

Bruits with both systolic and diastolic components suggest the turbulent blood flow of partial arterial occlusion.

See Table 11-3, Sounds in the Abdomen (p. 353).

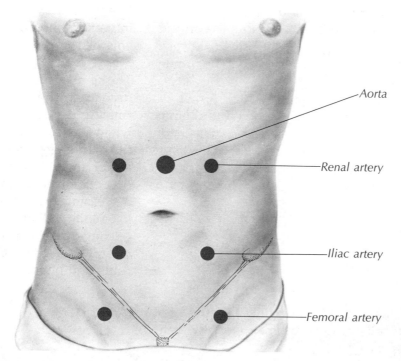

Aorta

Renal artery

Iliac artery

Femoral artery

If you suspect a liver tumor, gonococcal infection around the liver, or splenic infarction, listen over the liver and spleen for *friction rubs.*

See Table 11-3, Sounds in the Abdomen (p. 353).

Percussion

Percussion is useful for orientation to the abdomen, for measuring the liver and sometimes the spleen, and for identifying ascitic fluid, solid or fluid-filled masses, and air in the stomach and bowel. Although percussion for all these purposes is described in this section, some practitioners prefer to alternate percussion with palpation as they examine liver, spleen, and other areas of the abdomen. Either approach is satisfactory.

ORIENTATION. Percuss the abdomen lightly in all four quadrants to assess the distribution of tympany and dullness. Tympany usually predominates because of gas in the gastrointestinal tract, but normal fluid and feces here may also produce a duller sound. On each side note where abdominal tympany changes to the dullness of solid posterior structures. Check the suprapubic area for the dullness of a distended bladder or an enlarged uterus.

See Table 11-2, Protuberant Abdomens (p. 352).

Dullness in both flanks indicates further assessment for ascites (see pp. 347–348).

Lightly percuss the lower anterior chest, between lungs above and costal margins below. You will usually find on the right the dullness of liver and on the left the tympany that overlies the gastric air bubble and the splenic flexure of the colon.

Dullness above the left costal margin indicates need for a careful search for an enlarged spleen.

THE LIVER. In the right midclavicular line, starting at a level below the umbilicus (in an area of tympany, not dullness), lightly percuss upward toward the liver. Ascertain the lower border of liver dullness in the midclavicular line. Next, identify the upper border of liver dullness in the midclavicular line. Lightly percuss from lung resonance down toward liver dullness. Gently displace a woman's breast as necessary. The course of percussion is shown on the top of p. 337.

The span of liver dullness is increased when the liver is enlarged.

Now measure in centimeters the vertical span, or height, of liver dullness. Normal liver spans are shown on the bottom of page 337. They are generally greater in men than in women, in tall people than in short. If the liver seems to be enlarged, outline the lower edge by percussing in other areas.

The span of liver dullness is decreased when the liver is small. It may also be decreased when free air is present below the diaphragm, as from a perforated hollow viscus. Serial observations may show a decreasing span of dullness as a liver enlarged due to hepatitis or congestive heart failure improves or, less commonly, as fulminant hepatitis progresses.

Although percussion is probably the most accurate clinical method for estimating liver size, it typically results in underestimation of the true vertical span of the liver.

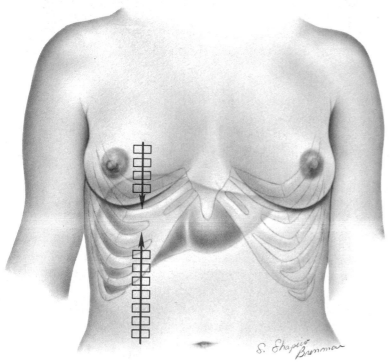

PERCUSSING LIVER SPAN

Liver dullness is commonly displaced downward in chronic obstructive pulmonary disease. Span, however, remains normal.

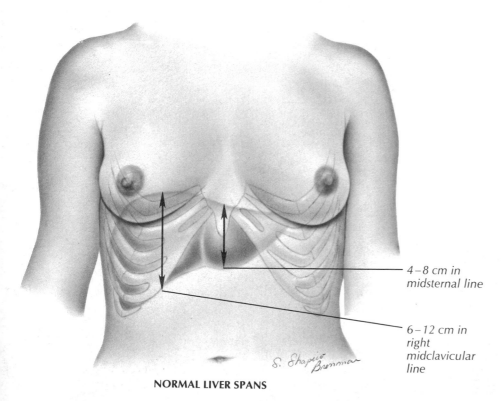

4–8 cm in midsternal line

6–12 cm in right midclavicular line

NORMAL LIVER SPANS

Dullness of a right pleural effusion or consolidated lung, if adjacent to liver dullness, may falsely increase the estimated liver size.

Gas in the colon may produce tympany in the right upper quadrant, obscure liver dullness, and falsely decrease the estimated liver size.

THE SPLEEN. The normal spleen lies in the curve of the diaphragm just posterior to the midaxillary line. A small oval area of splenic dullness can sometimes be found between pulmonary resonance above and abdominal tympany anteriorly, but searching for it is seldom worthwhile.

Percussion may give you a clue, however, to *splenomegaly,* an enlarged spleen. When a spleen enlarges, it does so anteriorly, downward, and medially, replacing the tympany of stomach and colon with the dullness of a solid organ. If you suspect splenomegaly, try two further maneuvers:

1. Percuss the lowest interspace in the left anterior axillary line. This area is usually tympanitic. Then ask the patient to take a deep breath, and percuss again. When spleen size is normal, the percussion note usually remains tympanitic.

A change in percussion note from tympany to dullness on inspiration suggests splenic enlargement. This is a positive *splenic percussion sign.* Dullness, however, may appear during inspiration even when spleen size is normal, thus giving a falsely positive sign.

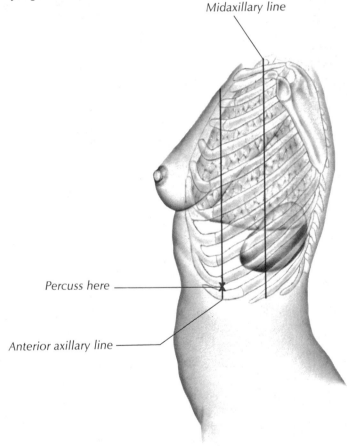

Midaxillary line

Percuss here

Anterior axillary line

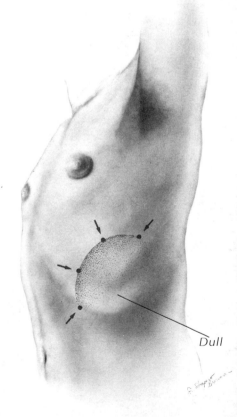

Dull

2. Percuss in several directions from resonance or tympany toward the estimated area of splenic dullness so that you can outline its edges. You cannot, of course, distinguish between the dullness of the posterior flank and that of the spleen.

Percussion as a method for estimating splenic size is impaired by the varying contents of stomach and colon, but it may suggest splenomegaly even before the organ becomes palpable. Further, it may help you to position your hands properly to feel for the splenic edge.

A large dull area suggests splenic enlargement.

Palpation

Light palpation is especially helpful in identifying muscular resistance, abdominal tenderness, and some superficial organs and masses. Its gentleness helps also to reassure and relax the patient.

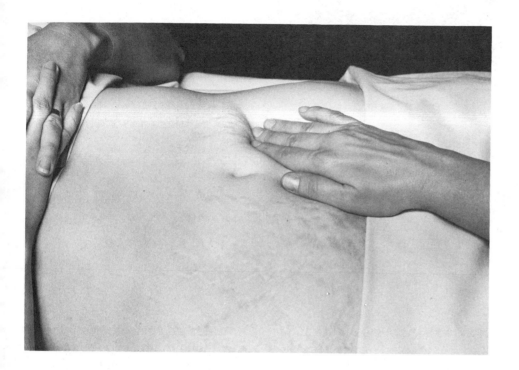

Keeping your hand and forearm on a horizontal plane, use the pads of your fingertips, with fingers together, in a light, gentle, dipping motion. Avoid short quick jabs. Moving smoothly, feel in all quadrants. Identify any organs or masses, any area of tenderness or increased resistance. If resistance is present, try to determine whether it is voluntary resistance or involuntary spasm: (1) Try all the maneuvers to relax the patient (see p. 333). (2) Feel for the relaxation of the rectus muscles that normally accompanies expiration. If the rigidity remains unaltered by all these maneuvers, it is probably involuntary.

Involuntary rigidity or spasm of the abdominal muscles indicates peritoneal inflammation.

Deep palpation is usually required to delineate abdominal masses. Again using the palmar surfaces of your fingers, feel in all four quadrants. Identify any masses and note their location, size, shape, consistency, tenderness, pulsations, and mobility (*e.g.*, with respiration or with the examining hand).

When deep palpation is difficult—because of obesity, for example, or muscular resistance—use two hands, one on top of the other. Exert pressure with the outside hand while concentrating on feeling with the inside hand.

Abdominal masses may be categorized in several ways: physiologic (pregnant uterus), inflammatory (diverticulitis of the colon or a pseudocyst of the pancreas), vascular (an aneurysm of the abdominal aorta), neoplastic (a myomatous uterus or a carcinoma of the colon or ovary), or obstructive (a distended bladder).

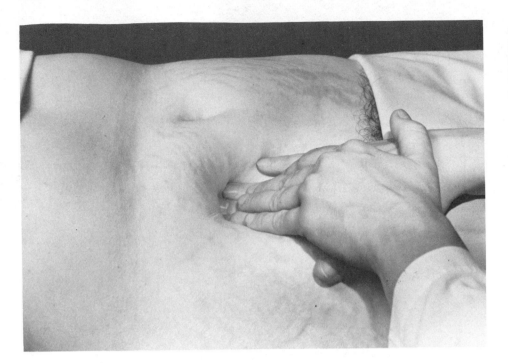

An obstructed, distended gallbladder may form an oval mass below the edge of the liver and merging with it. It is dull to percussion.

ASSESSMENT FOR PERITONEAL IRRITATION. Abdominal pain and tenderness, especially when associated with muscular spasm, suggest inflammation of the parietal peritoneum. Localize it as accurately as possible. First, even before palpation, *ask the patient to cough* and determine where the cough produced pain. Thus guided, *palpate gently with one finger* to map the tender area. Pain produced by light percussion has similar localizing value. These gentle maneuvers may be all you need to establish an area of peritoneal inflammation.

Abdominal pain on coughing or with light percussion suggests peritoneal inflammation. See Table 11-4, Tender Abdomens (pp. 354–355).

If not, *look for rebound tenderness.* Press your fingers in firmly and slowly, and then quickly withdraw them. If the withdrawal (not just the pressure) causes pain, you have elicited rebound tenderness.

Rebound tenderness suggests peritoneal inflammation.

Old age may blunt the manifestations of acute abdominal disease. Pain may be less severe, fever is often less pronounced, and signs of peritoneal inflammation such as muscular guarding and rebound tenderness may be diminished or even absent.

THE LIVER. Place your left hand behind the patient, parallel to and supporting the right 11th and 12th ribs. Remind the patient to relax on your hand if necessary. By pressing your left hand forward, the patient's liver is more easily felt in front.

Place your right hand on the patient's right abdomen lateral to the rectus muscle, with your fingertips well below the lower border of liver dullness.

Some examiners like to point their fingers up toward the patient's head, while others prefer a somewhat more oblique position. In either case, press gently in and up.

The liver below is palpable about 4 cm below the right costal margin in the midclavicular line.

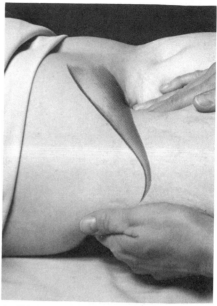

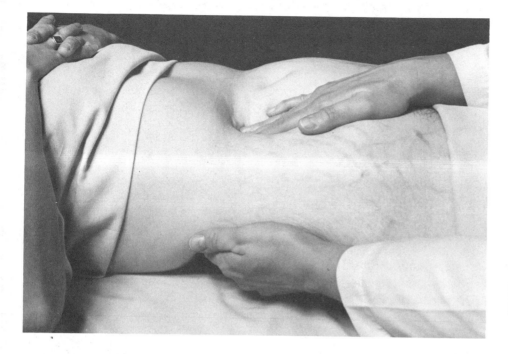

The edge of an enlarged liver may be missed by starting palpation too high in the abdomen.

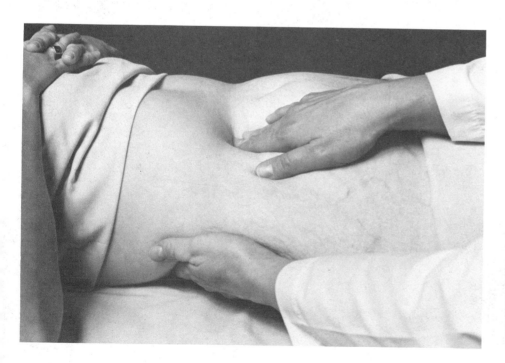

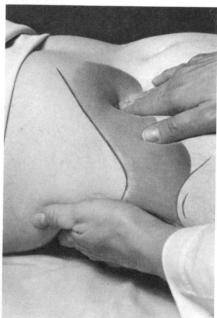

Ask the patient to take a deep breath. Try to feel the liver as it comes down to meet your fingertips. If you feel it, release the pressure of your palpating hand slightly so that the liver can slip under your finger pads and you can feel its anterior surface. Note any tenderness. If palpable at all, the edge of a normal liver is soft, sharp, and regular, its surface smooth. The normal liver may be slightly tender.

Firmness or hardness of the liver, bluntness or rounding of its edge, and irregularity of its contour suggest an abnormality of the liver. See Table 11-5, Liver Enlargement: Apparent and Real (pp. 356–357).

Try to trace the liver edge both laterally and medially. Palpation through the rectus muscles, however, is especially difficult. Describe or sketch the liver edge, and measure its distance from the right costal margin in the midclavicular line.

In order to feel the liver you may have to alter your pressure according to the thickness and resistance of the abdominal wall. If you cannot feel it, move your palpating hand closer to the costal margin and try again.

The liver may also be felt by the "hooking technique." Stand to the right of the patient's chest. Place both hands, side by side, on the right abdomen below the border of liver dullness. Press in with your fingers and up toward the costal margin. Ask the patient to take a deep breath.

The liver edge below is palpable with the finger pads of both hands.

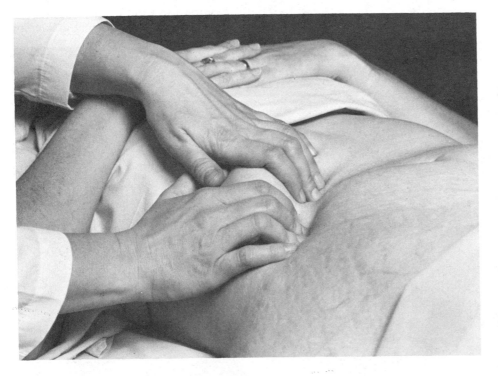

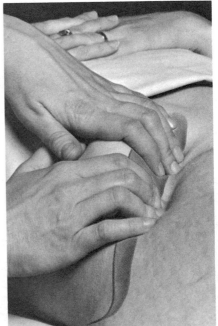

Some people, especially women, breathe primarily with their chests rather than with their diaphragms. It may be helpful to train such a patient to "breathe with the abdomen," thus bringing the liver, as well as the spleen and kidneys, into a palpable position during inspiration.

To check for liver tenderness when the organ is not palpable, place your left hand flat on the lower right rib cage and then gently strike your hand with the ulnar surface of your right fist. Ask the patient to compare the sensation with that produced by a similar maneuver on the left side.

Tenderness suggests inflammation, as in hepatitis.

THE SPLEEN. With your left hand, reach over and around the patient to support and press forward the lower left rib cage. With your right hand below the left costal margin, press in toward the spleen. Begin palpation low enough to be sure that you are below a possibly enlarged spleen. (If your hand is too close to the costal margin, furthermore, it is not sufficiently mobile to reach up under the rib cage.) Ask the patient to take a deep breath. Try to feel the tip or edge of the spleen as it comes down to meet your fingertips. Note any tenderness, assess the splenic contour, and measure the distance between the spleen's lowest point and the left costal margin.

An enlarged spleen may be missed if the examiner starts too high in the abdomen to feel the lower edge.

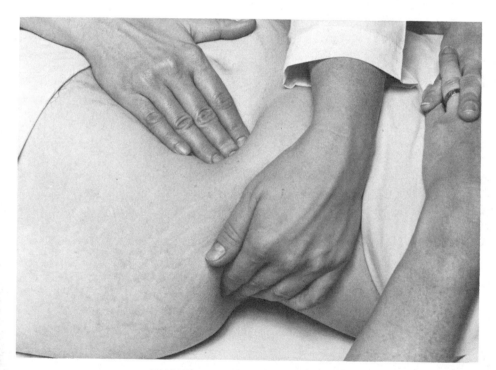

PALPATING SPLEEN — PATIENT SUPINE

If the spleen of an adult is palpable, it is probably considerably larger than normal. The spleen tip below is just palpable deep to the left costal margin.

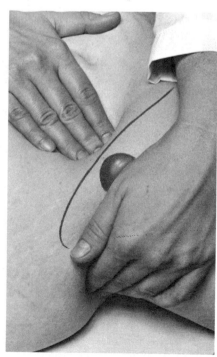

Repeat with the patient lying on the right side with legs somewhat flexed at hips and knees. In this position, gravity may bring the spleen forward and to the right into a palpable location.

The enlarged spleen below is palpable about 2 cm below the left costal margin on deep inspiration.

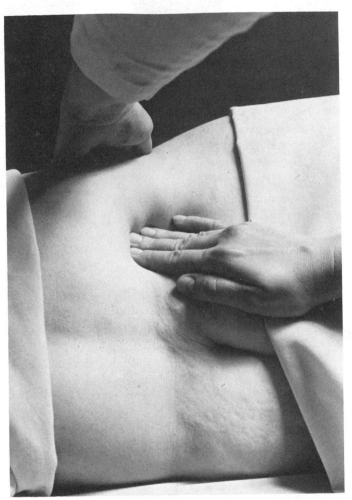

PALPATING SPLEEN—PATIENT LYING ON RIGHT SIDE

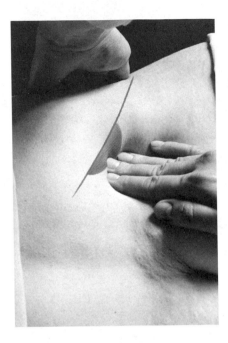

Marked and massive spleno-megaly are shown below.

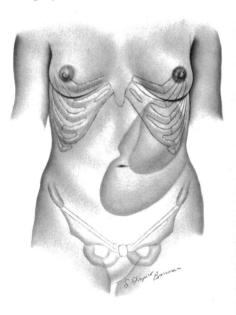

In assessment of a mass in the left flank, attributes that favor an enlarged spleen over an

THE KIDNEYS

The Right Kidney. Place your left hand behind the patient just below and parallel to the 12th rib, with your fingertips just reaching the costovertebral angle. Lift, trying to displace the kidney anteriorly. Place your right hand gently in the right upper quadrant, lateral and parallel to the rectus muscle. Ask the patient to take a deep breath. At the peak of inspiration, press your right hand firmly and deeply into the right upper quadrant, just below the costal margin, and try to "capture" the kidney between your two hands. Ask the patient to breathe out and then to stop breathing briefly. Slowly release the pressure of your right hand, feeling at the same

enlarged left kidney are a notch on the medial border, extension beyond the midline, dullness to percussion, and the ability to get your fingers deep to its medial and lower borders but not between the mass and the costal margin. Definitive differentiation, however, cannot usually be made on clinical criteria alone.

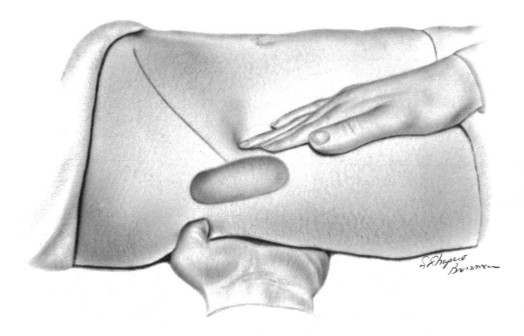

time for the kidney to slide back into its expiratory position. If the kidney is palpable, describe its size, contour, and tenderness.

A normal right kidney may be palpable, especially in thin, well relaxed women. It may or may not be slightly tender. The patient is usually aware of a capture and release. Occasionally a right kidney is located more anteriorly than usual and then must be distinguished from the liver. The edge of the liver, if palpable, tends to be sharper and to extend farther medially and laterally. It cannot be captured. The lower pole of the kidney is rounded.

The Left Kidney. To capture the left kidney move to the patient's left side. Use your right hand to lift from in back, and your left hand to feel deep in the left upper quadrant. Proceed as before.

Alternatively, try to feel for the left kidney by a method somewhat similar to feeling for the spleen. With your left hand reach over and around the

Causes of kidney enlargement include hydronephrosis, cysts, and tumors. Bilateral enlargement suggests polycystic disease.

In assessment of a mass in the left flank, attributes that favor an enlarged kidney over an enlarged spleen are the preservation of normal tympany in the left upper quadrant, and the

patient to lift the left loin, and with your right hand feel deep in the left upper quadrant. Ask the patient to take a deep breath, and feel for a mass.

A normal left kidney is rarely palpable.

Kidney Tenderness. Tenderness may be noted during abdominal palpation, but search for it also in each costovertebral angle. Pressure from your fingertips may be enough to reveal tenderness here, but, if not, use fist percussion. Place the ball of one hand in the costovertebral angle and strike it with the ulnar surface of your fist. Use force sufficient to cause a perceptible but painless jar or thud in a normal person.

ability to get your fingers between the mass and the costal margin but not deep to its medial and lower borders.

Pain with pressure or with fist percussion in the costovertebral angle suggests kidney infection, but it may also have a musculo-skeletal cause.

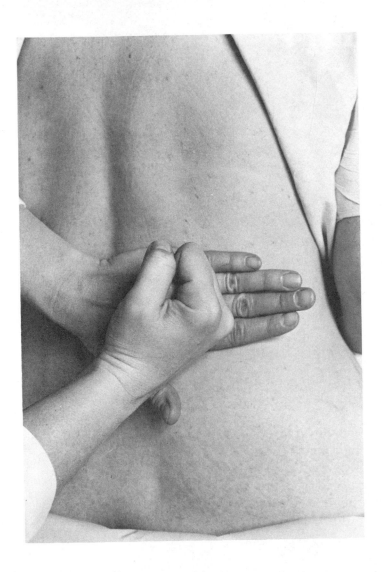

To save the patient needless exertion, integrate this maneuver with your examination of the back (see p. 122).

THE AORTA. Press firmly deep in the upper abdomen, slightly to the left of the midline, and identify the aortic pulsations. In persons over age 50 try to

In an older person a periumbili-cal or upper abdominal mass

assess the width of the aorta by pressing deeply in the upper abdomen with one hand on each side of the aorta, as illustrated. A normal adult aorta is not more than 2 cm wide. This measurement does not include the thickness of the abdominal wall.

with expansile pulsations strongly suggests an aortic aneurysm. A merely tortuous abdominal aorta, however, may be difficult to distinguish from an aneurysm on clinical grounds.

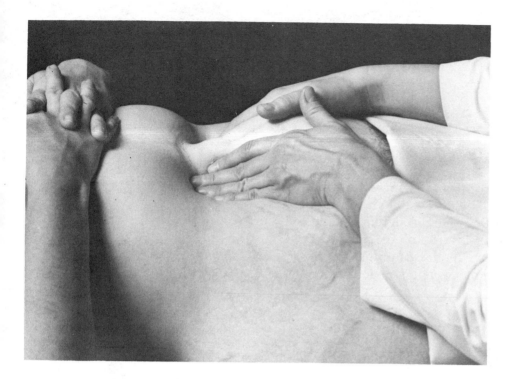

Special Maneuvers

TO ASSESS POSSIBLE ASCITES. A protuberant abdomen with bulging flanks suggests the possibility of ascitic fluid. Because ascitic fluid characteristically sinks with gravity while gas-filled loops of bowel float to the top, percussion gives a dull note in dependent areas of the abdomen. Look for such a pattern by percussing outward in several directions from the central area of tympany. Map the border between tympany and dullness.

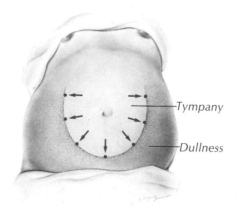

Two further maneuvers help to confirm the presence of ascites, although both signs may be misleading.

1. *Test for shifting dullness.* After mapping the borders of tympany and dullness, ask the patient to turn onto one side. Percuss and mark the

borders again. In a person without ascites the borders between tympany and dullness usually stay relatively constant.

In ascites, dullness shifts to the more dependent side, while tympany shifts to the top.

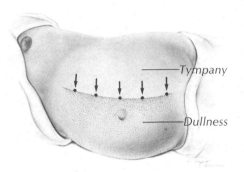

2. *Test for a fluid wave.* Ask the patient or an assistant to press the edges of both hands firmly down the midline of the abdomen. This pressure helps to stop the transmission of a wave through fat. While you tap one flank sharply with your fingertips, feel on the opposite flank for an impulse transmitted through the fluid. Unfortunately, this sign is often negative until ascites is obvious, and it is sometimes positive in people without ascites.

An easily palpable impulse suggest ascites.

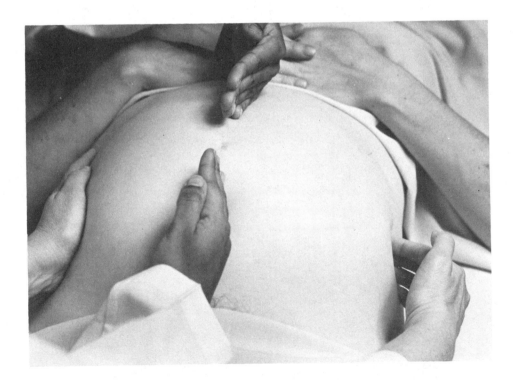

TO ASSESS POSSIBLE APPENDICITIS

1. Ask the patient to point to where the pain began and where it is now. Ask the patient to cough. Determine whether and where pain results.

1. The pain of appendicitis classically begins near the

umbilicus and then shifts to the right lower quadrant, where coughing increases it. Elderly patients report this pattern less frequently than younger ones.

2. Search carefully for an area of local tenderness.

2. Localized tenderness anywhere in the right lower quadrant, even in the right flank, may indicate appendicitis.

3. Feel for muscular rigidity.

3. Early voluntary guarding may be replaced by involuntary muscular rigidity.

4. Perform a rectal examination and, in women, a pelvic examination. These maneuvers may not help you to discriminate well between a normal and an inflamed appendix, but they may help to identify an inflamed appendix atypically located within the pelvic cavity. They may also suggest other causes of the abdominal pain.

4. Right-sided rectal tenderness may be caused by, for example, inflamed adnexa or an inflamed seminal vesicle, as well as by an inflamed appendix.

Some additional maneuvers are sometimes helpful.

5. Check the tender area for rebound tenderness. (If other signs are typically positive, you can save the patient unnecessary pain by omitting this test.)

5. Rebound tenderness suggests peritoneal inflammation, as from appendicitis.

6. Check for Rovsing's sign and for referred rebound tenderness. Press deeply and evenly in the *left* lower quadrant. Then quickly withdraw your fingers.

6. Pain in the *right* lower quadrant during *left*-sided pressure suggests appendicitis (a positive Rovsing's sign). So does right lower quadrant pain on quick withdrawal (referred rebound tenderness).

7. Look for a psoas sign. Place your hand just above the patient's right knee and ask the patient to raise the thigh against your hand. Alternatively, ask the patient to turn onto the left side. Then extend the patient's right leg at the hip. Flexion of the leg at the hip makes the psoas muscle contract; extension stretches it.

7. Increased abdominal pain on either maneuver constitutes a positive psoas sign, suggesting irritation of the psoas muscle by an inflamed appendix.

8. Look for an obturator sign. Flex the patient's right thigh at the hip, with the knee bent, and rotate the leg internally at the hip. This maneuver stretches the internal obturator muscle. (Internal rotation of the hip is illustrated on p. 437, lower right.)

8. Right hypogastric pain constitutes a positive obturator sign, suggesting irritation of the obturator muscle.

9. Look for cutaneous hyperesthesia. At a series of points down the abdominal wall gently pick up a fold of skin between your thumb and index finger, without pinching it. This maneuver should not normally be painful.

TO ASSESS POSSIBLE ACUTE CHOLECYSTITIS. When right upper quadrant pain and tenderness suggest acute cholecystitis, look for Murphy's sign. Hook your left thumb or the fingers of your right hand under the costal margin at the point where the lateral border of the rectus muscle intersects with the costal margin. Alternatively, if the liver is enlarged, hook your thumb or fingers under the liver edge at a comparable point below. Ask the patient to take a deep breath. Watch the patient's breathing and note the degree of tenderness.

TO ASSESS ABDOMINAL HERNIAS. If you suspect but do not see an umbilical or incisional hernia, ask the patient to raise both head and shoulders off the table.

Inguinal and femoral hernias (in both sexes) are discussed in the next chapter. They can give rise to important problems and must not be overlooked.

TO DISTINGUISH AN ABDOMINAL MASS FROM A MASS IN THE ABDOMINAL WALL. An occasional mass is in the abdominal wall rather than inside the abdominal cavity. Ask the patient either to raise the head and shoulders or to strain down, thus tightening the abdominal muscles. Feel for the mass again.

9. Localized pain with this maneuver, in all or part of the right lower quadrant, may accompany appendicitis.

A sharp increase in tenderness with a sudden stop in inspiratory effort constitutes a positive Murphy's sign of acute cholecystitis. Hepatic tenderness may also increase with this maneuver, but is usually less well localized.

The bulge of a hernia will usually appear with this action (see p. 351).

The cause of intestinal obstruction or peritonitis may be missed by overlooking a strangulated femoral hernia.

A mass in the abdominal wall remains palpable; an intra-abdominal mass is obscured by muscular tension.

Table 11-1

Table 11-1 Abdominal Hernias and Bulges

Abdominal hernias are almost always made more evident when the patient stands or raises the head and shoulders from a supine position.

UMBILICAL HERNIA

In young children an umbilical hernia is centrally located. In adults it is usually partially above the umbilicus.

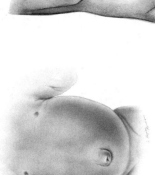

INFANT

ADULT

INCISIONAL HERNIA

A defect in the abdominal muscles may develop after a surgical incision.

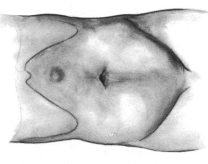

DIASTASIS RECTI

Not a true hernia, a diastasis recti is a separation of the two rectus abdominis muscles, often caused by pregnancy or obesity. The increased intra-abdominal pressure produced when the patient raises the head and shoulders causes a midline ridgelike bulge. It is of no clinical consequence.

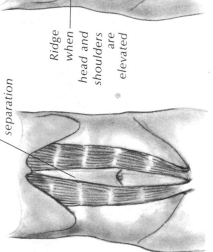

Ridge when head and shoulders are elevated

Palpable separation

HERNIA OF THE LINEA ALBA

This is a small, often tender, midline nodule usually located in the epigastrium and best discovered with the patient standing up. Its pain may mimic an ulcer. To find it, run the pad of your index finger down the linea alba.

Table 11-2

Table 11-2   Protuberant Abdomens

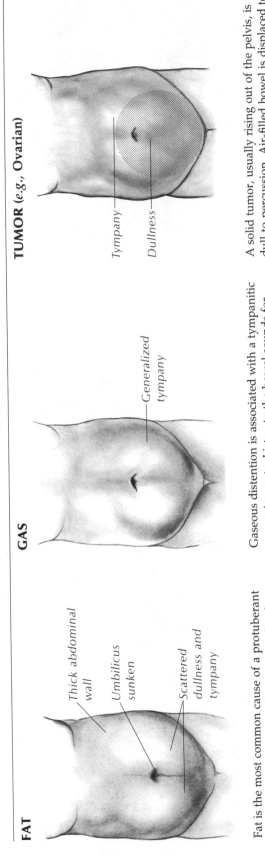

FAT

Thick abdominal wall

Umbilicus sunken

Scattered dullness and tympany

Fat is the most common cause of a protuberant abdomen and is associated with generalized obesity. The abdominal wall is thick. Additionally, fat in the mesentery and omentum contributes to abdominal size. The umbilicus may appear sunken. The percussion note is normal.

GAS

Generalized tympany

Gaseous distention is associated with a tympanitic percussion note. Listen to the bowel sounds for evidence of obstruction or ileus.

TUMOR (*e.g.,* Ovarian)

Tympany

Dullness

A solid tumor, usually rising out of the pelvis, is dull to percussion. Air-filled bowel is displaced to the periphery.

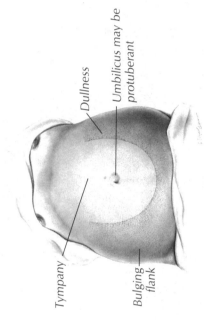

ASCITIC FLUID

Tympany

Bulging flank

Dullness

Umbilicus may be protuberant

Ascitic fluid seeks the lowest point in the abdomen, producing bulging flanks that are dull to percussion. The umbilicus may protrude. Turn the patient onto one side to detect the shift in position of the fluid level (shifting dullness).

PREGNANCY

Tympany

Dullness

Pregnancy is a common cause of a pelvic "tumor." Listen for the fetal heart with a fetoscope.

Table 11-3 Sounds in the Abdomen

BOWEL SOUNDS

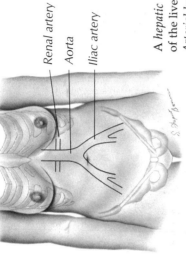

Bowel sounds may be:

1. Increased, as from diarrhea or early intestinal obstruction
2. Decreased, then absent, as in paralytic ileus and peritonitis. Before deciding that bowel sounds are absent, sit down and listen where shown for 2 min or even longer.

High-pitched tinkling sounds suggest intestinal fluid and air under tension in a dilated bowel. Rushes of high-pitched sounds coinciding with an abdominal cramp indicate intestinal obstruction.

BRUITS

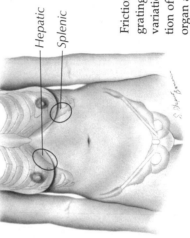

Renal artery
Aorta
Iliac artery

A *hepatic bruit* suggests carcinoma of the liver or alcoholic hepatitis. *Arterial bruits* with both systolic and diastolic components suggest partial occlusion of the aorta or large arteries.

VENOUS HUM

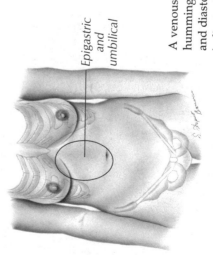

Epigastric and umbilical

A venous hum is rare. It is a soft humming noise with both systolic and diastolic components. It indicates increased collateral circulation between portal and systemic venous systems, as in hepatic cirrhosis.

FRICTION RUBS

Hepatic
Splenic

Friction rubs are rare. They are grating sounds with respiratory variation. They indicate inflammation of the peritoneal surface of an organ as from a liver tumor, gonococcal perihepatitis, recent liver biopsy, or splenic infarct. When a systolic bruit accompanies a hepatic friction rub, suspect carcinoma of the liver.

Table 11-3

Table 11-4

Table 11-4   Tender Abdomens

ABDOMINAL WALL TENDERNESS

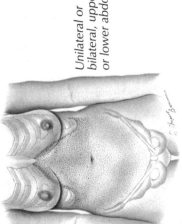

Superficial lesions

Muscle

Deep lesion

Tenderness may originate in the abdominal wall. When the patient raises head and shoulders, this tenderness persists, whereas tenderness from a deeper lesion (protected by the tightened muscles) decreases.

VISCERAL TENDERNESS

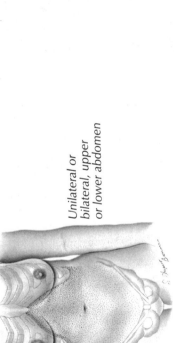

Normal aorta

Normal or spastic sigmoid colon

Enlarged liver

Normal cecum

The structures shown may be tender to deep palpation. Usually the discomfort is dull and there is no muscular rigidity or rebound tenderness. A reassuring explanation to the patient may prove quite helpful.

TENDERNESS FROM DISEASE IN THE CHEST AND PELVIS

ACUTE PLEURISY

Unilateral or bilateral, upper or lower abdomen

Abdominal pain and tenderness may be due to acute pleural inflammation. When unilateral it may mimic acute cholecystitis or appendicitis. Rebound tenderness and rigidity are less common; chest signs are usually present.

ACUTE SALPINGITIS

Frequently bilateral, the tenderness of acute salpingitis is usually maximal just above the inguinal ligaments. Rebound tenderness and rigidity may be present. On pelvic examination, motion of the uterus causes pain.

Table 11-4

TENDERNESS OF PERITONEAL INFLAMMATION

Tenderness associated with peritoneal inflammation is usually more severe than visceral tenderness. Muscular rigidity and rebound tenderness are frequently but not necessarily present. Examples follow:

ACUTE CHOLECYSTITIS

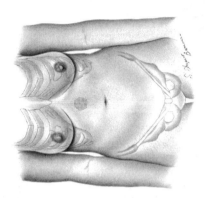

Signs are maximal in the right upper quadrant. Check for Murphy's sign (see p. 350).

ACUTE PANCREATITIS

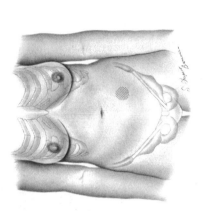

In acute pancreatitis epigastric tenderness and rebound tenderness are usually present but the abdominal wall may be soft.

ACUTE APPENDICITIS

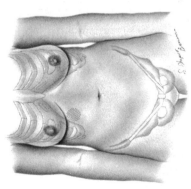

Just below the middle of a line joining the umbilicus and the anterior superior iliac spine

Right rectal tenderness

Right lower quadrant signs are typical of acute appendicitis but may be absent early in the course. The typical area of tenderness is illustrated. Explore other portions of the right lower quadrant as well as the right flank.

ACUTE DIVERTICULITIS

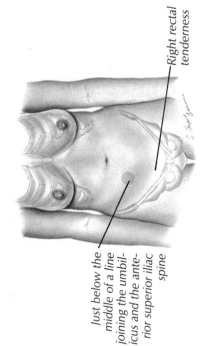

Acute diverticulitis most often involves the sigmoid colon and then resembles a left-sided appendicitis.

Table 11-5

Table 11-5   Liver Enlargement: Apparent and Real

A palpable liver does not necessarily indicate hepatomegaly (an enlarged liver) but more often results from a change in consistency—from the normal softness to an abnormal firmness or hardness, as in cirrhosis. Clinical estimates of liver size should be based on both percussion and palpation, although even then they are far from perfect.

DOWNWARD DISPLACEMENT OF THE LIVER BY A LOW DIAPHRAGM

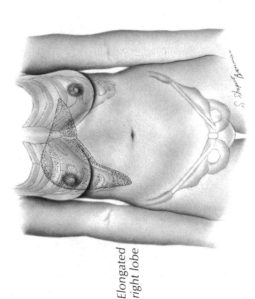

Upper border low

Height by percussion normal

This is a common finding (*e.g.,* in emphysema) when the diaphragm is low. The liver edge may be readily palpable well below the costal margin. Percussion, however, reveals a low upper edge also, and the total span or height is normal.

NORMAL VARIATIONS IN LIVER SHAPE

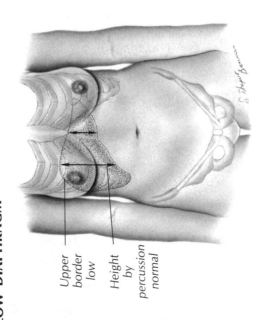

Elongated right lobe

In some persons, especially those with a lanky build, the liver tends to be somewhat elongated so that its right lobe is easily palpable as it projects downward toward the iliac crest. Such an elongation, sometimes called Riedel's lobe, represents a variation in shape, not an increase in liver volume or size. This variant illustrates the basic limitations of assessing liver size. We can only estimate the upper and lower borders of an organ that has three dimensions and differing shapes. Some error is unavoidable.

Table 11-5

SMOOTH LARGE NONTENDER LIVER

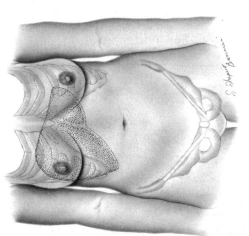

Cirrhosis may produce an enlarged liver with a firm nontender edge. The liver is not always enlarged in this condition, however, and many other diseases may produce similar findings.

SMOOTH LARGE TENDER LIVER

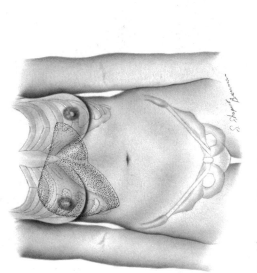

An enlarged liver with a smooth tender edge suggests inflammation, as in hepatitis, or venous congestion, as in right-sided heart failure.

LARGE IRREGULAR LIVER

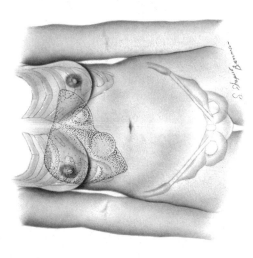

An enlarged liver that is firm or hard and has an irregular edge or surface suggests malignancy. There may be one or more nodules. The liver may or may not be tender.

Chapter 12
Male Genitalia and Hernias

Anatomy and Physiology

Review the anatomy of the male genitalia.

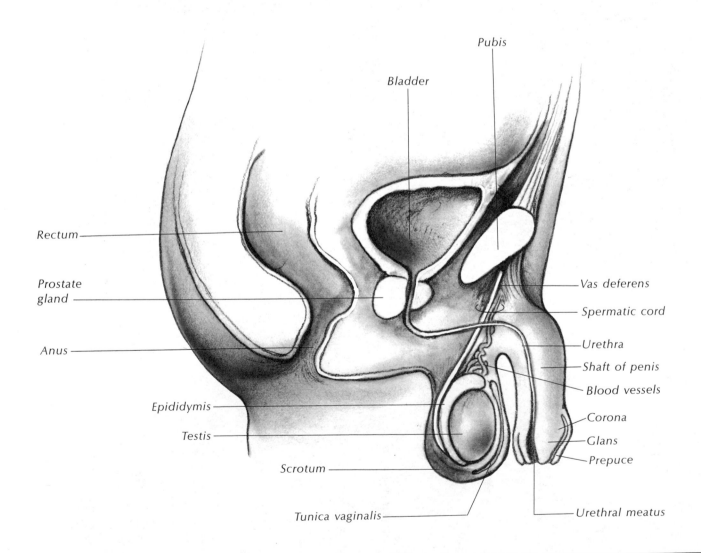

The shaft of the penis is formed by three columns of vascular erectile tissue bound together by fibrous tissue. At the end of the penis is the cone-shaped glans with its expanded base, or corona. Unless the person has been circumcised, the glans is covered by a loose, hoodlike fold of skin called the prepuce, or foreskin. The urethra is located ventrally in the shaft of the penis, within one of the vascular columns, and urethral abnormalities may sometimes be felt here. The urethra opens into the vertical, slitlike urethal meatus, located somewhat ventrally at the tip of the glans.

The scrotum is a loose, wrinkled pouch divided into two compartments, each of which contains a testicle. The testes are ovoid, somewhat rubbery structures, about 4.5 cm long in the adult, with a range from 3.5 cm to 5.5 cm. The left usually lies somewhat lower than the right. On the posterolateral surface of each testis is the softer, comma-shaped epididymis. It is most prominent along the superior margin of the testis. (The epididymis may be located anteriorly in 6% to 7% of males.) Surrounding the testis, except posteriorly, is the tunica vaginalis, a serous membrane enclosing a potential cavity.

The testes produce spermatozoa and testosterone. Testosterone stimulates the pubertal growth of the male genitalia, prostate, and seminal vesicles. It also stimulates the development of masculine secondary sex characteristics, including the beard, body hair, musculoskeletal development, and the enlarged larynx with its male voice.

The vas deferens, a cordlike structure, begins at the tail of the epididymis, ascends within the scrotal sac, and passes through the external inguinal ring on its way to the abdomen and pelvis. Behind the bladder it is joined by the duct from the seminal vesicle and enters the urethra within the prostate gland. Sperm thus pass from the testis and the epididymis through the vas deferens into the urethra. Secretions from the vasa deferentia, the seminal vesicles, and the prostate all contribute to the semen. Within the scrotum each vas is closely associated with blood vessels, nerves, and muscle fibers, with which it makes up the spermatic cord.

Lymphatics from the penile and scrotal surfaces drain into the inguinal nodes. When you find an inflammatory or possibly malignant lesion on these surfaces, assess the inguinal nodes especially carefully for enlargement or tenderness. The lymphatics of the testes, however, drain into the abdomen, where enlarged nodes are clinically undetectable. See page 410 for further discussion of the inguinal nodes.

Since hernias are relatively common, it is important to understand the anatomy of the groin. The basic landmarks are the anterior superior iliac spine, the pubic tubercle, and the inguinal ligament which runs between them. Find these on yourself or a colleague.

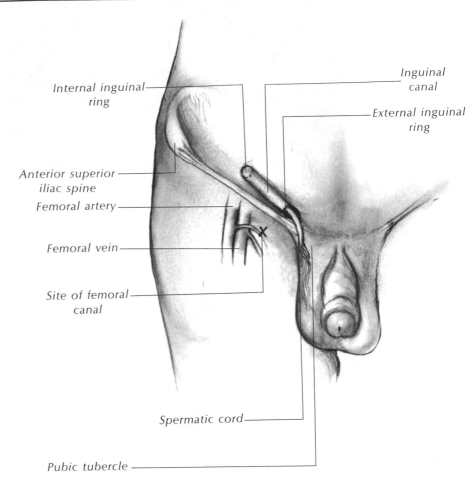

Internal inguinal ring

Inguinal canal

External inguinal ring

Anterior superior iliac spine

Femoral artery

Femoral vein

Site of femoral canal

Spermatic cord

Pubic tubercle

The inguinal canal, which lies above and approximately parallel to the inguinal ligament, forms a tunnel for the vas deferens as it passes through the abdominal muscles. The exterior opening of the tunnel—the external inguinal ring—is a triangular slitlike structure palpable just above and lateral to the pubic tubercle. The internal opening of the canal—or internal inguinal ring—is about 1 cm above the midpoint of the inguinal ligament. Neither canal nor internal ring is palpable through the abdominal wall. When loops of bowel force their way through weak areas of the inguinal canal they produce inguinal hernias, as illustrated on page 371.

Another potential route for a herniating mass is the femoral canal. This lies below the inguinal ligament. Although you cannot see it, you can estimate its location by placing your right index finger, from below, on the right femoral artery. Your middle finger will then overlie the femoral vein; your ring finger, the femoral canal. Femoral henias protrude here.

CHANGES WITH AGE

Important anatomic changes in the male genitalia accompany puberty and help to define its progress. A noticeable increase in the size of the testes constitutes the first reliable sign and usually begins between the ages of 9.5 years and 13.5 years. Next, pubic hair appears and the penis begins to grow. The complete change from preadolescent to adult form requires about 3 years, with a range from less than 2 years to almost 5 years.

By observing the pubic hair and the development of the penis, testes, and scrotum, you can assess sexual development according to the five stages described by Tanner. These are outlined and illustrated on page 361.

Sex Maturity Ratings in Boys

In assigning SMRs in boys, observe each of the three characteristics separately because they may develop at different rates. Record two separate ratings: pubic hair and genital. If the penis and testes differ in their stages, average the two into a single figure for the genital rating.

| | PUBIC HAIR | GENITAL | |
		PENIS	TESTES AND SCROTUM
STAGE 1	Preadolescent—no pubic hair except for the fine body hair (vellus hair) similar to that on the abdomen	Preadolescent—same size and proportions as in childhood	Preadolescent—same size and proportions as in childhood
STAGE 2	Sparse growth of long, slightly pigmented, downy hair, straight or only slightly curled, chiefly at the base of the penis	Slight or no enlargement	Testes larger; scrotum larger, somewhat reddened, and altered in texture
STAGE 3	Darker, coarser, curlier hair spreading sparsely over the pubic symphysis	Larger, especially in length	Further enlarged
STAGE 4	Coarse and curly hair, as in the adult; area covered greater than in stage 3 but not as great as in the adult and not yet including the thighs	Further enlarged in length and breadth, with development of the glans	Further enlarged; scrotal skin darkened
STAGE 5	Hair adult in quantity and quality, spread to the medial surfaces of the thighs but not up over the abdomen	Adult in size and shape	Adult in size and shape

(Illustrations through the courtesy of W.A. Daniel, Jr, Division of Adolescent Medicine, University of Alabama, Birmingham)

In about 80% of men, pubic hair spreads further up the abdomen in a triangular pattern pointing toward the umbilicus. Because this kind of spread, known as stage 6, is not completed until the mid-20s or later, however, it is not considered a pubertal change.

An average developmental sequence is diagrammed below. Note the rather wide age ranges for the start and completion of pubertal changes. Some normal boys may have completed their genital development while others of the same age have not yet begun. Boys often begin to experience ejaculation as they approach SMR 3, and sometimes mistake nocturnal emissions for the discharge of venereal disease. Discussion and explanation are indicated.

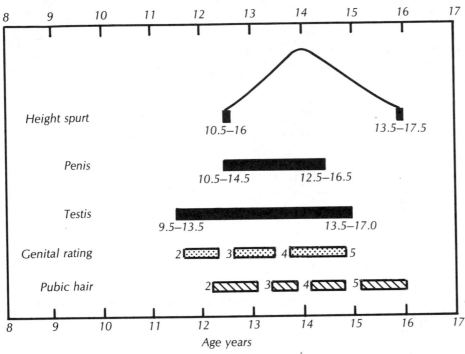

Numbers below the bars indicate the ranges in age within which certain changes occur. (Redrawn from Marshall WA, Tanner JM: Variations in the pattern of pubertal changes in boys. Arch Dis Child 45:22, 1970)

In elderly patients pubic hair may decrease and become gray. The penis decreases in size and the testicles hang lower in the scrotum. Although the testes often decrease in size with protracted, debilitating illnesses, they do not necessarily decrease with aging *per se.*

Techniques of Examination

GENERAL APPROACH

Many students—especially women but also men—feel anxious about examining a man's genitalia. "How will the patient react?" "Will he have an erection?" "Will he let me examine him?" These feelings are normal, and it is often helpful to talk them through with your instructor or another experienced clinician. In fact, a male patient, regardless of who examines him, does occasionally have an erection, though not very often, and is probably more embarrassed about it than you are. You should explain to him that this is a normal response, finish your examination, and proceed on with an unruffled demeanor. Occasionally, too, a man may refuse to be examined by a woman just as a woman sometimes refuses to allow a man to do a pelvic examination. Your own comfort with the procedures will minimize these difficulties, but you should respect the patient's wishes and rights.

A good genital examination can be done with the patient either standing or supine. To check for hernias or varicoceles, however, the patient should stand, and you should sit comfortably on a chair or stool. A gown conveniently covers the patient's chest and abdomen. If you suspect an infectious process, wear gloves. Expose the genitalia and groins.

ASSESSMENT OF SEXUAL DEVELOPMENT

Assess sexual maturation by noting the size and shape of the penis and testes, the color and texture of the scrotal skin, and the character and distribution of the pubic hair. Assessment of testicular size requires palpation (see. p. 365).

In adolescents, make two separate sex maturity ratings according to Tanner's stages: one for pubic hair, the other for genital development. If a boy's testes have increased in size to 2.5 cm or more, or if his pubic hair has reached stage 2, you can tell him that his sexual development has started. You may also use Tanner's diagrams to show your patient how he is developing, to review the wide range of normals for his age, and to answer any questions he may have.

Delayed puberty is often familial or related to chronic illness. It may also be due to abnormalities in the hypothalamus, anterior pituitary gland, or testes.

THE PENIS

Inspection

Inspect the penis, including:

1. The skin

See Table 12-1, Abnormalities of the Penis (p. 368).

2. The prepuce (foreskin). If it is present, retract it or ask the patient to retract it. This step is essential for the detection of many chancres and carcinomas. A cheesy, whitish material called smegma may normally accumulate under the foreskin.

Phimosis is a tight prepuce that cannot be retracted over the glans. Paraphimosis is a tight prepuce that, once retracted, gets caught behind the glans and cannot be returned. Edema ensues.

3. The glans

Look for any ulcers, scars, nodules, or signs of inflammation.

Balanitis (inflammation of the glans); balanoposthitis (inflammation of the glans and prepuce)

Check the skin around the base of the penis for excoriations or inflammation. Look for nits or lice at the bases of the pubic hairs.

Pubic or genital excoriations suggest the possibility of lice (crabs) or sometimes scabies.

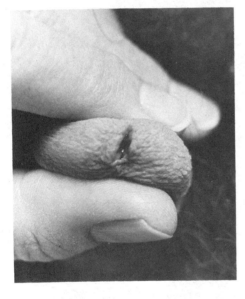

Note the location of the urethral meatus. Compress the glans gently between your index finger above and your thumb below. This maneuver should open the urethral meatus and allow you to inspect it for discharge. Normally there is none.

The discharge of gonococcal urethritis tends to be profuse and yellow, while that of nongonococcal urethritis tends to be scanty and white or clear. Definitive diagnosis, however, requires a Gram stain and culture.

If the patient has reported a discharge but you do not see any, ask him to strip, or milk, the shaft of the penis from its base to the glans. Alternatively, do it yourself. This maneuver may bring some discharge out of the urethral meatus for appropriate examination. Have a glass slide and culture materials ready.

Palpation

Palpate any abnormality of the penis, noting any tenderness or induration. Palpate the shaft of the penis between your thumb and first two fingers, noting any induration. Palpation of the shaft may be omitted in a young asymptomatic male patient.

Induration along the ventral surface of the penis suggests a urethral stricture or possibly a carcinoma. Tenderness of such an indurated area suggests periurethral inflammation secondary to a urethral stricture.

If you retracted the foreskin, replace it before proceeding on to the scrotum.

THE SCROTUM

Inspection

Inspect the contour of the scrotum, noting any lumps or swelling. Inspect the scrotal skin, noting any nodules, ulcers, excoriations, or signs of inflammation. Lift up the scrotum so that you can see its posterior surface as well.

Palpation

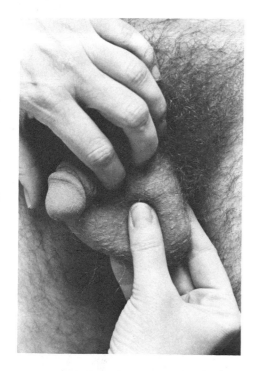

Between your thumb and first two fingers palpate each testis and epididymis.

Note their size, shape, consistency, and tenderness; feel for any nodules. Pressure on the testis normally produces a deep visceral pain.

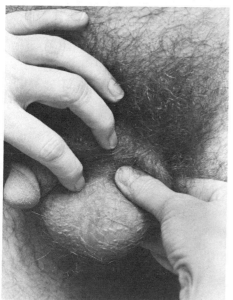

Identify each spermatic cord with its vas deferens, and palpate it between your thumb and fingers along its course from epididymis to superficial inguinal ring.

Note any nodules or swellings.

A poorly developed scrotum on one or both sides suggests cryptorchidism. Common scrotal swellings include indirect inguinal hernias, hydroceles, and scrotal edema. A tender, painful scrotal swelling occurs in acute epididymitis, acute orchitis, torsion of the spermatic cord, and strangulated hernia. A painless nodule in the testis must raise the question of testicular cancer.

See Table 12-2, Abnormalities in the Scrotum (pp. 369–370).

A varicocele (see p. 369) is best identified in this area.

Any swelling in the scrotum other than the testicles should be evaluated by transillumination. After darkening the room, shine the beam of a strong flashlight from behind the scrotum through the mass. Look for transmission of the light as a red glow.

Swellings containing serous fluid transilluminate (*i.e.,* light up with a red glow); those containing blood or tissue do not.

HERNIAS

Inspection

Inspect the inguinal and femoral areas carefully for bulges. While you continue your observation, ask the patient to strain down.

A bulge that appears on straining suggests a hernia.

Palpation

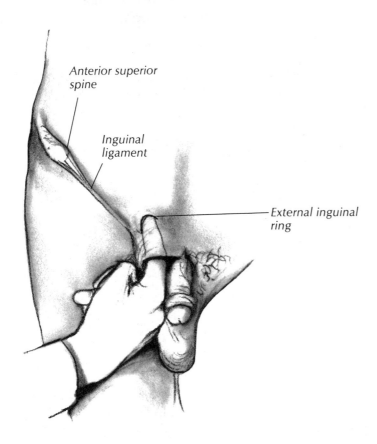

Anterior superior spine

Inguinal ligament

External inguinal ring

Using in turn your right hand for the patient's right side and your left hand for the patient's left side, invaginate loose scrotal skin with your index finger. Start at a point low enough to ensure full mobility of your finger. This may be the bottom of the scrotal sac. Follow the spermatic cord upward to above the inguinal ligament and find the triangular slitlike opening of the external inguinal ring. This is just above and lateral to the pubic tubercle. If the ring is somewhat enlarged, it may admit your index finger. If possible, gently follow the inguinal canal laterally in its oblique

See Table 12-3, Course and Presentation of Hernias in the Groin (p. 371)

See Table 12-4, Differentiation of Hernias in the Groin (p. 372).

course. With your finger located either at the external ring or within the canal, ask the patient to strain down or cough. Note any palpable herniating mass as it touches your finger.

Inspect and palpate the anterior thigh in the region of the femoral canal. Ask the patient to strain down again or cough. Note any swelling or tenderness.

If you find a large scrotal mass and suspect that it may be a hernia, ask the patient to lie down. The mass may return to the abdomen by itself. If not—

1. Can you get your fingers above the mass in the scrotum?

2. Listen to the mass with a stethoscope for bowel sounds.

If you can, suspect a hydrocele.

Bowel sounds may be heard over a hernia, but not over a hydrocele.

If the findings suggest a hernia, gently try to reduce it (return it to the abdominal cavity) by sustained pressure with your fingers. Do not attempt this maneuver if the mass is tender or the patient reports nausea and vomiting.

History may be helpful here. The patient can usually tell you what happens to his swelling on lying down and may be able to demonstrate how he reduces it himself. Remember to ask him.

A hernia is *incarcerated* when its contents cannot be returned to the abdominal cavity. A hernia is *strangulated* when the blood supply to the entrapped contents is compromised. Suspect strangulation in the presence of tenderness, nausea, and vomiting.

HERNIAS IN WOMEN

Both femoral and indirect inguinal hernias occur in women too. The techniques are basically the same as for men. To feel an indirect inguinal hernia, however, palpate in the labia majora and upward to just lateral to the pubic tubercles.

Table 12-1

Table 12-1   Abnormalities of the Penis

HYPOSPADIAS

Hypospadias is a congenital displacement of the urethral meatus to the inferior surface of the penis. A groove extends from the actual urethral meatus to its normal location on the tip of the glans.

SYPHILITIC CHANCRE

A syphilitic chancre usually appears as an oval or round, dark red, painless erosion or ulcer with an indurated base. Nontender enlarged inguinal lymph nodes are typically associated. Chancres may be multiple and when secondarily infected may be painful. They may then be mistaken for the lesions of herpes.

GENITAL HERPES

A cluster of small vesicles, followed by shallow, painful, nonindurated ulcers on red bases, suggests a herpes simplex infection. The lesions may occur anywhere on the penis. Usually there are fewer lesions when the infection recurs.

VENEREAL WART
(*Condyloma acuminatum*)

A variant of the ordinary wart, these are rapidly growing warty excrescences.

CARCINOMA OF THE PENIS

Carcinoma may present as an indurated nodule or ulcer that is usually nontender. Limited almost completely to men who are not circumcised in childhood, it may be masked by the prepuce. Any persistent penile sore must be considered suspicious.

PEYRONIE'S DISEASE

In Peyronie's disease there are palpable nontender hard plaques just beneath the skin, usually along the dorsum of the penis. The patient complains of crooked, painful erections.

Table 12-2

Table 12-2 Abnormalities in the Scrotum

HYDROCELE

Fingers can get above mass

A hydrocele is a nontender, fluid-filled mass that occupies the space within the tunica vaginalis. The examining fingers can get above the mass within the scrotum. The mass transilluminates.

SCROTAL HERNIA

Fingers cannot get above mass

A hernia located within the scrotum is usually an indirect inguinal hernia. Since it comes through the external inguinal ring, the examining fingers cannot get above it in the scrotum.

TUMOR OF THE TESTIS

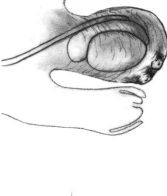

EARLY

LATE

A tumor of the testis usually appears as a painless nodule. It does not transilluminate. Any nodule within the testis must raise the suspicion of malignancy.

As a testicular neoplasm grows and spreads, it may seem to replace the entire organ. The testicle characteristically feels heavier than normal.

SPERMATOCELE OR CYST OF THE EPIDIDYMIS

A painless, movable cystic mass just above the testis, a spermatocele or cyst of the epididymis transilluminates.

VARICOCELE

Varicocele refers to varicose veins of the spermatic cord, usually found on the left. It feels like a soft "bag of worms" separate from the testis and slowly collapses when the scrotum is elevated in the supine patient. Infertility may be associated.

TUBERCULOUS EPIDIDYMITIS

The chronic inflammation of tuberculosis produces a firm enlargement of the epididymis, sometimes tender, with thickening or beading of the vas deferens.

SEBACEOUS CYSTS

These are firm, yellowish, nontender, cutaneous cysts up to about 1 cm in diameter. They are common and frequently multiple.

Continued

Table 12-2

Table 12-2 (Cont'd.)

ACUTE ORCHITIS	ACUTE EPIDIDYMITIS	TORSION OF THE SPERMATIC CORD

An acutely inflamed testis is painful, tender, and swollen. The testis may be difficult to distinguish from the epididymis. The scrotum may be reddened. Look for evidence of postpubertal mumps or other less common infectious causes.

An acutely inflamed epididymis is tender and swollen and may be difficult to distinguish from the testis. The scrotum may be reddened, and the vas deferens may also be inflamed. Epididymitis occurs chiefly in adults. Coexisting urinary tract infection or prostatitis supports the diagnosis.

Torsion, or twisting, of the testicle on its spermatic cord produces an acutely painful, tender, and swollen organ that is retracted upward in the scrotum. The scrotum becomes red and edematous. There is no associated urinary infection. Torsion, most common in adolescents, is a surgical emergency because of obstructed circulation.

SMALL TESTIS	CRYPTORCHIDISM	SCROTAL EDEMA

Adult testes are considered small when they are less than 3.5 cm long. Small firm testes (usually less than 2 cm long) suggest Klinefelter's syndrome. Small soft testes suggest atrophy, associated with several conditions (*e.g.,* cirrhosis, myotonia dystrophica, administration of estrogens, and hypopituitarism). Atrophy may also follow orchitis (*e.g.,* from mumps).

An undeveloped scrotum suggests cryptorchidism (an undescended testicle), as shown on the left in a fifteen-year-old. The testis and epididymis are not palpable in the scrotal sac. When this condition persists, it eventually leads to testicular atrophy on the involved side(s) and increases the risk of testicular cancer.

The scrotal skin may become taut with pitting edema. Scrotal edema is usually associated with generalized edema, as in chronic congestive heart failure or the nephrotic syndrome.

Table 12-3

Table 12-3 Course and Presentation of Hernias in the Groin

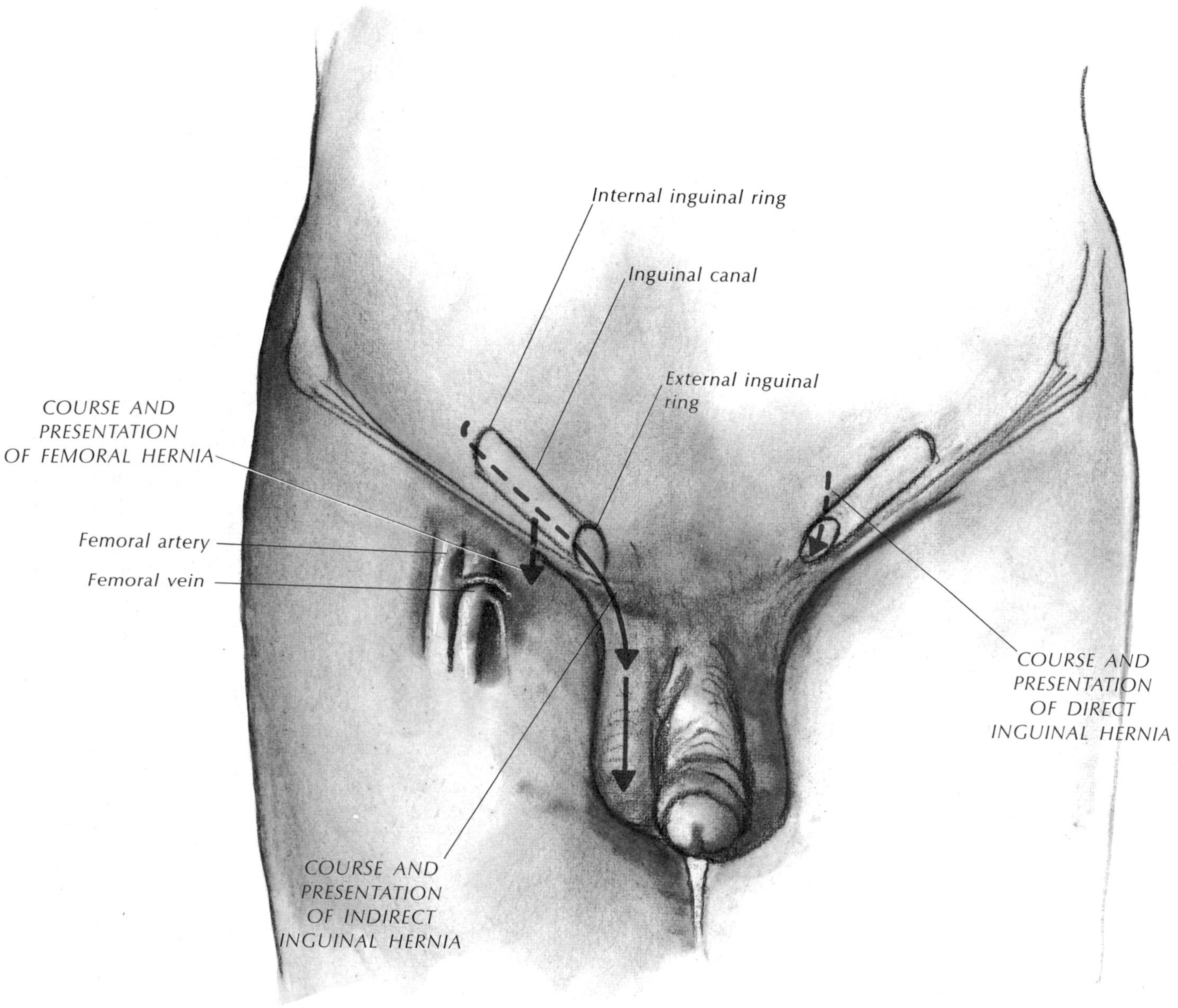

Internal inguinal ring

Inguinal canal

External inguinal ring

COURSE AND PRESENTATION OF DIRECT INGUINAL HERNIA

COURSE AND PRESENTATION OF INDIRECT INGUINAL HERNIA

COURSE AND PRESENTATION OF FEMORAL HERNIA

Femoral artery

Femoral vein

Table 12-4

Table 12-4 Differentiation of Hernias in the Groin

Differentiation among these hernias is not always clinically possible. Understanding their features, however, improves your observation.

	INGUINAL		FEMORAL
	INDIRECT	**DIRECT**	
FREQUENCY	Most common, all ages, both sexes	Less common	Least common
AGE AND SEX	Often in children, may be in adults	Usually men over age 40, rare in women	More common in women than in men
POINT OF ORIGIN	Above inguinal ligament, near its midpoint (the internal inguinal ring)	Above inguinal ligament, close to the pubic tubercle (near the external inguinal ring)	Below the inguinal ligament; appears more lateral than an inguinal hernia and may be hard to differentiate from lymph nodes
COURSE	Often into the scrotum	Rarely into the scrotum	Never into the scrotum
(With the examining finger in the inguinal canal during straining or cough)	The hernia comes down the inguinal canal and touches the fingertip.	The hernia bulges anteriorly and pushes the side of the finger forward.	The inguinal canal is empty.

Chapter 13
Female Genitalia

Anatomy and Physiology

Review the anatomy of the external female genitalia, or vulva, including the mons pubis, a hair-covered fat pad overlying the symphysis pubis; the labia majora, rounded folds of adipose tissue; the labia minora, thinner pinkish red folds that extend anteriorly to form the prepuce; and the clitoris. The vestibule is the boat-shaped fossa between the labia minora. In its posterior portion lies the vaginal opening or introitus, which in virgins may be hidden by the hymen. The term perineum, as commonly used clinically, refers to the tissues between the introitus and anus.

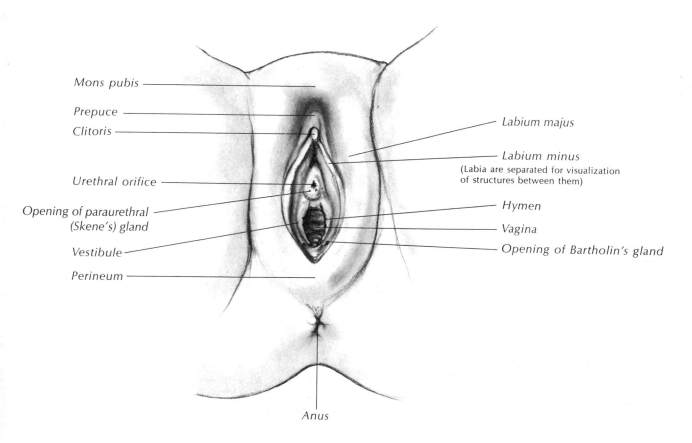

Mons pubis

Prepuce

Clitoris

Labium majus

Labium minus
(Labia are separated for visualization
of structures between them)

Urethral orifice

Opening of paraurethral
(Skene's) gland

Hymen

Vagina

Vestibule

Opening of Bartholin's gland

Perineum

Anus

The urethral orifice (urethral meatus) opens into the vestibule between the clitoris and vagina. Just posterior to it on either side can sometimes be discerned the openings of the paraurethral or Skene's glands. The openings of Bartholin's glands are located posteriorly on either side of the vaginal opening, but are not usually visible. Bartholin's glands themselves are situated more deeply.

The vagina is a hollow tube extending between urethra and rectum upward and back. It terminates in the cup-shaped fornix. At almost right angles to it sits the uterus, a flattened, pear-shaped, fibromuscular structure. The uterus has two parts: the body (or corpus) and the cervix, which are joined together by the isthmus. The convex upper surface of the body is called the fundus of the uterus. The lower part of the uterus, the cervix, protrudes into the vagina, dividing the fornix into anterior, posterior, and lateral fornices. A round or slitlike depression, the external os of the cervix, marks the opening into the endocervical canal and uterine cavity.

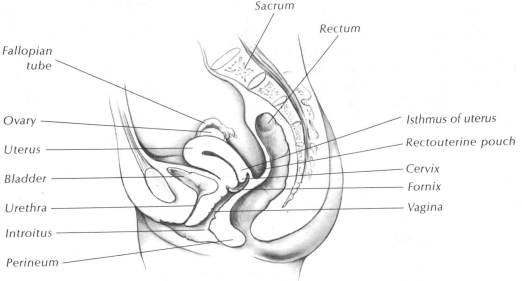

Location of Bartholin's glands

CROSS SECTION, SIDE VIEW

From each side of the fundus extends a fallopian tube, the fringed, funnel-shaped end of which curves toward the ovary. An ovary is an almond-shaped structure that varies considerably in size but averages about 3.5 × 2 × 1.5 cm from adulthood through menopause. The ovaries are often palpable on pelvic examination during a woman's reproductive years, but normal tubes cannot be felt. The term adnexa refers to the ovaries, tubes, and supporting tissues.

The ovaries have two primary functions: the production of ova and the secretion of hormones, including estrogen, progesterone, and testosterone. Increased hormonal secretions during puberty stimulate the growth of the uterus and its endometrial lining. They enlarge the vagina and thicken its epithelium. They also stimulate the development of secondary sex characteristics, including the breasts and pubic hair.

The parietal peritoneum extends downward behind the uterus into a cul de sac called the rectouterine pouch (or pouch of Douglas). You can just reach this area on rectal examination.

Lymph from the vulva and the lower third of the vagina drains to the inguinal nodes, but that from the internal genitalia, including the upper third of the vagina, flows into pelvic and abdominal lymph nodes which are not palpable clinically. Lymph from the middle third of the vagina can go in either direction.

CHANGES WITH AGE

During the pubertal years the vulva and internal genitalia grow and change to their adult proportions. Assessment of sexual maturity in girls, as classified by Tanner, depends not on internal examination, however, but on the growth of pubic hair and the development of breasts. Tanner's stages, or sex maturity ratings, as they relate to pubic hair are shown below; those relating to breasts are shown on page 313.

Sex Maturity Ratings in Girls: Pubic Hair

STAGE 1 Preadolescent—no pubic hair except for the fine body hair (vellus hair) similar to that on the abdomen

STAGE 2 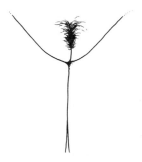 STAGE 3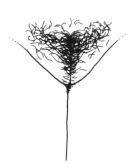

Sparse growth of long, slightly pigmented, downy hair, straight or only slightly curled, chiefly along the labia

Darker, coarser, curlier hair, spreading sparsely over the pubic symphysis

STAGE 4 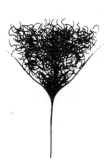 STAGE 5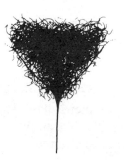

Coarse and curly hair as in adults; area covered greater than in stage 3 but not as great as in the adult and not yet including the thighs

Hair adult in quantity and quality, spread on the medial surfaces of the thighs but not up over the abdomen

(Illustrations through the courtesy of W.A. Daniel, Jr., Division of Adolescent Medicine, University of Alabama, Birmingham)

A girl's first sign of puberty is usually the appearance of breast buds. Sometimes, however, pubic hair appears first. On the average these changes start at around 11 years of age, with a range from 8 to 13 years for breast buds, 8 to 14 years for pubic hair. The transformation from preadolescent to adult form takes about 3 years, with a range of 1.5 to 6 years. Menarche tends to occur during breast stage 3 or 4, at ages ranging from 10 to 16.5 years according to Tanner's studies (summarized below). The age of menarche in the United States is a little earlier, roughly from 9 to 16 years.

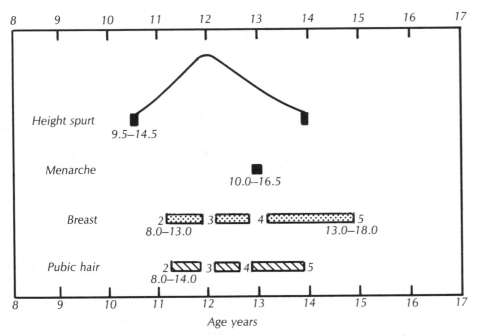

Numbers below the bars indicate the ranges in age within which certain changes occur. (Redrawn from Marshall WA, Tanner JM: Variations in the pattern of pubertal changes in boys. Arch Dis Child 45:22, 1970)

As in boys, there is a wide range of normal in pubertal development. Some girls may have completed the development of their secondary sex characteristics while others of the same age have not yet begun.

In 10% or more of women pubic hair spreads further up the abdomen in a triangular pattern, pointing toward the umbilicus. This spread can be classified as stage 6 but, because it is usually not completed until the mid-20s or later, it is not considered a pubertal change.

Just before menarche there is a physiologic increase in vaginal secretion — a normal change that sometimes worries a girl or her mother. As menses become established, increased secretions, or leukorrhea, coincide with ovulation. They also accompany sexual arousal. These normal kinds of discharges must be differentiated from those of infectious processes.

Ovarian function usually starts to diminish during a woman's 40s, and menstrual periods cease on the average between the ages of 45 and 52, sometimes earlier and sometimes later. Pubic hair becomes sparse as well as gray. With the decline of estrogenic stimulus the labia and clitoris become smaller. The vagina narrows and shortens and its mucosa becomes thin, pale, and dry. The uterus and ovaries diminish in size.

Techniques of Examination

GENERAL APPROACH

Most students feel anxious, embarrassed, or uncomfortable when first examining the genitalia of another person. These feelings are normal, and it may be useful to talk them through with your instructor or another experienced clinician. At the same time, patients bring to the examination their own concerns. Some women have had painful, embarrassing, or even demeaning experiences during previous examinations while others may be facing with apprehension their first examination. A patient's reactions and behavior give you important clues to these feelings and to her attitudes toward sexuality. If she adducts her thighs, pulls away, or expresses negative feelings during the examination, you can gently confront her as you would during the interview. "I notice you are having some trouble relaxing . . . or seem disgusted. . . . Is it just being here or is it the same way at home? . . . or during intercourse?" Behavior that seems to present an annoying obstacle to your examination may become the key to understanding your patient's problem.

A patient who has never had a pelvic examination is often fearful of it, embarrassed, and ignorant of what to expect. Try to make the experience one in which she learns about both her body and the examination itself and becomes more comfortable with them. Before she undresses, explain the relevant anatomy with the help of three-dimensional models. Show her the speculum and other equipment and encourage her to handle them. During the examination, then, she can better understand your explanations and procedures. It is especially important not to hurt the patient during her first encounter.

Indications for a pelvic examination during adolescence include menstrual abnormalities such as amenorrhea, excessive bleeding, or dysmenorrhea, unexplained abdominal pain, vaginal discharge, the prescription of contraceptives, bacteriological and cytological studies in a sexually active girl, and the patient's own desire for assessment. Rape and maternal exposure to diethylstilbestrol during pregnancy require special evaluation for which specialty references should be consulted.

At any age, getting the patient to relax is essential for an adequate examination. Sensitivity to her feelings may help here. In addition,

1. Ask the patient to empty her bladder before the examination.
2. Drape her appropriately. Some patients are more comfortable when drapes cover their thighs and knees. Others prefer to watch both the practitioner and the examination itself and object to drapes that obscure their view. A girl or woman may wish to use a mirror to see her own genitalia during the examination. Ask the patient which method she prefers.

3. The patient's arms should be at her sides or folded across her chest — not over her head, since this last position tends to tighten the abdominal muscles.

4. Explain in advance each step of the examination and tell the patient what she may feel. Avoid any sudden or unexpected movements. When beginning palpation or using a speculum, it may be helpful to make initial contact not on the genitalia themselves but on the upper inner thigh.

5. Have warm hands and a warm speculum.

6. Monitor your examination when possible by watching the patient's face. Depressing the center of the drape onto the patient's abdomen allows you to maintain eye contact while you are seated.

7. Finally, of course, be as gentle as possible.

Wear a glove on the hand you use for internal examination or, if you suspect an infectious process, on both hands. During the bimanual examination, an ungloved abdominal hand makes palpation easier.

EQUIPMENT. You should have within reach a good light, a vaginal speculum of appropriate size, water-soluble lubricant, and materials for bacteriologic cultures and Papanicolaou smears. Specula are made of metal or plastic and come in two basic shapes. Graves specula are usually best for sexually active women. They are available in small, medium, and large sizes. The narrow-bladed Pedersen speculum is useful for a patient with a relatively small introitus, such as a virgin or an elderly woman, and is often more comfortable for other patients as well.

Before using a speculum become thoroughly familiar with how to open and close its blades, lock the blades in an open position, and release them again. Although the instructions in this chapter refer to a metal speculum, you can easily adapt them to a plastic one by handling the speculum before using it. Plastic specula typically make a loud click when locked or released. Forewarning the patient about this click helps to avoid unnecessary surprise.

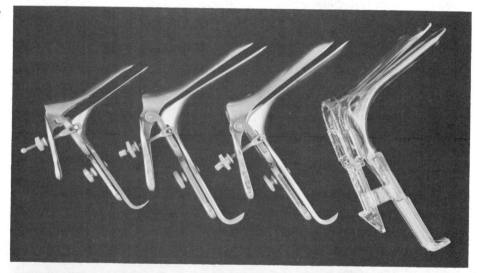

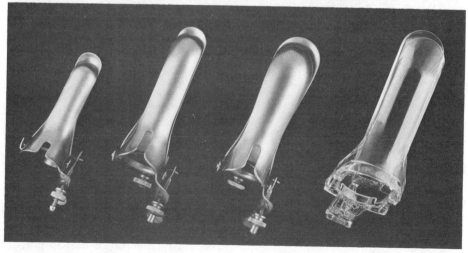

Specula, from left to right: small metal Pedersen, medium metal Pedersen, medium metal Graves, and large plastic Pedersen

Male examiners are customarily attended by female assistants. Female examiners may or may not prefer to work alone but should be similarly attended if the patient is emotionally disturbed.

POSITION. Drape the patient appropriately and then assist her into the lithotomy position. Help her to place first one heel and then the other into the stirrups. She may be more comfortable with shoes on than with bare feet. Then ask her to move toward the end of the examining table until her buttocks extend slightly beyond the edge. Her thighs should be flexed and abducted. A pillow should support her head.

EXTERNAL EXAMINATION

ASSESS THE SEXUAL MATURITY OF AN ADOLESCENT PATIENT. You can assess pubic hair during either the abdominal or the pelvic examination. Note its character and distribution, and rate it according to Tanner's stages described on page 375.

Delayed puberty is often familial or related to chronic illness. It may also be due to abnormalities in the hypothalamus, anterior pituitary gland, or ovaries.

INSPECT THE PATIENT'S EXTERNAL GENITALIA. Seat yourself comfortably and inspect the mons pubis, labia, and perineum. With your gloved hand, separate the labia and inspect:

Excoriations or itchy, small, red maculopapules suggest pediculosis pubis (lice or crabs). Look for nits or lice at the bases of the pubic hairs.

The labia minora

The clitoris

Enlarged clitoris in masculinizing conditions

The urethral orifice

Urethral caruncle, prolapse of the urethral mucosa

The vaginal opening or introitus

See Table 13-1, Lesions of the Vulva (p. 388).

Note any inflammation, ulceration, discharge, swelling, or nodules. If there are any lesions, palpate them.

Syphilitic chancre, sebaceous cyst

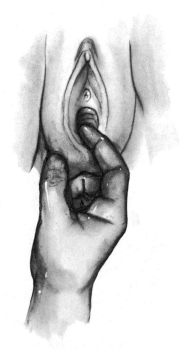

If there is a history or appearance of labial swelling, check Bartholin's glands. Insert your index finger into the vagina near the posterior end of the introitus. Place your thumb outside the posterior part of the labium majus. On each side in turn palpate between your finger and thumb for swelling or tenderness. Note any discharge exuding from the duct opening of the gland. If any is present, culture it.

A Bartholin's gland may become acutely or chronically infected and then produces a swelling. See Table 13-2, Bulges and Swellings of Vulva and Vagina (p. 389).

PALPATING BARTHOLIN'S GLAND

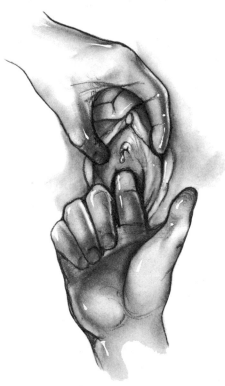

If you suspect urethritis or inflammation of the paraurethral glands, insert your index finger into the vagina and milk the urethra gently from inside outward. Note any discharge from or about the urethral orifice. If any is present, culture it.

MILKING THE URETHRA

INTERNAL EXAMINATION

LOCATE THE CERVIX. Insert your index finger into the vagina and identify the firm, rounded surface of the cervix. Locating the cervix manually will help you to find it more easily with a speculum. This maneuver also helps you to assess the size of the introitus and guides your choice of speculum. You may need to lubricate your finger with water but do not use other lubricants.

ASSESS THE SUPPORT OF THE VAGINAL OUTLET. With the labia separated by your middle and index fingers, ask the patient to strain down. Note any bulging of the vaginal walls.

Cystocele and rectocele. See Table 13-2, Bulges and Swellings of Vulva and Vagina (p. 389).

INSERT THE SPECULUM. Select a speculum of appropriate size and shape, and lubricate and warm it with warm water. (Other lubricants may interfere with cytological or other studies but may be used if no such tests are planned.) If you have your speculum ready during assessment of the vaginal outlet, you can ease speculum insertion and increase your efficiency by proceeding to this next maneuver while the patient is still straining down.

Place two fingers at or just inside the introitus and gently press down on the perineal body. With your other hand introduce the closed speculum past your fingers at a 45° angle downward. The blades should be held obliquely and the pressure exerted toward the posterior vaginal wall in order to avoid the more sensitive anterior wall and urethra. Be careful not to pull on the pubic hair nor to pinch the labia with the speculum.

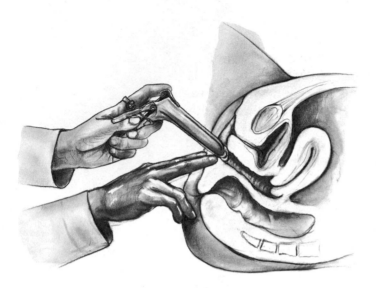

After the speculum has entered the vagina, remove your fingers from the introitus. Rotate the blades of the speculum into a horizontal position, maintaining the pressure posteriorly, and insert the speculum to its full length.

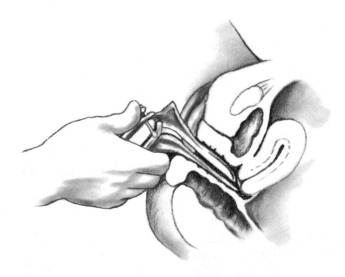

INSPECT THE CERVIX. Open the blades and maneuver the speculum, if necessary, so that the cervix comes into full view. When the uterus is retroverted, the cervix points more anteriorly than illustrated. If you have difficulty finding such a cervix, withdraw the speculum slightly and position it more anteriorly (*i.e.,* more horizontally).

See retroversion of the uterus, page 396.

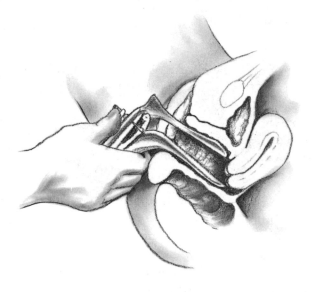
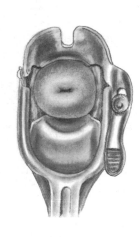

Inspect the cervix and its os. Note the color of the cervix, its position, and any ulcerations, nodules, masses, bleeding, or discharge.

Purplish color in pregnancy

Secure the speculum with the blades open by tightening the thumb screw.

See Table 13-3, Variations and Abnormalities of the Cervix (pp. 390–391).

OBTAIN SPECIMENS FOR CERVICAL CYTOLOGY (PAPANICOLAOU SMEARS). Specimens from three sites are described here. Clinicians and pathologists vary in their preferences as to the numbers and sites of cytologic specimens. All agree on a cervical scrape and also use one or both of the other two methods.

1. *Endocervical Swab.* Insert the end of a cotton applicator stick into the cervical os. Roll it between your thumb and index finger, clockwise and counterclockwise. Remove it. Smear a glass slide with the cotton swab, gently, in a painting motion. (Rubbing hard on the slide will destroy the cells.) Either place the slide into an ether-alcohol fixative at once, or spray it promptly with a special fixative.

A yellowish discharge on the endocervical swab suggests a mucopurulent cervicitis, which is commonly caused by *Chlamydia trachomatis.*

2. *Cervical Scrape.* Place the longer end of the scraper into the os of the cervix. Press, turn, and scrape in a full circle. Prepare a second slide as before.

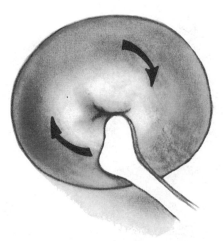

3. *Vaginal Pool.* Roll a cotton applicator stick in the posterior fornix and prepare a third slide as before. If the vaginal mucosa is dry, as it may be in an elderly woman, for example, moisten the cotton tip with saline before gathering the specimen.

If the cervix has been removed, do a vaginal pool and a scrape from the cuff of the vagina.

INSPECT THE VAGINA. Withdraw the speculum slowly while observing the vagina. As the speculum clears the cervix, release the thumb screw and maintain the open position of the speculum with your thumb. Close the blades as the speculum emerges from the introitus, avoiding both excessive stretching and pinching of the mucosa. During withdrawal inspect the vaginal mucosa, noting its color and any inflammation, discharge, ulcers, or masses.

See Table 13-4, Inflammations Of and Around the Vagina (pp. 392–393).

Cancer of the vagina

PERFORM A BIMANUAL EXAMINATION. Lubricate the index and middle fingers of your gloved hand, and from a *standing position* insert them into the vagina, again exerting pressure primarily posteriorly. Your thumb should be abducted, your ring and little fingers flexed into your palm. Pressing inward on the perineum with your flexed fingers causes little if any discomfort and allows you to position your palpating fingers correctly. Note any nodularity or tenderness in the vaginal wall, including the region of the urethra and bladder anteriorly.

Stool in the rectum may simulate a rectovaginal mass, but unlike a tumor mass can usually be dented by digital pressure. Rectovaginal examination confirms the distinction.

Identify the cervix, noting its position, shape, consistency, regularity, mobility, and tenderness. Normally the cervix can be moved somewhat without pain. Palpate the fornix around the cervix.

See Table 13-5, Changes in Pregnancy (p. 394).

Pain on movement of the cervix, together with adnexal tenderness, suggests pelvic inflammatory disease.

Place your abdominal hand about midway between the umbilicus and symphysis pubis. While you elevate the cervix and uterus with your pelvic hand, press your abdominal hand in and down, trying to grasp the uterus between your two hands. Note its size, shape, consistency, and mobility, and identify any tenderness or masses.

See Table 13-6, Abnormalities and Displacements of the Uterus (pp. 395–396).

Uterine enlargement suggests pregnancy or benign or malignant tumors.

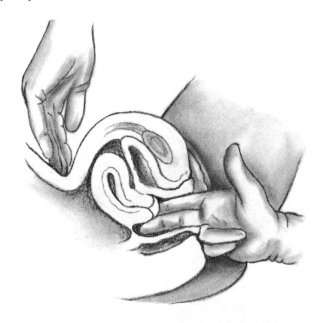

Now slide both fingers of your pelvic hand into the anterior fornix and palpate the body of the uterus between your hands. In this position your pelvic hand can feel the anterior surface of the uterus, and your abdominal hand can feel part of the posterior surface.

If you cannot feel the uterus with either of these maneuvers, it may be tipped posteriorly (retrodisplaced). In this case slide your pelvic fingers into the posterior fornix and feel for the uterus butting against your fingertips. An obese or poorly relaxed abdominal wall may also prevent you from feeling the uterus even when it is located anteriorly.

Next, place your abdominal hand on the right lower quadrant, your pelvic hand in the right lateral fornix. Press your abdominal hand in and down, trying to push the adnexal structures toward your pelvic hand. Try to identify the right ovary or any adjacent adnexal masses. By moving your hands slightly, slide the adnexal structures between your fingers, if possible, and note their size, shape, consistency, mobility, and tenderness. Repeat the procedure on the left side.

Nodules on the uterine surfaces suggest myomas (see p. 395).

See retroversion and retroflexion of the uterus (p. 396).

Three to five years after menopause the ovaries have usually atrophied and are no longer palpable. If you can feel an ovary in a postmenopausal woman, consider an abnormality such as a cyst or a tumor.

Adnexal masses include ovarian cysts and tumors, the swollen fallopian tube(s) of pelvic inflammatory disease, and a tubal pregnancy. A uterine myoma may simulate an adnexal mass. See Table 13-7, Adnexal Masses (p. 397).

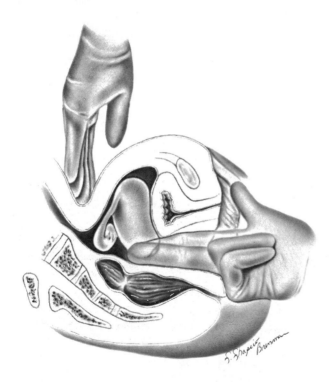

Normal ovaries are somewhat tender. They are usually palpable in slender, relaxed women but are difficult or impossible to feel in others who are obese or poorly relaxed.

Withdraw your fingers. Lubricate your gloves again if necessary. (See note on using lubricant, p. 386.) Then slowly reintroduce your index finger into the vagina, your middle finger into the rectum. Ask the patient to strain down as you do this so that her anal sphincter will relax. Tell her that this examination may make her feel as if she has to move her bowels but that she will not. Repeat the maneuvers of the bimanual examination, giving special attention to the region behind the cervix that may be accessible only to the rectal finger. Rectovaginal palpation is especially valuable in assessing a retrodisplaced uterus, as illustrated.

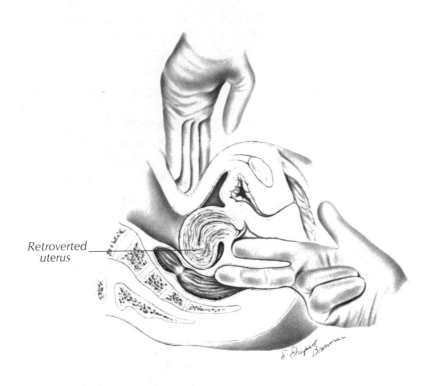

Retroverted uterus

Proceed to the rectal examination (see Chap. 14). After your examination, wipe off the external genitalia and anus or offer the patient some tissue with which to do it herself.

A NOTE ON THE SMALL INTROITUS. Many virginal vaginal orifices will readily admit a single examining finger. Modify your technique so as to use your index finger only. A small Pedersen speculum or even a nasal speculum may make inspection possible. When the vaginal orifice is even smaller, a fairly good bimanual examination can be performed by placing one finger in the rectum rather than in the vagina.

An imperforate hymen occasionally delays menarche. Be sure to check for this possibility when menarche seems unduly late in relation to the development of a girl's breasts and pubic hair.

Similar techniques may be indicated in elderly women in whom the introitus has become tight.

A NOTE ON USING LUBRICANT. If you use a large tube of lubricant during a pelvic or rectal examination, you may inadvertently contaminate it by touching the tube with your gloved fingers after touching the patient. To avoid this problem, let the lubricant drop onto your gloved fingers without allowing contact between the tube and the gloves. If you or your assistant should inadvertently contaminate the tube, discard it. Small disposable tubes for use with one patient circumvent this problem.

THE RISK OF SPREADING INFECTION BETWEEN VAGINA AND RECTUM. Gonorrhea may infect the rectum as well as the female genitalia. This fact, together with the high prevalence of sexually transmitted diseases, has led to the recommendation that gloves be changed between vaginal and rectal examination in order to avoid spreading infection. In order to avoid fecal soiling, gloves should always be changed if for some reason the practitioner examines the vagina after the rectum.

Table 13-1

Table 13-1 Lesions of the Vulva

SEBACEOUS CYST	VENEREAL WART (Condyloma Acuminatum)	SECONDARY SYPHILIS (Condyloma Latum)

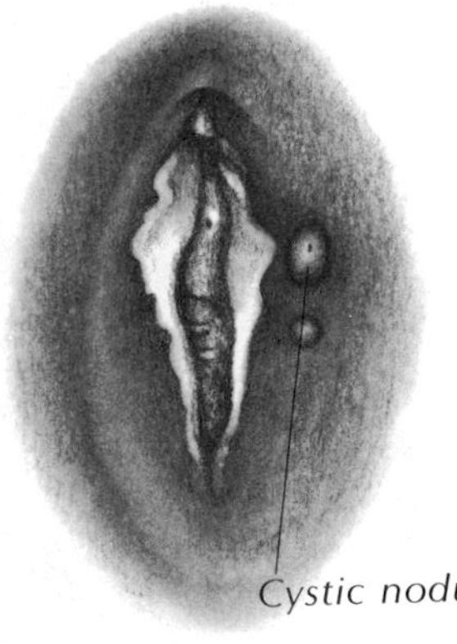

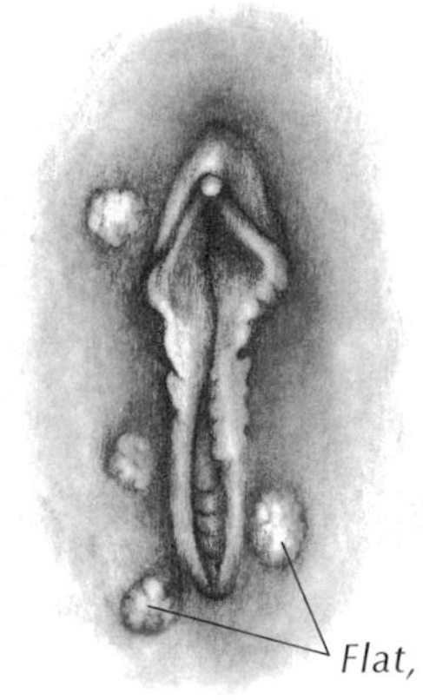

Cystic nodule in skin

Warts

Flat, gray papules

Small, firm, round cystic nodules in the labia suggest sebaceous cysts. They are sometimes yellowish in color. Look for the dark punctum marking the blocked opening of the gland.

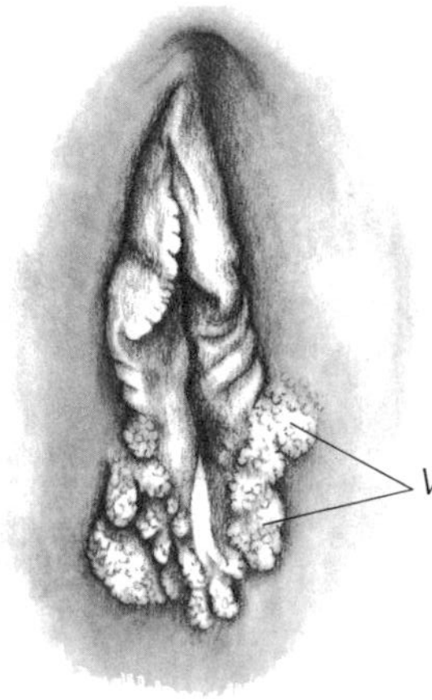

Warty lesions on the labia and within the vestibule suggest condylomata acuminata. Like warts elsewhere, they are reactions to a viral infection.

Slightly raised, flat, round or oval papules covered by a gray exudate suggest condylomata lata. These constitute one manifestation of secondary syphilis and are contagious.

SYPHILITIC CHANCRE	GENITAL HERPES	CARCINOMA OF THE VULVA

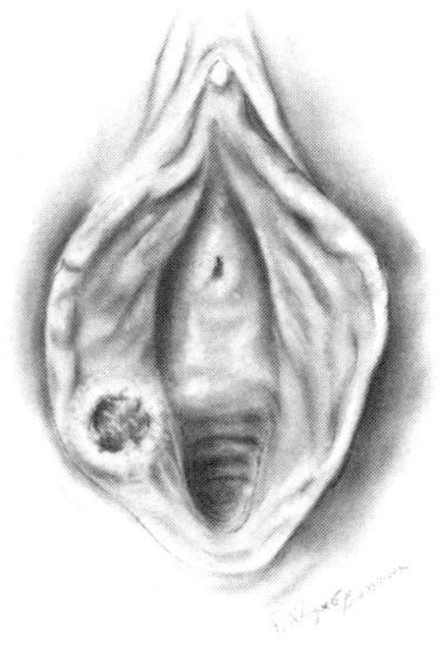

Shallow ulcers on red bases

A firm, painless ulcer suggests the chancre of primary syphilis. Since most chancres in women develop internally, they often go undetected.

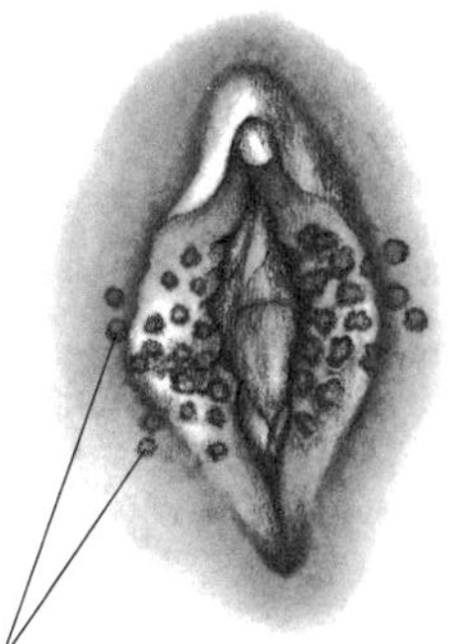

Shallow, small, painful ulcers on red bases suggest a herpes infection. Initial infection may be extensive, as illustrated here. Recurrent infections are usually confined to a small local patch.

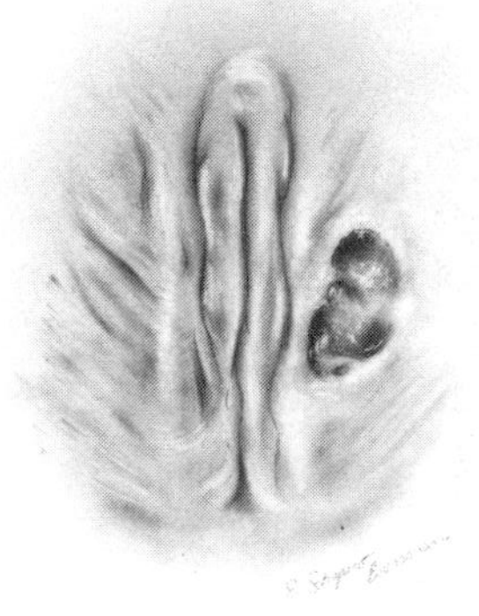

An ulcerated or raised red vulvar lesion in an elderly woman may indicate vulvar carcinoma.

Table 13-2

Table 13-2 Bulges and Swellings of Vulva and Vagina

CYSTOCELE

A cystocele is present when the anterior wall of the vagina, together with the bladder above it, bulges into the vagina and sometimes out the introitus. Look for the bulging vaginal wall as the patient strains down.

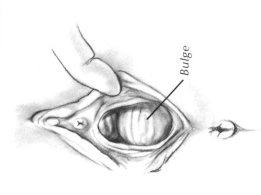

Bulge

RECTOCELE

A rectocele is formed by the anterior and downward bulging of the posterior vaginal wall together with the rectum behind it. To identify it, spread the patient's labia and ask her to strain down.

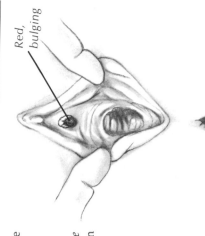

Bulge

INFLAMMATION OF BARTHOLIN'S GLAND

Inflammation of Bartholin's glands may be acute or chronic. Causes include gonococci, *Chlamydia trachomatis*, and other organisms. Acutely, it appears as a tense, hot, very tender abscess. Look for pus coming out of the duct or erythema around the duct opening. Chronically, a nontender cyst occupies the posterior labium. It may be large or small.

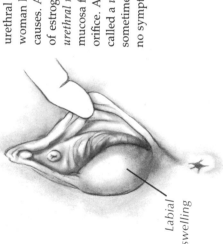

Labial swelling

PROLAPSED URETHRAL MUCOSA AND URETHRAL CARUNCLE

A small red swelling in the area of the urethral orifice in a postmenopausal woman has two reasonably common causes. Atrophic changes due to lack of estrogen may lead to *prolapse of the urethral mucosa*. The reddened swollen mucosa forms a rosette around the orifice. A small red polypoid mass, called a *urethral caruncle*, may sometimes develop. It usually causes no symptoms but may bleed.

Red, bulging

Table 13-3

Table 13-3 Variations and Abnormalities of the Cervix

NORMAL NULLIPAROUS CERVIX

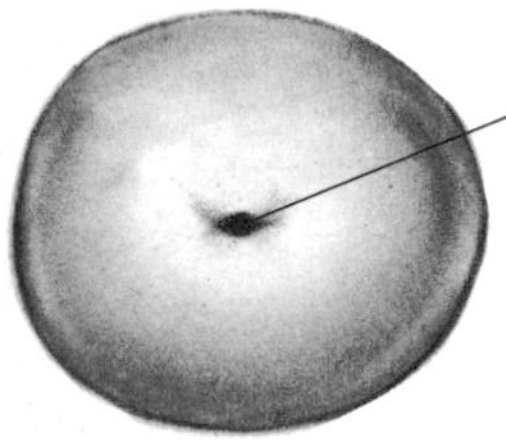

Round or oval

NORMAL PAROUS CERVIX

Slitlike

The nulliparous cervical os is small and either round or oval. The cervix is covered by smooth pink epithelium.

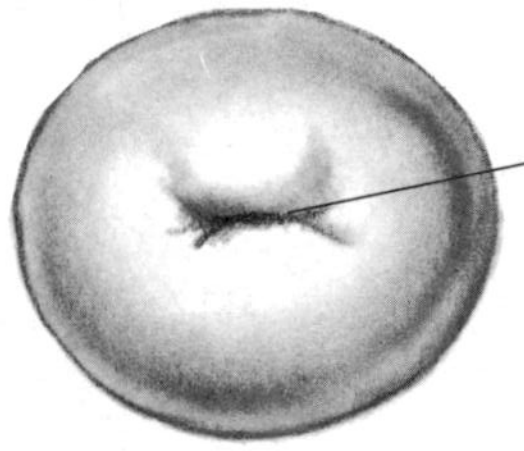

After childbirth, the cervical os presents a slitlike appearance.

LACERATIONS OF THE CERVIX

UNILATERAL TRANSVERSE	BILATERAL TRANSVERSE	STELLATE

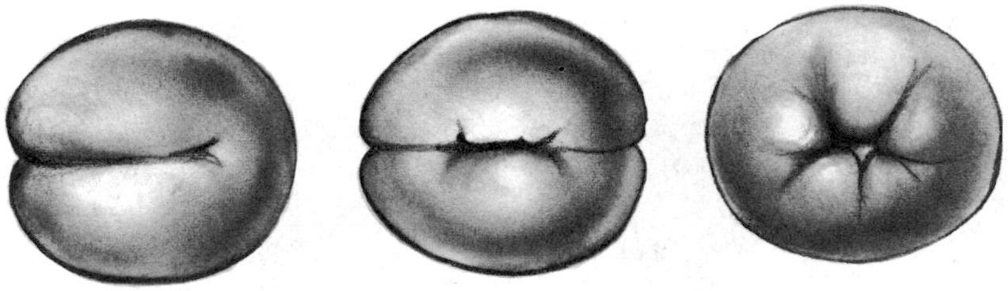

The trauma of difficult deliveries may tear the cervix, producing permanent transverse or stellate lacerations.

Table 13-3

ECTROPION (*Erosion*)

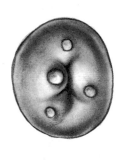

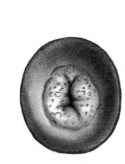

The mucosa around the central os is at times a plush red rather than the usual shiny pink. It may bleed easily when touched. This appearance is usually due to an ectropion (*i.e.*, the presence of columnar epithelium like that lining the cervical canal). An ectropion is not abnormal but may be indistinguishable from early carcinoma without further study (*e.g.*, by cytology, colposcopy, or biopsy). The term erosion is also used for this condition but is misleading because the mucosa has not actually eroded away.

NABOTHIAN OR RETENTION CYSTS

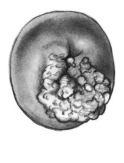

Retention or nabothian cysts may accompany or follow chronic cervicitis. Variable in size, single or multiple, they appear as translucent nodules on the cervical surface.

CERVICAL POLYP

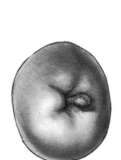

Cervical polyps usually arise from the endocervical canal, becoming visible when they protrude through the cervical os. They are bright red, soft, and rather fragile. When only the tips are seen they cannot be clinically differentiated from polyps originating in the endometrium.

CARCINOMA OF THE CERVIX

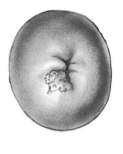

Carcinoma of the cervix usually begins at or near the cervical os. It often has a hard granular surface that bleeds easily. In later stages an extensive irregular cauliflower type of growth may develop. Early carcinomas are clinically indistinguishable from ectropions and may even be present in a cervix that appears normal.

Table 13-4

Table 13-4 Inflammations Of and Around the Vagina

Trichomonas vaginitis illustration labeled "Red spots" and "Inflamed mucosa"

Monilia vaginitis illustration labeled "White patches" and "Inflamed mucosa"

	TRICHOMONAS VAGINITIS*	MONILIA (Candida) VAGINITIS*
DISCHARGE	Thin or thick; white, yellowish, or green; often bubbly; often pooled in the vaginal fornix; profuse; malodorous	May be thin but is characteristically thick, white, and curdy; not so profuse as in Trichomonas vaginitis
VULVA	May be reddened, especially the vestibule and labia minora. Pruritus, though possibly present, is not usually so severe as in Monilia infection.	Often reddened, itchy, sometimes swollen, varying in extent from the vestibule alone to extension outward to involve the labia and the skin around them. Vulvar changes may occur without vaginal inflammation.
URETHRITIS	Usually absent, but a Trichomonas urethrocystitis occurs occasionally	Absent
BARTHOLIN'S GLAND INFECTION	Absent	Absent
VAGINAL MUCOSA	In acute infection the mucosa is red and inflamed, with red granular or petechial spots in the fornix. In mild or chronic infections the mucosa may look normal.	In severe cases red and inflamed, with white or grayish, often tenacious patches of discharge. May bleed when plaques of discharge are scraped off. In mild cases the vaginal mucosa may look normal.
CERVIX	May show red spots ("strawberry" spots)	May show patches of discharge

* Many patients show less typical signs. Definitive diagnosis depends on identification of the causative organism.

Table 13-4

	EARLY GONORRHEA*	**NONSPECIFIC VAGINITIS** (Associated with Gardnerella Vaginalis)	**ATROPHIC VAGINITIS** (Associated with Aging)
	Purulent exudate from os; Urethritis and Skene's gland infection; Bartholin's gland infection		Small introitus; Small cervix; Atrophic mucosa
DISCHARGE	Greenish yellow	Gray, thin, homogeneous, malodorous, occasionally somewhat frothy; not so profuse as in Trichomonas or Monilia infections, may be minimal	Variable in color, consistency, and amount. May be whitish, gray, yellow, green, or blood-tinged; thick or watery; rarely profuse
VULVA	May be inflamed	Usually normal	Atrophic
URETHRITIS	Often present. The urethral orifice is red and swollen. Pus may be milked from the urethra and sometimes from Skene's glands.	Absent	Absent
BARTHOLIN'S GLAND INFECTION	May be present	Absent	Absent
VAGINAL MUCOSA	Usually normal in the adult	Usually normal; occasionally may be red or swollen	Atrophic, dry, pale, though may become reddened and develop petechiae, ecchymoses, and superficial erosions. May show filmy adhesions. Bleeds easily.
CERVIX	May be inflamed; pus exudes from os	Normal	Small

* Many patients show less typical signs. Definitive diagnosis depends on identification of the causative organism. *Chlamydia trachomatis* may cause an infection with a clinical picture similar to gonorrhea. It is suggested by a yellowish endocervical exudate.

Table 13-5

Table 13-5 Changes in Pregnancy

6th WEEK FROM THE LAST MENSTRUAL PERIOD

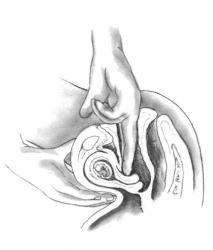

The isthmus of the uterus softens. Its soft consistency contrasts with the firm cervix below and the somewhat doughy or elastic uterus above. This phenomenon is called Hegar's sign. It is the first clinical manifestation of pregnancy but is not absolutely diagnostic. The uterine fundus tends to feel more globular and may become asymmetrical at the site of fetal implantation.

2nd MONTH

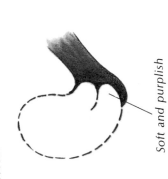

Soft and purplish

The cervix itself softens. In consistency it begins to resemble lips rather than a nose. Its color and that of the adjacent vaginal mucosa become purplish.

3rd THROUGH 10th MONTHS

(Read from the bottom up.)

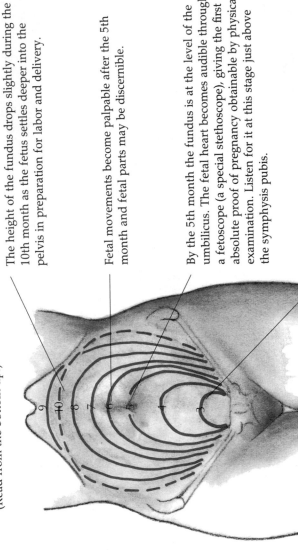

The height of the fundus drops slightly during the 10th month as the fetus settles deeper into the pelvis in preparation for labor and delivery.

Fetal movements become palpable after the 5th month and fetal parts may be discernible.

By the 5th month the fundus is at the level of the umbilicus. The fetal heart becomes audible through a fetoscope (a special stethoscope), giving the first absolute proof of pregnancy obtainable by physical examination. Listen for it at this stage just above the symphysis pubis.

By the 3rd month, the uterus has become globular in shape and first rises above the symphysis pubis.

Table 13-6

Table 13-6 Abnormalities and Displacement of the Uterus

MYOMAS OF THE UTERUS *(Fibroids)*

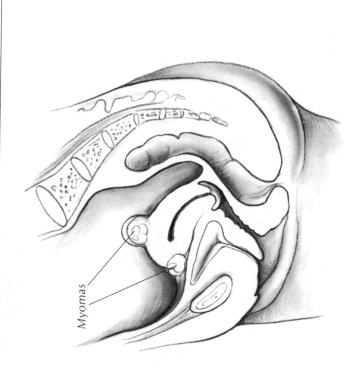

Myomas

Myomas are very common, benign, uterine tumors. They may be single or multiple and vary greatly in size, occasionally reaching massive proportions. They feel like firm, irregular nodules in continuity with the uterine surface. Occasionally a myoma projecting laterally can be confused with an ovarian mass; a nodule projecting posteriorly can be mistaken for a retroflexed uterus. Submucous myomas project toward the endometrial cavity and are not themselves palpable, although they may be suspected because of an enlarged uterus.

Continued

PROLAPSE OF THE UTERUS

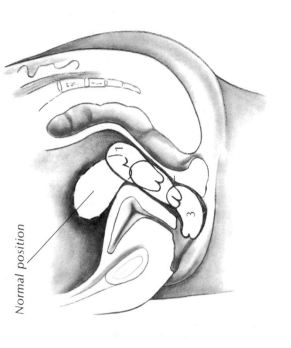

Normal position

Prolapse of the uterus results from weakness of the supporting structures of the pelvic floor and is often associated with a cystocele and rectocele. In progressive stages the uterus becomes retroverted and descends down the vaginal canal to the outside. In first degree prolapse the cervix is still well within the vagina. In second degree, it is at the introitus. In third degree prolapse, also called procidentia uteri, the cervix and vagina are outside the introitus.

Table 13-6

Table 13-6 (Cont'd.)

RETROVERSION OF THE UTERUS

RETROFLEXION OF THE UTERUS

MODERATE

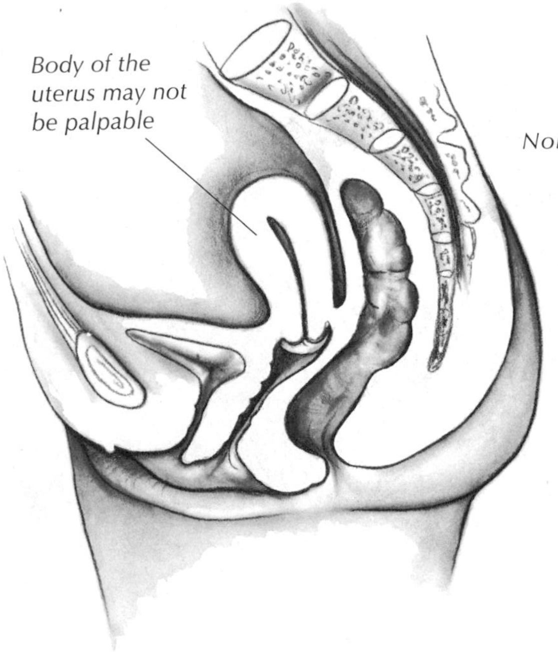

Body of the uterus may not be palpable

MARKED

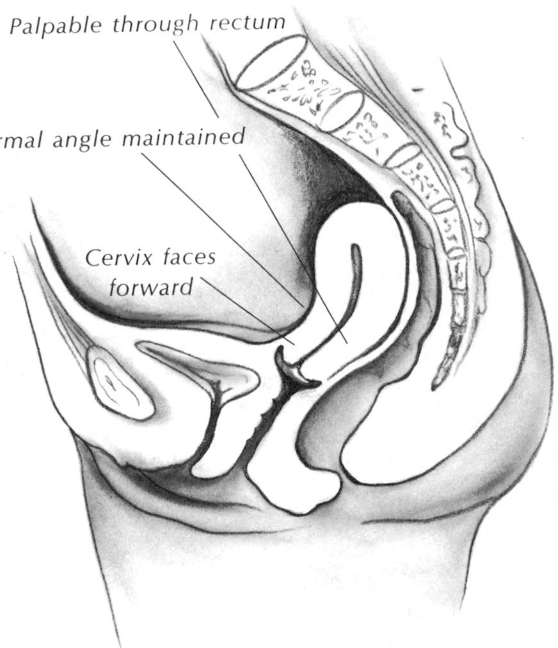

Palpable through rectum

Normal angle maintained

Cervix faces forward

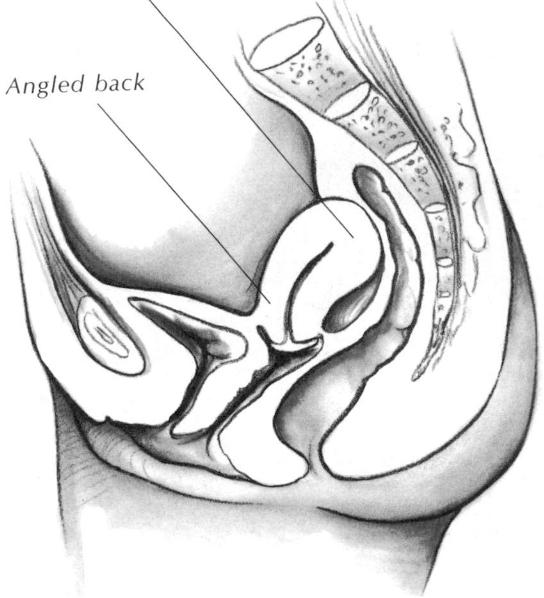

May be palpable through rectum

Angled back

Retroversion of the uterus refers to a tilting backward of the entire uterus, including both body and cervix. It is a common variant occurring in about 1 out of 5 women. Early clues on pelvic examination are a cervix that faces forward and a uterine body that cannot be felt by the abdominal hand. In moderate retroversion, shown on the left, the body may not be palpable with either hand. In marked retroversion, shown on the right, the body can be felt posteriorly, either through the posterior fornix or through the rectum. A retroverted uterus is usually both mobile and asymptomatic. Occasionally such a uterus is fixed and immobile, held in place by conditions such as endometriosis or pelvic inflammatory disease.

Retroflexion of the uterus refers to a backward angulation of the body of the uterus in relationship to the cervix. The cervix maintains its usual position. The body of the uterus is often palpable through the posterior fornix or through the rectum.

Table 13-7

Table 13-7   Adnexal Masses

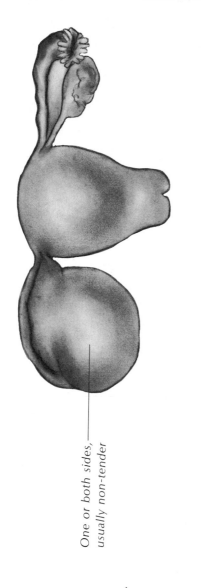

One or both sides, usually non-tender

OVARIAN CYSTS AND TUMORS

Ovarian cysts and tumors may be detected as adnexal masses on one or both sides. Later they may grow up out of the pelvis. Cysts tend to be smooth and compressible, tumors more solid and often nodular. Uncomplicated cysts and tumors are not usually tender.

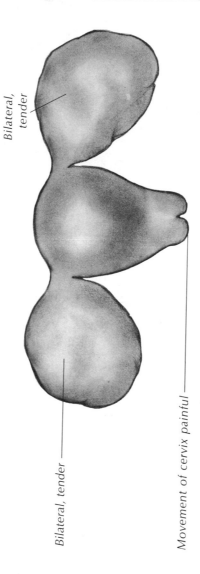

Bilateral, tender

Bilateral, tender

Movement of cervix painful

PELVIC INFLAMMATORY DISEASE

(*Salpingitis or Salpingo–Oophoritis*)

Acute pelvic inflammatory disease is associated with very tender, bilateral adnexal masses, although pain and muscle spasm usually make it impossible to delineate them. Movement of the cervix produces pain. *Chronic* pelvic inflammatory disease is manifested by bilateral, tender, usually irregular, and fairly fixed adnexal masses.

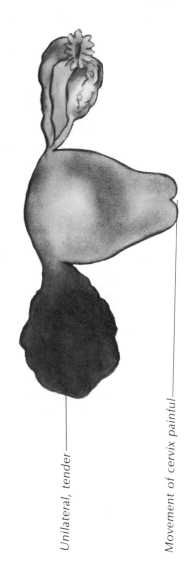

Unilateral, tender

Movement of cervix painful

RUPTURED TUBAL PREGNANCY

A ruptured tubal pregnancy spills blood into the peritoneal cavity, causing severe abdominal pain and tenderness. Guarding and rebound tenderness are sometimes associated. A unilateral adnexal mass may be palpable, but tenderness often prevents its detection. Faintness, syncope, nausea, vomiting, tachycardia, and shock may be present, reflecting the hemorrhage. There may be a prior history of amenorrhea or other symptoms of a pregnancy.

Chapter 14
The Anus, Rectum, and Prostate

Anatomy and Physiology

The gastrointestinal tract terminates in a short segment, the anal canal. Its external margin is poorly demarcated, but generally the skin of the anal canal can be distinguished from the surrounding perianal skin by its moist, hairless appearance. The anal canal is normally held in a closed position by action of the voluntary external muscular sphincter and the involuntary internal sphincter, the latter an extension of the muscular coat of the rectal wall.

The direction of the anal canal on a line roughly between anus and umbilicus should be carefully noted. Unlike the rectum above it the canal is liberally supplied by somatic sensory nerves, and a poorly directed finger or instrument will produce pain.

The anal canal is demarcated from the rectum superiorly by a serrated line marking the change from skin to mucous membrane. This anorectal junction (often called the pectinate or dentate line) also denotes the boundary between somatic and visceral nerve supplies. It is readily visible on proctoscopic examination but is not palpable.

Above the anorectal junction, the rectum balloons out and turns posteriorly into the hollow of the coccyx and sacrum, forming almost a right angle with the anal canal. In the male, the prostate gland is palpable anteriorly as a rounded, heart-shaped structure about 2.5 cm in length. Its two lateral lobes are separated by a shallow median sulcus or groove. The seminal vesicles, shaped like rabbit ears above the prostate, are not normally palpable.

Through the anterior wall of the female rectum the uterine cervix can usually be felt.

The rectal wall contains three inward foldings, called valves of Houston. The lowest of these can sometimes be felt, usually on the patient's left.

Most of the rectum that is accessible to digital examination does not have a peritoneal surface. The anterior rectum usually does, however, and you may reach it with the tip of your examining finger. You may thus be able to identify the tenderness of peritoneal inflammation or the nodularity of peritoneal metastases.

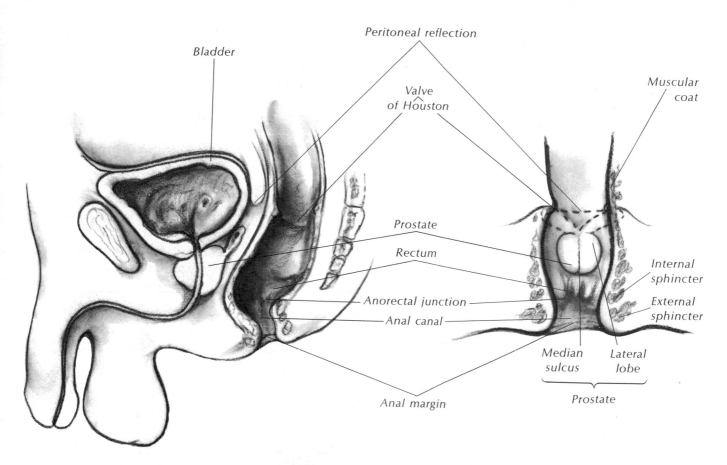

CROSS SECTION, SIDE VIEW

ANTERIOR WALL

ANUS AND RECTUM—MALE

Techniques of Examination

For most patients the rectal examination is probably the least popular segment of the entire physical examination. It may cause discomfort for the patient, perhaps embarrassment, but, if skillfully done, should not be truly painful in most circumstances. Although you may choose to omit a rectal examination in adolescents who have no relevant complaints, you should do one in adult patients. In middle-aged and older persons omission risks missing an asymptomatic carcinoma. A successful examination requires gentleness, slow movement of your finger, a calm demeanor, and an explanation to the patient of what he or she may feel.

MALE

The anus and rectum may be examined with the patient in one of several positions. For most purposes, the side-lying position is satisfactory and allows good visualization of the perianal and sacrococcygeal areas. This is the position described below. The lithotomy position may help you to reach a cancer high in the rectum. It also permits a bimanual examination, enabling you to delineate a pelvic mass. Some clinicians prefer to examine a patient while he stands with his hips flexed and his upper body resting across the examining table.

No matter how you position the patient, your examining finger cannot reach the full length of the rectum. If a rectosigmoid cancer is suspected, direct visualization by proctosigmoidoscopy is necessary.

Ask the patient to lie on his left side with his buttocks close to the edge of the examining table near you. Flexing the patient's hips and knees, especially in the top leg, stabilizes his position and improves visibility. Drape the patient appropriately and adjust the lighting for good visualization of the anus and surrounding area. Put a glove on your right hand. With your left hand spread the buttocks apart.

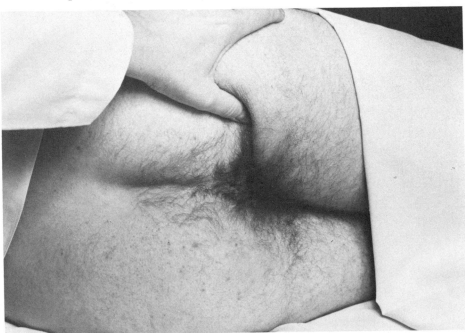

Inspect the sacrococcygeal and perianal areas for lumps, ulcers, inflammation, rashes, or excoriations. Adult perianal skin is normally more pigmented and somewhat coarser than the skin over the buttocks. Palpate any abnormal areas, noting lumps or tenderness.

Lubricate your gloved index finger, explain to the patient what you are going to do, and tell him that the examination may make him feel as if he were moving his bowels but that he will not do so. Ask him to strain down. Inspect the anus, noting any lesions.

As the patient strains, place the pad of your lubricated and gloved index finger over the anus. As the sphincter relaxes, gently insert your fingertip into the anal canal, in a direction pointing toward the umbilicus.

Anal and perianal lesions include hemorrhoids, venereal warts, herpes, syphilitic chancre, and carcinoma. A perianal abscess produces a painful, tender, indurated, and reddened mass. Pruritus ani causes swollen, thickened, fissured skin with excoriations.

Soft pliable tags of redundant skin at the anal margin are common. Though sometimes due to past anal surgery or previously thrombosed hemorrhoids, they are often unexplained.

See Table 14-1, Abnormalities of the Anus, Surrounding Skin, and Rectum (pp. 403–404).

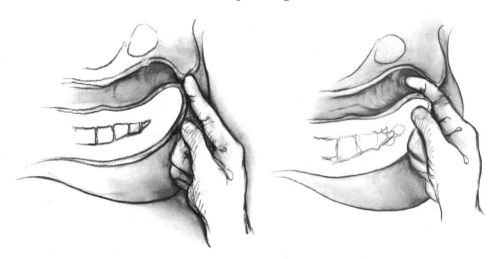

If you feel the sphincter tighten, pause, reassure the patient, and, when in a moment the sphincter relaxes, proceed. Occasionally severe tenderness prevents you from examining the anus. Do not try to force it. Instead place your fingers on both sides of the anus, gently spread the orifice, and ask the patient to strain down. Look for a lesion such as an anal fissure.

Note:

The sphincter tone of the anus. Normally the muscles of the anal sphincter close snugly around your finger.

Tenderness

Induration

Irregularities or nodules

Sphincter tightness in anxiety, inflammation, or scarring; laxity in some neurologic diseases

Induration may be due to inflammation, scarring, or malignancy.

Insert your finger farther into the rectum so that you can examine as much of the rectal wall as possible. Palpate in sequence the right lateral, posterior, and left lateral surfaces, noting any induration, nodules, or irregularities.

Cancer of the rectum (see p. 404)

Then turn your hand so that your finger can examine the anterior surface and the prostate gland. Tell the patient that you are going to feel his prostate gland and that it may make him want to urinate but he will not. Identify the lateral lobes of the prostate, and the median sulcus between them. Note the size, shape, and consistency of the prostate, feel for any nodules, and note any tenderness.

See Table 14-2, Abnormalities of the Prostate (p. 405).

If possible, extend your finger above the prostate to the region of the seminal vesicles and peritoneal cavity. Note nodules or tenderness.

A rectal "shelf" of peritoneal metastases (see p. 404)

Rectal lesions just beyond your fingertip can sometimes be felt by asking the patient to strain down again. Use this maneuver if there is any suspicion of cancer.

Gently withdraw your finger, and wipe the patient's anus or give him tissues to do it himself. Note the color of any fecal matter on your glove, and test it for occult blood.

FEMALE

The rectum is usually examined after the female genitalia, while the patient is in the lithotomy position. This position is essential for bimanual palpation. If a rectal examination alone is indicated, the lateral position offers a satsifactory alternative and affords much better visualization of the perianal and sacrococcygeal areas.

The technique is basically similar to that described for males. The cervix is usually readily felt through the anterior rectal wall. Sometimes a retroverted uterus is also palpable. Neither of these, nor a tampon, should be mistaken for a tumor.

Table 14-1

Table 14-1   Abnormalities of the Anus, Surrounding Skin, and Rectum

PILONIDAL CYST AND SINUS

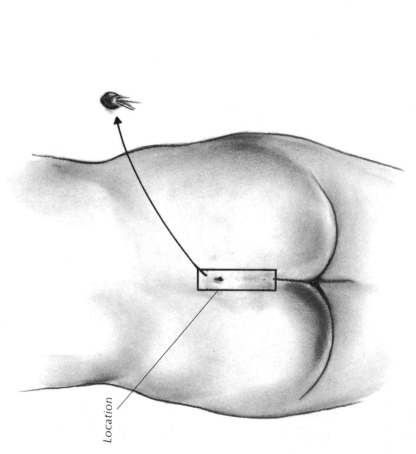

Location

A pilonidal cyst is a fairly frequent, probably congenital abnormality located in the midline superficial to the coccyx or lower sacrum. It is clinically identified by the opening of a sinus tract. This opening may exhibit a small tuft of hair and be surrounded by a halo of erythema. Although pilonidal cysts are generally asymptomatic, except perhaps for slight drainage, abscess formation and secondary sinus tracts may complicate the picture.

Continued

ANORECTAL FISTULA

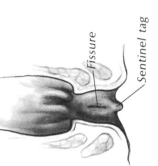

Opening

Fistula

An anorectal fistula is an inflammatory tract or tube that opens at one end into the anus or rectum and at the other end onto the skin surface (as shown here) or into another viscus. An abscess usually antedates such a fistula. Look for the fistulous opening or openings anywhere in the skin around the anus.

ANAL FISSURE

Fissure

Sentinel tag

An anal fissure is a very painful oval ulceration of the anal canal, found most commonly in the midline posteriorly, less commonly in the midline anteriorly. Its long axis lies longitudinally. Inspection may show a swollen "sentinel" skin tag just below it, and gentle separation of the anal margins may reveal the lower edge of the fissure. The sphincter is spastic; the examination painful. Local anesthesia may be required.

Table 14-1 (Cont'd.)

EXTERNAL HEMORRHOIDS

External hemorrhoids are dilated hemorrhoidal veins that originate below the pectinate line and are covered with skin. They seldom produce symptoms unless thrombosis occurs. This causes acute local pain that is increased by defecation and by sitting. A tender, swollen, bluish, ovoid mass is visible at the anal margin.

Thrombosed

INTERNAL HEMORRHOIDS

Internal hemorrhoids are an enlargement of the normal vascular cushions that are located above the pectinate line. Here they are not usually palpable. Sometimes, especially during defecation, internal hemorrhoids may cause bright red bleeding. They may also prolapse through the anal canal and appear as reddish, moist, protruding masses, typically located in one or more of the positions illustrated.

ANTERIOR

POSTERIOR

PROLAPSED HEMORRHOIDS

PROLAPSE OF THE RECTUM

On straining for a bowel movement the rectal mucosa, with or without its muscular wall, may prolapse through the anus, appearing as a doughnut or rosette of red tissue. A prolapse involving only mucosa is relatively small and shows radiating folds, as illustrated. When the entire bowel wall is involved, the prolapse is larger and covered by concentrically circular folds.

POLYPS OF THE RECTUM

Polyps of the rectum are fairly common. Varying considerably in size and number, they can develop on a stalk (pedunculated) or lie close to the mucosal surface (sessile). They are soft and may be difficult or impossible to feel even when in reach of the examining finger. Proctoscopy is usually required for diagnosis, as is biopsy for the differentiation of benign from malignant lesions.

Sessile

Pedunculated

CARCINOMA OF THE RECTUM

Asymptomatic carcinoma of the rectum makes routine rectal examination mandatory for virtually all adults. As noted above, polypoid masses may be malignant. Another common form is the firm, nodular, rolled edge of an ulcerated malignancy.

Rolled nodular edge

PERITONEAL METASTASES

SIDE VIEW

ANTERIOR WALL

Palpable rectal shelf

Widespread peritoneal metastases from any source may develop in the area of the peritoneal reflection anterior to the rectum. A firm to hard nodular rectal "shelf" may be just palpable with the tip of the examining finger.

Table 14-2

Table 14-2 Abnormalities of the Prostate

THE NORMAL PROSTATE GLAND

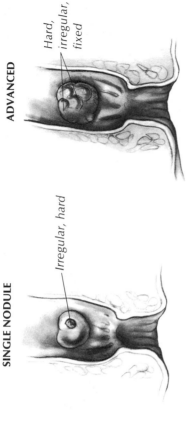

Smooth, elastic, symmetrical

As palpated through the anterior rectal wall, the normal prostate is a rounded, heart-shaped structure about 2.5 cm in length, projecting less than 1.0 cm into the rectal lumen. The median sulcus can be felt between the two lateral lobes. Only the posterior surface of the prostate is palpable. Anterior lesions, including those that may obstruct the urethra, may not be detectable by physical examination.

CARCINOMA OF THE PROSTATE

SINGLE NODULE

Irregular, hard

ADVANCED

Hard, irregular, fixed

A hard, irregular nodule, producing asymmetry of the gland and a variation in its consistency, is especially suggestive of carcinoma. Prostatic stones and chronic inflammation can produce similar findings, and differential diagnosis often depends upon biopsy. Later in its course the carcinoma grows in size, obliterates the median sulcus, and may extend beyond the confines of the gland, producing a fixed, hard, irregular mass.

BENIGN PROSTATIC HYPERTROPHY

A very common condition in men over 50 years of age, benign prostatic hypertrophy feels like a firm, smooth, symmetrical, and slightly elastic enlargement of the gland. It may bulge more than 1.0 cm into the rectal lumen. The hypertrophied tissue tends to obliterate the median sulcus.

PROSTATITIS

ACUTE

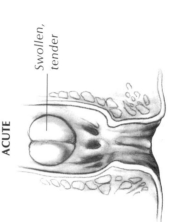

Swollen, tender

The acutely inflamed prostate gland is swollen, tender, and often somewhat asymmetrical.

The gland of chronic prostatitis is variable: it may (1) feel normal, (2) be somewhat enlarged, tender, and boggy, or (3) contain scattered firm areas of fibrosis.

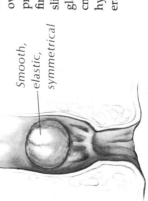

Chapter 15
The Peripheral Vascular System

Anatomy and Physiology

ARTERIES

The carotid arteries have been described in Chapters 7 and 9, the abdominal aorta in Chapter 11. This section will focus on the arteries supplying the arms and legs.

In the arms, arterial pulses are clinically accessible in two or perhaps three locations: (1) the *brachial artery* just medial to the biceps tendon and muscle at and above the elbow, (2) the *radial artery,* and (3) the less easily felt *ulnar artery* at the wrist.

The radial and ulnar arteries are interconnected by two vascular arches within the hand. Circulation to the hand and fingers is thereby doubly protected against possible arterial occlusion.

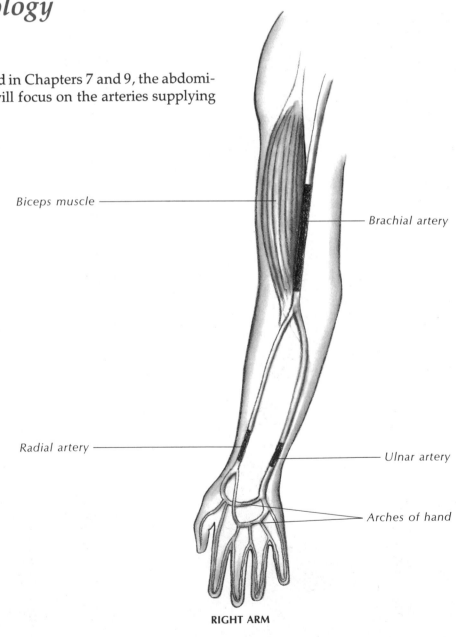

Biceps muscle

Brachial artery

Radial artery

Ulnar artery

Arches of hand

RIGHT ARM

Pulses in the legs can be identified in the following locations: the *femoral artery,* below the inguinal ligament midway between the anterior superior iliac spine and symphysis pubis; the *popliteal artery,* behind the knee; the *dorsalis pedis artery,* on the dorsum of the foot; and the *posterior tibial artery,* just behind the medial malleolus.

Like the hand, the foot is protected by an interconnecting arch between the two chief arterial branches supplying it.

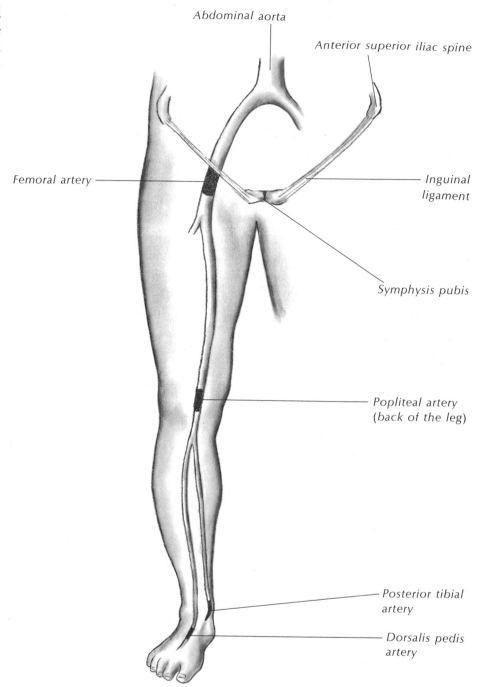

RIGHT LEG

VEINS

The jugular veins have been discussed in Chapters 7 and 9. They are the principal veins from the head and, together with veins from the arms and upper trunk, drain into the superior vena cava. Veins from the legs and lower trunk drain into the inferior vena cava. Since venous disease most commonly affects the legs, special attention should be paid to the structure and function of the leg veins.

The *deep veins* of the legs carry about 90% of the venous return from the lower extremities. They are well supported by surrounding tissues.

In contrast, the *superficial veins* are located subcutaneously, and are supported relatively poorly. The superficial veins include (1) the *great saphenous vein*, which originates on the dorsum of the foot, passes just in front of the medial malleolus, and then continues up the medial aspect of the leg to join the deep venous system (the femoral vein) below the inguinal ligament; and (2) the *small saphenous vein*, which begins at the side of the foot and passes upward along the back of the leg to join the deep system in the popliteal space. Anastomotic channels join the two saphenous veins, and *communicating*, or *perforating*, *veins* connect the saphenous system with the veins of the deep system along its entire course.

Deep, superficial, and communicating veins all have thin valves along their courses, about 10 cm to 12 cm apart. These are so arranged that venous blood can flow from the superficial to the deep system and toward the heart but not in the opposite directions. Muscular activity provides the driving force behind venous blood flow. As muscles contract in walking, for example, blood is squeezed upward against gravity and kept from falling back by competent valves.

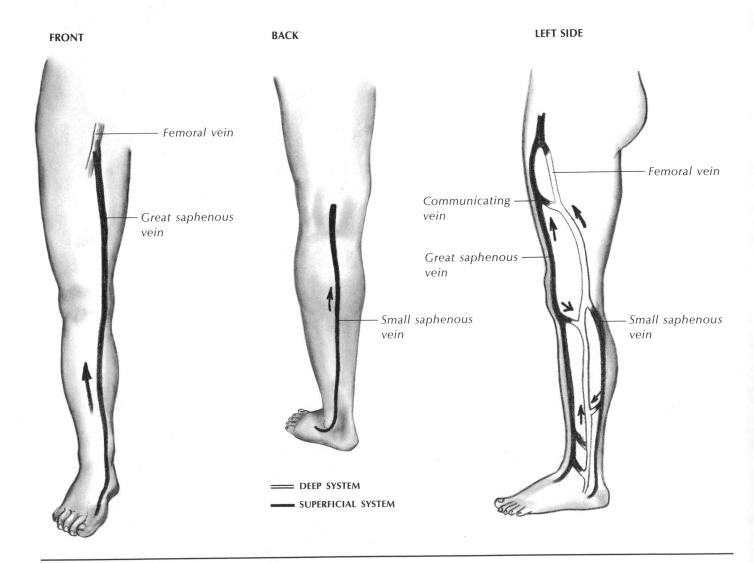

FRONT

BACK

LEFT SIDE

Femoral vein

Great saphenous vein

Small saphenous vein

Communicating vein

Great saphenous vein

Femoral vein

Small saphenous vein

DEEP SYSTEM
SUPERFICIAL SYSTEM

THE LYMPHATIC SYSTEM AND LYMPH NODES

The lymphatic system consists of a series of channels that begin peripherally in blind lymphatic capillaries. These capillaries remove excess fluid from the tissues. The lymph so formed is carried centrally through lymphatic vessels and collecting ducts to empty into the venous system at the root of the neck. In its passage, lymph is filtered through lymph nodes that are interposed along the way.

The lymphatics draining the head and neck have been described in Chapter 7, the lymph nodes of the axilla in Chapter 10.

Recall that the axillary lymph nodes drain most of the arm. Lymphatics from the ulnar surface of the forearm, the little and ring fingers, and the adjacent surface of the middle finger drain first into the *epitrochlear node.* This node is located on the medial surface of the arm above the elbow. Most of the rest of the arm sends lymphatics directly to the axillary nodes. Some lymphatics may go directly to the infraclaviculars.

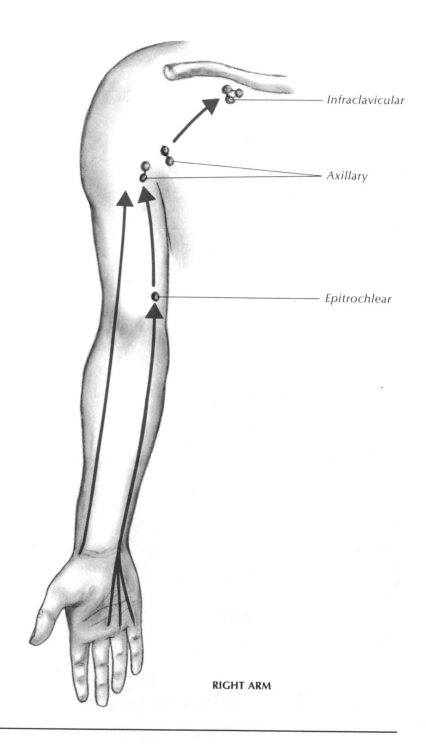

Infraclavicular

Axillary

Epitrochlear

RIGHT ARM

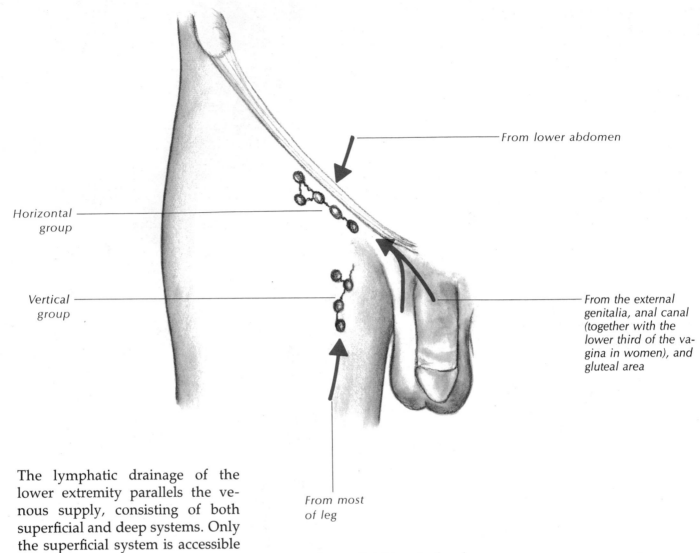

From lower abdomen

Horizontal
group

Vertical
group

From the external
genitalia, anal canal
(together with the
lower third of the va-
gina in women), and
gluteal area

From most
of leg

The lymphatic drainage of the lower extremity parallels the venous supply, consisting of both superficial and deep systems. Only the superficial system is accessible to physical examination. There are two groups of *superficial inguinal nodes*. The *vertical group* lies close to the upper portion of the great saphenous vein and drains a corresponding area of the leg. In contrast, lymphatics from the portion of the leg drained by the small saphenous vein (*i.e.,* the heel and outer aspect of the foot) drain into the deep system at the level of the popliteal space. Lesions in this area, therefore, are not usually associated with palpable inguinal lymph nodes.

A *horizontal group* of superficial nodes lies just below the inguinal ligament. This group drains the skin of the lower abdominal wall, the external genitalia (excluding the testes), the anal canal, the lower vagina, and the gluteal area.

FLUID EXCHANGE AND THE CAPILLARY BED

Blood circulates from arteries to veins through the capillary bed. Here fluids diffuse across the capillary membrane, maintaining a dynamic equilibrium between the vascular and interstitial spaces. Blood pressure (or hydrostatic pressure) within the capillary bed, especially near the arteriolar end, forces fluid out into the tissue spaces. In effecting this movement, it is aided by the relatively weak osmotic attraction of proteins within the tissues (interstitial colloid osmotic pressure) and is opposed by the hydrostatic pressure of the tissues.

As blood continues through the capillary bed toward the venous end its hydrostatic pressure falls, and another force gains dominance. This is the colloid osmotic pressure of plasma proteins, which pulls fluid back into the vascular tree. Net flow of fluid, which was directed outward on the arteriolar side of the capillary bed, reverses itself and turns inward on the venous side. Lymphatic capillaries, which also play an important role in this equilibrium, remove excessive fluid, including protein, from the interstitial space.

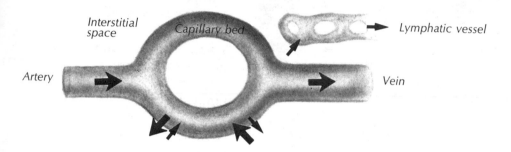

Lymphatic dysfunction or disturbances in hydrostatic or osmotic forces can all disrupt this equilibrium. The most common clinical result is the increased interstitial fluid known as edema. (See Table 15-3, Mechanisms and Patterns of Edema, pp. 422–423.) Secondary renal and hormonal forces that increase total body water and salt in most edematous states will not be discussed here.

CHANGES WITH AGE

Aging itself brings relatively few clinically important changes to the peripheral vascular system. Although arterial and venous disorders, especially atherosclerosis, do afflict older people more frequently, they probably cannot be considered part of the aging process. Age lengthens the arteries, makes them tortuous, and typically stiffens their walls, but these changes develop with or without atherosclerosis and therefore lack diagnostic specificity. Loss of arterial pulsations is not a part of normal aging, however, and demands careful evaluation. Skin may get thin and dry with age, nails may grow more slowly, and hair on the legs often becomes scant. Since these changes are common they are not specific for arterial insufficiency, although they are classically associated with it.

Techniques of Examination

Although this chapter focuses on the peripheral vascular system, you should integrate this examination with your assessment of the skin and of the musculoskeletal and neurological systems. See Chapter 4 for a method of doing this. Throughout your assessment compare one side with the other.

ARMS

Inspect both arms from the fingertips to the shoulders. Note:

　Their size and symmetry
　The color and texture of the skin
　　and nail beds
　The venous pattern
　Edema

With the pads of your index and middle fingers, *palpate the radial pulse* on the flexor surface of the wrist laterally. Compare the volume of the pulses on each side.

If you suspect arterial insufficiency, palpate also for the ulnar and brachial pulses. Feel for the *ulnar pulse* on the flexor surface of the wrist medially.

Feel for the *brachial pulse* in the groove between the biceps and triceps muscles above the elbow. Alternatively, feel for it at the elbow, just medial to the biceps tendon (as described on p. 270).

Pulses may be described as normal, diminished, or absent. A finer numerical classification is based on a 0 to 4 scale:

　0 — completely absent
　1 — markedly impaired
　2 — moderately impaired
　3 — slightly impaired
　4 — normal

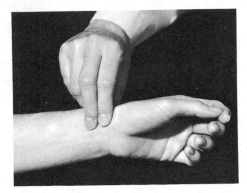

Radial pulse

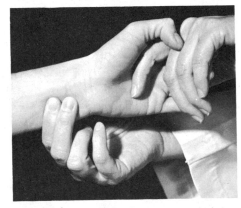

Ulnar pulse

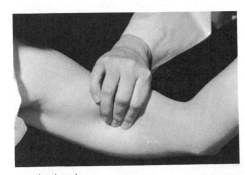

Brachial pulse

Lymphedema of the arm and hand may follow radical mastectomy with axillary node dissection. Edema of the arm with prominent veins suggests venous obstruction.

Arterial occlusion in the arms is much less common than in the legs. If pulses are markedly diminished or absent, however, consider thromboangiitis obliterans (Buerger's disease), scleroderma, or, possibly, a cervical rib.

The normal ulnar artery is often not palpable. To assess its patency and that of the arteries distal to the wrist use the *Allen test.* The patient should rest with hands in the lap, palms up. Place your thumbs lightly over both radial arteries and ask the patient to clench both fists tightly. Clenching blanches the skin of the palms. Now compress the radial arteries firmly with your thumbs, occluding arterial flow, and ask the patient to open both hands into a relaxed, partly flexed position. Observe the color of the palms. Normally they should turn pink promptly, indicating normal flow through the ulnar arteries, interconnecting arches, and distal branches. Repeat, occluding the ulnar arteries.

Persistence of pallor when one artery is manually compressed indicates occlusion of the other artery or its more distal branches and interconnections.

Opening the hands into full extension may itself cause persisting pallor and a falsely positive Allen test.

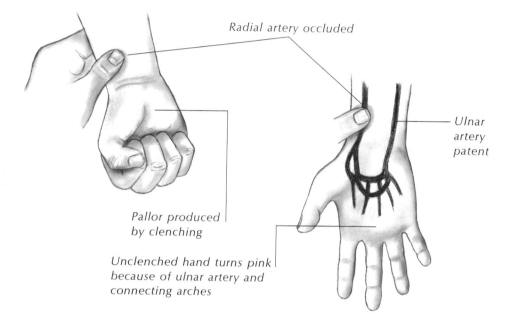

Radial artery occluded

Ulnar artery patent

Pallor produced by clenching

Unclenched hand turns pink because of ulnar artery and connecting arches

Medial aspect of left arm

Right hand of examiner

Palpate for the *epitrochlear node.* With the patient's elbow flexed to about 90° and the forearm supported by your hand, reach around behind the arm and feel in the groove between the biceps and triceps muscles, about 3 cm above the medial epicondyle. If a node is present, note its size, consistency, and tenderness.

An enlarged epitrochlear node may be secondary to a lesion in its drainage area or may be associated with generalized lymphadenopathy.

Medial epicondyle of humerus

LEGS

The patient should be lying down and draped so that the external genitalia are covered and the legs fully exposed. A good examination is impossible through stockings or socks!

Inspect both legs from the groin and buttocks to the feet. Note:

See Table 15-1, Chronic Insufficiency of Arteries and Veins (p. 420).

Their size and symmetry
The color and texture of the skin and nail beds, and the hair distribution on the lower legs, feet, and toes
Pigmentation, rashes, scars, and ulcers
The venous pattern and evidence of venous enlargement
Edema

See Table 15-2, Common Ulcers of the Feet and Ankles (p. 421).

Palpate the superficial inguinal lymph nodes, both the horizontal and the vertical groups. Note their size, consistency, and tenderness. (Small, mobile, nontender inguinal nodes are frequently present.)

Tenderness suggests lymphadenitis.

Note any tenderness in the region of the femoral vein.

Venous tenderness together with other signs of venous obstruction suggests iliofemoral thrombophlebitis.

Palpate the pulses in order to assess the arterial circulation.

1. *The femoral pulse.* Press deeply, below the inguinal ligament and about midway between the anterior superior iliac spine and the symphysis pubis. As in deep abdominal palpation, the use of two hands, one on top of the other, may facilitate this examination, especially in obese patients.

Significant decrease or absence of arterial pulses in the legs is most commonly due to arteriosclerosis obliterans. When a pulse is diminished or absent, it indicates partial or complete arterial occlusion proximally. A decreased or absent femoral pulse, for example, suggests disease at the aortic or iliac level. All pulses distal to the occlusion are typically affected. Chronic arterial occlusion causes intermittent claudication (pp. 86–87), postural color changes (pp. 418–419), and trophic changes in the skin (p. 420).

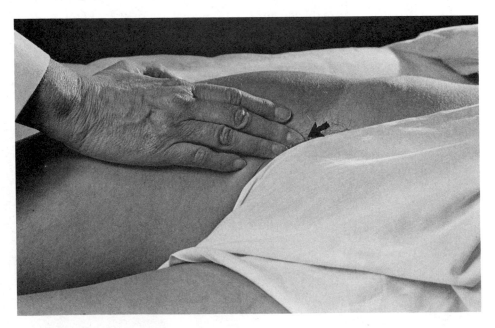

An exaggerated, widened femoral pulse suggests a femoral aneurysm.

2. *The popliteal pulse.* The patient's knee should be somewhat flexed, the leg relaxed. Place the fingertips of both hands so that they just meet in the midline behind the knee and press them deeply into the popliteal fossa. The popliteal pulse is frequently more difficult to find than other pulses. It is deeper and feels more diffuse.

Arteriosclerosis obliterans most commonly obstructs arterial circulation in the thigh. The femoral pulse is then normal, the popliteal decreased or absent.

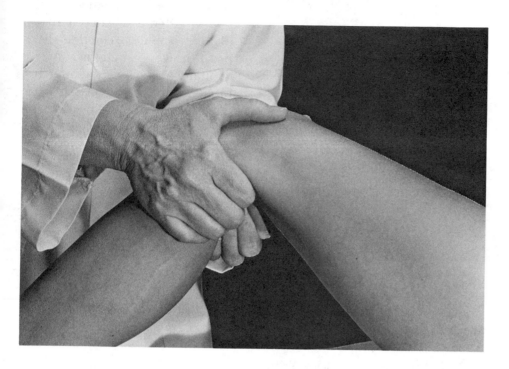

If you cannot feel the popliteal pulse with this approach, try feeling for it with the patient prone. Flex the patient's knee to about 90°, let the lower leg relax against your shoulder or upper arm, and press your two thumbs deeply into the popliteal fossa.

An exaggerated, widened popliteal pulse suggests an aneurysm of the popliteal artery.

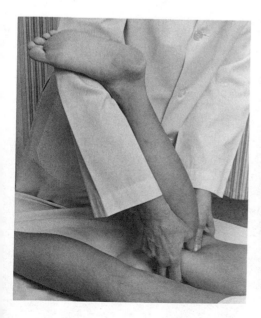
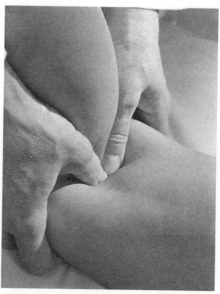

3. *The dorsalis pedis pulse.* Feel the dorsum of the foot (not the ankle) just lateral to the extensor tendon of the great toe. If you cannot feel a pulse, explore the dorsum of the foot more laterally.

4. *The posterior tibial pulse.* Curve your fingers behind and slightly below the medial malleolus of the ankle. (This pulse may be hard to feel in a fat or edematous ankle.)

Decreased or absent foot pulses (assuming a warm environment) with normal femoral and popliteal pulses suggest occlusive disease in the lower popliteal artery or its branches—a pattern often associated with diabetes mellitus. The dorsalis pedis, however, may be congenitally absent or may branch higher in the ankle. Search more laterally on the dorsum of the foot for another pulse.

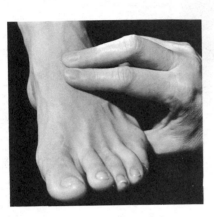
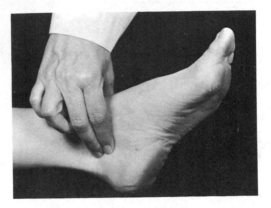

Note: Some pulses may be difficult to feel. Here are some aids: (1) Keep your own body and examining hand comfortable; awkward positions decrease your tactile sensitivity. (2) Place your hand properly and linger there, varying the pressure of your fingers to pick up a weak pulsation. If unsuccessful, then explore the area deliberately. Avoid flitting about. (3) Do not confuse the patient's pulse with your own pulsating fingertips. If you are unsure, count your own heart rate and compare it with the patient's. The rates are usually different. Your carotid pulse is convenient for this comparison.

Using the backs of your fingers, *note the temperature of the feet and legs,* comparing one side with the other. Bilateral coldness is most often due to a cold environment or anxiety.

Coldness, especially when unilateral or associated with other signs, suggests arterial insufficiency, an inadequate arterial circulation.

Look for edema of the legs and *check for pitting edema.* Press firmly but gently with your thumb for at least 5 seconds behind each medial malleolus, over the dorsum of each foot, and over the shins. Look for pitting, a depression in the skin caused by your pressure. The severity of edema is often graded on a 4-point scale from slight to very marked, but the scale is not well standardized.

See Table 15-3, Mechanisms and Patterns of Edema (pp. 422–423).

See Table 15-4, Some Peripheral Causes of Edema (p. 424).

If you note edema involving much of one leg, look for other signs that might suggest deep iliofemoral thrombophlebitis. These include an in-

A painful swollen leg with an increased venous pattern,

crease in the venous pattern of the leg and a diffuse reddish cyanosis of the leg.

Palpate the calf for signs of deep phlebitis. The patient's leg should be flexed at the knee and relaxed. With your fingertips gently compress the calf muscles against the tibia and search for any tender areas. Feel for any increased firmness or tension of the muscles.

Look for any signs of superficial phlebitis, such as redness or discoloration overlying the saphenous veins. If you see any or suspect phlebitis, palpate for tenderness or cords.

Ask the patient to stand, and *inspect the saphenous system for varicosities.* The standing posture allows any varicosities to fill with blood and makes them visible. You can easily miss them when the patient is in a supine position. Feel for any varicosities, noting any signs of thrombophlebitis.

increased warmth, and a normal or faintly reddish cyanotic hue suggests iliofemoral thrombophlebitis.

Tenderness, increased firmness, and tension suggest deep thrombophlebitis in the calf. Unfortunately, however, phlebitis here usually has no signs.

A tender, indurated, subcutaneous cord with warmth, redness, or discoloration indicates superficial thrombophlebitis.

Varicose veins are dilated and tortuous. Their walls may feel somewhat thickened.

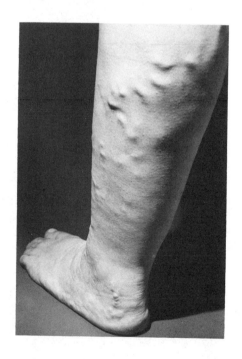

SPECIAL MANEUVERS

EVALUATING THE COMPETENCY OF VENOUS VALVES IN VARICOSE VEINS. Assessing the competency of valves in varicose veins tests the functional sufficiency of the venous system. Two tests are useful:

Incompetent valves increase the hydrostatic pressure in the lower legs and lead to venous insufficiency.

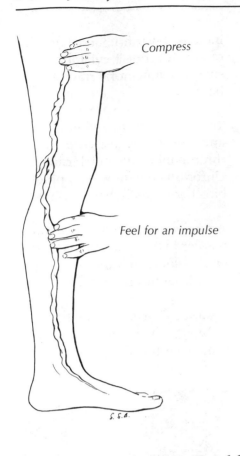

Compress

Feel for an impulse

S. S. B.

1. *The manual compression test.* With the fingertips of one hand, feel the dilated vein. With your other hand compress the vein firmly at least 20 cm higher in the leg. Feel for an impulse transmitted to your lower hand. Competent saphenous valves should block the transmission of any impulse.

A palpable transmitted impulse indicates incompetency of the valve(s) in that portion of the vein between your two hands.

2. *The retrograde filling (Trendelenburg) test.* This test helps to assess valvular competency in the communicating veins as well as in the saphenous system. Elevate the patient's leg to 90° to empty it of venous blood. Place a tourniquet around the upper thigh, tightly enough to occlude the great saphenous vein without occluding the femoral artery. Ask the patient to stand. Watch for venous filling. Normally the saphenous vein fills slowly from below, taking about 35 seconds, as blood flows from arteries through the capillary bed into the venous system.

See Table 15-5, The Retrograde Filling Test for Incompetent Venous Valves (p. 425).

Rapid filling of superficial veins while the tourniquet is applied indicates incompetent valves in the communicating veins. Blood flows quickly in a retrograde direction from the deep to the superficial saphenous system.

After the patient has stood for 20 seconds, release the tourniquet and look for any sudden effect on venous filling. Normally there is none, since competent valves block retrograde flow.

Sudden additional filling of superficial veins after the release of the tourniquet indicates incompetent valves in the saphenous vein. Blood flows backward, unchecked by valves.

POSTURAL COLOR CHANGES OF CHRONIC ARTERIAL INSUFFICIENCY. If pain or diminished pulses suggest arterial insufficiency, look for postural color changes. Raise both legs to about 60° until maximal pallor of the feet develops—usually within a minute. Slight pallor is normal in light-skinned persons. Then ask the patient to sit up with legs dangling down. Comparing both feet, note the time required for

Marked pallor on elevation, delayed color return and venous filling, and rubor on dependency indicate chronic arterial insufficiency. Absence of color changes when arterial pulses

1. Return of pinkness to the skin, normally about 10 seconds or less

2. Filling of the veins of the feet and ankles, normally about 15 seconds. Look for any unusual rubor (dusky redness) or cyanosis of the dependent feet. Color changes may be difficult to see in black persons. Look at the soles of the feet if necessary. Good tangential lighting may help you to visualize the veins.

are diminished suggests that good collateral circulation has developed around an arterial occlusion. When veins are incompetent, dependent rubor and the timing of color return and venous filling are not reliable tests of arterial insufficiency.

EVALUATING THE BEDFAST PATIENT. People who are confined to bed, especially when they are emaciated, elderly, or have neurologic impairment, are particularly susceptible to skin damage and ulceration. *Pressure sores* result when sustained compression obliterates arteriolar and capillary blood flow to the skin. Sores may also result from the shearing forces created by bodily movements. When a person slides down in bed from a partially sitting position, for example, or is dragged rather than lifted up from a supine position, the movements may distort the soft tissues of the buttocks and close off the arteries and arterioles within.

The assessment of every susceptible patient should include careful inspection of the skin overlying the sacrum, buttocks, greater trochanters, knees, and heels. Roll the patient onto one side to get a good view of the sacrum and buttocks.

Local redness of the skin warns of impending necrosis, although some deep pressure sores develop without antecedent redness. Ulcers may be seen.

Use this position also to evaluate a patient for *sacral edema.* Press firmly for at least 5 seconds in the sacral area and look for any pitting. If you find it, check other areas higher on the back.

Dependent edema may accumulate in the back of a bed patient and not be apparent in the legs.

Table 15-1

Table 15-1 Chronic Insufficiency of Arteries and Veins

	CHRONIC ARTERIAL INSUFFICIENCY (Advanced)	CHRONIC VENOUS INSUFFICIENCY (Advanced)
PAIN	Intermittent claudication, progressing to rest pain	None to an aching pain on dependency
PULSES	Decreased or absent	Normal, though may be difficult to feel through edema
COLOR	Pale, especially on elevation; dusky red on dependency	Normal, or cyanotic on dependency. Petechiae, then brown pigmentation appear with chronicity.
TEMPERATURE	Cool	Normal
EDEMA	Absent or mild; may develop as the patient tries to relieve rest pain by lowering the leg	Present, often marked
SKIN CHANGES	Thin, shiny, atrophic skin; loss of hair over foot and toes; nails thickened and ridged (trophic changes)	Often brown pigmentation around the ankles, stasis dermatitis, and possible thickening of the skin and narrowing of the leg as scarring develops
ULCERATION	If present, involves toes or points of trauma on feet	If present, develops at sides of ankle, especially medially
GANGRENE	May develop	Does not develop

Arterial image labels: No edema; Skin shiny, atrophic; Nails thick, ridged; Ulcer of toe

Venous image labels: Edema; Brown pigment; Ulcer of ankle

Table 15-2

Table 15-2 Common Ulcers of the Feet and Ankles

	CHRONIC VENOUS INSUFFICIENCY	ARTERIAL INSUFFICIENCY	TROPHIC ULCER
LOCATION	Inner, sometimes outer ankle	Toes, feet, or possibly in areas of trauma (*e.g.,* the shin)	Pressure points in areas with diminished sensation, as in diabetic polyneuropathy
SKIN SURROUNDING THE ULCER	Pigmented, sometimes fibrotic	No callus or excess of pigment, may be atrophic	Calloused
PAIN	Not severe	Often severe, unless neuropathy masks it	Absent (and therefore the ulcer may go unnoticed)
ASSOCIATED GANGRENE	Absent	May be present	In uncomplicated trophic ulcer, absent
ASSOCIATED SIGNS	Edema, pigmentation, stasis dermatitis, and, possibly, cyanosis of the foot on dependency	Decreased pulses, trophic changes, pallor of the foot on elevation, dusky or cyanotic rubor on dependency	Decreased sensation, ankle jerks absent

Table 15-3

Table 15-3   Mechanisms and Patterns of Edema

Causes of edema may be divided roughly into two groups: (1) *general or systemic causes*, including congestive heart failure, hypoalbuminemia, and excessive renal retention of salt and water; and (2) *local causes*, such as venous stasis, lymphatic stasis, and prolonged dependency. Increased capillary permeability may be either local or general in distribution.

	MECHANISM OF EDEMA	DISTRIBUTION OF EDEMA	OTHER SIGNS MAY INCLUDE—
RIGHT-SIDED CONGESTIVE HEART FAILURE 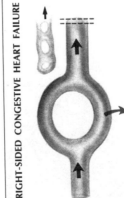	Decreased ability of the heart to accept venous blood increases the hydrostatic pressure in the veins and capillaries, producing congestion and loss of fluid into the tissues.	Edema first appears in the dependent areas of the body where hydrostatic pressure is highest (*i.e.*, the feet and the legs). When the patient is bedridden, the low back is dependent.	Increased jugular venous pressure, an enlarged and often tender liver, an enlarged heart, S₃
HYPOALBUMINEMIA 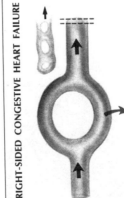	Decreased colloid osmotic pressure in the plasma allows excessive fluid to escape into the interstitial space. Causes include cirrhosis, the nephrotic syndrome, and severe malnutrition.	Edema may appear first in the loose subcutaneous tissues of the eyelids, especially after the patient lies down at night, but may also show first in the feet and legs. In cirrhosis, ascites often appears first. When cirrhosis is more advanced, edema may become generalized.	Signs of chronic liver disease such as ascites, spider angiomas, and jaundice. Signs of the nephrotic syndrome vary with its causes. Serum albumin is low, of course.
EXCESSIVE RENAL RETENTION OF SALT AND WATER 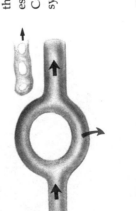	The kidneys may initiate edema by retaining excessive amounts of salt and water, some of which pass into the interstitial space. Drugs such as corticosteroids, estrogens, and some antihypertensives may be responsible.	Edema usually starts in the dependent areas and may become generalized.	Usually none

Table 15-3

	Mechanism	Location	Clinical Features
VENOUS STASIS SECONDARY TO OBSTRUCTION OR INSUFFICIENCY 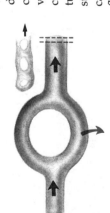	Thrombophlebitis may block venous drainage. Venous valves may be damaged by thrombophlebitis or become incompetent because of varicose veins. Less commonly, veins may be compressed from the outside, as by a tumor or fibrosis. In any case hydrostatic pressure rises in the veins and capillaries, producing excessive loss of fluid into the tissues.	Edema is limited to the area of blockage, often one leg or, less commonly, both legs or an arm. A blocked superior vena cava may cause edema in the entire upper part of the body.	Local swelling and increased tissue turgor. When large veins such as the superior vena cava or the iliofemoral veins are involved, an increased venous pattern of dilated veins may be visible. Tenderness sometimes accompanies phlebitis. Signs of venous insufficiency
LYMPHATIC STASIS (LYMPHEDEMA) 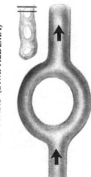	Lymph channels may be congenitally abnormal or they may be obstructed by tumor, fibrosis, or inflammation.	Local, often involving one or both legs. Lymphedema of an arm may follow radical mastectomy.	Indurated skin in the involved area. Except in the early phases, lymphedema is characteristically nonpitting.
ORTHOSTATIC EDEMA 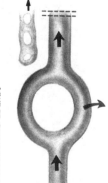	Prolonged sitting or standing, without sufficient muscular activity to promote venous flow, increases the pressure in the veins and capillaries and thus increases the flow of fluid into the interstitial spaces.	The dependent areas (*e.g.*, the legs)	None. Get a good history, including long bus or train trips. People who get up after prolonged bedrest are at first especially susceptible to orthostatic edema.
INCREASED CAPILLARY PERMEABILITY 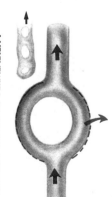	When capillary permeability increases, protein leaks into the interstitial spaces and, by increasing the interstitial colloid osmotic pressure, draws excessive fluid with it. Causes vary, including burns, snake bite, and allergy.	Usually local, depending on the cause; may be general	Variable

Table 15-4

Table 15-4 Some Peripheral Causes of Edema

	ORTHOSTATIC EDEMA	LYMPHEDEMA	LIPEDEMA	CHRONIC VENOUS INSUFFICIENCY
	Pitting — *Foot swollen*	*No pitting* — *Skin thick* — *Foot swollen*	*No pitting* — *Foot spared*	*Pitting* — *Pigment* — *Ulcer* — *Advanced*
PROCESS	Edema from prolonged sitting or standing	Lymphatic obstruction	Fatty deposition in legs	Deep venous obstruction or valvular incompetence
NATURE OF EDEMA	Soft, pits on pressure	Soft early, becomes hard and nonpitting	Minimal if any	Soft, pits on pressure, later may become brawny (hard)
SKIN THICKENING	Absent	Marked	Absent	Occasional
ULCERATION	Absent	Rare	Absent	Common
PIGMENTATION	Absent	Absent	Absent	Common
FOOT INVOLVEMENT	Present	Present	Absent	Present
BILATERALITY	Always	Often	Always	Occasionally

Table 15-5

Table 15-5 The Retrograde Filling Test for Incompetent Venous Valves

	NORMAL	SAPHENOUS VEIN INCOMPETENT AND COMMUNICATING VEINS INCOMPETENT	SAPHENOUS VEIN INCOMPETENT BUT COMMUNICATING VEINS COMPETENT
ON STANDING WITH THE TOURNIQUET FASTENED	Slow venous filling from below	Rapid filling through communicating veins	Slow venous filling from below
ON RELEASE OF THE TOURNIQUET	No additional filling from above	Sudden additional filling from above	Sudden additional filling from above

Chapter 16
The Musculoskeletal System

Anatomy and Physiology

This section will review briefly the structure and function of joints and will describe the anatomical landmarks of several clinically important joints. Identify these landmarks first on yourself or on a fellow student. Range of motion at each joint varies greatly with age and health. The figures given here are intended to be general guides, not absolute standards.

STRUCTURE AND FUNCTION OF JOINTS

A typical *freely movable joint* is diagrammed at the right.

Note that the bones themselves do not touch each other within a joint but are covered by articular cartilage that forms a cushion between the bony surfaces. At the margins of the articular cartilage is attached the synovial membrane. This membrane is pouched or folded to allow for joint movement. It encloses the synovial cavity and secretes into it a small amount of viscous lubricating fluid—the synovial fluid.

The synovial membrane is surrounded by a fibrous joint capsule, which in turn is strengthened by ligaments extending from bone to bone.

Some joints, such as those between the vertebral bodies illustrated here, are *slightly movable joints.* Here the bones are separated not by a synovial cavity but by a fibrocartilaginous disc. At the center of each disc is the nucleus pulposus, fibrogelatinous material that forms a cushion or shock absorber between the vertebral bodies.

Bursae are disc-shaped, fluid-filled synovial sacs that occur at points of friction around joints and facilitate movement. They lie between the skin and the convex surface of a bone or joint (*e.g.*, the prepatellar bursa, p. 435) or in areas where tendons or muscles rub against bone, ligaments, or other tendons or muscles (*e.g.*, the subacromial bursa, p. 431).

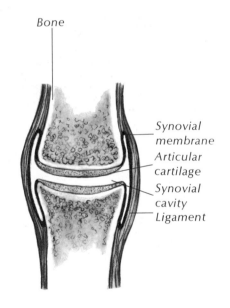

Bone

Synovial membrane
Articular cartilage
Synovial cavity
Ligament

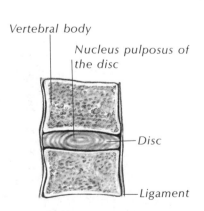

Vertebral body

Nucleus pulposus of the disc

Disc

Ligament

SPECIFIC JOINTS

TEMPOROMANDIBULAR JOINT. The temporomandibular joint forms the articulation between mandible and skull. Feel for it just in front of the tragus of each ear as the jaw is opened and closed.

WRISTS AND HANDS. At the wrist identify the bony tips of the radius (laterally) and the ulna (medially). On the dorsum of the wrist, palpate the groove of the radiocarpal or wrist joint.

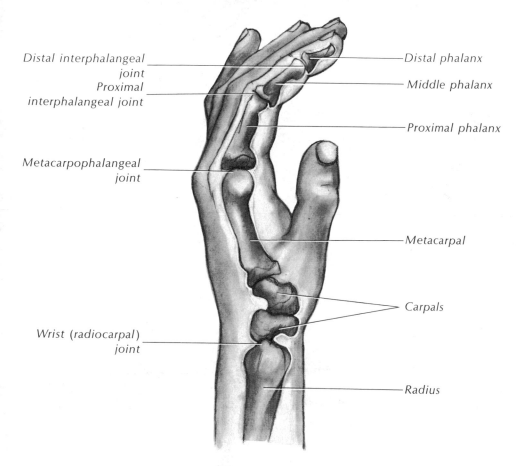

Distal interphalangeal joint
Proximal interphalangeal joint
Metacarpophalangeal joint
Wrist (radiocarpal) joint

Distal phalanx
Middle phalanx
Proximal phalanx
Metacarpal
Carpals
Radius

The carpal bones within the hand cannot be readily identified clinically. However, palpate each of the five metacarpals and the proximal, middle, and distal phalanges. (The thumb lacks a middle phalanx.) Flex the hand somewhat and find the groove marking the metacarpophalangeal joint of each finger. It is distal to the knuckle and can be felt best on either side of the extensor tendon.

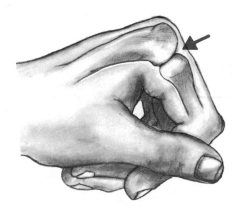

Many tendons pass across the wrist and hand to insert on the fingers. Through much of their course these tendons travel in synovial sheaths or tunnels. Although not normally palpable, these sheaths may become swollen or inflamed.

Illustrated below and at the right is the *range of motion at the wrists:*

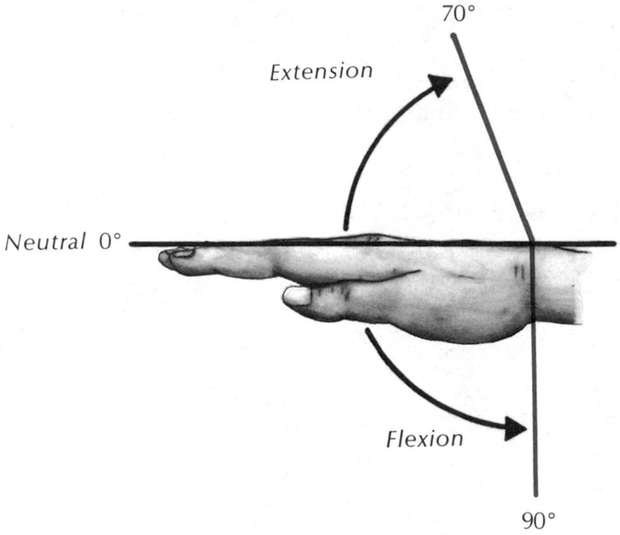

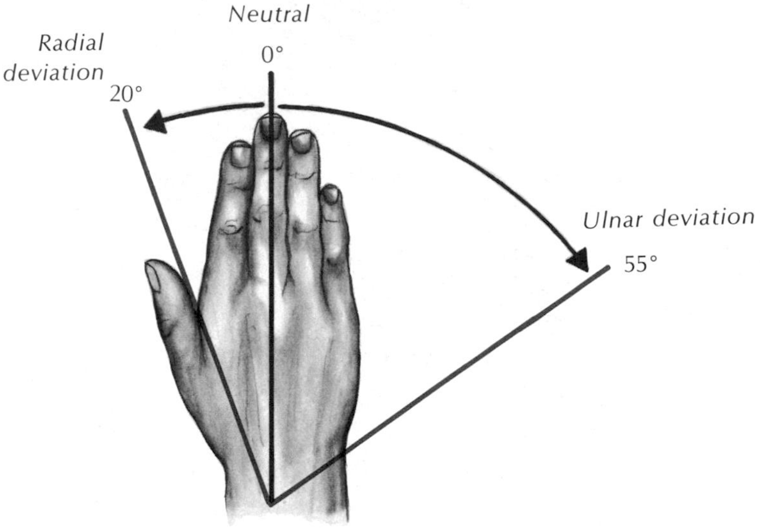

Extension

70°

Neutral 0°

Flexion

90°

Radial deviation

Neutral 0°

20°

Ulnar deviation

55°

And *at the joints of the fingers:*

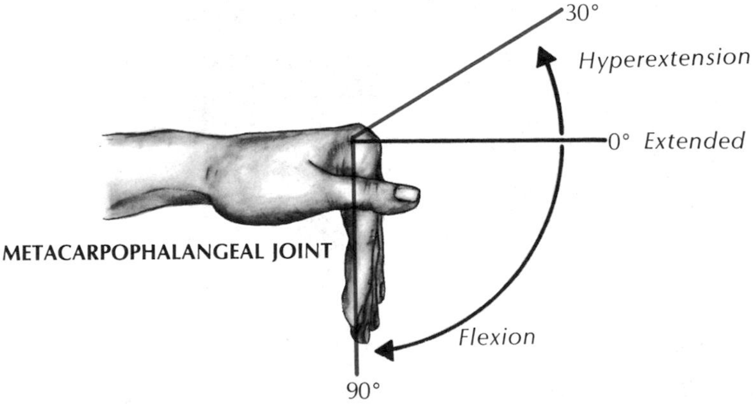

30°

Hyperextension

0° *Extended*

METACARPOPHALANGEAL JOINT

Flexion

90°

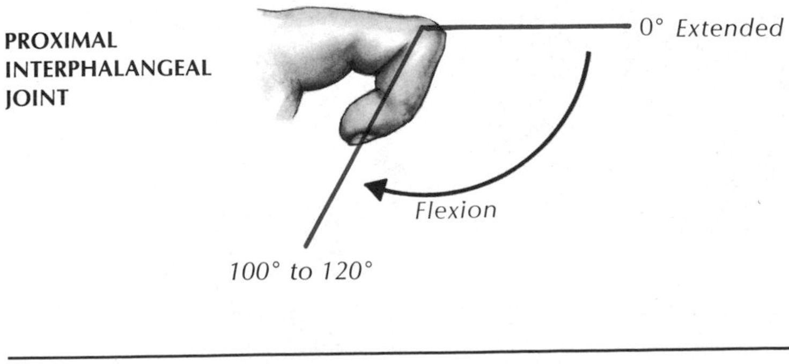

PROXIMAL INTERPHALANGEAL JOINT

0° *Extended*

Flexion

100° *to* 120°

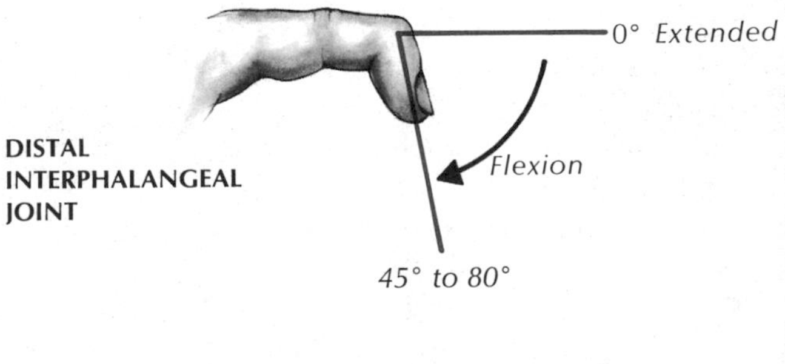

DISTAL INTERPHALANGEAL JOINT

0° *Extended*

Flexion

45° *to* 80°

ELBOWS. Identify the medial and lateral epicondyles of the humerus and the olecranon process of the ulna. A bursa lies between the olecranon process and the skin. The synovial membrane is most accessible to examination between the olecranon and the epicondyles. Neither bursa nor synovium is normally palpable, however.

The sensitive ulnar nerve can be felt posteriorly between olecranon and medial epicondyle.

Movements at the elbow are illustrated below.

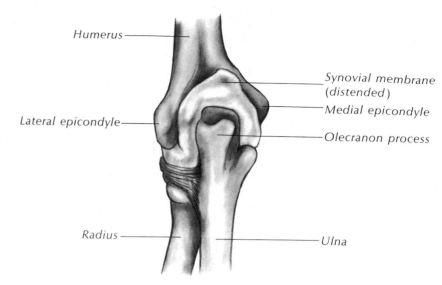

LEFT ELBOW—POSTERIOR VIEW

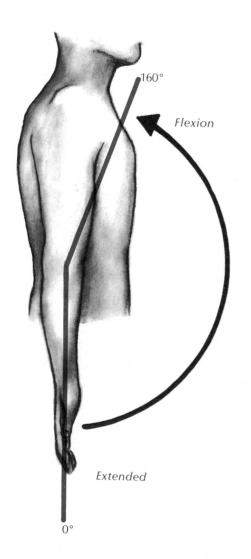

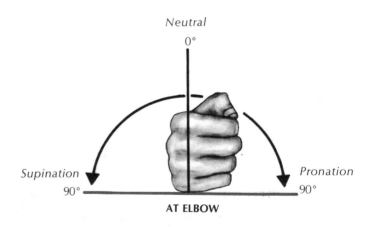

Pronation and supination of the forearm take place at the two radioulnar joints, one at the elbow and one at the wrist.

SHOULDERS AND ENVIRONS. Identify the following landmarks: (1) the manubrium of the sternum, (2) the sternoclavicular joint, and (3) the clavicle. With your fingers trace the clavicle laterally—over its medial two thirds, which is convex, and its lateral third, which is concave. Now, from behind, follow the bony spine of the scapula laterally and upward until it becomes the *acromion*, the summit of the shoulder. Its upper surface is rough and slightly convex. Identify the anterior surface, or tip, of the acromion and mark it with ink. With your index finger on top of the acromion, just behind its tip, press medially to find the slightly elevated ridge that marks the distal end of the clavicle. This junction marks the acromioclavicular joint (shown by the arrow). Now, from the top of the acromion again, move your finger laterally and down a short step to the next bony prominence, the *greater tubercle of the humerus.* Mark this with ink. Now sweep your finger medially a few centimeters until you feel a large bony prominence, the *coracoid process* of the scapula. Mark this also. These three points—(1) the tip of the acromion, (2) the greater tubercle of the humerus, and (3) the coracoid process—orient you to the anatomy of the shoulder.

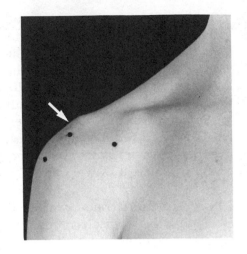

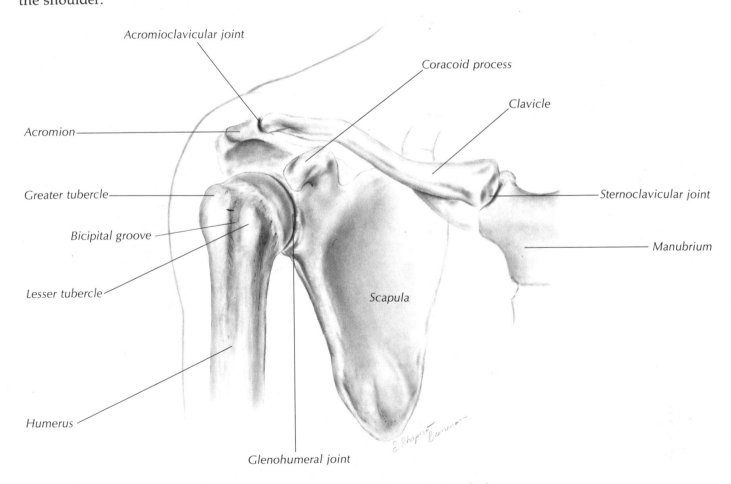

Acromioclavicular joint

Coracoid process

Clavicle

Acromion

Greater tubercle

Sternoclavicular joint

Bicipital groove

Manubrium

Lesser tubercle

Scapula

Humerus

Glenohumeral joint

Rotate the arm externally and find the tendinous cord that runs just medial to the greater tubercle. Roll it under your fingers. This is the tendon of the long head of the biceps. It runs in the bicipital groove between greater and lesser tubercles.

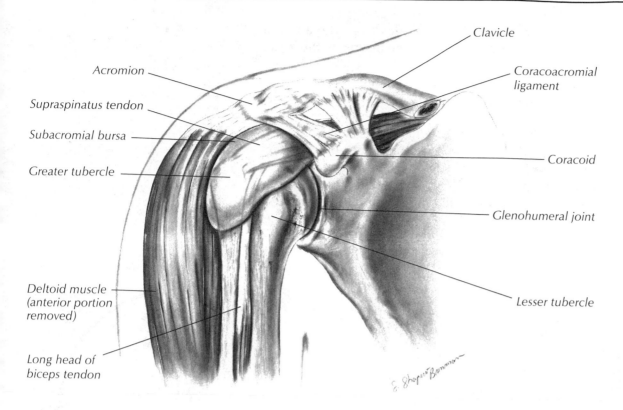

The glenohumeral joint, between the scapula and humerus, is deeply situated and not normally palpable. Its fibrous capsule is reinforced by the tendons of four muscles, which together are called the *rotator cuff*. The supraspinatus, which runs above the joint, and the infraspinatus and teres minor, which cross it posteriorly, all insert on the greater tubercle of the humerus.

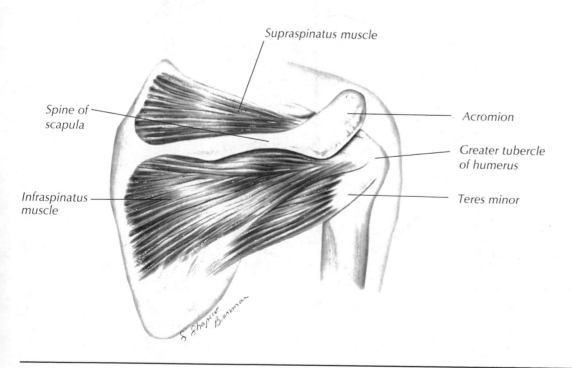

The subscapularis (not illustrated), which originates from the anterior surface of the scapula, crosses the joint anteriorly and inserts on the lesser tubercle.

The arch formed by the acromion, the coracoid, and the coracoacromial ligament protects the glenohumeral joint. Deep to this arch and extending anterolaterally under the deltoid muscle lies the subacromial bursa. It overlies the supraspinatus tendon. Although you cannot normally feel either the bursa or the supraspinatus tendon, tenderness originating there can be found just below the tip of the acromion. Extending the shoulder brings more of their rounded surfaces under your palpating fingers.

The normal *range of motion at the shoulder* is illustrated below.

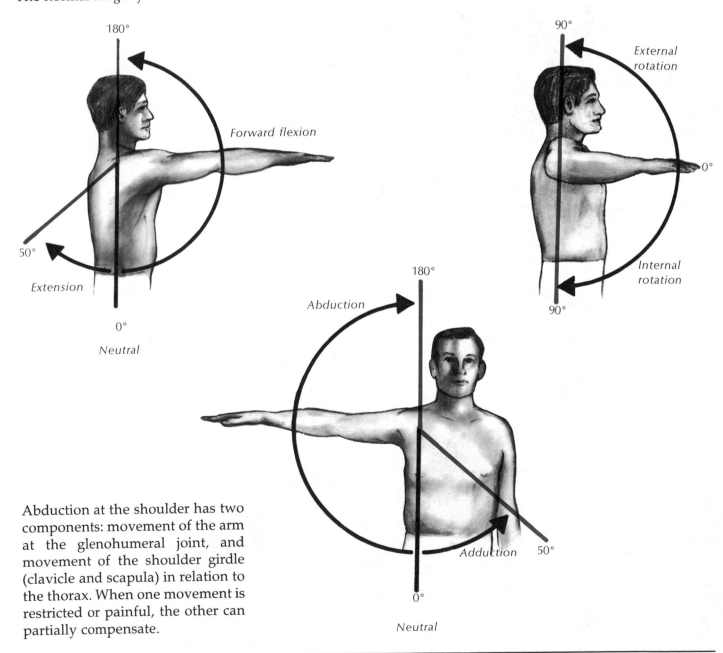

Abduction at the shoulder has two components: movement of the arm at the glenohumeral joint, and movement of the shoulder girdle (clavicle and scapula) in relation to the thorax. When one movement is restricted or painful, the other can partially compensate.

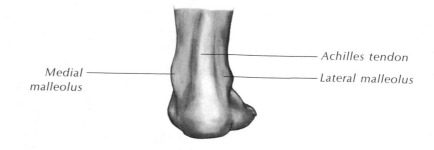

ANKLES AND FEET. The principal landmarks of the ankle are (1) the medial malleolus, the bony prominence at the distal end of the tibia, and (2) the lateral malleolus, the distal end of the fibula. Ligaments extend from each malleolus onto the foot. The strong Achilles tendon inserts on the heel posteriorly.

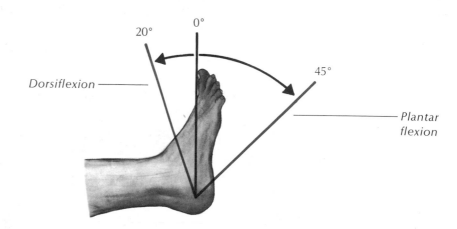

Motions at the ankle joint itself (the tibiotalar joint) are limited to dorsiflexion and plantar flexion.

Inversion and eversion of the foot are functions of the subtalar (talocalcaneal) and transverse tarsal joints.

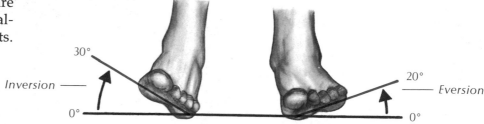

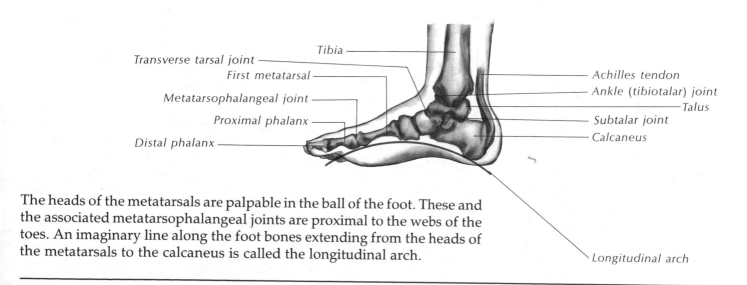

The heads of the metatarsals are palpable in the ball of the foot. These and the associated metatarsophalangeal joints are proximal to the webs of the toes. An imaginary line along the foot bones extending from the heads of the metatarsals to the calcaneus is called the longitudinal arch.

THE KNEE. The knee joint involves three bones: the femur, the tibia, and the patella (or kneecap). It also has three articular surfaces: two between femur and tibia (the medial and lateral compartments of the tibiofemoral joint) and one between patella and femur (the patellofemoral compartment). Landmarks in and around the knee will orient you to this complicated joint.

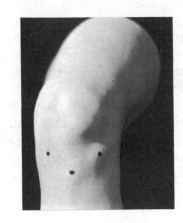

Identify the flat medial surface of the tibia—the shin. Follow its anterior border upward to the tibial tuberosity. Mark this point with a dot of ink. Now follow the medial border of the tibia upward until it merges into a bony prominence—the medial condyle of the tibia. This is somewhat higher than the tibial tuberosity. In a comparable location on the other side of the knee, find a similar prominence—the lateral condyle. Mark both condyles with ink. These three points form an isosceles triangle. On the lateral surface of the knee, somewhat below the level of the lateral tibial condyle, find the head of the fibula.

Now bring your fingertips firmly down the medial surface of the thigh along a line analogous to the inner seam of a pant leg. Your fingers will run up against an abrupt bony prominence, the adductor tubercle of the femur. Just below this is the medial epicondyle of the femur. The lateral epicondyle can be found comparably situated on the other side. The patella rests on the anterior articulating surface of the femur, roughly midway between the epicondyles. It lies within the tendon of the quadriceps muscle. This tendon continues below as the patellar tendon and inserts on the tibial tuberosity.

With the knee flexed about 90° you can press your thumbs—one on each side of the patellar tendon—into the groove of the tibiofemoral joint. Note that the patella lies just above this joint line. As you press downward you can feel the edges of the tibial plateaus, the upper surfaces of the tibia. Follow them medially, then laterally until you are stopped by the converging femur and tibia. The medial and lateral

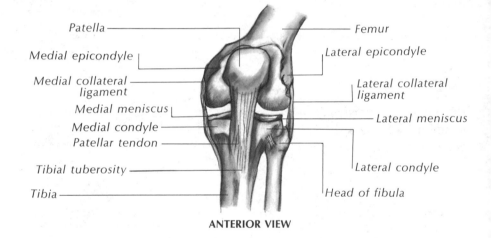

ANTERIOR VIEW

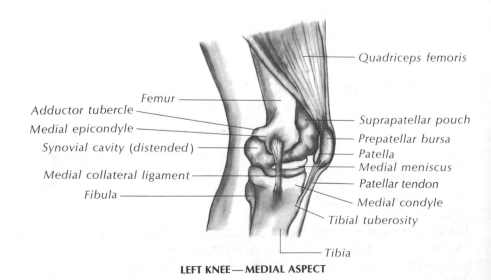

LEFT KNEE—MEDIAL ASPECT

menisci, crescent-shaped fibrocartilaginous pads that lie on the tibial plateaus, form cushions between tibia and femur. Although they are not palpable, they may cause tenderness here when injured. By moving your thumbs upward and medially toward the top of the patella you can follow the articulating surface of the femur, and identify the margins of the joint.

Two collateral ligaments, one on each side of the knee, give it medial and lateral stability. To feel the lateral collateral ligament, cross one leg so that the ankle rests on the opposite knee and find the firm cord that runs from the lateral epicondyle of the femur to the head of the fibula. The medial collateral ligament is not palpable. Two cruciate ligaments (not illustrated) cross obliquely within the knee and give it anteroposterior stability.

The soft tissue in front of the joint space, on either side of the patellar tendon, is the infrapatellar fat pad.

Several bursae lie near the knee. The prepatellar bursa lies between the patella and the overlying skin while the superficial infrapatellar bursa lies anterior to the patellar tendon.

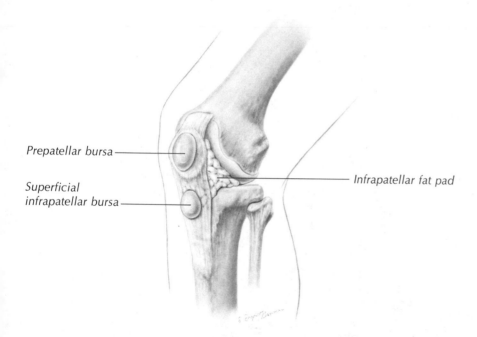

Prepatellar bursa

Superficial
infrapatellar bursa

Infrapatellar fat pad

Above the patella the quadriceps muscle, when contracted, can be identified. Observe the normal concavities on both sides of the patella and also above it. Occupying these areas is the synovial cavity of the knee joint, including its extension up behind the quadriceps, which is called the suprapatellar pouch. Although the synovium is not normally detectable here, these areas may become swollen and tender when the joint is inflamed.

The principal *movements of the knee* are extension, flexion, and sometimes hyperextension.

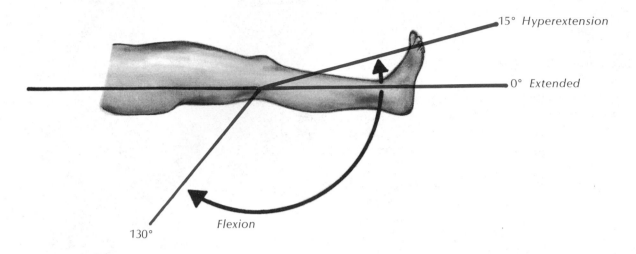

15° *Hyperextension*

0° *Extended*

Flexion

130°

PELVIS AND HIPS. The hip joint lies deep and is not directly palpable. The greater trochanter of the femur can be felt about a palm's breadth below the iliac crest. The superficial trochanteric bursa lies on the posterolateral surface of the greater trochanter.

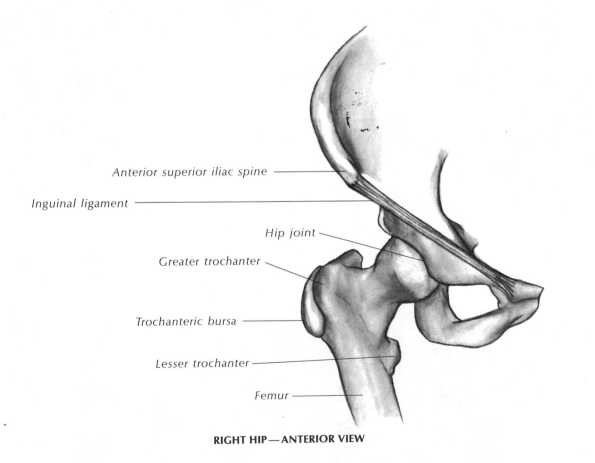

Anterior superior iliac spine

Inguinal ligament

Hip joint

Greater trochanter

Trochanteric bursa

Lesser trochanter

Femur

RIGHT HIP—ANTERIOR VIEW

Movements of the hip are illustrated below.

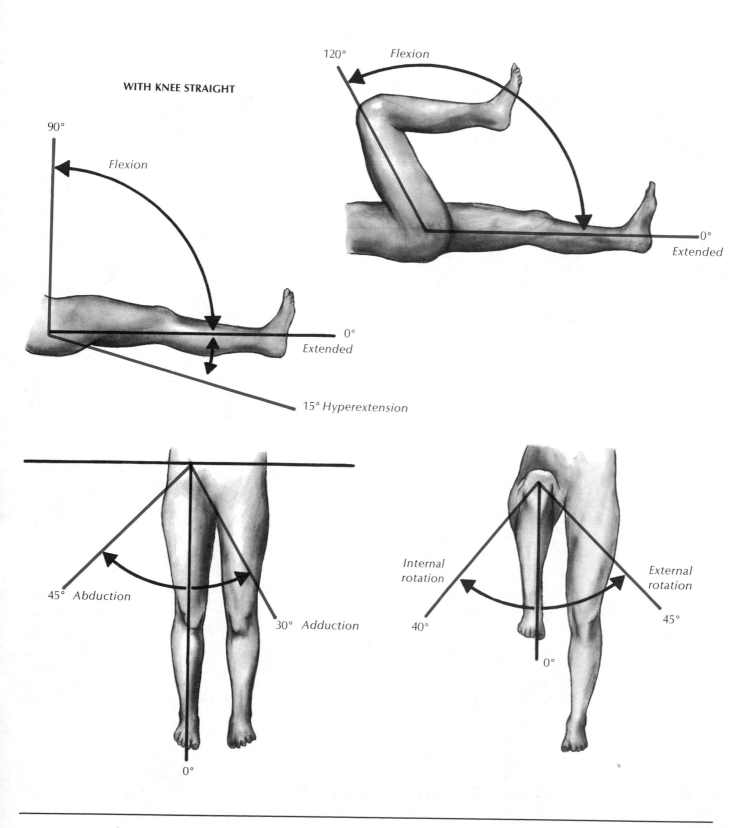

WITH KNEE FLEXED

120° *Flexion*

0°
Extended

WITH KNEE STRAIGHT

90°

Flexion

0°
Extended

15° *Hyperextension*

45° *Abduction*

30° *Adduction*

0°

Internal rotation

External rotation

40°

45°

0°

SPINE. Viewing the patient from behind, identify the following land-marks: (1) the spinous processes, which become more evident on forward flexion, (2) the paravertebral muscles on either side of the midline, (3) the scapulae, (4) the iliac crests, and (5) the posterior superior iliac spines, usually marked by skin dimples. The spinous processes of C7 and often T1 are unusually prominent. A line between the iliac crests crosses the spinous process of L4.

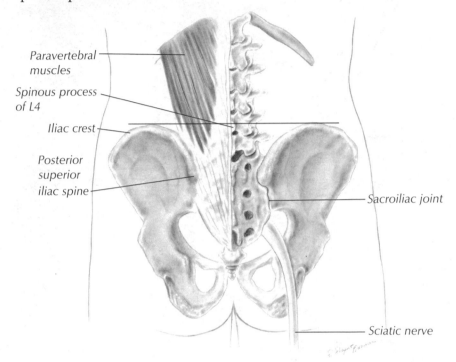

Paravertebral muscles

Spinous process of L4

Iliac crest

Posterior superior iliac spine

Sacroiliac joint

Sciatic nerve

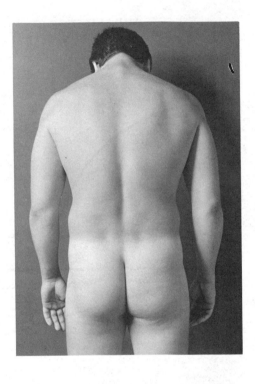

Viewed laterally, the spine has cervical and lumbar concavities and a thoracic convexity. The sacral curve forms a second convexity.

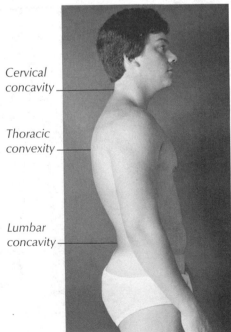

Cervical concavity

Thoracic convexity

Lumbar concavity

The most mobile portion of the spine is the neck. Flexion and extension occur chiefly between the head and the 1st cervical vertebra, rotation occurs primarily between the 1st and 2nd vertebrae, and lateral bending involves the cervical spine from the 2nd to the 7th vertebra.

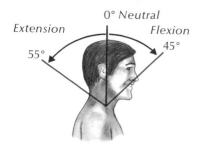

Extension 0° Neutral Flexion
55° 45°

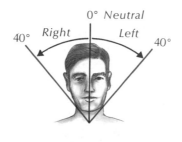

0° Neutral
40° Right Left 40°

LATERAL BENDING

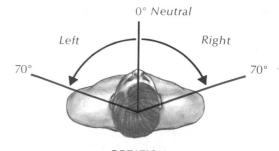

0° Neutral
Left Right
70° 70°

ROTATION

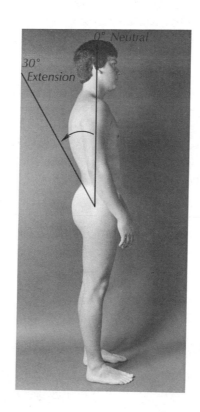

0° Neutral
30° Extension

Movements of the rest of the spine (*i.e.*, from the sacrum to the base of the neck) are more difficult to measure than those in the neck and are subject to considerable individual variation. What looks like spinal flexion takes place partly at the hips. For this reason, and because people differ in the length of their limbs, flexion cannot be accurately estimated by noting the distance of their fingertips from the floor. As the patient flexes forward, watch the lumbar area. Its normal concavity should flatten out.

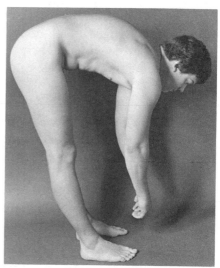

FLEXION

LATERAL BENDING
0°
35° To the left | To the right 35°

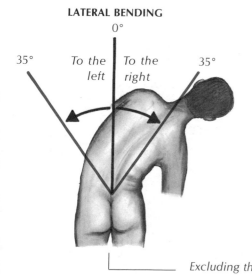

ROTATION
0° 0°
To the left To the right
30° 30°

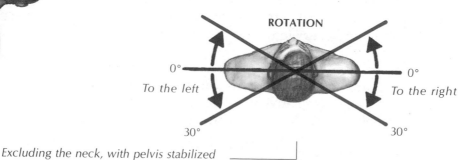

Excluding the neck, with pelvis stabilized

CHANGES WITH AGE

The musculoskeletal system changes importantly during adolescence — in size, proportion, and strength. Between the approximate ages of 12.5 and 15 years boys undergo an adolescent growth spurt, gaining an average of 8 inches in height and over 40 pounds in weight. On the average the growth spurt in girls occurs about 2 years earlier and is smaller in magnitude. Bodily proportions change in fairly regular sequence: the legs elongate, the hips and chest widen, the shoulders broaden, and finally the trunk lengthens and the chest deepens. Shoulders broaden more in boys, while in girls an increase in the bony pelvis produces relatively greater widening of the hips. Muscles increase in size and strength, especially in boys. For illustrations of these changes see page 126.

As in sexual maturation, adolescents vary widely in their musculoskeletal development. Those who mature relatively late in relation to their peers face competitive disadvantages even though they are entirely normal. Adolescent changes in height, musculoskeletal development, and sex maturity correlate well with each other and provide a better basis for counselling teenagers than does a normative concept based on chronological age alone.

Musculoskeletal changes continue through the adult years. Soon after maturity adults begin to lose height subtly, and significant shortening becomes obvious in old age. Most loss of height occurs in the trunk as intervertebral discs become thinner and the vertebral bodies shorten or even collapse because of osteoporosis. Flexion at the knees and hips may contribute to the shortened stature. The limbs of an elderly person thus tend to look long in proportion to the trunk.

The alterations in discs and vertebrae contribute too to the kyphosis of aging and increase the anteroposterior diameter of the chest, especially in women. For illustrations of these changes see page 127.

Skeletal muscles decrease in bulk and power. The hands of an aged person often look thin and bony because the small muscles of the hands have atrophied. Look for such muscular wasting in the backs of the hands where atrophy of the dorsal interosseous muscles leaves concavities or grooves. As illustrated on the facing page, this change is often most evident between thumb and hand (1st and 2nd metacarpals) but may also be seen between the other metacarpals. Atrophy of small muscles may also flatten the thenar and hypothenar eminences of the palms.

Although this kind of wasting would suggest neurologic disease in a younger person, it is normal in many elderly persons, and strength, although somewhat diminished, is relatively well maintained. Arm and leg muscles also show atrophy, sometimes exaggerating the apparent size of the joints.

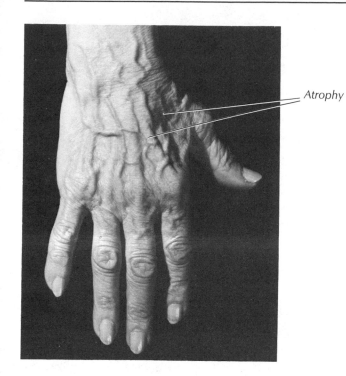

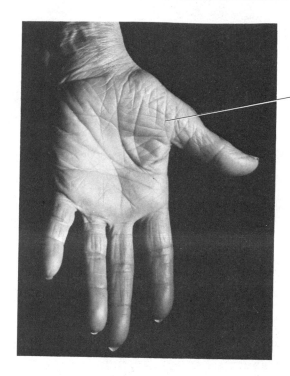

Atrophy

Flattening
of mild
atrophy

Range of motion diminishes with age, partly because of osteoarthritis, a condition that usually accompanies the repetitive and accumulated stresses of the passing years.

Techniques of Examination

GENERAL APPROACH

While examining the musculoskeletal system, direct your attention not only to structure but also to function. During the interview you should have evaluated the patient's abilities to carry out normal activities of daily living. Keep these functional abilities in mind too during your physical examination.

In your initial survey of the patient you have assessed general appearance, bodily proportions, and ease of movement. Now, using inspection and palpation, you will examine individual joints or groups of joints, their range of motion, and the tissues surrounding them.

Note particularly:

1. Any *limitation* in the normal *range of motion* or any unusual *increase* in the *mobility* of a joint (instability). Range of motion varies among individuals and decreases with aging.

    Decreased range of motion in arthritis, inflammation of tissues around the joint, fibrosis in or around a joint, or bony fixation (ankylosis)

2. Any *signs of inflammation* such as:

    Swelling in or around the joint. Swelling may involve the synovial membrane, which then feels boggy, or doughy, to your fingers, or may be produced by excessive synovial fluid within the joint space. Swelling sometimes originates not in the joint itself but in tissues around it, such as bones, tendons, tendon sheaths, bursae, and fat. Trauma to any of these structures may also cause swelling.

    Palpable bogginess, or doughiness, of the synovial membrane indicates synovitis. Palpable joint fluid indicates an effusion in the joint. Synovitis and joint fluid often coexist.

    Tenderness in or around the joint. Try to define the specific anatomic structure that is tender. Trauma may also cause tenderness.

    Arthritis, tendonitis, bursitis, osteomyelitis

    Increased *heat.* Use the backs of your fingers to compare the joint with the symmetrical joint on the opposite side or, if both joints are involved, with the tissues near them.

    Tenderness and warmth over a thickened synovium suggest rheumatoid arthritis.

    Redness of the overlying skin. This is the least common sign of inflammation near the joints.

    Redness of the skin over a tender joint suggests septic or gouty arthritis, or possibly rheumatic fever.

3. *Crepitus (Crepitation),* a palpable or even audible crunching or grating produced by movement of a joint or tendon. Crepitus is more significant when it is associated with other symptoms or signs than when it exists by itself. Cracking or snapping sounds, which result from movement of tendons or ligaments over bone, may occur in normal joints such as the knees.

    Fine, soft crepitus may be felt over inflamed joints. Coarser crepitus suggests roughened articular cartilages, as in an inflamed joint or osteoarthritis. A creaking leathery crepitus may arise in inflamed tendon sheaths.

4. *Deformities,* including:

Those produced by a restriction in the range of motion at a joint

Flexion deformity of the hip (see p. 452)

Malalignment of articulating bones

Ulnar deviation of the fingers in rheumatoid arthritis (see p. 458); bowlegs

An abnormality in the relationship between two articulating surfaces

Dislocation, a complete loss of contact between the two surfaces, and subluxation, a partial loss of contact

5. The *condition of the surrounding tissues,* including muscle atrophy, subcutaneous nodules, and skin changes

Subcutaneous nodules in rheumatoid arthritis or rheumatic fever

6. *Muscular strength.* Testing of muscular strength is described in Chapter 17.

Muscular weakness and atrophy in rheumatoid arthritis

7. *Symmetry* of involvement. Note whether arthritic changes involve several joints symmetrically on both sides of the body or affect only one or perhaps two joints.

Involvement of only one joint increases the likelihood of bacterial arthritis. Rheumatoid arthritis typically involves several joints, symmetrically distributed.

When handling a person with painful joints, be gentle and move slowly. Often patients can move more comfortably by themselves. Let them show you how they manage.

The detail with which you examine the musculoskeletal system will vary widely from patient to patient. In an asymptomatic adolescent, for example, simple inspection of bodily proportions and major joints, together with careful assessment of the spine, may suffice. This chapter will describe a fairly detailed examination such as you might perform on a patient with joint complaints.

Scoliosis is an important problem in adolescents, especially girls, and is frequently asymptomatic in its early stages.

WITH THE PATIENT SITTING UP

HEAD AND NECK

To palpate the temporomandibular joint, place the tip of your index finger just in front of the tragus of each ear and ask the patient to open the mouth. The tips of your fingers should drop into the joint spaces as the mouth opens. Observe the range of motion, feel for swelling, and note any tenderness. Snapping or clicking may be felt and heard in normal people.

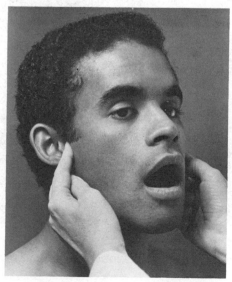

Swelling, tenderness, and decreased range of motion suggest arthritis.

Inspect the neck for deformities and abnormal posture.

Palpate the spinous processes of the cervical spine and the related soft tissues, including the trapezius muscles, the muscles between the scapulae, and the sternomastoids. Identify any areas of tenderness.

Test the range of motion by asking the patient to:

Touch chin to chest (flexion)

Touch chin to each shoulder (rotation)

Touch each ear to the corresponding shoulder without raising the shoulder (lateral bending)

Put the head back (extension)

See Table 2-18, Pain in the Neck (p. 91). Late ankylosing spondylitis may cause an immobile neck with a characteristic deformity. The head and neck are thrust forward, contrasting with a kyphotic thorax.

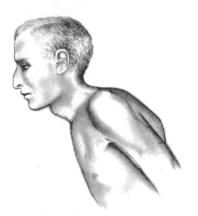

HANDS AND WRISTS

Test the range of motion of the fingers and wrists by asking the patient to:

1. Make a fist with each hand, thumb across the knuckles, and then extend and spread the fingers.

Conditions that impair range of motion include arthritis, inflammation of the tendon sheaths (tenosynovitis), and fibrosis in the palmar fascia (Dupuytren's contracture). See Table 16-1, Swellings and Deformities of the Hands (pp. 458–460).

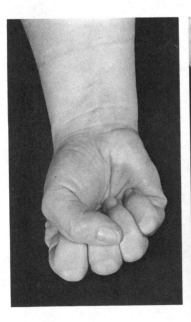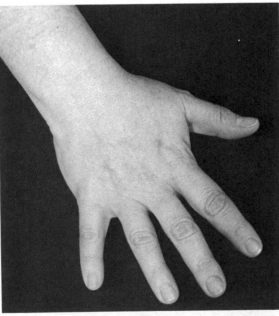

A person should be able to make tight fists and extend and spread the fingers smoothly and easily.

2. Flex and extend the wrists, and with palms down turn the hands laterally and medially (ulnar and radial deviation). Because grip is strongest when the wrist is partly extended, impaired extension is especially important.

Inspect the hands and wrists, noting any swelling, redness, nodules, deformity, or muscular atrophy.

Osteoarthritis of the distal interphalangeal joints appears as hard dorsolateral nodules called Heberden's nodes.

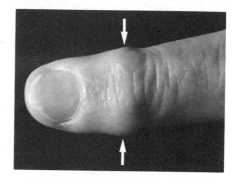

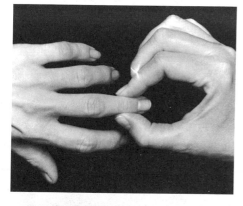

Palpate the medial and lateral aspects of each interphalangeal joint between your thumb and index finger, noting any swelling, bogginess, bony enlargement, or tenderness.

The proximal interphalangeal joints are affected less often. Rheumatoid arthritis commonly involves the proximal joints.

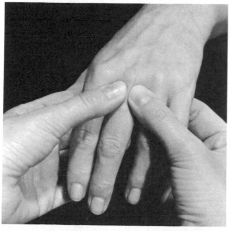

With your thumbs palpate the metacarpophalangeal joints, just distal to and on each side of the knuckle.

Note any swelling, bogginess, or tenderness.

Rheumatoid arthritis often involves the metacarpophalangeal joints; osteoarthritis rarely does.

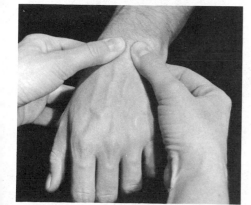

Palpate each wrist joint, with your thumbs on the dorsum of the wrist, your fingers beneath it. Note any swelling, bogginess, or tenderness.

Swelling suggests rheumatoid arthritis if it is bilateral and lasts for several weeks.

Gonococcal infection may involve the wrist joint (arthritis) or the tendon sheaths at the wrist (gonococcal tenosynovitis).

ELBOWS

Test the range of motion by asking the patient to bend and straighten the elbows. With arms at sides and elbows flexed (so that shoulder movements cannot simulate those of the forearm), ask the patient to turn palms up (supination) and down (pronation).

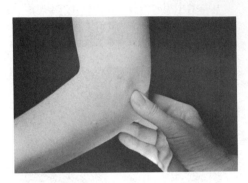

Support the patient's forearm with your opposite hand so that the elbow is flexed to about 70°. Inspect and palpate the elbow, including the extensor surface of the ulna and the olecranon process, noting any nodules or swelling. Palpate the groove on either side of the olecranon as illustrated, noting any thickening, swelling, or tenderness.

Press on the lateral and medial epicondyles, noting any tenderness.

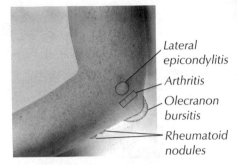

Lateral epicondylitis
Arthritis
Olecranon bursitis
Rheumatoid nodules

See Table 16-2, Swollen or Tender Elbows (p. 461).

SHOULDERS AND ENVIRONS

Test the range of motion by asking the patient to (1) raise both arms to a vertical position at the sides of the head, (2) place both hands behind the neck, with elbows out to the side (external rotation and abduction), and (3) place both hands behind the small of the back (internal rotation). By cupping your hand over the shoulder during these movements, note any crepitus.

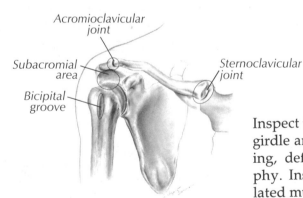

Acromioclavicular joint
Subacromial area
Bicipital groove
Sternoclavicular joint

Inspect the shoulders and shoulder girdle anteriorly, noting any swelling, deformity, or muscular atrophy. Inspect the scapulae and related muscles posteriorly.

If there is a history of shoulder pain, ask the patient to show you just where it is. Palpate for tenderness of (1) the sternoclavicular joint, (2) the acromioclavicular joint, (3) the subacromial area, and (4) the bicipital groove.

The most common cause of shoulder pain is rotator cuff tendinitis (the impingement syndrome). See Table 16-3, Painful Shoulders (pp. 462–463).

WITH THE PATIENT LYING DOWN

ANKLES AND FEET

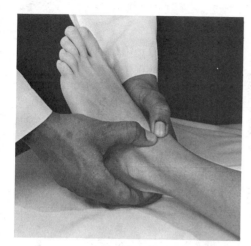

Inspect all surfaces of the ankles and feet, noting any deformities, nodules, or swellings, and any calluses or corns.

See Table 16-4, Abnormalities of the Feet and Toes (pp. 464–465).

With your thumbs palpate the anterior aspect of the ankle joint, noting any bogginess, swelling, or tenderness.

Localized tenderness in arthritis of the ankle

Feel along the Achilles tendon for nodules and tenderness.

Rheumatoid nodules; tenderness of Achilles tendinitis or bursitis

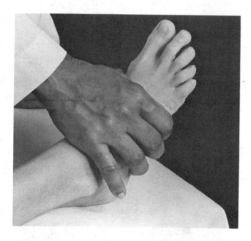

Test for tenderness of the metatarsophalangeal joints by compressing the forefoot between your thumb and fingers. Exert your pressure just proximal to the heads of the 1st and 5th metatarsals.

Tenderness on compression of the metatarsophalangeal joints is an early sign of rheumatoid arthritis. Acute inflammation of the first metatarsophalangeal joint suggests gout.

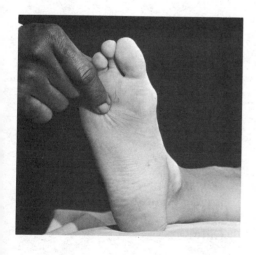

To evaluate the metatarsophalangeal joints individually, firmly palpate the heads of the five metatarsals and the grooves between them with your thumb and index finger. Place your thumb on the dorsum of the foot and your index finger on the plantar surface. Note any tenderness.

Pain and tenderness, called metatarsalgia, have many causes.

Check the range of motion in ankles and feet:

1. Dorsiflex and plantar flex the foot at the ankle (the tibiotalar joint).

2. Stabilize the ankle with one hand, grasp the heel with the other, and invert and evert the foot at the subtalar joint.

These four maneuvers help to identify which joints of an arthritic foot are involved.

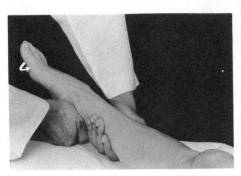

INVERSION

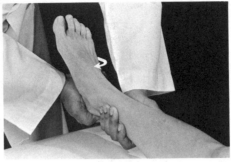

EVERSION

An arthritic joint is frequently painful when moved in any direction, while a ligamentous sprain produces maximal pain when the ligament is stretched. For example, in a common form of sprained ankle, inversion and plantar flexion of the foot cause pain while eversion and dorsiflexion are relatively pain-free.

3. Stabilize the heel and invert and evert the forefoot, thereby testing the transverse tarsal joint.

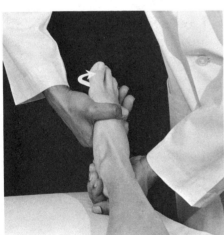

INVERSION

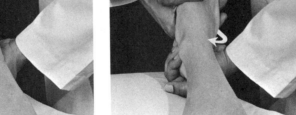

EVERSION

4. Flex the toes at the metatarsophalangeal joints.

KNEES AND HIPS

Inspect the *knees*, noting their alignment and any deformity. Note any atrophy of the quadriceps muscles. Look for loss of the normal hollows around the patella (an early sign of swelling in the knee joint and suprapatellar pouch), and note any other swelling in or around the knee.

Bowlegs (genu varum), knock knees (genu valgum), or flexion contracture (inability to extend fully)

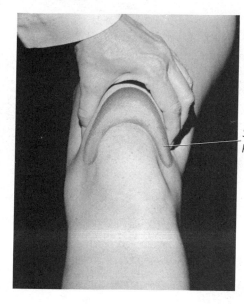

Suprapatellar
pouch

Swelling above and adjacent to the patella suggests synovial thickening or fluid in the knee joint.

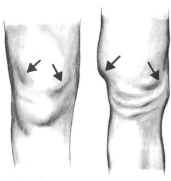

Moderate
swelling

Marked
swelling

Try to palpate any thickening or swelling in the suprapatellar pouch and along the sides of the patella. Starting about 10 cm above the superior border of the patella (well above the pouch), feel the soft tissues between your thumb and fingers. Move your hand distally in progressive steps, trying to identify the pouch. Continue your palpation along the sides of the patella. Note any tenderness or any warmth greater than that of surrounding tissues. The synovial membrane of the suprapatellar pouch and knee joint is not normally palpable.

Thickening, bogginess, tenderness, and warmth in these areas indicates synovial inflammation. Nontender effusions are common in osteoarthritis.

Bursitis causes a more localized swelling, as in prepatellar bursitis (housemaid's knee).

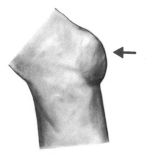

If you suspect a small amount of fluid in the knee joint:

LOOK FOR A BULGE SIGN

1. With the ball of your hand milk the medial aspect of the knee firmly upward two or three times to displace any fluid.

2. Then press or tap the knee just behind the lateral margin of the patella.

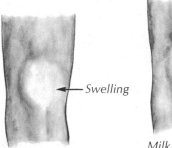

— Swelling

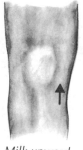

Milk upward

A bulge of returning fluid indicates an effusion within the

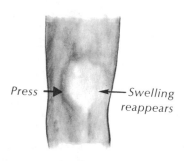

Press — — Swelling reappears

3. Watch for a bulge of returning fluid in the hollow medial to the patella. Normally none is seen.

knee joint. You can thus detect very small amounts of fluid, but a bulge sign may be absent when a large amount of fluid is present under pressure.

TRY TO BALLOTTE A "FLOATING PATELLA." Firmly grasp the thigh just above the patella with one hand, thus forcing fluid out of the suprapatellar pouch into the space between the patella and femur. With the fingers of your other hand, push the patella sharply back against the femur. Feel for a palpable tap. In the absence of fluid none is felt because the patella is already snug against the femur.

When the patella is separated from the femur by excessive joint fluid, the sharp backward thrust makes it collide against the femur with a palpable tap. Ballottement is a less sensitive test than the procedure to detect a bulge sign, but it is useful when larger amounts of fluid are present.

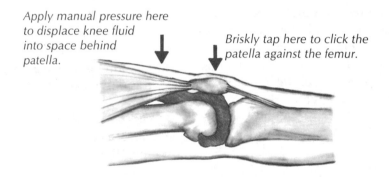

Apply manual pressure here to displace knee fluid into space behind patella.

Briskly tap here to click the patella against the femur.

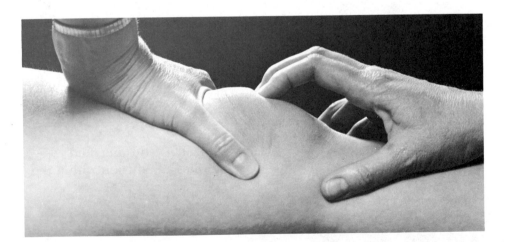

To examine the patellofemoral compartment of the knee joint, compress the patella and move it against the underlying femur. Then push the patella distally and ask the patient to tighten the knee against the table, thus contracting the quadriceps. Note any pain or crepitus with these maneuvers. Crepitus alone has little significance.

Pain and crepitus occur in osteoarthritis and in chondromalacia patellae, a similar condition that affects younger people.

Now flex the patient's knee to about 90° so that you can better palpate the tibiofemoral joint. The patient's foot should rest on the examining table. With your thumbs press into the joint and palpate along the tibial margins

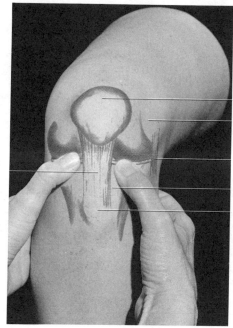

Patella
Lateral epicondyle
Lateral collateral ligament
Tibia
Tibial tuberosity
Patellar tendon

from the patellar tendon toward each side of the knee. Then palpate along the course of each collateral ligament. Identify any points of tenderness. Note any irregular bony ridges along the joint margins.

In an adolescent with knee pain, press on the tibial tuberosity and note any swelling or tenderness.

Palpation of the posterior aspects of the knees is best done when the patient stands (see p. 454).

Tenderness from damaged menisci or collateral ligaments. The fat pad, when injured, may also be tender.

Bony ridges along the joint margins may be felt in osteoarthritis.

A tender, swollen tibial tuberosity in an adolescent suggests Osgood–Schlatter disease.

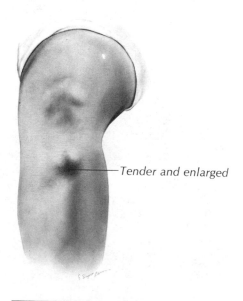

Tender and enlarged

RANGE OF MOTION AT KNEES AND HIPS. Ask the patient to bend each knee in turn up to the chest and pull it firmly against the abdomen.

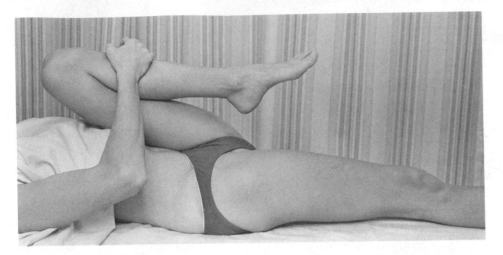

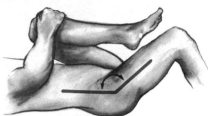

Flexion of the opposite thigh indicates a flexion deformity of that hip.

Observe the degree of flexion at the hip and knee. In addition, note whether the opposite thigh remains on the table and thus can fully extend.

To test rotation of the hip, flex the leg to 90° at hip and knee, stabilize the thigh with one hand, grasp the ankle with the other, and swing the lower leg—medially for external rotation at the hip, and laterally for internal rotation.

Restriction of internal rotation is an especially sensitive indicator of hip disease such as arthritis. External rotation is often restricted also.

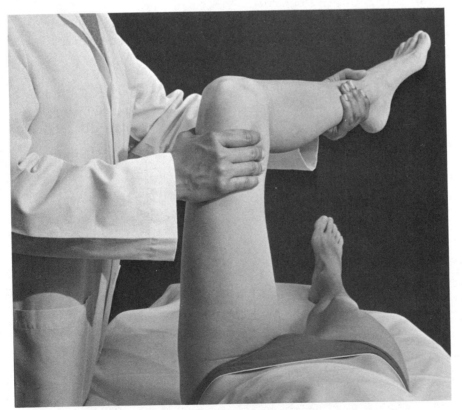

EXTERNAL ROTATION

Rotation may also be tested with the patient's legs extended. From the foot of the table grasp the ankle and rotate the leg internally and externally. Judge the range of movement by watching the patella. Rotation in this position is normally somewhat less than with the hip flexed to 90°.

To abduct the hip, stabilize the pelvis by pressing down on the opposite anterior superior iliac spine with one hand. With the other hand grasp the ankle and abduct the extended leg until you feel the iliac spine move. This movement marks the limit of hip abduction.

Restricted abduction is common in hip disease.

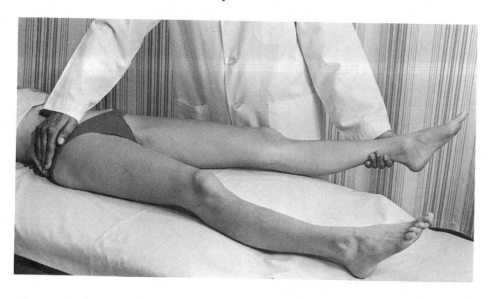

Alternatively, stand at the foot of the table, grasp both ankles, and abduct both extended legs at the hips.

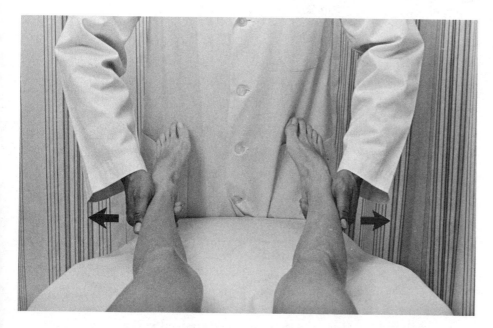

This method allows easy comparison of the two sides when movements are restricted.

WITH THE PATIENT STANDING

THE SPINE

The gown should allow adequate visualization of the patient's spine.

From the side inspect the spinal profile, noting the cervical, thoracic, and lumbar curves.

See Table 16-5, Abnormal Spinal Curvatures (pp. 466–467).

From behind the patient inspect the spine for lateral curves. Look for any differences in the heights of the shoulders, the iliac crests, and the skin creases below the buttocks. Note whether an imaginary line dropped from the spinous process of T1 falls, as it should, through the gluteal cleft.

Unequal heights of the iliac crests (a pelvic tilt) suggest unequal lengths of the legs. Such a tilt is abolished by placing supports under one foot. Scoliosis and adduction or abduction deformities of the hip may also cause a tilt.

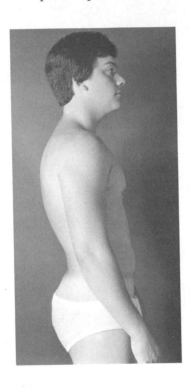
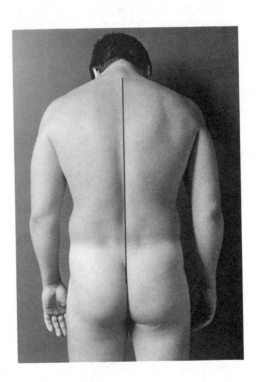

Note any deformities of the knees, any swellings in the popliteal spaces, or other deformities such as flat feet.

Bowlegs, knock-knees, popliteal swelling of a Baker's cyst (usually a swollen bursa)

Check the range of motion in the spine:

Ask the patient to bend forward to touch the toes (flexion). Note the smoothness and symmetry of movement, the range of motion, and the curve in the lumbar area. As flexion proceeds, the lumbar concavity should flatten out.

Paravertebral muscle spasm and ankylosing spondylitis may prevent flattening; the lumbar concavity persists.

Sit down, stabilize the patient's pelvis with your hands, and ask the patient to (1) bend sideways (lateral bending), (2) bend backwards toward you

Decreased spinal mobility in osteoarthritis and ankylosing

(extension), and (3) twist the shoulders one way and then the other (rotation).

From a sitting or standing position, palpate the spinous processes with your thumb. In the lower lumbar area determine whether one spinous process seems unusually prominent in relation to the one above it. Identify any tenderness.

You may also wish to percuss the spine for tenderness by thumping it (not too roughly) with the ulnar surface of your fist.

Inspect and palpate the paravertebral muscles for tenderness and spasm. Palpate for tenderness in any other areas that are suggested by the patient's symptoms. Try to identify the underlying structures involved. A skin dimple usually overlies the posterior iliac spine and guides you toward the sacroiliac area.

spondylitis, among other conditions

A spinous process of L5 or possibly L4 that feels unusually prominent in relation to the one above it suggests spondylolisthesis of the prominent vertebra.

Percussion may produce pain when osteoporosis, malignancy, or infection involves the spine.

A paravertebral muscle in spasm looks prominent, feels tight, and is usually tender.

Remember that tenderness in the costovertebral angles may signify kidney infection rather than a musculoskeletal problem.

Herniated intervertebral discs, most common between L5 and S1 or between L4 and L5, may produce tenderness of the spinous processes, the intervertebral joints, the paravertebral muscles, the sacrosciatic notch, and the sciatic nerve.

Rheumatoid arthritis may also cause tenderness of the intervertebral joints. Ankylosing spondylitis may produce sacroiliac tenderness.

See Table 2-17, Low Back Pain (p. 90).

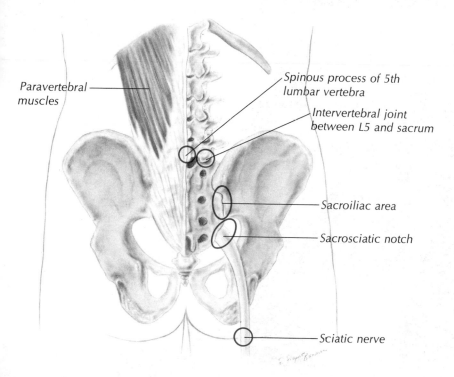

Paravertebral muscles

Spinous process of 5th lumbar vertebra

Intervertebral joint between L5 and sacrum

Sacroiliac area

Sacrosciatic notch

Sciatic nerve

See pages 456–457 for further testing of low back pain with leg radiation.

SPECIAL MANEUVERS

FOR THE CARPAL TUNNEL SYNDROME. Pain and numbness in the hand, especially at night, suggest compression of the median nerve in the carpal tunnel. This tunnel is a narrow channel in the palm of the hand, between the carpal bones dorsally and a band of more superficial fascia ventrally.

Through the tunnel run the flexor tendons and the median nerve. Two clinical tests are used:

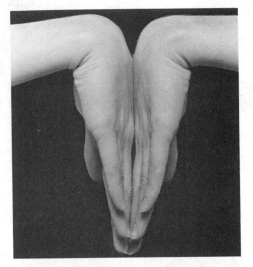

Phalen's Test. Hold the patient's wrists in acute flexion for 60 seconds. Alternatively, ask the patient to press the back of both hands together to form right angles.

If numbness and tingling develop over the distribution of the median nerve (*e.g.*, the palmar surface of the thumb, and the index, middle, and part of the ring fingers) the sign is positive, suggesting the carpal tunnel syndrome.

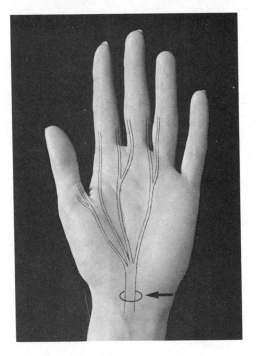

Tinel's Sign. With your finger percuss lightly over the course of the median nerve in the carpal tunnel at the spot indicated by the arrow.

Tingling or electric sensations in the distribution of the median nerve constitute a positive test, suggesting the carpal tunnel syndrome.

FOR LOW BACK PAIN WITH RADIATION INTO THE LEG. If the patient has noted low back pain that radiates down the leg, check straight leg raising on each side in turn. Raise the patient's relaxed and straightened leg until pain occurs. Then dorsiflex the foot.

Record the degree of elevation at which pain occurs, the quality and distribution of the pain, and the effects of dorsiflexion. Tightness and mild discomfort in the hamstrings with these maneuvers are common and do not indicate radicular pain.

Sharp pain radiating from the back down the leg in an L5 or S1 distribution (radicular pain) suggests tension or compression of the nerve root(s), often caused by a herniated lumbar disc. Dorsiflexion of the foot increases the pain. Increased pain in the affected leg when

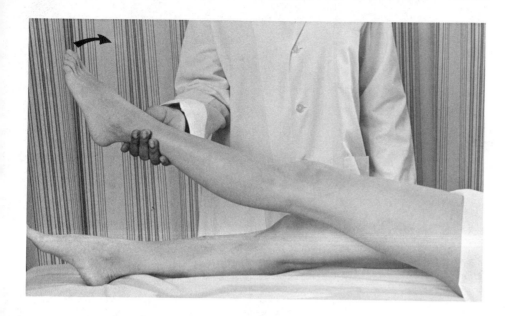

the opposite leg is raised strongly confirms radicular pain and constitutes a positive *crossed straight leg-raising sign.*

MEASURING THE LENGTH OF LEGS. If you suspect that the patient's legs are unequal in length, measure them. Get the patient relaxed in the supine position and symmetrically aligned with legs extended. With a tape, measure the distance between anterior superior iliac spine and the medial malleolus. The tape should cross the knee on its medial side.

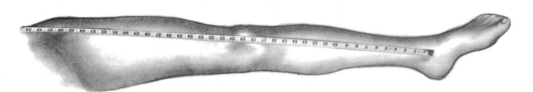

DESCRIBING LIMITED MOTION OF A JOINT. Although precise measurement of motion is not routinely necessary, limitations can be described in degrees. Pocket goniometers are available for this purpose. In the two examples shown below, the red lines indicate the range of the patient's movement and the black lines show the normal range.

Your observations may be described in several ways. The numbers in parentheses are suitably abbreviated recordings.

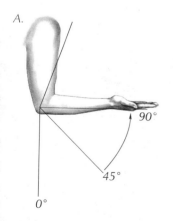

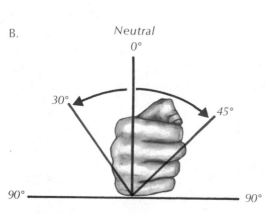

A. The elbow flexes from 45° to 90° (45° → 90°),

-or-

The elbow has a flexion deformity of 45° and flexes farther to 90° (45° → 90°).

B. Supination at elbow = 30° (0° → 30°)
Pronation at elbow = 45° (0° → 45°)

Table 16-1

Table 16-1   Swellings and Deformities of the Hands

OSTEOARTHRITIS (Degenerative Joint Disease)

Nodules on the dorsolateral aspects of the distal interphalangeal joints, called Heberden's nodes, are due to the bony overgrowth of osteoarthritis. Usually hard and painless, they affect the middle-aged or elderly and often, although not always, are associated with arthritic changes in other joints. Flexion and deviation deformities may develop. Similar nodules on the proximal interphalangeal joints, called Bouchard's nodes, are less common. The metacarpophalangeal joints are spared.

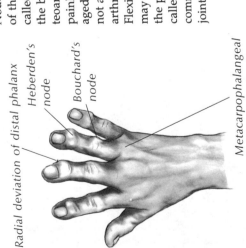

Radial deviation of distal phalanx

Heberden's node

Bouchard's node

Metacarpophalangeal joints uninvolved

ACUTE RHEUMATOID ARTHRITIS

Tender, painful, stiff joints characterize rheumatoid arthritis. Symmetrical involvement on both sides of the body is typical. The proximal interphalangeal, metacarpophalangeal, and wrist joints are frequently affected; the distal interphalangeal joints are rarely so. Patients with acute disease often have fusiform or spindle-shaped swelling of the proximal interphalangeal joints.

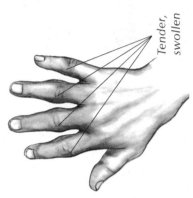

Tender, swollen

CHRONIC RHEUMATOID ARTHRITIS

As the arthritic process continues and worsens, chronic swelling and thickening of the metacarpophalangeal and proximal interphalangeal joints appear. Range of motion becomes limited and the fingers may deviate toward the ulnar side. The interosseous muscles atrophy. The fingers may show "swan neck" deformities (*i.e.*, hyperextension of the proximal interphalangeal joints with fixed flexion of the distal interphalangeal joints). Less common is a boutonniere deformity (*i.e.*, persistent flexion of the proximal interphalangeal joint with hyperextension of the distal interphalangeal joint).

Rheumatoid nodules may accompany either the acute or the chronic stage.

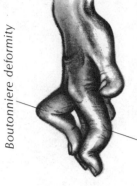

Boutonniere deformity

Swan neck deformity

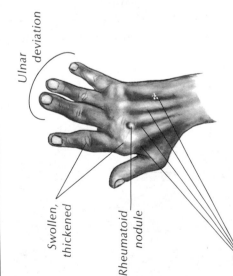

Ulnar deviation

Swollen, thickened

Rheumatoid nodule

Muscular atrophy

Table 16-1

CHRONIC TOPHACEOUS GOUT

The deformities that develop in longstanding chronic tophaceous gout can sometimes mimic those of rheumatoid and osteoarthritis. Joint involvement is usually not so symmetrical as in rheumatoid arthritis. Acute inflammation may be present. Knobby swellings around the joints sometimes ulcerate and discharge white chalklike urates.

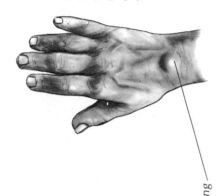

Swollen

Knobby swelling

Draining tophus

GANGLION

Ganglia are cystic, round, usually nontender swellings located along tendon sheaths or joint capsules. The dorsum of the hand and wrist is a frequent site of involvement. Flexion of the wrist makes ganglia more prominent; extension tends to obscure them. Ganglia may also develop elsewhere on the hands, wrists, ankles, and feet.

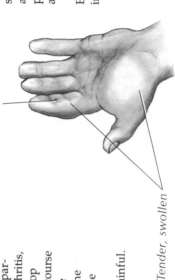

Cystic swelling

TENDON SHEATH AND PALMAR SPACE INFECTIONS

ACUTE TENOSYNOVITIS

Infection of the flexor tendon sheaths (acute tenosynovitis) may follow local injury, even of apparently trivial nature. Unlike arthritis, tenderness and swelling develop not in the joint but along the course of the tendon sheath, from the distal phalanx to the level of the metacarpophalangeal joint. The finger is held in slight flexion; attempts to extend it are very painful.

ACUTE TENOSYNOVITIS AND THENAR SPACE INVOLVEMENT

If the infection progresses, it may escape the bounds of the tendon sheath to involve one of the adjacent fascial spaces within the palm. Infections of the index finger and thenar space are illustrated.

Early diagnosis and treatment are important.

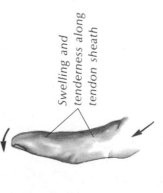

Puncture wound

Tender, swollen

Pain on extension

Swelling and tenderness along tendon sheath

Finger held in slight flexion

Continued

Table 16-1

Table 16-1 (Cont'd.)

FELON

Injury to the fingertip may result in infection in the enclosed fascial spaces of the finger pad. Severe pain, localized tenderness, swelling, and dusky redness are characteristic. Early diagnosis and treatment are important.

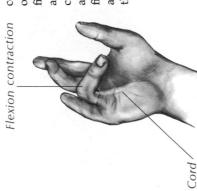

Puncture wound

Swollen, tender, dusky red

DUPUYTREN'S CONTRACTURE

The first sign of a Dupuytren's contracture is a thickened plaque overlying the tendon of the ring finger and possibly the little finger at the level of the distal palmar crease. Subsequently the skin in this area puckers, and a thickened fibrotic cord develops between palm and finger. Flexion contracture of the fingers may gradually ensue.

Flexion contraction

Cord

THENAR ATROPHY

Muscular atrophy localized to the thenar eminence suggests a disorder of the median nerve or its components. Pressure on the nerve at the wrist is a common cause (the carpal tunnel syndrome). Hypothenar atrophy suggests an ulnar nerve disorder.

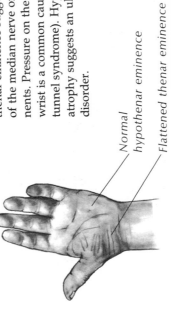

Normal hypothenar eminence

Flattened thenar eminence

Table 16-2

Table 16-2 Swollen or Tender Elbows

OLECRANON BURSITIS

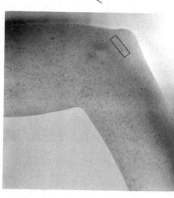

Olecranon bursitis

Swelling and inflammation of the olecranon bursa may result from trauma or may be associated with rheumatoid or gouty arthritis. The swelling is superficial to the olecranon process.

ARTHRITIS OF THE ELBOW

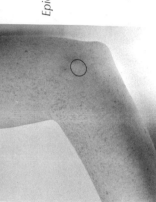

Arthritis

Synovial inflammation or fluid is best felt in the grooves between the olecranon process and the epicondyles on either side. Palpate for a boggy, soft, or fluctuant swelling and for tenderness.

RHEUMATOID NODULES

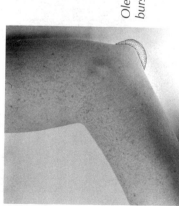

Rheumatoid nodules

Subcutaneous nodules may develop at pressure points along the extensor surface of the ulna in patients with rheumatoid arthritis. They are firm and nontender, and are not attached to the overlying skin. They may or may not be attached to the underlying periosteum. Although they may develop in the area of the olecranon bursa, they often occur more distally.

EPICONDYLITIS

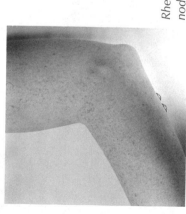

Epicondylitis

Lateral epicondylitis (tennis elbow) follows repetitive extension of the wrist or pronation–supination of the forearm. Pain and tenderness develop at the lateral epicondyle and possibly in the extensor muscles close to it. When the patient tries to extend the wrist against resistance, pain increases.

Medial epicondylitis (pitcher's or Little League elbow) follows repetitive wrist flexion, as in throwing. Tenderness is maximal at the medial epicondyle. Wrist flexion against resistance increases the pain.

Table 16-3

Table 16-3 Painful Shoulders

ROTATOR CUFF TENDINITIS
(Impingement Syndrome)

When the arm is raised, the rotator cuff may impinge against the under surface of the acromion and the coracoacromial ligament. Repeated impingement of this kind, as in throwing or swimming, can cause edema and hemorrhage followed by inflammation and fibrosis, most often involving the supraspinatus tendon. Acute, recurrent, or chronic pain may result, often aggravated by activity. Sharp catches of pain may occur as the arm is elevated into an overhead position. When the supraspinatus tendon is involved, tenderness is maximal just below the tip of the acromion. The patients tend to be young (teens to 40 years) and are often, though not necessarily, athletically active.

ROTATOR CUFF TEARS

Shoulder-shrugging effort

Limited abduction

Normal abduction

Repeated impingement (or other conditions) may weaken the rotator cuff and eventually cause partial or complete tears in it, usually after the age of 40 years. Injury, such as falling, may precipitate a tear. Manifestations include weakness, atrophy of the supraspinatus and infraspinatus muscles, pain, and tenderness. In a complete tear of the supraspinatus tendon (illustrated), active abduction at the glenohumeral joint is severely impaired. Efforts to abduct the arm produce a characteristic shoulder-shrugging instead.

CALCIFIC TENDINITIS

Calcific tendinitis refers to a degenerative process in the tendon that is associated with the deposition of calcium salts. Like rotator cuff tendinitis it usually involves the supraspinatus tendon. Acute, disabling attacks of shoulder pain may occur, usually in patients over 30 years of age and more often in women. The arm is held close to the side, and all motions are severely limited by pain. Tenderness is maximal below the tip of the acromion. The subacromial bursa, which overlies the supraspinatus tendon, may become involved in the inflammation. Chronic, less severe pain may also occur.

Table 16-3

BICIPITAL TENDINITIS	ACROMIOCLAVICULAR ARTHRITIS	ADHESIVE CAPSULITIS *(Frozen Shoulder)*
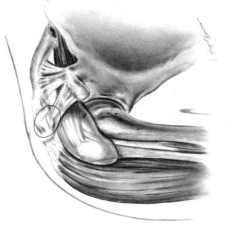		

Inflammation of the long head of the biceps tendon and its sheath causes anterior shoulder pain that may resemble rotator cuff tendinitis and may coexist with it. This tendon, like the cuff, may suffer impingement injury. Tenderness is maximal in the bicipital groove. By externally rotating and abducting the arm you can more easily separate this area from the subacromial tenderness of supraspinatus tendinitis. With the patient's arm at the side, elbow flexed to 90°, ask the patient to supinate the forearm against your resistance. Increased pain in the bicipital groove confirms this condition.

Acromioclavicular arthritis is not a common cause of shoulder pain. When present it is usually the result of direct injury to the shoulder girdle with resulting degenerative changes. Tenderness is localized over the acromioclavicular joint. Although motion in the glenohumeral joint is not painful, as it is in many other painful conditions of the shoulder, movements of the scapula, such as shoulder-shrugging, are.

Adhesive capsulitis refers to a mysterious fibrosis of the glenohumeral joint capsule, manifested by diffuse, dull, aching pain in the shoulder and progressive restriction of motion, but usually no localized tenderness. The condition is usually unilateral and occurs in persons aged 50 to 70. There is often an antecedent painful disorder of the shoulder or possibly another condition (such as myocardial infarction) that has decreased shoulder movements. The course is chronic, lasting months to years, but the disorder often resolves spontaneously, at least partially.

Table 16-4

Table 16-4   Abnormalities of the Feet and Toes

ACUTE GOUTY ARTHRITIS	HALLUX VALGUS	FLAT FEET

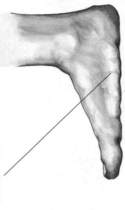

Medial border becomes convex

Sole touches floor

Signs of flat feet may be apparent only when the patient stands, or they may become permanent. The longitudinal arch flattens so that the sole approaches or touches the floor. The normal concavity on the medial side of the foot becomes convex. Tenderness may be present from the internal malleolus down along the medial-plantar surface of the foot. Swelling may develop anterior to the malleoli. Inspect the shoes for excess wear on the inner side of the soles and heels.

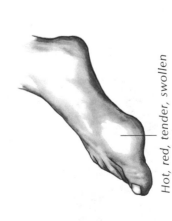

In hallux valgus the great toe is abnormally abducted in relationship to the first metatarsal, which itself is deviated medially. The head of the first metatarsal may enlarge on its medial side and a bursa may form at the pressure point. This bursa may become inflamed.

Hot, red, tender, swollen

The metatarsophalangeal joint of the great toe is often the first joint involved in acute gouty arthritis. It is characterized by a very painful and tender, hot, dusky red swelling that extends beyond the margin of the joint. It is easily mistaken for a cellulitis.

Table 16-4

INGROWN TOENAIL	HAMMER TOE	CORN
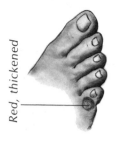 *Red, tender* *Granulation tissue*	*Hyperextended* *Flexed*	*Red, thickened*
The sharp edge of the great toenail may dig into and injure the skin fold, resulting in inflammation and infection. A tender, reddened, overhanging nail fold, sometimes with granulation tissue and purulent discharge, results.	Most commonly involving the second toe, a hammer toe is characterized by hyperextension at the metatarsophalangeal joint with flexion at the proximal interphalangeal joint. A corn frequently develops at the pressure point over the proximal interphalangeal joint.	A corn is a painful conical thickening of skin that results from recurrent pressure on normally thin skin. The apex of the cone points inward and causes pain. Corns characteristically occur over bony prominences (*e.g.,* the 5th toe). When located in moist areas (*e.g.,* at pressure points between the 4th and 5th toes), they are called soft corns.

CALLUS	PLANTAR WART	NEUROTROPHIC ULCER
	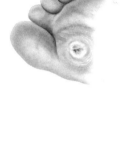	
Like a corn, a callus is an area of greatly thickened skin that develops in a region of recurrent pressure. Unlike a corn, however, a callus involves skin that is normally thick, such as the sole, and is usually painless. If a callus is painful, suspect an underlying plantar wart.	A plantar wart is a common wart (verruca vulgaris) located in the thickened skin of the sole. It may look somewhat like a callus or even be covered by one. Look for the characteristic small dark spots that give a stippled appearance to a wart. Normal skin lines stop at the wart's edge.	When pain sensation is diminished or absent (as in diabetic neuropathy, for example), neurotrophic ulcers may develop at pressure points on the feet. Although often deep, infected, and indolent, they are painless. Callus formation about the ulcer is diagnostically helpful. Like the ulcer itself, it results from chronic pressure.

Table 16-5

Table 16-5 Abnormal Spinal Curvatures

NORMAL SPINAL CURVATURES 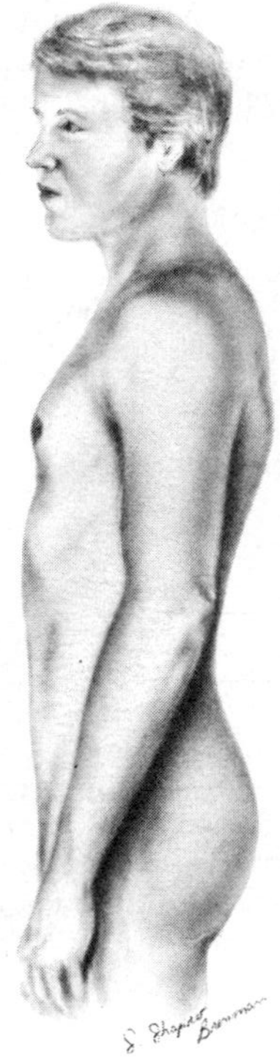	FLATTENING OF THE LUMBAR CURVE 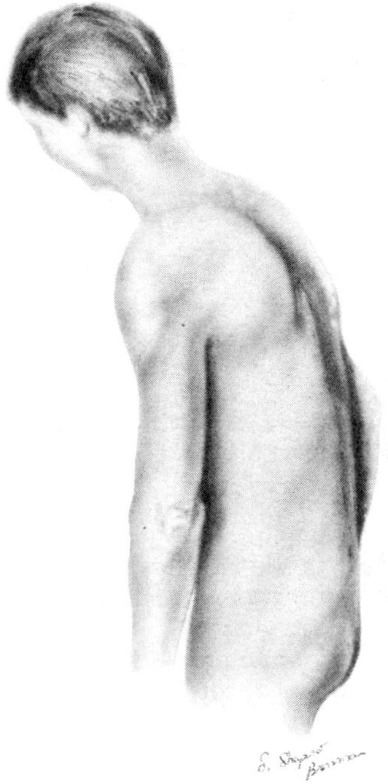	LUMBAR LORDOSIS 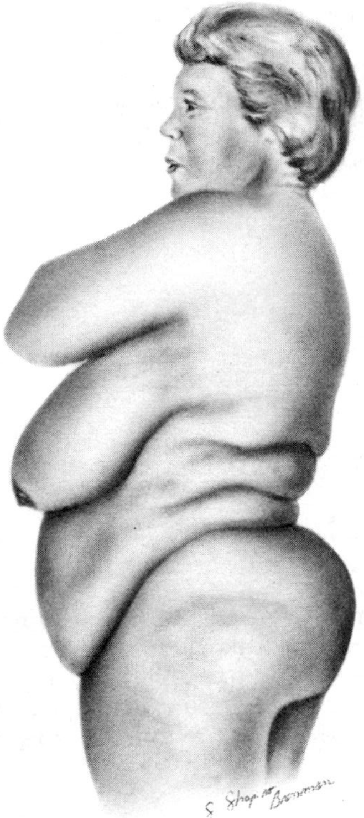	KYPHOSIS 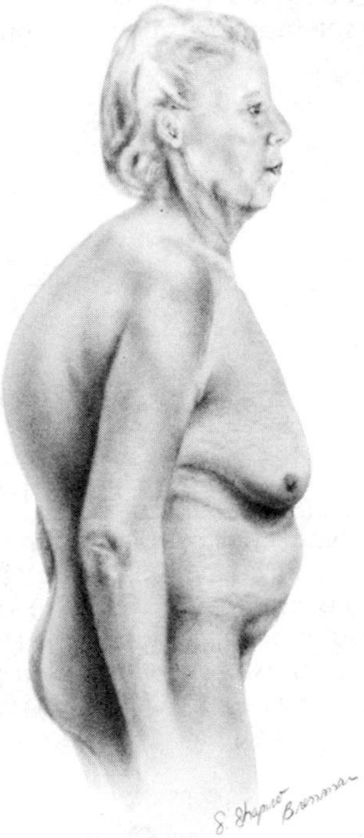

Note the gentle curves of the normal spine—concavities in the cervical and lumbar regions and a convexity in the thorax.

When you see flattening of the lumbar curve, look for muscle spasm in the lumbar area and for decreased spinal mobility. This combination of signs suggests the possibility of a herniated lumbar disc or, especially in men, ankylosing spondylitis.

Lordosis—an accentuation of the normal lumbar curve—develops to compensate for the protuberant abdomen of pregnancy or marked obesity (as illustrated here). It may also compensate for kyphosis and flexion deformities of the hips. A deep midline furrow may be seen between the lumbar paravertebral muscles.

Kyphosis—a rounded thoracic convexity—is common in aging, especially in women. In adolescent patients consider Scheuermann's disease.

Table 16-5

GIBBUS	LIST	SCOLIOSIS

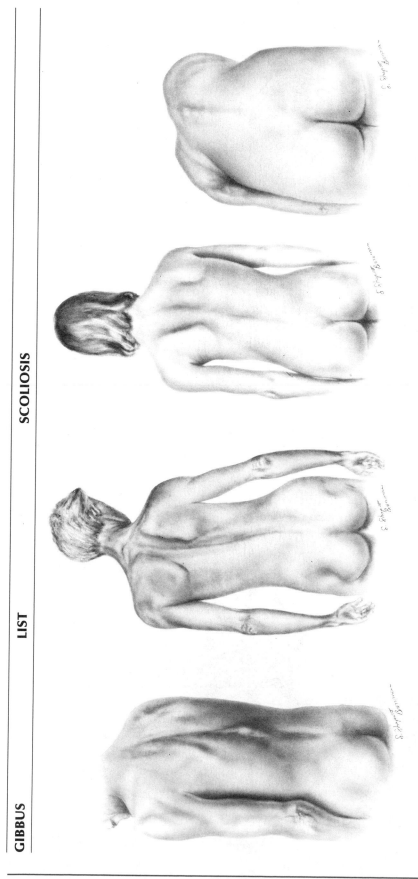

Gibbus is an angular deformity of a collapsed vertebra. Causes include metastatic cancer and tuberculosis of the spine.

List is a lateral tilt of the spine. When a plumb line dropped from the spinous process of T1 falls to one side of the gluteal cleft, a list is present. Causes include a herniated disc and painful spasms of the paravertebral muscles. Scoliosis (a lateral curve of the spine) is inherent in a list but has not been fully compensated for by a spinal deviation in the opposite direction.

Scoliosis—a lateral curvature of the spine—is shown here with a thoracic convexity to the right. Scoliosis may be structural, as illustrated, or functional, when it compensates for other abnormalities such as unequal leg lengths. Structural scoliosis is typically associated with rotation of the vertebrae upon each other, and the rib cage is accordingly deformed. When the patient bends forward, structural scoliosis is accentuated, the chest wall on the side of the thoracic convexity is prominent, and the scapula is elevated. Functional scoliosis does not involve vertebral rotation and disappears with forward flexion.

Chapter 17
The Nervous System

Anatomy and Physiology

This section deals briefly with some of the anatomy and physiology that relate directly to the neurologic examination. After a short description of the brain, it discusses the spinal cord and the simplest level of nervous response—the reflex arc. It then summarizes the motor pathways that initiate voluntary action, coordinate movements, and maintain posture and balance. Sensory pathways are considered next, and then the cranial nerves with both their motor and their sensory functions. The section concludes with variations in neurologic findings that are associated with age.

THE BRAIN

The brain has three regions: the brain stem, the cerebrum, and the cerebellum.

The brain stem is continuous with the spinal cord. It is traditionally divided into four sections: the diencephalon, the midbrain, the pons, and the medulla.

The paired cranial nerves 2 through 12 emerge from the brain stem. Their involvement by pathologic processes sometimes helps to localize neurologic lesions. The relationships of the cranial nerves to the four parts of the brain stem are summarized in the diagram on the right. The functions of the cranial nerves are summarized on pages 477–478.

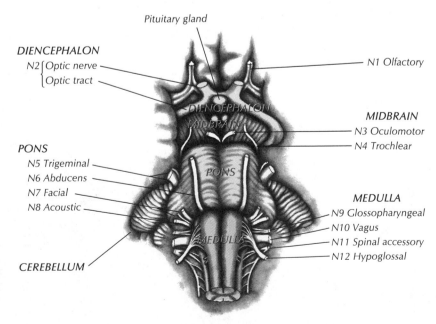

Pituitary gland

DIENCEPHALON
N2 { Optic nerve
Optic tract

N1 Olfactory

MIDBRAIN
N3 Oculomotor
N4 Trochlear

PONS
N5 Trigeminal
N6 Abducens
N7 Facial
N8 Acoustic

MEDULLA
N9 Glossopharyngeal
N10 Vagus
N11 Spinal accessory
N12 Hypoglossal

CEREBELLUM

The cerebral hemispheres comprise the greatest mass of brain tissue. Their outer layers are formed by the cellular gray matter known as the cerebral cortex.

Consciousness depends upon interaction between intact cerebral hemispheres and the upper brain stem, where arousal or activating mechanisms reside. Either extensive disease of the cerebral cortex or lesions of the brain stem may impair consciousness to the point of coma.

The cerebellum is primarily concerned with coordination.

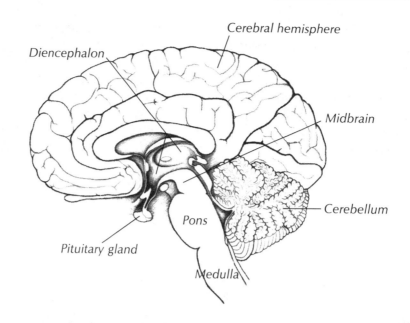

THE SPINAL CORD AND REFLEX ARC

The spinal cord is a cylindrical mass of nervous tissue that is encased within the bony vertebral column. It contains long tracts that connect the brain with the peripheral nervous system, and it also mediates reflex activity.

A reflex is an involuntary bodily response involving three basic components: a receiving apparatus, a nerve center, and a responding apparatus. Deep tendon (muscle stretch) reflexes in the arms and legs illustrate this fundamental organization.

To elicit a deep tendon reflex one briskly taps the tendon of a partially stretched muscle. By stretching the muscle farther, such a tap stimulates special sensory endings in the muscle and generates an impulse that travels up each of many *sensory* nerve fibers* to the spinal cord. Each sensory fiber travels with other sensory and motor nerve fibers in a *peripheral nerve.*

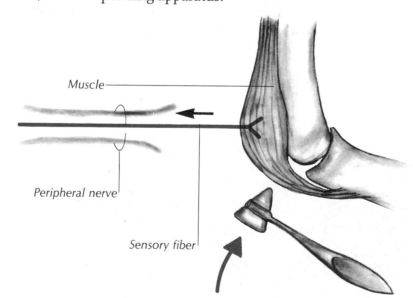

* The word "sensory," as used here, does not necessarily imply conscious sensation, although many authors prefer to use the term in this restricted sense. It would be more precise to use the term "afferent," indicating the direction in which the nerve impulse travels (*i.e.,* toward the spinal cord or brain). The term "efferent" (away from the cord or brain) would then be used instead of "motor."

A peripheral nerve may carry nerve fibers supplying a fairly large area of the body. As the nerve fibers approach the cord, they are reorganized on a segmental basis into 31 pairs of *spinal nerves* (8 cervical, 12 thoracic, 5 lumbar, 5 sacral, and 1 coccygeal). Within the vertebral canal, each spinal nerve separates into posterior (dorsal) and anterior (ventral) roots. The *posterior root* contains the sensory fibers. The sensory nerve impulse for the deep tendon reflex is carried on through the sensory fiber into the spinal cord where it synapses with a *motor neuron,* or *anterior horn cell.*

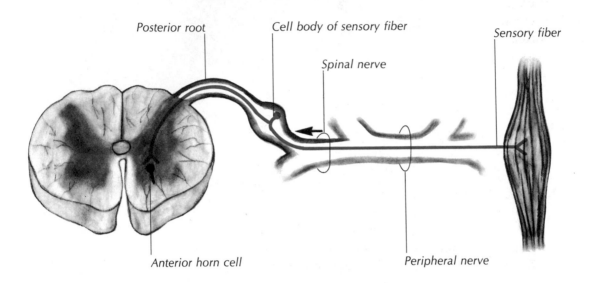

Posterior root — Cell body of sensory fiber — Sensory fiber — Spinal nerve — Anterior horn cell — Peripheral nerve

After stimulation across the synapse, an impulse is then transmitted down the motor neuron, traversing in turn the motor *anterior nerve root,* the spinal nerve, and the peripheral nerve. By transmitting an impulse across the neuromuscular junction, it then stimulates the muscle to a brisk contraction, completing the reflex arc.

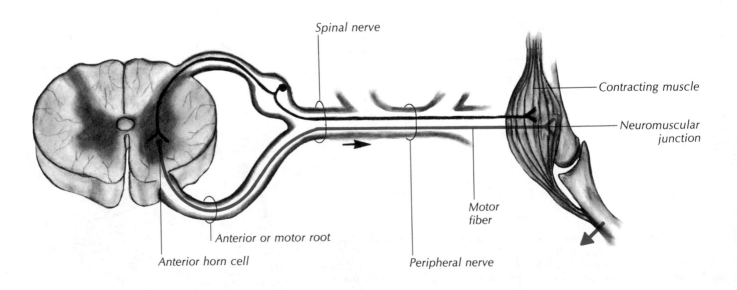

Spinal nerve — Contracting muscle — Neuromuscular junction — Motor fiber — Anterior or motor root — Anterior horn cell — Peripheral nerve

A deep tendon reflex is thus dependent on (1) intact sensory (afferent) nerve fibers, (2) functional synapses in the spinal cord, (3) intact motor (efferent) nerve fibers, (4) functional neuromuscular junctions, and (5) competent muscle fibers.

A single deep tendon reflex characteristically involves only a few spinal segments together with their sensory and motor fibers. An abnormality in such a reflex, therefore, helps to localize a pathologic lesion. You should know the segmental levels of the following deep tendon reflexes:

Biceps reflex	Cervical 5,6
Supinator (brachioradialis) reflex	Cervical 5,6
Triceps reflex	Cervical 6,7,8
Knee reflex	Lumbar 2,3,4
Ankle reflex	Lumbar 5, Sacral 1,2

Reflexes may be initiated by stimulating skin as well as muscle. Stroking the skin of the abdomen, for example, produces a localized muscular twitch. These superficial (cutaneous) reflexes (and the spinal segments from which they come) include:

Abdominal reflexes—upper	Thoracic 8,9,10
—lower	Thoracic 10,11,12
Plantar responses	Lumbar 4,5, Sacral 1,2

MOTOR PATHWAYS

Higher motor pathways of three kinds impinge on the anterior horn cells: (1) the corticospinal (pyramidal) tract, (2) the extrapyramidal system, and (3) the cerebellar system.

1. *The corticospinal (pyramidal) tract.** Voluntary movements originate in the motor cortex of the brain. Fibers from nerve cells there travel down through the corticospinal tract to the brain stem. Here most of them cross over to the opposite side and then continue down the spinal cord, where they synapse with anterior horn cells or with intermediate neurons. The corticospinal tracts not only mediate voluntary movement but also integrate skilled, complicated, or delicate movements by grading the motor responses and by stimulating selected muscular actions while inhibiting others. They also carry impulses

---

* Strictly speaking the corticospinal tract, the pyramidal tract, and upper motor neurons are not synonymous, but clinically the terms are often used interchangeably.

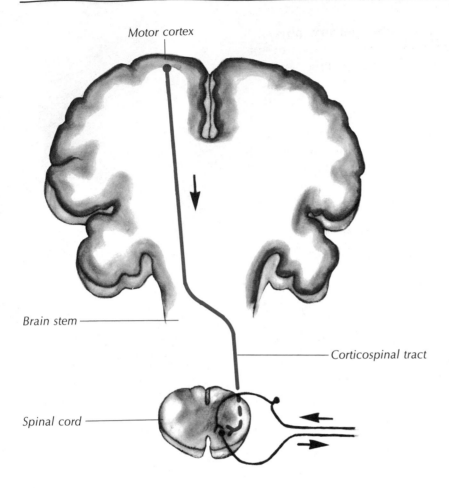

Motor cortex

Brain stem

Corticospinal tract

Spinal cord

that inhibit muscle tone, the slight tension maintained by a normal muscle even when it is relaxed. Fibers similar to corticospinal fibers connect with motor nerve cells in the cranial nerves and are then termed corticobulbar. Both corticospinal and corticobulbar neurons are often called "upper motor neurons."

2. *The extrapyramidal system.* This exceedingly complex system includes motor pathways between the cerebral cortex, basal ganglia, brain stem, and spinal cord but is outside the corticospinal (pyramidal) tract system. It helps to maintain muscle tone and to control body movements, especially gross automatic movements such as walking.

3. *The cerebellar system.* The cerebellum receives both sensory and motor input and coordinates muscular activity, maintains equilibrium, and helps to control posture.

All three of these higher motor pathways affect motor activity only through the lower motor neurons—sometimes called the "final common pathway." Any movement, whether initiated voluntarily in the cortex, "automatically" in the basal ganglia, or reflexly in the sensory receptors, must ultimately be translated into action via the anterior horn cells, the lower motor neurons. A lesion in any of these areas will produce effects on movement or reflex activity.

The type and distribution of motor deficit produced help the examiner to determine where the causative lesion might be. A cerebellar lesion produces incoordination, for example, while disease of the basal ganglia increases muscle tone and diminishes the automatic movements associated with walking. Neither causes paralysis. In contrast, lesions of both upper and lower motor neurons cause weakness or paralysis.

Upper and lower motor neuron lesions may be distinguished by their different effects on muscle size, muscle tone, reflex activity, and involuntary movements. When lower motor neurons are interrupted, the affected muscles lose both bulk and tone, reflexes disappear, and spontaneous fine movements known as fasciculations may develop. In contrast, when upper motor neurons are interrupted, muscle bulk is not affected except possibly through disuse. Both muscle tone and deep tendon reflexes increase because the normal inhibitory action on them is lost, and no fasciculations develop. Abdominal reflexes disappear in both kinds of lesions, but the plantar responses differ. They disappear in lower motor neuron lesions, but in upper motor neuron disease they change from flexor to extensor responses (see Table 17-5, p. 521).

SENSORY PATHWAYS

Sensory impulses not only participate in reflex activity, as previously described, but also give rise to conscious sensation.

Sensation is initiated by stimulation of sensory receptors located in skin, mucous membranes, muscles, tendons, and viscera. An impulse generated by one of these receptors travels along a sensory nerve fiber toward the spinal cord. In its course it usually travels with other sensory and motor nerve fibers in a peripheral nerve. The peripheral nerve is reorganized centrally on a segmental basis, divides into posterior and anterior roots, and enters the spinal cord. The sensory nerve fiber follows the posterior (or dorsal) root. After entry into the spinal cord, the sensory impulse proceeds along one of two courses: (1) the spinothalamic tracts, or (2) the posterior columns.

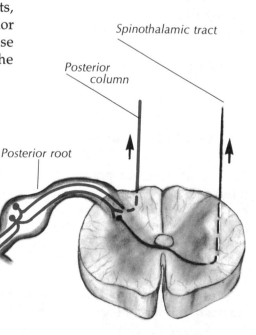

Spinothalamic tract

Posterior column

Posterior root

Sensory receptors

Spinal nerve

Peripheral nerve

Within one or two spinal segments from their entry into the cord, fibers conducting the sensations of *pain* and *temperature* pass into the posterior horn of the spinal cord and synapse with secondary sensory neurons. These secondary neurons then cross to the opposite side just anterior to the central canal and pass upward in the lateral spinothalamic tract of the cord.

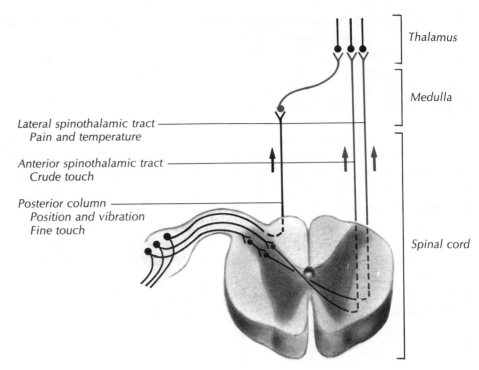

Lateral spinothalamic tract —
Pain and temperature

Anterior spinothalamic tract —
Crude touch

Posterior column —
Position and vibration
Fine touch

Thalamus

Medulla

Spinal cord

Fibers conducting the sensations of *position* and *vibration* pass directly into the *posterior columns* of the cord and travel upward to the medulla, where they then synapse with secondary sensory neurons. These secondary neurons also cross over to the other side, where they and the spinothalamic tracts continue on to the thalamus.

Nerve fibers carrying the sensation of *light touch* take one of two pathways. Some fibers conduct *fine touch* — touch that is accurately localized and finely discriminating. These fibers travel in the posterior column together with fibers that carry position and vibration sense. A second group transmits *crude touch* — a sensation perceived as light touch but without accurate localization. These fibers synapse in the posterior horn with secondary neurons that cross to the opposite side and ascend in the anterior spinothalamic tract to the thalamus. Because touch impulses originating on one side of the body travel up both sides of the cord, touch sensation is often preserved despite partial damage to the cord.

At the thalamic level, the general quality of sensation is perceived (*e.g.*, pain, cold, pleasant and unpleasant), but fine distinctions are not made. For full perception, a third group of sensory neurons carries impulses from synapses in the thalamus to the sensory cortex of the brain. Here stimuli are localized and discriminations made between them.

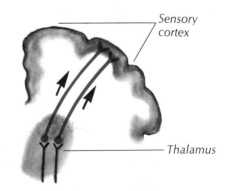

Sensory cortex

Thalamus

Lesions at different points in the sensory pathways produce different kinds of sensory loss. Patterns of sensory loss, together with their associated motor findings, are therefore helpful in figuring out where the causative lesions might be. A lesion in the sensory cortex may not impair the perception of pain, touch, and position, for example, but does impair finer discriminations. A person so affected cannot appreciate the size, shape, or texture of an object by feeling it and therefore cannot identify it. Loss of position and vibration sense with preservation of other sensations points to disease of the posterior columns, while the loss of all sensations from the waist down, together with paralysis and hyperactive reflexes in the legs, indicates transection of the spinal cord (see Table 17-6, pp. 522–523).

A knowledge of dermatomes also aids in localizing neurologic lesions. A dermatome is the band of skin innervated by the sensory nerve root of a single spinal segment. Dermatome patterns are mapped in the next two figures. Their levels are considerably more variable than the diagrams suggest, and dermatomes overlap each other. The sensory nerves from each side of the body overlap slightly across the midline.

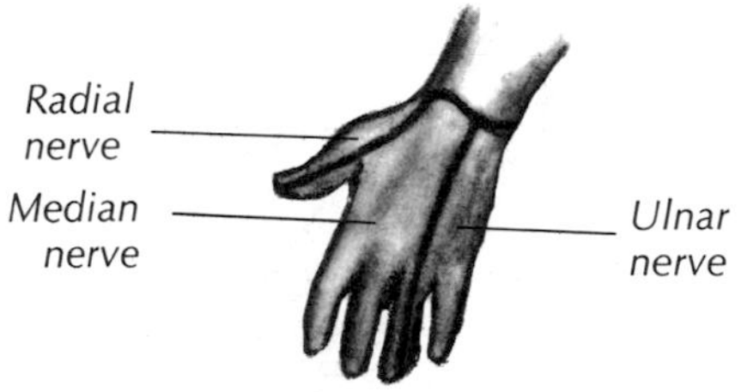
Radial nerve
Median nerve
Ulnar nerve

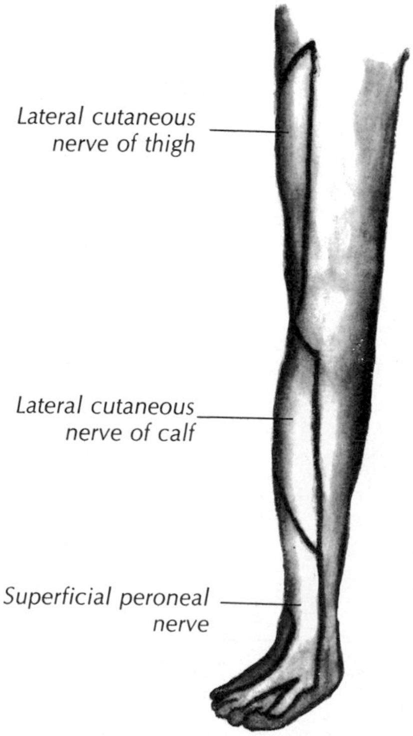
Lateral cutaneous nerve of thigh
Lateral cutaneous nerve of calf
Superficial peroneal nerve

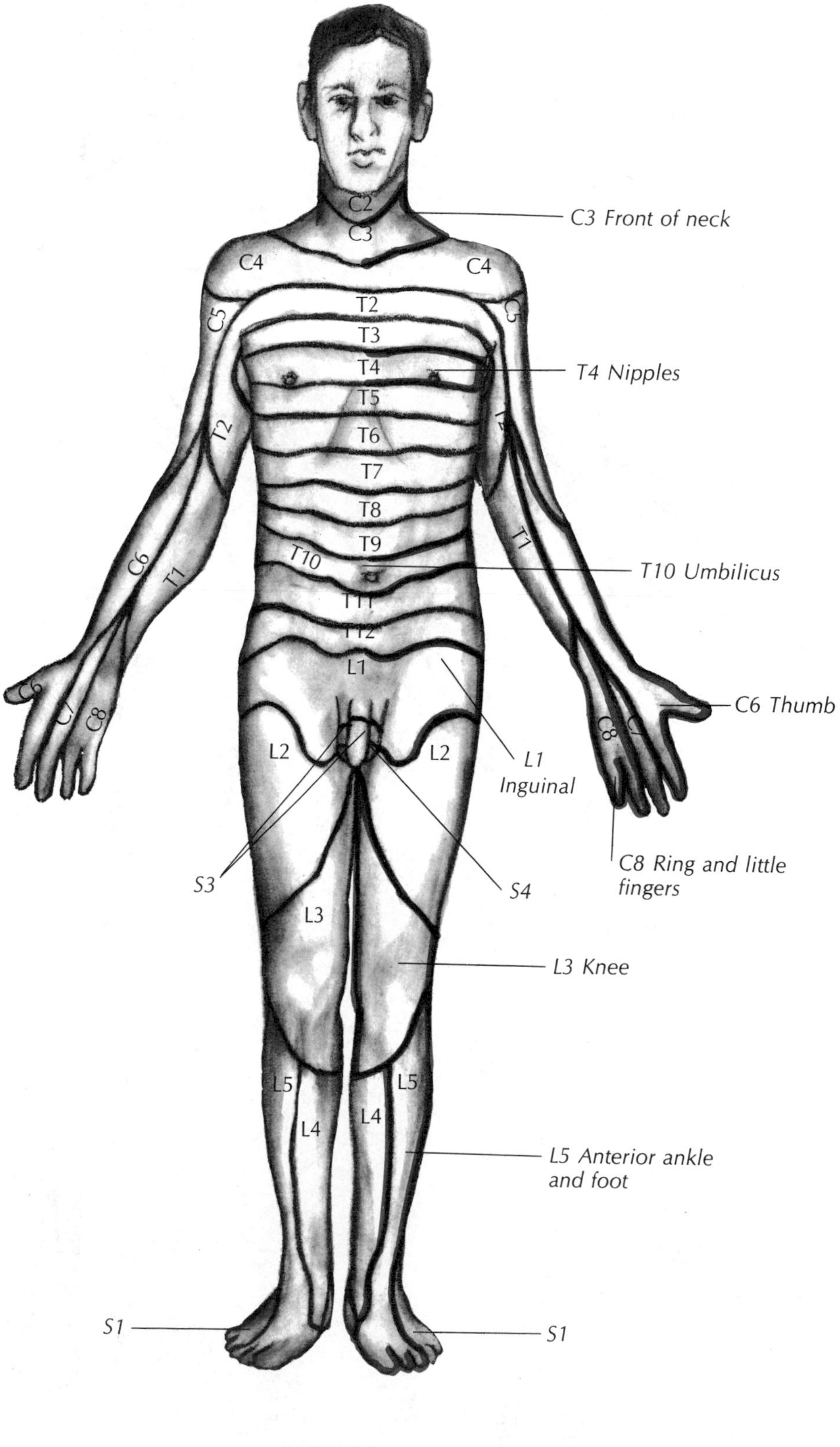
C2
C3
C3 Front of neck
C4
C4
C5
C5
T2
T3
T4
T5
T6
T7
T8
T9
T10
T11
T12
L1
T4 Nipples
T2
T1
T1
C6
T10 Umbilicus
C6
C7
C8
C8
C6 Thumb
L2
L2
L1 Inguinal
S3
S4
C8 Ring and little fingers
L3
L3 Knee
L5
L5
L4
L4
L5 Anterior ankle and foot
S1
S1

ANTERIOR

Do not try to memorize all the dermatomes. It is useful, however, to remember the locations of some, such as those outlined in red on the right side of the diagrams. The distribution of a few key peripheral nerves is shown in the inserts on the left.

(Figures on pages 475 and 476 are adapted from Haymaker W, Woodhall B: Peripheral Nerve Injuries, 2nd ed, pp 26, 28, 40, 43. Philadelphia, W B Saunders, 1953)

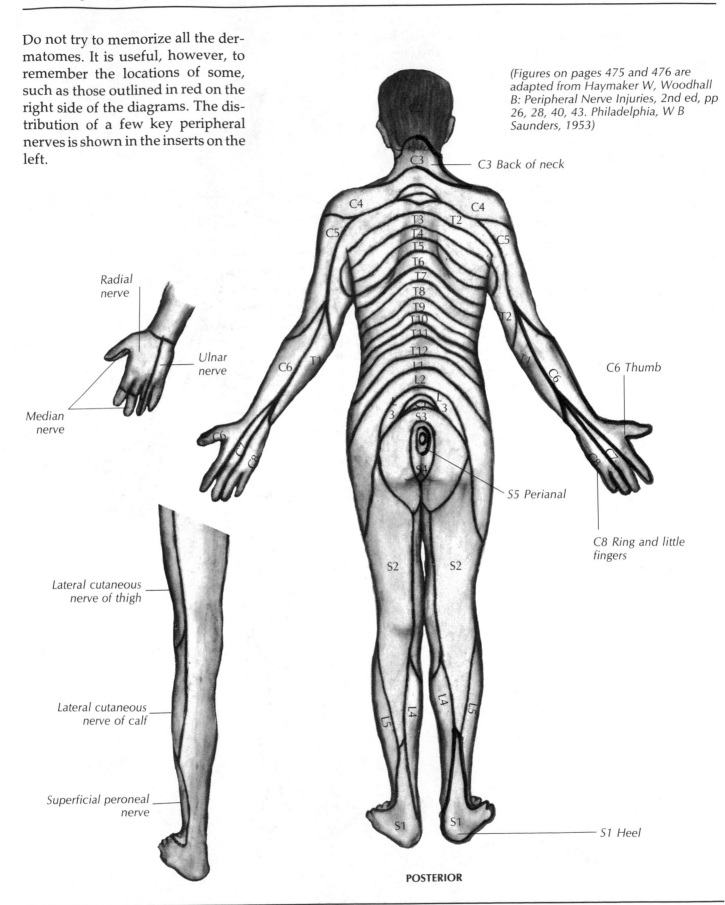

Radial nerve

Ulnar nerve

Median nerve

C3 Back of neck

C6 Thumb

S5 Perianal

C8 Ring and little fingers

Lateral cutaneous nerve of thigh

Lateral cutaneous nerve of calf

Superficial peroneal nerve

S1 Heel

POSTERIOR

THE CRANIAL NERVES

Nerves that emerge from the central nervous system within the head rather than from the vertebral column are called cranial nerves. There are 12 pairs. Functions of the cranial nerves most relevant to physical examination are summarized below.

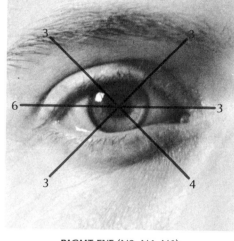

RIGHT EYE (N3, N4, N6)

NO.	NERVE	FUNCTION
N1	Olfactory	Sense of smell
N2	Optic	Vision
N3	Oculomotor	Pupillary constriction, elevation of the upper eyelid, and most of the extraocular movements
N4	Trochlear	Downward, inward movement of the eye
N6	Abducens	Lateral deviation of the eye
N5	Trigeminal	*Motor*—temporal and masseter muscles (jaw clenching), also lateral movement of the jaw

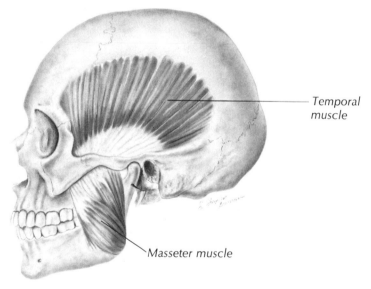

Temporal muscle

Masseter muscle

N5 MOTOR

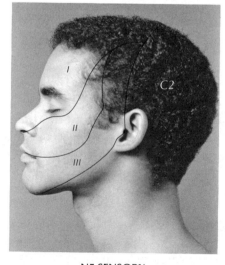

N5 SENSORY

Sensory—facial. The nerve has three divisions: I. ophthalmic, II. maxillary, and III. mandibular.

N7	Facial	*Motor*—muscles of the face, including those of the forehead and around the eyes and mouth
		Sensory—taste for salty, sweet, sour, and bitter substances on the anterior ⅔ of the tongue
N8	Acoustic	Hearing (cochlear division) and balance (vestibular division)
N9	Glossopharyngeal	*Sensory*—posterior portions of the eardrum and ear canal, the pharynx, and the posterior tongue, including taste (salty, sweet, sour, bitter)
		Motor—pharynx

Continued

NO.	NERVE	FUNCTION
N10	Vagus	*Sensory*—pharynx and larynx
		Motor—palate, pharynx, and larynx
N11	Spinal accessory	*Motor*—the sternomastoid and upper portion of the trapezius

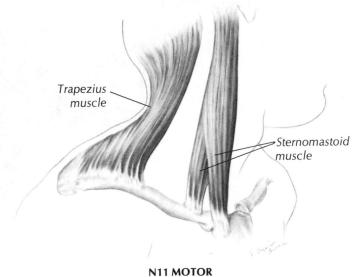

Trapezius muscle

Sternomastoid muscle

N11 MOTOR

N12	Hypoglossal	*Motor*—tongue

CHANGES WITH AGE

In assessing the nervous system of an elderly person it is sometimes difficult to distinguish the changes of normal aging from those of age-related or other diseases. Some findings that you would consider abnormal in younger people, however, occur often enough in the elderly that you may attribute them to aging alone. Alterations in hearing, vision, extraocular movements, and pupillary size, shape, and reactivity have been described in Chapter 7 (see pp. 161–162).

Muscular strength and agility begin to wane fairly early in adult life, as the relatively brief careers of professional athletes illustrate. Elderly persons move and react more slowly than younger ones. Muscle bulk decreases, and about half of elderly people will show some degree of muscular atrophy in their hands (see pp. 488–489). Grip, though diminished, remains relatively strong. Ankle reflexes may be symmetrically decreased or absent, even when reinforced. Less commonly, knee reflexes are similarly affected. Abdominal reflexes may diminish or disappear, and partly because of musculoskeletal changes in the feet the plantar responses become less obvious and more difficult to interpret. Vibration sense is frequently decreased or lost in the feet and ankles. Less commonly, position sense may diminish or disappear. Falls become increasingly common among the aged for reasons that include neurologic disease, orthostatic hypotension, arthritis, and a poorly understood deterioration in postural stability. Aged people occasionally become tremulous. Head, jaw, lips, or hands may tremble at a rate and amplitude suggesting Parkinson's disease, but without its muscular rigidity.

If changes such as those described are accompanied by other neurologic abnormalities, or if atrophy and reflex changes are asymmetrical, you should search for an explanation other than age alone.

Techniques of Examination

GENERAL APPROACH

Appropriate neurologic examination varies widely. In apparently healthy young adults simple screening is adequate. Screening procedures for the motor and sensory systems are included in this chapter and summarized in Chapter 4. If a person has symptoms such as headache, weakness, sensory changes, or loss of consciousness, however, you should evaluate the nervous system in greater depth. This chapter presents a practicable and reasonably inclusive neurologic examination. Be aware that many other techniques may be useful in specific situations. Consult textbooks of neurology as the need arises.

For efficiency you should integrate certain portions of your neurologic assessment with other parts of your examination. Make an initial survey of mental status and speech, for example, during the interview. Assess at least some of the cranial nerves as you examine the head and neck, and inspect the arms and legs for neurologic abnormalities while you also evaluate the peripheral vascular and musculoskeletal systems. Chapter 4 provides an outline for this kind of integrated approach. Think about and describe your findings, however, in terms of the nervous system as a unit.

Organize your thinking into five categories: (1) mental status and speech, (2) cranial nerves, (3) the motor system, (4) the sensory system, and (5) reflexes.

For abnormalities of mental status and speech, see Chapter 3, *Mental Status.*

THE CRANIAL NERVES

FIRST CRANIAL NERVE (OLFACTORY). Test the *sense of smell* by presenting the patient with familiar and nonirritating odors. First be sure that each nasal passage is open by compressing one side of the nose and asking the patient to sniff through the other. The patient should then close both eyes. Occlude one nostril and under the other hold one of several substances such as cloves, coffee, soap, or vanilla. Ask if the patient smells anything and, if so, what. Test the other side. A person should normally perceive odor on each side and can often identify it.

Bilateral decrease or loss of smell has many causes, including nasal disease, excessive smoking, and the use of cocaine. It may be congenital. Unilateral loss of smell without nasal disease suggests a lesion in the frontal lobe of the brain.

SECOND CRANIAL NERVE (OPTIC). Test *visual acuity.* (See pp. 163–164.)

Inspect the *optic fundi* ophthalmoscopically, with special attention to the optic discs. (See pp. 171–176.)

Optic atrophy, papilledema

Determine the *visual fields* by confrontation. (See pp. 164–165.)

See Table 7-2, Visual Field Defects (p. 188).

Now test for *extinction of vision* on one side. With both the patient's eyes open, wiggle your fingers simultaneously in both upper temporal quadrants. Your fingers should be outside the binocular field of vision. The stimulus on the patient's left side is thus seen only by the left eye and that

Perception of movement on only one side suggests extinc-

on the right only by the right eye, as diagrammed below. Ask the patient to point to your movements. Both stimuli should be seen. Repeat in the lower temporal quadrants. This test is designed to detect extinction, a subtle suppression of vision when the vision itself, as evaluated directly by confrontation, is normal. Patterns of abnormality resemble homonymous hemianopsias and quadrantic defects.

tion, signifying a lesion of the parietal or occipital cortex. Below, for example, the only stimuli perceived are those on the patient's right. Those on the left are extinguished.

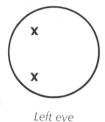 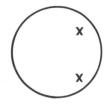

Left eye   *Right eye*

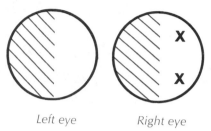

Left eye   *Right eye*

THIRD, FOURTH, AND SIXTH CRANIAL NERVES (OCULOMOTOR, TROCHLEAR, AND ABDUCENS). (See pp. 169–171.) Inspect the size and shape of the pupils, and compare one side with the other. Test the *pupillary reactions to light* and, if these are abnormal, examine the *near response* also.

See Table 7-7, Pupillary Abnormalities (pp. 193–194).

Test the *extraocular movements* in the six cardinal fields of gaze, and look for loss of conjugate movements in any of the six directions. Check convergence of the eyes. Identify any nystagmus, noting the field of gaze in which it appears, the plane in which movements occur (*e.g.,* horizontal, vertical), and the direction of the quick and slow components.

See Table 7-8, Deviations of the Eyes (p. 195).

See Table 17-1, Nystagmus (pp. 512–513).

Look for ptosis of the upper eyelids. A slight difference in the width of the palpebral fissures may be noted in about one third of all normal people.

Ptosis in 3rd nerve palsy, Horner's syndrome, myasthenia gravis

FIFTH CRANIAL NERVE (TRIGEMINAL)

Motor. While palpating the temporal and masseter muscles in turn, ask the patient to clench the teeth. Note the strength of muscle contraction.

Weak or absent contraction of the temporal and masseter muscles on one side suggests a lesion of the 5th cranial nerve. Bilateral weakness may result from upper or lower motor neuron involvement. When the patient has no teeth, this test may be difficult to interpret.

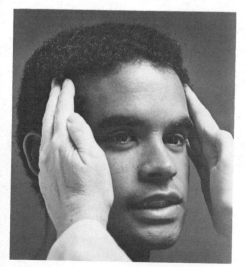

PALPATING TEMPORAL MUSCLES

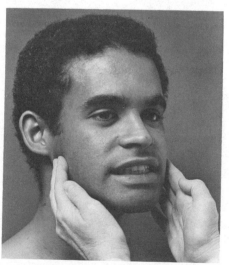

PALPATING MASSETER MUSCLES

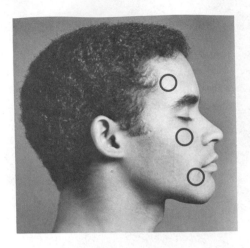

Sensory. With the patient's eyes closed, test the forehead, cheeks, and jaw on each side for *pain* sensation. Suggested areas are indicated by the circles. Use a safety pin, occasionally substituting the blunt end for the point as a stimulus. Ask the patient to report whether it is "sharp" or "dull" and to compare sides. (*Note:* You have tested for pain only in areas touched with the point of the pin. The dull end is a check on the patient's reliability.)

Unilateral decrease or loss of facial sensation suggests a lesion of the 5th cranial nerve or of interconnecting higher sensory pathways. Such a sensory loss may also be associated with a conversion reaction.

If you find an abnormality, confirm it by testing *temperature* sensation. Use two test tubes filled with hot and cold water. Touch the skin and ask the patient to identify "hot" or "cold."

Then test for *light touch,* using a fine wisp of cotton. Ask the patient to respond whenever you touch the skin.

Test *the corneal reflex.* Ask the patient to look up and away from you. Approaching from the other side, out of the patient's line of vision, and avoiding the eyelashes, touch the cornea (not the conjunctiva) lightly with a fine wisp of cotton.

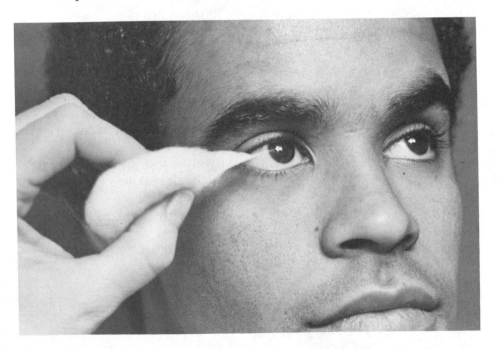

Look for blinking of the eyes, the normal reaction to this stimulus. (The sensory limb of this reflex is carried in the 5th cranial nerve, the motor response in the 7th.)

Absence of blinking suggests a lesion of the 5th cranial nerve. A lesion of the 7th cranial nerve (the nerve to the muscles that close the eyes) may also impair this reflex. Use of contact lenses frequently diminishes or abolishes this reflex.

SEVENTH CRANIAL NERVE (FACIAL). Inspect the face, both at rest and during conversation with the patient. Note any asymmetry (*e.g.,* of the nasolabial folds), and observe any tics or other abnormal movements. Ask the patient to:

Flattening of the nasolabial fold and drooping of the lower eyelid suggest facial weakness.

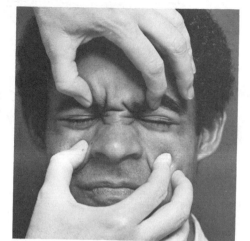

1. Raise both eyebrows
2. Frown
3. Close both eyes tightly so that you cannot open them. Test muscular strength by trying to open them.

4. Show both upper and lower teeth
5. Smile
6. Puff out both cheeks

A lower motor neuron lesion, such as Bell's palsy, affects both the upper and the lower face; an upper motor neuron (or central) lesion affects mainly the lower face. See Table 17-2, Types of Facial Paralysis (pp. 514–515).

In unilateral facial paralysis, the mouth is pulled away from the paralyzed side when the patient smiles or shows the teeth.

Note any weakness or asymmetry.

EIGHTH CRANIAL NERVE (ACOUSTIC). Assess *hearing.* If hearing loss is present, (1) test for *lateralization,* and (2) compare *air and bone conduction.* (See pp. 178–179.)

See Table 7-15, Patterns of Hearing Loss (pp. 210–211).

Specific tests of *vestibular function* are seldom included in the usual neurologic examination, although nystagmus may indicate vestibular dysfunction. Consult textbooks of neurology or otolaryngology as the need arises.

NINTH AND TENTH CRANIAL NERVES (GLOSSOPHARYNGEAL AND VAGUS). Listen to the patient's *voice.* Is it hoarse or does it have a nasal quality?

Hoarseness in vocal cord paralysis; a nasal voice in paralysis of the palate

Ask the patient to say "ah" or to yawn as you watch the *movements of the soft palate and pharynx.* The soft palate normally rises symmetrically, the uvula remains in the midline, and each side of the posterior pharynx moves medially, like a curtain. A normal uvula is sometimes slightly curved.

The palate fails to rise with a bilateral lesion of the vagus nerve. In unilateral paralysis, one side of the palate fails to rise and, together with the uvula, is pulled toward the normal side. (See p. 219.)

Warn the patient that you are going to test the *gag reflex.* Stimulate the back of the throat lightly on each side in turn and note the gag reflex. It may be symmetrically diminished or absent in some normal people.

Unilateral absence of this reflex suggests a lesion of the 9th or perhaps the 10th cranial nerve.

ELEVENTH CRANIAL NERVE (SPINAL ACCESSORY). From behind, look for atrophy or fasciculations in the trapezius muscles, and compare one

Weakness with atrophy and fasciculations indicates lower

483

side with the other. Ask the patient to shrug both shoulders upward against your hands. Note the strength and contraction of the trapezii.

motor neuron disease. When the trapezius is paralyzed, the shoulder droops and the scapula is displaced downward and laterally.

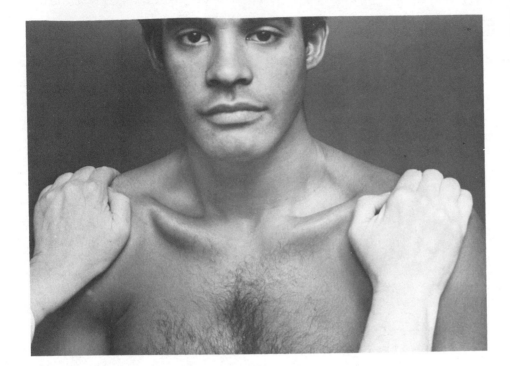

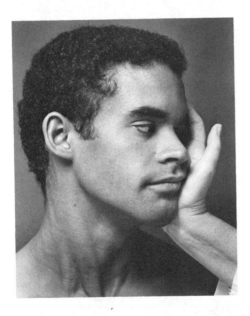

Ask the patient to turn the head to each side against your hand. Observe the contraction of the opposite sternomastoid and note the force of the movement against your hand.

A supine patient with bilateral weakness of the sternomastoids has difficulty raising the head off the pillow.

TWELFTH CRANIAL NERVE (HYPOGLOSSAL). Inspect the patient's tongue as it lies on the floor of the mouth. Look for any fasciculations. Some coarser restless movements are often seen in a normal tongue.

Atrophy and fasciculations suggest lower motor neuron disease.

Ask the patient to stick out the tongue. Look for asymmetry, atrophy, or deviation from the midline. Ask the patient to move the tongue from side to side, and note the symmetry of the movement.

The tongue, when protruded forward, deviates toward the paralyzed side. (See p. 218.)

THE MOTOR SYSTEM

By inspecting the patient during other parts of the examination you should already have gathered at least some tentative information with which to assess the motor system. This section describes additional screening procedures and outlines the organization of motor assessment.

Screening Procedures, Including Gait

Ask the patient to *walk* across the room or, preferably, down the hall, then turn, and come back. Observe posture, balance, swinging of the arms, and movements of the legs. Normally balance is easy, the arms swing at the sides, and turns are smoothly accomplished.

A gait that lacks coordination, with reeling and instability, is called ataxic. Ataxia may be due to cerebellar disease, loss of position sense, or intoxication. See Table 17-3, Abnormalities of Gait and Posture (pp. 514 – 515).

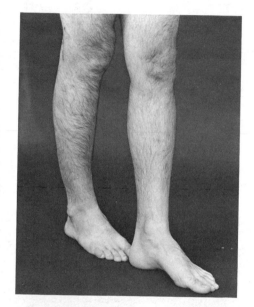

Then ask the patient to walk *heel-to-toe* in a straight line—a pattern called *tandem walking.*

Tandem walking may reveal an ataxia not previously obvious.

Now ask the patient to walk *on the toes* and then *on the heels*—sensitive tests respectively for plantar flexion and dorsiflexion of the ankles, as well as for balance.

Walking on toes and heels may reveal distal muscular weakness in the legs. Further, weak dorsiflexion is a sensitive test for upper motor neuron weakness.

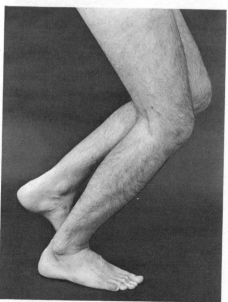

Ask the patient, if reasonably young and healthy, to *hop in place* on each foot in turn. Hopping involves the proximal muscles of the legs as well as the distal ones and requires both good position sense and normal cerebellar function.

Difficulty with hopping may be due to weakness, lack of position sense, or cerebellar dysfunction.

Then ask the patient to do a *shallow knee bend,* first on one leg, then on the other.

Difficulty here suggests proximal weakness (extensors of the hip), weakness of the quadriceps (the extensor of the knee), or both.

In older and less robust patients, watching how they *rise from a sitting position*, without arm support, is a more suitable screening maneuver than hopping and knee bends. Stepping up onto a sturdy stool is similarly useful.

People with proximal muscle weakness involving the pelvic girdle and legs have difficulty rising from a chair and stepping up onto a stool.

To screen the arms, ask the patient to hold the arms straight forward, palms up, and then to close both eyes and maintain this position for 20 to 30 seconds. A normal person can hold this position well. Stand close enough to protect the patient from falling. Alternatively, the patient may sit during this test.

The tendency of one forearm to pronate suggests a mild hemiparesis; downward drift of the arm with flexion of fingers and elbow may also occur. These movements are called a *pronator drift*, shown below.

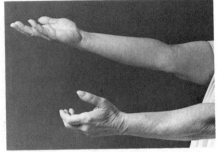

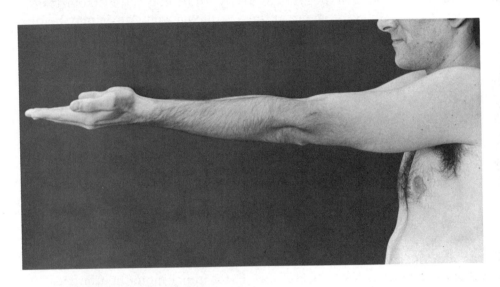

A sideward or upward drift, sometimes with searching, writhing movements of the hands, suggests loss of position sense.

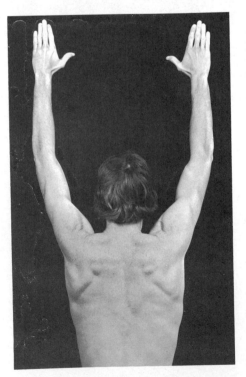

Now, instructing the patient to keep the arms up and eyes shut, as shown above, tap the arms briskly downward. The arms will normally return smoothly to the horizontal position. This response requires muscular strength, coordination, and a good sense of position.

A weak arm is easily displaced and often remains so. When position sense is lacking, the patient may not recognize the displacement and, if told to correct it, does so poorly. In cerebellar incoordination the arm returns to its original position but with overshooting and bounces.

Then ask the patient to raise both arms overhead with palms forward for 20 to 30 seconds. Again, observe the maintenance of this position. Try to force the arms down to the sides against the patient's resistance. Note any weakness.

Drifting or weakness on one side suggests hemiparesis. Shoulder girdle disease may also cause drifting or weakness.

Ask the patient to lower both arms slowly forward and down to the sides. Watch the scapulae for *winging,* a backward displacement away from the chest wall.

When the serratus anterior muscle is weak, the medial border of the scapula juts backward, simulating a wing.

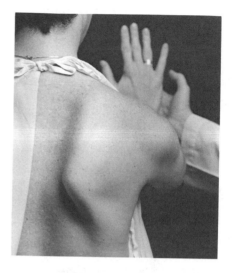

Alternatively, look for winging as the patient pushes with arms extended forward against a wall or against your hand. In very thin but normal people the scapulae may look somewhat winged in the absence of weakness.

Some winging may also accompany weakness of the trapezius.

To test the *grip,* ask the patient to squeeze two of your fingers as hard as possible and not let them go. (To avoid getting hurt by hard squeezes, place your own middle finger on top of your index finger.) You should normally have difficulty removing your fingers from the patient's grip.

A weak grip may be due to either upper or lower motor neuron disease. It may also result from painful disorders of the hands.

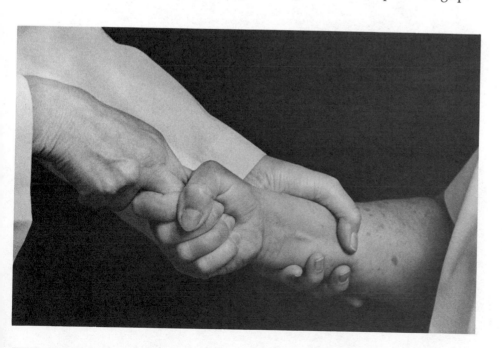

If you have noted poor balance during these screening maneuvers, perform a *Romberg test* in order to evaluate its cause. Ask the patient to stand with feet together and without support from the arms. Note the patient's ability to maintain an upright posture, first with eyes open and then with eyes closed for 20 to 30 seconds. Stand close enough to give support should the patient's balance falter. Normally only minimal swaying occurs. (This test may be combined with that for pronator drift.)

In cerebellar ataxia the patient has difficulty standing with feet together whether the eyes are open or closed. In ataxia due to loss of position sense, vision compensates for the sensory loss. The patient can stand fairly well with eyes open but loses balance when they are closed, thus demonstrating a *positive Romberg sign.*

Further Motor Assessment

Although the exact sequence in which you make your observations may vary, keep in mind the basic components of the motor assessment: muscle bulk, muscle tone, muscle strength, coordination, and involuntary movements.

INSPECTION. Inspect the muscles of the limbs and the trunk, noting their *bulk* and *contours*, the presence of *involuntary movements*, or any *abnormalities of bodily position (posture)*.

When looking for atrophy, pay particular attention to the shoulder and pelvic girdles and the hands. The thenar and hypothenar eminences should be full and convex, and the spaces between the metacarpals, where the dorsal interosseous muscles lie, should be full or only slightly depressed. Atrophy of hand muscles may occur with normal aging, however, as shown on the right.

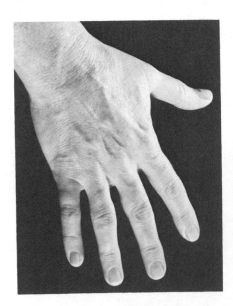

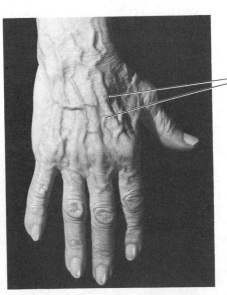

Atrophy

Muscular *atrophy* refers to a loss of muscle bulk (wasting). It results from lower motor neuron disease and disease of the muscle itself. *Hypertrophy* refers to an increase in bulk with proportionate strength, while increased bulk with diminished strength is called *pseudohypertrophy* (seen in the Duchenne form of muscular dystrophy).

Hand of a 44-year-old woman   Hand of an 84-year-old woman

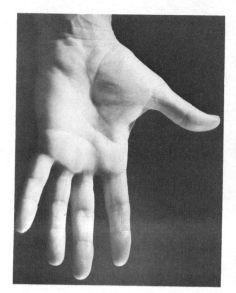

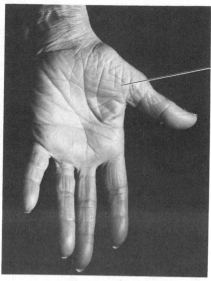

Flattening of mild atrophy

Hand of a 44-year-old woman

Hand of an 84-year old woman

Flattening of the thenar and hypothenar eminences and concavities or furrowing between the metacarpals suggest atrophy. Localized atrophy of the thenar and hypothenar eminences suggests damage to the median and ulnar nerves respectively.

Be alert for fasciculations (fine, flickering, irregular movements) in atrophic muscles. A tap on the muscle with a reflex hammer may stimulate them.

Other causes of muscular atrophy include disuse of the muscles, rheumatoid arthritis, and protein-calorie malnutrition.

If you see any involuntary movements, note their location, quality, rate, rhythm, amplitude, and relation to posture, activity, fatigue, emotion, or other factors. If you note an abnormality of bodily position (such as persisting flexion of an elbow or external rotation at the hip), observe the parts of the body involved and the nature of the deviation.

The presence of fasciculations supports lower motor neuron disease as the cause of atrophy.

See Table 17-4. Involuntary Movements (pp. 518–520). For examples of abnormal positions see page 524.

ASSESSMENT OF MUSCLE TONE. When a normal muscle with an intact nerve supply is voluntarily relaxed, it maintains a slight residual tension known as muscle tone. This can be best assessed by feeling the muscle's resistance to passive stretch. Persuade the patient to relax. Take one hand with yours and, while supporting the elbow, flex and extend the patient's fingers, wrist, and elbow, and put the shoulder through a moderate range of motion. With practice, these actions can be combined into a single smooth movement. On each side note muscle tone—the resistance offered to your movements. Tense patients may show increased resistance. You will learn the feel of normal resistance only with repeated practice.

Resistance to passive stretch is decreased when the reflex arc is interrupted by a lesion affecting the sensory or the lower motor neuron. It may also be decreased in muscular and cerebellar disease and in the acute stages of a spinal cord injury or cerebrovascular accident.

If you suspect decreased resistance, hold the forearm and shake the hand loosely back and forth. Normally the hand moves back and forth freely but is not completely floppy.

Marked floppiness indicates hypotonic (flaccid) muscles.

If resistance is increased, determine whether it varies as you move the limb or whether it persists throughout the range of movement and in both directions, *e.g.,* during both flexion and extension. Feel for any jerkiness in the resistance.

Increased resistance that varies, commonly worse at the extremes of the range, is called *spasticity.* High resistance,

To assess muscle tone in the legs support the patient's thigh with one hand, grasp the foot with the other, and flex and extend the patient's knee and ankle on each side. Note the resistance to your movements.

followed by sudden relaxation as the limb is moved, is called *clasp-knife spasticity.* Spasticity indicates upper motor neuron disease. Resistance that persists throughout the range and in both directions is called *lead-pipe rigidity.* A superimposed ratchetlike jerkiness is *cogwheel rigidity.* Both kinds of rigidity may be felt in parkinsonism.

TESTING MUSCLE STRENGTH. Normal individuals vary widely in their strength, and your standard of normal, while admittedly rough, should allow for such variables as age, sex, and muscular training. A person's dominant side is usually stronger than the other side. Keep this difference in mind when you compare sides.

You usually test muscle strength by asking the patient to move actively against your resistance or to resist your movement. Watch for muscular contraction and feel for the strength exerted. Some muscles may be too weak to overcome resistance. You can then test them against gravity alone or with gravity eliminated. When the forearm rests in a pronated position, for example, dorsiflexion at the wrist can be tested against gravity alone. When the forearm is midway between pronation and supination, dorsiflexion at the wrist can be tested with gravity eliminated. Finally, you may be able to see or feel a weak muscular contraction even if it fails to move the body part.

Impaired strength is called weakness or paresis. Absence of strength is called paralysis. *Hemiparesis* refers to weakness of one half of the body; *hemiplegia* refers to paralysis of one half of the body. *Paraplegia* means paralysis of the legs; *quadriplegia* means paralysis of all four limbs.

Muscle strength may be graded on a 0 to 5 scale:

See Table 17-5, Differentiation of Motor Dysfunctions (p. 521).

0 — No muscular contraction detected
1 — A barely detectable flicker or trace of contraction
2 — Active movement of the body part with gravity eliminated
3 — Active movement against gravity
4 — Active movement against gravity and some resistance
5 — Active movement against full resistance without evident fatigue. This is normal muscle strength.

Described below are methods of testing some major muscle groups, the spinal levels for which are shown in parentheses. To localize lesions in the spinal cord or the peripheral nervous system more precisely, however, very discrete testing may be necessary. For these specialized methods, refer to detailed texts of neurology.

At the elbow test flexion (C5,6) and extension (C6,7,8) by having the patient pull and push against your hand.

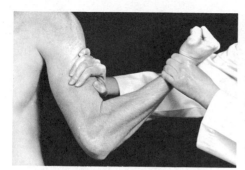

FLEXION

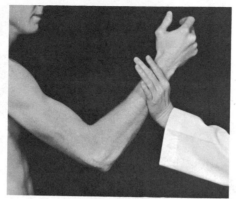

EXTENSION

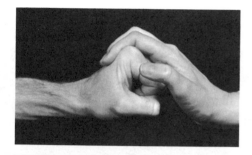

Test extension at the wrist (C6,7,8, radial nerve) by asking the patient to make a fist and resist your pulling it down.

Weakness of dorsiflexion is seen in lower motor neuron disease (*e.g.*, radial nerve damage) and upper motor neuron disease (*e.g.*, hemiplegia).

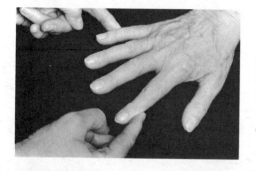

Position the patient's hand with palm down and fingers spread. Instructing the patient not to let you move the fingers, try to force them together. This effort tests finger abduction (C8, T1, ulnar nerve).

Weak finger abduction in ulnar nerve disorders

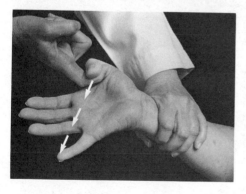

The patient should now try to touch the tip of the little finger with the thumb, against your resistance. This effort tests opposition of the thumb (C8, T1, median nerve).

Weak opposition of the thumb in median nerve disorders such as the carpal tunnel syndrome

Assessment of muscle strength of the trunk may already have been made in other segments of the examination. It includes:

1. Flexion, extension, and lateral bending of the trunk
2. Excursion of the rib cage and diaphragm during respiration

Test flexion at the hip (L2,3,4) by placing your hand on the patient's thigh and asking the patient to raise the leg against it.

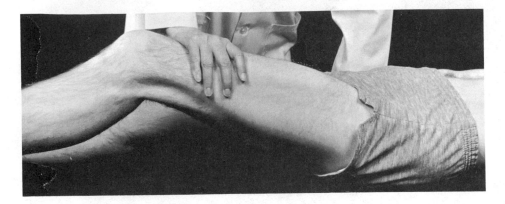

Test abduction at the hips (L2,3,4). Place your hands firmly on the bed outside the patient's knees. Ask the patient to spread both legs against your hands.

Symmetrical weakness of the proximal muscles suggests a myopathy; symmetrical weakness of distal muscles suggests a polyneuropathy.

Test adduction at the hips (L4,5, S1). Place your hands firmly on the bed between the patient's knees. Ask the patient to bring the legs together.

Text extension at the knee (L2,3,4) by supporting the knee in flexion and asking the patient to straighten the leg against your hand.

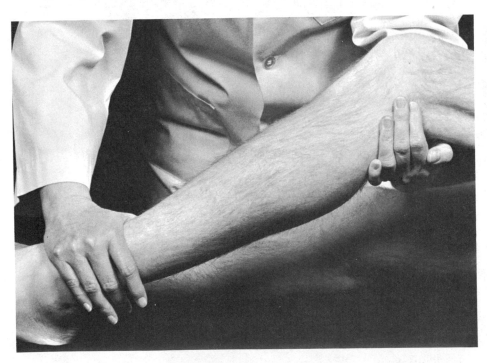

Test flexion at the knee (L4,5, S1,2). Place the patient's leg so that the knee is flexed with the foot resting on the bed. Tell the patient to keep the foot down as you try to straighten the leg.

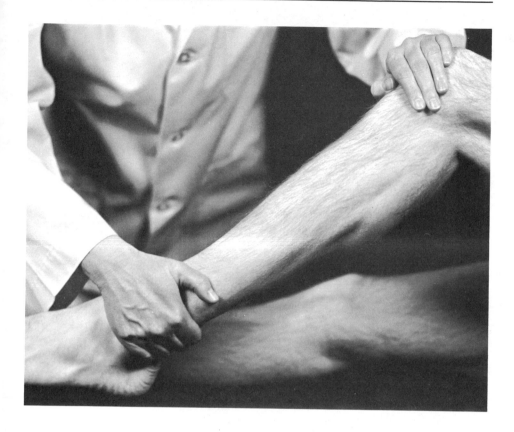

At the ankle, test dorsiflexion (L4,5, S1) and plantar flexion (mainly S1,2) by asking the patient to pull up and push down against your hand.

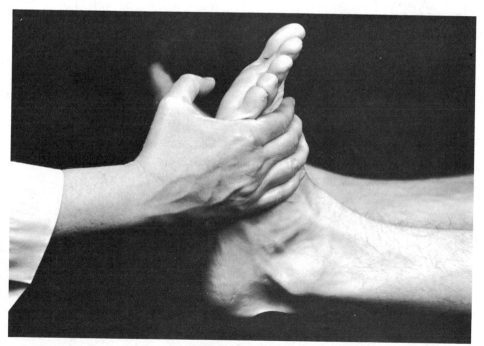

DORSIFLEXION

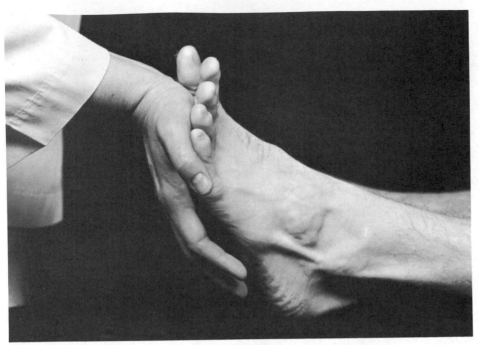

PLANTAR FLEXION

ASSESSING COORDINATION. During the motor screening examination you have already done a preliminary assessment of coordination. Now test it further by two methods. The sitting position is preferable for testing the arms.

1. *Rapid Alternating Movements.* Show the patient how to strike one hand on the thigh, raise the hand, turn it over, and then strike the back of the hand down on the same place. Urge the patient to repeat these alternating movements as rapidly as possible.

   Observe the speed, rhythm, and smoothness of the movements. Repeat with the other hand. The nondominant hand often performs somewhat less well.

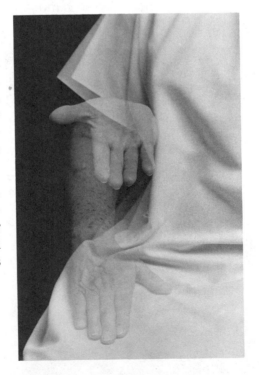

In cerebellar disease one movement cannot be followed quickly by its opposite and movements are slow, irregular, and clumsy. This abnormality is called *dysdiadochokinesis.* Upper motor neuron weakness and extrapyramidal disease may also impair rapid alternating movements, but not in the same manner.

Show the patient how to tap the distal joint of the thumb with the tip of the index finger, again as rapidly as possible.

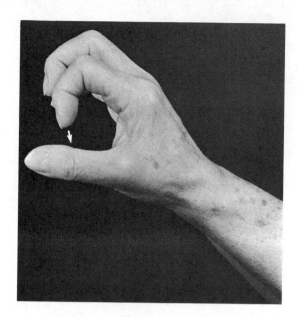

2. *Point-to-Point Testing.* Ask the patient to touch your index finger and then his or her nose alternately several times. Move your finger about so that the patient has to alter directions and extend the arm fully to reach it. Observe the accuracy and smoothness of movements and watch for any tremor.

In cerebellar disease movements are clumsy, unsteady, and inappropriately varying in their speed, force, and direction. The finger may initially overshoot its mark but finally reaches it fairly well. Such movements are termed *dysmetria.* An intention tremor may appear toward the end of the movement (see p. 518).

Now hold your finger in one place so that the patient can touch it with one arm and finger outstretched. Ask the patient to raise the arm overhead and lower it again to touch your finger. After several repeats, ask the patient to close both eyes and try several more times. Repeat on the other side. Normally a person can touch the examiner's finger successfully with eyes open or closed. These maneuvers test position sense and the functions of both the labyrinth and the cerebellum.

Cerebellar disease causes incoordination that may get worse with eyes closed. Inaccuracy that appears with eyes closed suggests loss of position sense. Repetitive and consistent deviation to one side (referred to as *past pointing*), worse with the eyes closed, suggests cerebellar or vestibular disease.

To assess the legs the patient should be lying down.

1. *Rapid Alternating Movements.* Ask the patient to tap your hand as quickly as possible with the ball of each foot in turn. Note any slowness or awkwardness. The feet normally perform less well than the hands.

2. *Point-to-Point Testing.* Ask the patient to place one heel on the opposite knee, and then run it down the shin to the big toe. Note the

In cerebellar disease the heel may overshoot the knee and

smoothness and accuracy of the movements. Repetition with the patient's eyes closed tests for position sense. Repeat on the other side.

then oscillate from side to side down the shin. When position sense is lost, the heel is lifted too high and the patient tries to look. With eyes closed, performance is poor.

THE SENSORY SYSTEM

Evaluation of the sensory system involves testing each kind of sensation: pain, temperature (perhaps), light touch, vibration, position, and discriminative sensations. In a patient with no neurologic symptoms or signs, a few *screening procedures* may be selected from the more detailed examination described below. These include (1) assessment of pain and vibration sense in the hands and feet, (2) brief comparison of light touch over the arms and legs, and (3) assessment of stereognosis.

Other patients need a *more complete evaluation.* Because sensory testing quickly fatigues many patients and then produces unreliable results, conduct the examination as efficiently as possible. Pay special attention to those areas (1) where there are symptoms such as numbness or pain, (2) where there are motor or reflex abnormalities that suggest a lesion of the spinal cord or peripheral nervous system, and (3) where there are trophic changes (*e.g.,* absent or excessive sweating, atrophic skin, or cutaneous ulceration). Repeated testing at another time is often required to confirm abnormalities.

Meticulous sensory mapping helps to establish the level of a spinal cord lesion and to determine the location of a more peripheral lesion, such as in a nerve root, in a major peripheral nerve, or in one of its branches.

PATTERNS OF SENSORY TESTING

1. Compare symmetrical areas on the two sides of the body, including the arms, legs, and trunk.

   Hemisensory loss due to a lesion in the spinal cord or higher pathways

2. When testing pain, temperature, and touch, also compare the distal with the proximal areas of the extremities. Further, scatter the stimuli so as to sample most of the dermatomes and major peripheral nerves (see pp. 475–476). One suggested pattern includes both shoulders (C4), the inner and outer aspects of the forearms (C6 and T1), the thumbs and little fingers (C6 and C8), the fronts of both thighs (L2), the medial and lateral aspects of both calves (L4 and L5), the little toes (S1), and each buttock medial to its midline (S3).

   Symmetrical distal sensory loss suggests a polyneuropathy.

3. When testing vibration and position, first test the fingers and toes. If these are normal you may safely assume that more proximal areas will also be normal.

4. Vary the pace of your testing so that the patient does not merely respond to your repetitive rhythm.

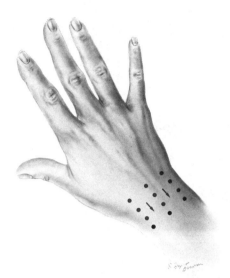

5. When you detect an area of sensory loss or hypersensitivity, map out its boundaries in detail. Stimulate first at a point of reduced sensation and move outward by progressive steps until the patient detects the change. An example is shown at right.

Here pain, together with all other sensation, is lost at a sharp line around the wrist. This distribution of sensory loss does not fit any organic pattern such as peripheral nerve or dermatome. It is characteristic of the "glove and stocking" sensory loss associated with a conversion reaction. In polyneuropathy, the demarcation of sensory loss is less distinct.

By identifying the distribution of sensory abnormalities and the kinds of sensations affected, you can infer where the causative lesion might be. Any motor deficit or reflex abnormality, of course, also helps in this localizing process.

See Table 17-6, Patterns of Sensory Loss (pp. 522–523).

SENSORY TESTS. Ask the patient to close both eyes. Test sensation on the arms, trunk, and legs, using the following stimuli:

1. *Pain.* Use a sharp safety pin, occasionally substituting the blunt end for the point as a stimulus. Stimulating in patterns suggested above, ask the patient, "Is this sharp or dull?" or, when you are making comparisons with a sharp stimulus, "Does this feel the same as this?" Use as light a stimulus as the patient can perceive, and try not to draw blood.

   The risk, if any, of transmitting blood-borne infections with a safety pin has not been ascertained. Some clinicians are now using large, disposable splinters of wood made by twisting a tongue blade lengthwise or breaking an applicator stick. These must be sharp enough to make them clearly distinguishable from a dull object. All such tools, including any pin that has drawn blood, must be safely discarded.

2. *Temperature.* (This is often omitted if pain sensation is normal, but include it if there is any question.) Use two test tubes, filled with hot and cold water. Touch the skin and ask the patient to identify "hot" or "cold."

3. *Light touch.* With a fine wisp of cotton touch the skin lightly, avoiding pressure. Ask the patient to respond whenever a touch is felt, and to compare one area with another. Callaused skin is normally relatively insensitive and should be avoided.

4. *Vibration.* Use a relatively low-pitched tuning fork, preferably of 128 Hz. Tap it on the heel of your hand and place it firmly over a distal interphalangeal joint of the patient's finger and over the interphalangeal joint of the big toe. Ask what the patient feels. If you are uncertain

Analgesia refers to absence of pain sensation, *hypalgesia* to decreased sensitivity to pain, and *hyperalgesia* to increased sensitivity.

Anesthesia is absence of touch sensation, *hypesthesia* is decreased sensitivity, and *hyperesthesia* is increased sensitivity.

Vibration sense is often the first sensation to be lost in a peripheral neuropathy. Common causes include diabetes and

whether it is pressure or vibration, ask the patient to tell you when the vibration stops, and then touch the fork to stop it. If vibration sense is impaired, proceed to more proximal bony prominences (*e.g.*, wrist and elbow or medial malleolus, patella, anterior superior iliac spine, spinous processes, and clavicles).

alcoholism. Vibration sense is also lost in posterior column disease. It is here where testing vibration sense in the trunk may be useful in estimating the level of a cord lesion. Remember that aging may also be associated with decreased vibration sense.

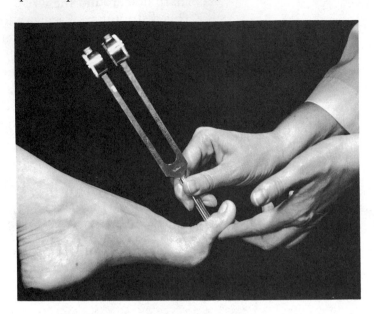

5. *Position.* Grasp the patient's big toe, holding it by its sides between your thumb and index finger, and then pull it away from the other 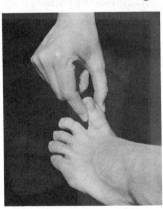 toes so as to avoid friction. (These precautions prevent extraneous tactile stimuli from indicating to the patient a change of position that might not otherwise be detected.) Show what you mean by "up" and "down" as you move the patient's toe clearly upward and downward. Then, with the patient's eyes closed, ask for an "up" or "down" response as you move the toe in a small arc.

Loss of position sense, like loss of vibration sense, suggests either posterior column disease or a lesion of the peripheral nerve or root.

Repeat several times on each side, avoiding simple alternation of the stimuli. If position sense is impaired, move proximally to test it at the ankle joint. In a similar fashion test position in the fingers, moving proximally if indicated to the metacarpophalangeal joints, wrist, and elbow.

6. *Discriminative sensations.* Several additional maneuvers test the ability of the sensory cortex to correlate, analyze, and interpret sensations. Because discriminative sensations are dependent on touch and position sense they are useful only when these sensations, when tested directly, are either normal or only slightly impaired.

When touch and position sense are normal or only slightly impaired, a disproportionate decrease in or loss of discriminative sensations suggests disease

Screen a patient with stereognosis, and proceed on to the other methods if indicated. The patient's eyes should be closed during all these maneuvers.

of the sensory cortex. Stereognosis, number identification, and two-point discrimination are also impaired by posterior column disease.

a. *Stereognosis.* Stereognosis refers to the ability to identify an object from its size and shape. Place in the patient's hand a familiar object such as a coin, paper clip, key, pencil, or cotton ball, and ask the patient to tell you what it is. Normally a patient will manipulate it skillfully and identify it correctly. Asking the patient to distinguish ''heads'' from ''tails'' on a coin is a sensitive test of stereognosis.

Astereognosis refers to the inability to recognize objects placed in the hand.

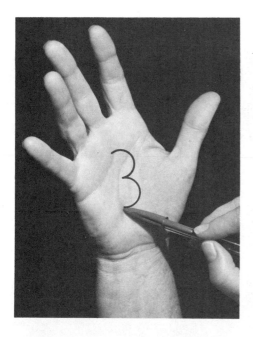

b. *Number identification (graphesthesia).* When motor impairment, arthritis, or other conditions prevent the patient from manipulating an object well enough to identify it, test the ability to identify numbers. With the blunt end of a pen or pencil, draw a large number in the patient's palm. A normal person can identify most such numbers.

The inability to recognize numbers, like astereognosis, suggests a lesion in the sensory cortex.

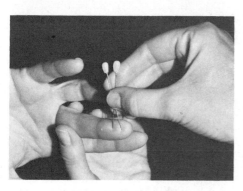

c. *Two-point discrimination.* Using the sides of two pins or the two ends of an opened paper clip, touch a finger pad in two places simultaneously. Alternate the double stimulus irregularly with a one-point touch. This stimulus should not cause pain.

Find the minimal distance at which the patient can discriminate one from two points (normally less than 5 mm on the finger pads). This test may be used on other parts of the body but normal distances vary widely from one body region to another.

Lesions of the sensory cortex increase the distance between two recognizable points.

d. *Point localization.* Briefly touch a point on the patient's skin. Then ask the patient to open both eyes and point to the place touched. Normally a person can do so accurately. This test, together with that for extinction, is especially useful on the trunk and legs.

Lesions of the sensory cortex impair the ability to localize points accurately.

e. *Extinction.* Simultaneously stimulate corresponding areas on both sides of the body. Ask where the patient feels your touch. Normally both stimuli are felt.

With lesions of the sensory cortex, only one stimulus may be recognized. The stimulus on the side opposite the damaged cortex is extinguished.

REFLEXES

To *elicit a deep tendon reflex,* persuade the patient to relax, position the limbs properly and symmetrically, and strike the tendon briskly, using a wrist movement. Your strike should be quick and direct, not glancing. You may use either the pointed or the flat end of the hammer. The pointed end is useful in striking small areas, such as your finger as it overlies the biceps tendon, while the flat end gives the patient less discomfort over the brachioradialis. Hold the reflex hammer between your thumb and index finger so that it swings freely within the limits set by your palm and other fingers. Note the speed, force, and amplitude of the reflex response. Always compare one side with the other.

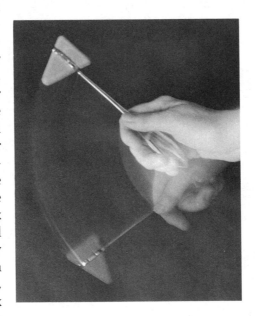

Reflexes are usually graded on a 0 to 4+ scale:

4+ Very brisk, hyperactive; often indicative of disease; often associated with clonus (rhythmic oscillations between flexion and extension)
3+ Brisker than average; possibly but not necessarily indicative of disease
2+ Average; normal
1+ Somewhat diminished; low normal
0 No response

Reflex response depends partly on the force of your stimulus. Use no more force than you need to provoke a definite response. Differences between sides are usually easier to assess than symmetrical changes. Symmetrically diminished or absent reflexes may be found in some normal people.

Hyperactive reflexes suggest upper motor neuron disease. Sustained clonus confirms it. Reflexes may be diminished or absent when sensation is lost, when the relevant spinal segments are damaged, or when the lower motor neurons are damaged. Diseases of muscles and neuromuscular junctions may also decrease reflexes.

If the patient's reflexes are symmetrically diminished or absent, use *reinforcement,* a technique involving isometric contraction of other muscles that may increase reflex activity. In testing arm reflexes, for example, ask the patient to clench the teeth or to squeeze one thigh with the opposite hand. If leg reflexes are diminished or absent, reinforce them by asking the patient to lock fingers and pull one hand against the other. Tell the patient to pull just before you strike the tendon.

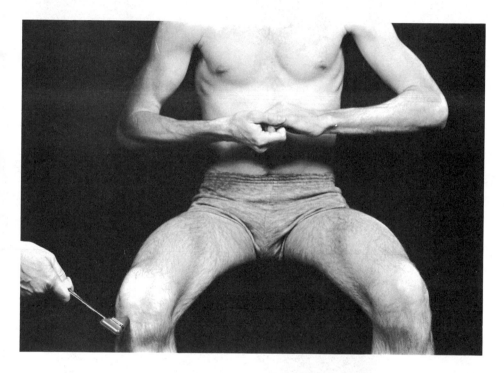

THE BICEPS REFLEX (C5, C6). The patient's arms should be partially flexed at the elbows with palms down. Place your thumb or finger firmly on the biceps tendon. Strike with the reflex hammer so that the blow is aimed directly through your digit toward the biceps tendon.

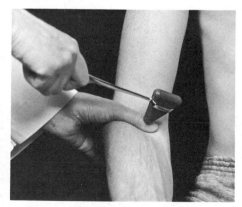
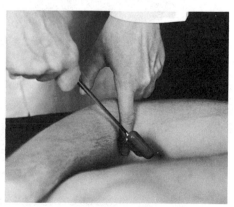

PATIENT SITTING   **PATIENT LYING DOWN**

Observe flexion at the elbow, and watch for and feel the contraction of the biceps muscle.

THE TRICEPS REFLEX (C6, C7, C8). Flex the patient's arm at the elbow, with palm toward the body, and pull it slightly across the chest. Strike the triceps tendon above the elbow. Use a direct blow from directly behind it. Watch for contraction of the triceps muscle and extension at the elbow.

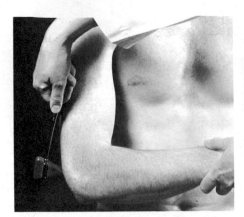

PATIENT SITTING

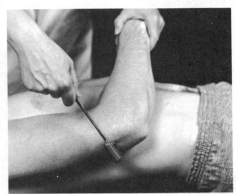

PATIENT LYING DOWN

When it is difficult to get a sitting patient relaxed for a triceps reflex, an alternate method may help. Support the upper arm as illustrated, and ask the patient to let it go limp as if it were "hung up to dry." Then strike the triceps tendon.

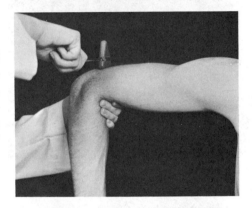

THE SUPINATOR OR BRACHIORA-DIALIS REFLEX (C5, C6). The patient's forearm should rest on the abdomen or in the lap, palm down. Strike the radius about 1 to 2 inches above the wrist. Observe flexion and supination of the forearm.

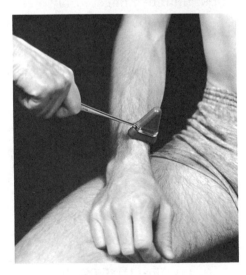

THE ABDOMINAL REFLEXES. Test the abdominal reflexes by lightly but briskly stroking each side of the abdomen, above (T8, T9, T10) and below (T10, T11, T12) the umbilicus, in the directions illustrated. Use a key, the

Abdominal reflexes may be absent in both upper and lower motor neuron disorders.

opposite end of a cotton-tipped applicator, or a tongue blade twisted so that it is split longitudinally. Note the contraction of the abdominal muscles and deviation of the umbilicus toward the stimulus. Obesity may mask an abdominal reflex. In this situation, use your finger to retract the patient's umbilicus away from the side to be stimulated. Feel with your retracting finger for the muscular contraction.

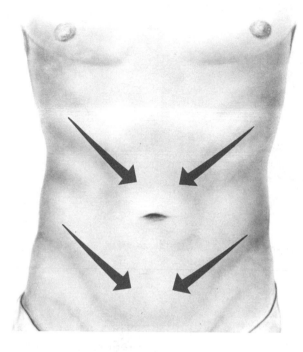

THE KNEE REFLEX (L2, L3, L4). The patient may be either sitting or lying down as long as the knee is flexed. Briskly tap the patellar tendon just below the patella. Note contraction of the quadriceps with extension at the knee.

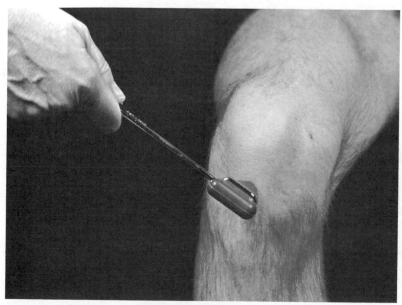

PATIENT SITTING

Two methods are useful in examining the supine patient. Supporting both knees at once, as shown below on the left, allows you to assess small differences between knee reflexes by repeated testing of one and then the other. Sometimes, however, supporting both legs is uncomfortable for both the examiner and the patient. A comfortable alternative method by which your supporting arm is in turn supported by the patient's opposite leg is shown below on the right. Some patients are better able to relax with this method.

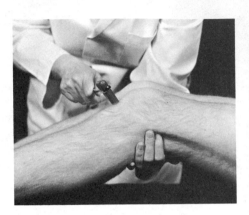 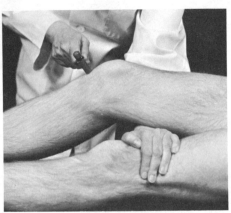

THE ANKLE REFLEX (S1, S2). With the leg somewhat flexed at the knee, dorsiflex the foot at the ankle. Persuade the patient to relax. Strike the Achilles tendon. Watch for plantar flexion at the ankle. Note also the speed of relaxation after muscular contraction.

The slowed relaxation phase of reflexes in hypothyroidism is often easily seen and felt in the ankle reflex.

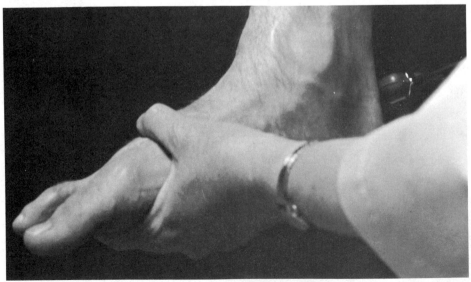

PATIENT SITTING

When the patient is lying down, flex one leg at both hip and knee and rotate it externally so that it rests across the opposite shin. Then dorsiflex the foot at the ankle and strike the Achilles tendon.

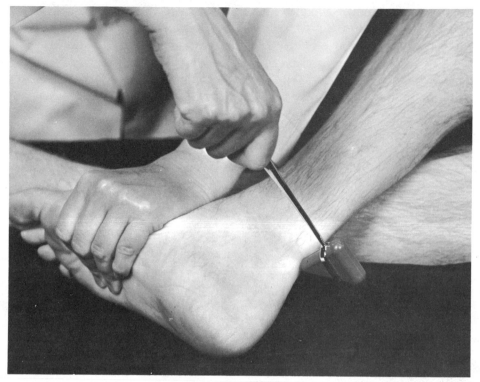

PATIENT LYING DOWN

THE PLANTAR RESPONSE (L4, L5, S1, S2). With a moderately sharp object such as a key, stroke the lateral aspect of the sole from the heel to the ball of the foot, curving medially across the ball. Use the lightest stimulus that will provoke a response. Note movement of the toes, normally flexion.

Dorsiflexion of the great toe with fanning of the other toes (Babinski response) indicates upper motor neuron disease. It

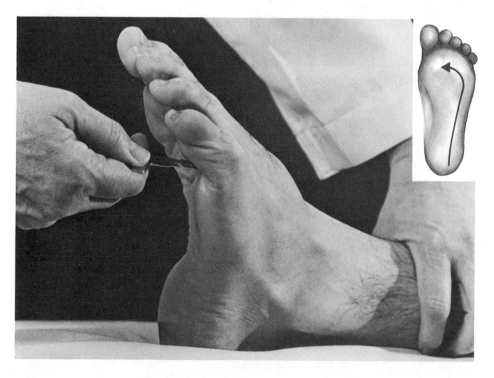

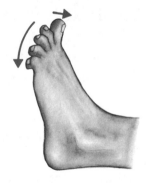

may also occur in unconscious states associated with drug and alcohol intoxication or following an epileptic seizure.

Some patients withdraw from this stimulus by flexing the hip and knee. Hold the ankle, if necessary, to complete your observation. It is sometimes difficult to distinguish withdrawal from a Babinski response.

If the reflexes are hyperreactive, test for *ankle clonus.* Support the knee in a partly flexed position. With your other hand dorsiflex and plantar flex the foot a few times while encouraging the patient to relax, and then sharply dorsiflex the foot and maintain it in dorsiflexion. Look and feel for rhythmic oscillations between dorsiflexion and plantar flexion. A few clonic beats may be seen in normal persons, especially when a patient is tense or has exercised.

A marked Babinski response is occasionally accompanied by reflex flexion at hip and knee.

Sustained clonus indicates upper motor neuron disease.

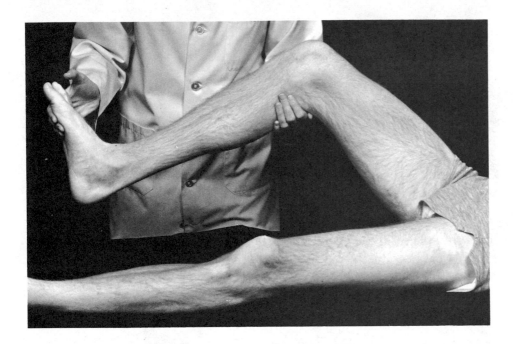

Clonus may also be elicited at other joints. A sharp downward displacement of the patella, for example, may elicit patellar clonus in the extended knee.

SPECIAL MANEUVERS

MENINGEAL SIGNS. Testing for meningeal signs is not part of a routine examination but should be done when you suspect inflammation of the meninges, by infection (meningitis), for example, or by blood (as in subarachnoid hemorrhage). (See also pp. 555–556 and 589.)

With the patient recumbent, place your hands behind the patient's head and flex the neck forward, until the chin touches the chest if possible. Note resistance or pain. Watch also for flexion of the patient's hips and knees in reaction to your maneuver (*Brudzinski's sign*).

Pain in the neck and resistance to flexion suggest meningeal inflammation but may be due to arthritis or neck injury. Flexion of hips and knees suggests meningeal inflammation.

Flex one of the patient's legs at hip and knee, and then straighten the knee. Note resistance or pain (*Kernig's sign*).

Resistance to straightening the knee and pain in the low back and posterior thigh suggest meningeal inflammation or possibly compression of a nerve root.

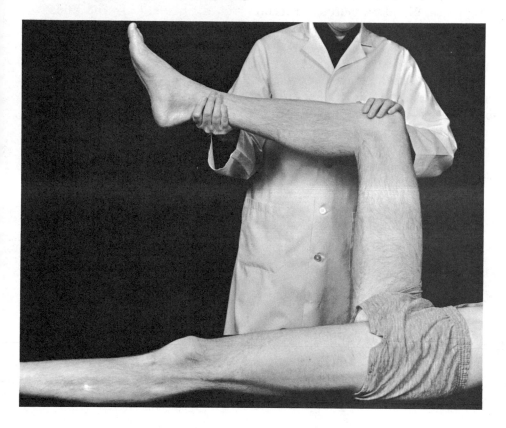

FRONTAL RELEASE SIGNS. When you suspect widespread disease of the brain, because of bilateral hyperactive reflexes and Babinski responses, for example, or because of signs of dementia (see p. 116), look for frontal release signs. These include:

1. The *grasp reflex*. While you are talking with the patient, insert your fingers between the patient's thumb and fingers and gently touch or stroke the palm with them.

   Slow flexion of the patient's fingers, often with closure around your fingers, constitutes a positive grasp reflex. Family members may mistake this reflex for a conscious response.

2. The *snout reflex*. Sweep a tongue depressor briskly and lightly across the lips from side to center. Alternatively, tap the lips lightly with a reflex hammer.

   Puckering and protrusion of the lips constitute a positive snout reflex.

3. The *sucking reflex*. Use the same stimulus as in the snout reflex.

   Sucking movements of the lips, tongue, and jaw constitute a positive sucking reflex.

All three of these reflexes are normal in early infancy but not in later life.

These three reflexes suggest diffuse brain disease, often involving the frontal lobes.

THE STUPOROUS OR COMATOSE PATIENT. Survey the patient quickly. Make sure that the airway is clear, and look for evidence of bleeding and shock. Assess the vital signs, including pulse, blood pressure, and rectal temperature. (Laboratory studies and emergency management are beyond the scope of this text.)

Without neglecting further observations of the patient, make every effort possible to get a history from relatives or friends or from witnesses to the developing illness. Try to determine the speed with which unconsciousness developed; any premonitory symptoms, precipitating factors, or previous episodes; the duration of the unconsciousness; and the appearance and behavior of the patient during it. A history of past medical or psychiatric illnesses is also useful.

Despite the atmosphere of emergency, take several minutes and carefully observe:

The rate and rhythm of respirations

See Table 8-1, Abnormalities in Rate and Rhythm of Breathing (p. 245).

Posture and motor activity, noting especially position in bed

See Table 17-7, Abnormal Postures in the Comatose Patient (p. 524).

The position of head and eyes, and any spontaneous movements

Any odors

Any abnormalities of the skin, including color, moisture, evidence of bleeding disorders, and needlemarks or other lesions

Jaundice, cyanosis, cherry red color of carbon monoxide poisoning

As you go on with your examination, take two *important precautions:*

1. If there is any question of trauma to the head or neck, do not bend the neck until x-ray examination has ruled out a fracture of the cervical spine.
2. In examining the ocular fundi do not dilate the pupils with a mydriatic solution. It could mask important eye signs.

Proceed to a *general and neurologic examination,* with special attention to the following:

Examine the head carefully for signs of trauma.

Bruises, lacerations, local swelling

Test for meningeal signs.

Meningitis, subarachnoid hemorrhage

Examine the eyes, especially:

The fundi

Papilledema, hypertensive retinopathy

The pupils and their reaction to light

The extraocular movements, if possible

See Table 7-7, Pupillary Abnormalities (pp. 193–194). In deep coma, the presence of pupillary reflexes favors a metabolic cause; their absence favors a structural cause.

The corneal reflexes

Inspect the ears and nose.

Watch for facial asymmetry.

Blood or cerebrospinal fluid in the nose or ears suggests a skull fracture; otitis media suggests a possible brain abscess.

Inspect the mouth and throat.

Tongue injury suggests a seizure.

Examine the heart, lungs, and abdomen.

Complete a neurologic examination, insofar as you are able.

Four additional maneuvers may be especially helpful:

1. *Assess the response to stimuli,* increasing the strength of the stimulus as follows:

   a. Give a simple command.
   b. Call the patient's name.
   c. Produce pain — for example, by pressing the bony ridges above the eyes, or by pinching the sides of the neck or the inner portions of upper arms and thighs. Start gently.

   Avoidance movements persist in stupor and light coma but are lost in deeper coma.

   Observe how strong a stimulus is required to produce a response. Note whether:

   a. Motor responses are confined to one side of the body

   Motor responses confined to one side suggest paralysis of the other side.

   b. Stimuli from both sides or only one side of the body produce a response

   When a stimulus on one side of the body produces a response but a similar stimulus on the opposite side does not, suspect a sensory deficit on the latter side.

2. *Look for flaccid paralysis*, as in acute hemiplegia, by grasping each arm below the wrist and raising it to a vertical position. Note the position of the hand, usually only slightly flexed at the wrist.

The hemiplegia of sudden cerebral accidents is usually flaccid at first. A flaccid hand droops limply to form a right angle with the wrist.

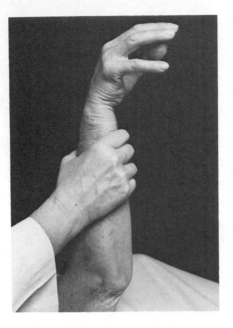
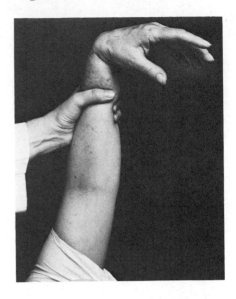

Then lower the arms to about 12 or 18 inches off the bed and drop them. Watch the way they fall. A normal arm drops, but somewhat slowly.

A flaccid arm drops rapidly, like a flail.

Flex the patient's knees and support them on your arm. Then extend one leg at a time at the knee and drop it to the bed. Compare the speed with which each leg in turn falls.

In hemiplegia the flaccid leg falls more rapidly.

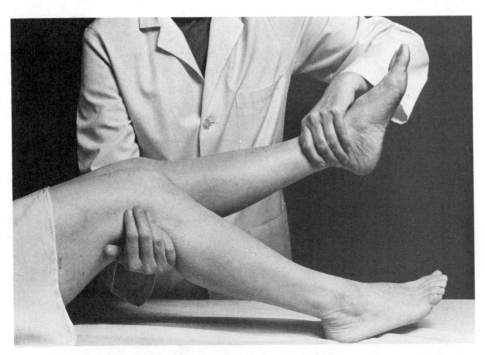

Flex the legs so that the heels rest on the bed and release them. The normal leg returns slowly to its original position.

In hemiplegia the flaccid leg falls rapidly into extension with external rotation at the hip.

3. *Test the oculocephalic reflex (doll's eye movements).* Holding open the upper eyelids so that you can see the eyes, turn the head quickly first to one side, then to the other. Flex the neck forward, and then extend it.

In a comatose patient with an intact brain stem, the patient's eyes move in the opposite direction as if still gazing ahead in their initial position (doll's eye movements).

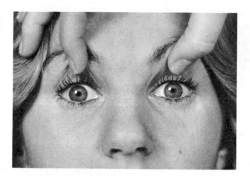 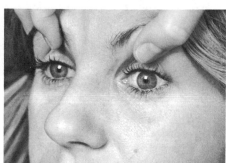

Observe the eye movements.

Unless consciously fixing their gaze, fully conscious patients move their eyes unpredictably or only slightly in a direction opposite to your movement. As illustrated above, for example, you have turned the patient's head to her right, and her eyes have moved slightly to her left.

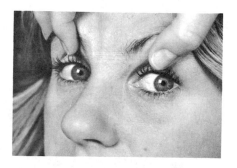

Loss of doll's eye movements in a comatose patient suggests a lesion of midbrain or pons, or very deep coma.

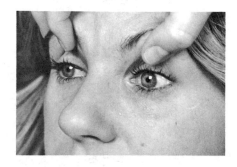

4. *Test the oculovestibular reflex with caloric stimulation.* Make sure that the eardrums are intact and the canals clear. Elevate the head to 30°. With a large syringe, inject icewater through a small catheter that is lying in (but not plugging) the ear canal. Watch for eye movements. The normal awake patient responds with nystagmus, with the quick jerking component moving away from the irrigated ear. Although a few milliliters of ice water often produce a response in a normal person, you may need to use up to 200 ml in a comatose patient. Repeat on the opposite side, waiting 3 to 5 minutes if necessary for the first response to disappear.

A comatose patient with an intact brain stem responds by conjugate deviation of the eyes toward the irrigated ear. Loss of this reflex (no response to stimulation) suggests a brain stem lesion.

Table 17-1

Table 17-1 Nystagmus

Nystagmus is a rhythmic oscillation of the eyes. Analogous to a tremor in other parts of the body, it is essentially a disorder of ocular posture. Its causes are multiple, including impairment of vision in early life, disorders of the labyrinth and the cerebellar system, and drug toxicity. Nystagmus occurs normally when a person watches a rapidly moving object (*e.g.*, a passing train). Observe the three characteristics of nystagmus listed below and on the following page. Then refer to textbooks of neurology for differential diagnosis.

DIRECTION OF THE QUICK AND SLOW COMPONENTS

EXAMPLE: NYSTAGMUS TO THE LEFT—

A SLOW DRIFT TO THE RIGHT, THEN A QUICK JERK

TO THE LEFT IN EACH EYE

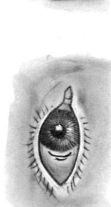

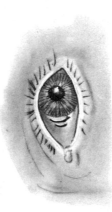

Nystagmus is usually quicker in one direction than in the other, and is then defined by its quicker phase. For example, if the eyes jerk quickly to the patient's left and drift back slowly to the right, the patient is said to have nystagmus to the left.

Occasionally nystagmus consists only of coarse oscillations without quick and slow components. It is then said to be *pendular*.

PLANE OF THE MOVEMENTS

HORIZONTAL NYSTAGMUS

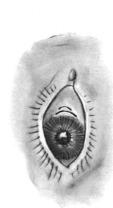

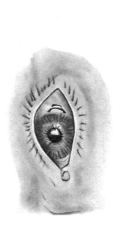

The movements of nystagmus may occur in one or more planes (*i.e.*, horizontal, vertical, or rotary). It is the plane of the movements, not the direction of the gaze, that defines this variable.

VERTICAL NYSTAGMUS

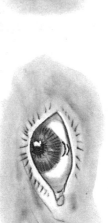

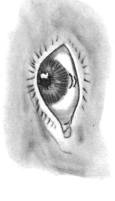

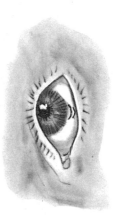

ROTARY NYSTAGMUS

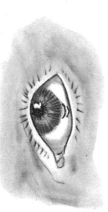

Table 17-1

FIELD OF GAZE IN WHICH NYSTAGMUS APPEARS
EXAMPLE: NYSTAGMUS ON RIGHT LATERAL GAZE

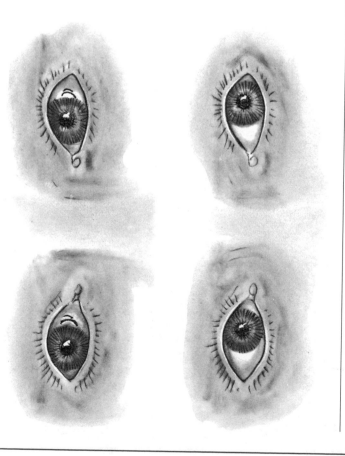

Although nystagmus may be present in all fields of gaze, it may instead appear or become accentuated only on deviation of the eyes (*e.g.,* to the side or upward). On extreme lateral gaze the normal person may show a few beats resembling nystagmus. Avoid making assessments in such extreme positions, and observe for nystagmus only within the field of full binocular vision.

Table 17-2

Table 17-2 Types of Facial Paralysis

Facial weakness or paralysis may result either (1) from a lesion of the facial nerve itself, anywhere from its origin in the pons to its periphery in the face, or (2) from a lesion involving the upper motor neurons anywhere between the cortex and the pons. A lesion of the facial nerve (the lower motor neuron), exemplified here by a Bell's palsy, is compared with an upper motor neuron lesion, exemplified by a hemiplegia. Note their different effects on the upper part of the face, by which they can be distinguished.

LOWER MOTOR NEURON PARALYSIS

Damage to the right facial nerve paralyzes the entire right side of the face, including the forehead.

CLOSING EYES

Eye does not close; eyeball rolls up

Flat nasolabial fold

RAISING EYEBROWS

Forehead not wrinkled; eyebrow not raised

Paralysis of lower face

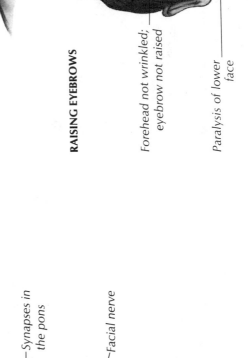

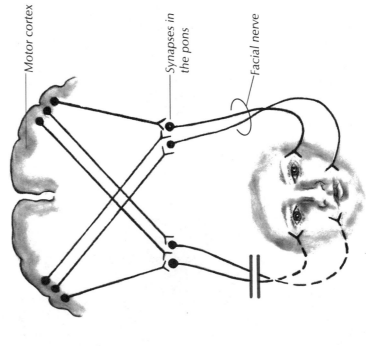

Motor cortex

Synapses in the pons

Facial nerve

Table 17-2

UPPER MOTOR NEURON PARALYSIS

The lower part of the face is normally controlled by upper motor neurons located on only one side of the cortex—the opposite side. Left-sided damage to these upper motor neurons, as in a stroke, paralyzes the right lower face. The upper face, however, is controlled by upper motor neurons from both sides of the cortex. Even though the upper motor neurons on the left are destroyed, others on the right remain and the right upper face continues to function fairly well.

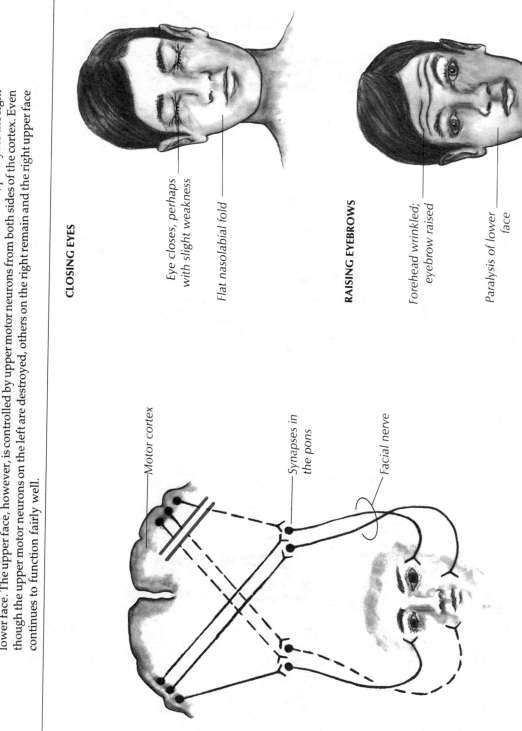

Motor cortex

Synapses in the pons

Facial nerve

CLOSING EYES

Eye closes, perhaps with slight weakness

Flat nasolabial fold

RAISING EYEBROWS

Forehead wrinkled; eyebrow raised

Paralysis of lower face

Table 17-3

Table 17-3 Abnormalities of Gait and Posture

	SPASTIC HEMIPARESIS	SCISSORS GAIT	STEPPAGE GAIT
UNDERLYING DEFECT	Associated with unilateral upper motor neuron disease, as with a stroke	Associated with bilateral spastic paresis of the legs	Associated with foot drop, usually secondary to lower motor neuron disease
DESCRIPTION	One arm is held immobile and close to the side, with elbow, wrist, and interphalangeal joints flexed. The leg is extended, with plantar flexion of the foot. On walking, the patient either drags the foot, often scraping the toe, or circles it stiffly outward and forward (circumduction).	The gait is stiff. Each leg is advanced slowly and the thighs tend to cross forward on each other at each step. The steps are short. The patient appears to be walking through water.	The patient either drags the feet or lifts them high, with knees flexed, and brings them down with a slap onto the floor, thus appearing to be walking up stairs. The patient is unable to walk on the heels. The steppage gait may involve one or both sides.

Table 17-3

	SENSORY ATAXIA	CEREBELLAR ATAXIA	PARKINSONIAN GAIT	GAIT OF OLD AGE
UNDERLYING DEFECT	Associated with loss of position sense in the legs, as from polyneuropathy or posterior column damage	Associated with disease of the cerebellum or associated tracts	Associated with the basal ganglia defects of Parkinson's disease	
DESCRIPTION	The gait is unsteady and wide-based (with feet wide apart). The patient throws the feet forward and outward and brings them down, first on the heel and then on the toes, with a double tapping sound. The patient watches the ground for guidance while walking. With eyes closed, the patient cannot stand steadily with feet together (positive Romberg sign) and the staggering gait worsens.	The gait is staggering, unsteady, and wide-based, with exaggerated difficulty on the turns. The patient cannot stand steadily with feet together, whether eyes are open or closed.	The posture is stooped, with head and neck forward and hips and knees slightly flexed. Arms are flexed at elbows and wrists. The patient is slow in getting started. Steps are short and often shuffling. Arm swings are decreased and the patient turns around stiffly—"all in one piece."	Speed, balance, and grace decrease with aging. Steps become short, uncertain, and even shuffling. The legs may be flexed at hips and knees. A cane may bolster lost confidence.

Table 17-4

Table 17-4 Involuntary Movements

TREMORS

Tremors are relatively rhythmic oscillatory movements which may be roughly subdivided into three groups: resting (or static) tremors, intention tremors, and postural tremors.

RESTING (OR STATIC) TREMORS

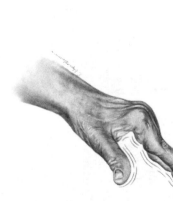

These tremors are most prominent at rest, and may decrease or disappear with voluntary movement. Illustrated is the common, relatively slow, fine, pill-rolling tremor of parkinsonism, about 5 per second.

INTENTION TREMORS

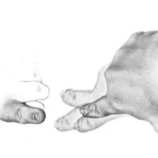

Intention tremors, absent at rest, appear with activity and often get worse as the target is neared. Causes include disorders of cerebellar pathways, as in multiple sclerosis.

POSTURAL TREMORS

These tremors appear when the affected part is actively maintaining a posture. Examples include the fine, rapid tremor of hyperthyroidism and the tremors of anxiety and fatigue. Some postural tremors are familial.

ASTERIXIS

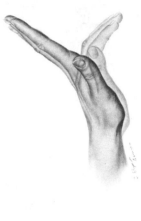

Asterixis is a postural tremor characterized by nonrhythmic, flapping movements of wide amplitude. The extended wrist or fingers flex suddenly and briefly, then return to their original position. Watch 1–2 minutes for this sign while the patient holds both arms forward, with hands cocked up and fingers spread. Causes include liver failure, renal failure, and pulmonary insufficiency.

Table 17-4

TICS

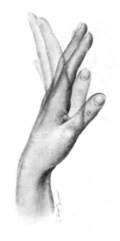

Tics are brief, repetitive, stereotyped, coordinated movements occurring at irregular intervals. Examples include repetitive winking, grimacing, and shoulder shrugging.

ATHETOSIS

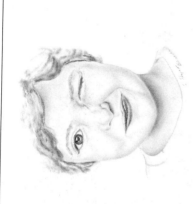

Athetoid movements are slower and more twisting and writhing than chorea, and have a larger amplitude. They most commonly involve the face and distal extremities. Athetosis is often associated with spasticity. Causes include cerebral palsy.

CHOREA

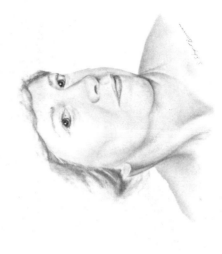

Choreiform movements are brief, rapid, jerky, irregular, and unpredictable movements which occur at rest or interrupt normal coordinated movements. Unlike tics, they seldom repeat themselves. The face, head, lower arms, and hands are often involved. Causes include Sydenham's chorea (with rheumatic fever) and Huntington's disease.

DYSTONIA

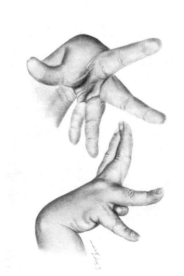

Dystonic movements are somewhat similar to athetosis, but often involve larger portions of the body, including the trunk. Grotesque, twisted postures may result. Causes include drugs such as phenothiazines, dystonia musculorum deformans, and, as illustrated, spasmodic torticollis.

Continued

Table 17-4

Table 17-4 (Cont'd.)

MYOCLONUS

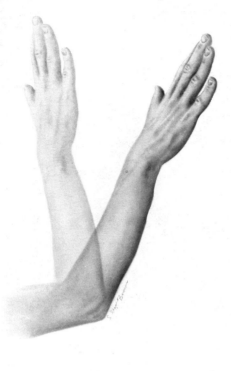

Myoclonic movements are sudden, brief, rapid, unpredictable jerks, usually involving the limbs or trunk. They may be single or repetitive. Myoclonus may occur in a normal person who is falling asleep, but is also associated with a variety of neurologic disorders.

FASCICULATIONS

Fasciculations are fine, rapid, flickering or twitching movements originating in relatively small groups of muscle fibers (fascicles, or muscle bundles). They vary irregularly in frequency and extent, but rarely move a joint. When seen in muscles that are undergoing atrophy, they indicate lower motor neuron disease.

ORAL–FACIAL DYSKINESIAS

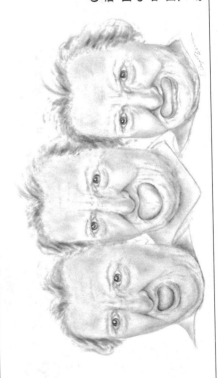

Oral–facial dyskinesias are repetitive, bizarre movements that chiefly involve the face, mouth, jaw, and tongue: grimacing, pursing of the lips, protrusions of the tongue, opening and closing of the mouth, and deviations of the jaw. The hands may show lesser involvement. These movements may be a late complication of psychotropic drugs such as phenothiazines, and have then been termed *tardive* (late) dyskinesias. They also occur in longstanding psychoses, in some elderly individuals, and in some edentulous persons.

Table 17-5

Table 17-5   Differentiation of Motor Dysfunctions

	LOWER MOTOR NEURON DISORDERS	UPPER MOTOR NEURON DISORDERS	PARKINSONISM (an Extrapyramidal Disorder)	CEREBELLAR DISORDERS
DESCRIPTION	Muscle strength, tone, and reflexes are decreased or lost. Deficits are limited to areas supplied by the spinal segment(s), root(s), or nerve(s) involved. In peripheral polyneuropathy, weakness is more prominent distally.	Weakness involves whole groups of muscles such as the abductors and extensors of the arms and the flexors of the legs. Deep tendon reflexes and muscle tone, in contrast to strength, are increased.	Movements are diminished and slowed, with little or no real weakness. Muscle tone is increased, causing rigidity which, when marked, may impair the deep tendon reflexes. A resting tremor is typical.	Balance and coordination are impaired, as manifested by dysarthria, an ataxic gait, intention tremors, and poor performance of rapid alternating movements and point-to-point tests. Muscle tone is decreased.
MUSCLE BULK	Atrophy	Normal, or mild atrophy due to disuse	Normal	Normal
INVOLUNTARY MOVEMENTS	Often fasciculations	No fasciculations	Resting tremors	Intention tremors
MUSCLE TONE	Decreased to absent	Increased, spastic	Increased, rigid	Decreased
MUSCLE STRENGTH	Decreased or lost	Decreased or lost	Normal or slightly decreased	Normal or slightly decreased
COORDINATION	Unimpaired although limited by weakness. Finger tapping on the thumb is accurate within the limits of residual strength.	Slowed and limited by weakness. Fine movements such as finger tapping are particularly impaired, but without cerebellar deficits.	Relatively unimpaired, although movements are slowed and often tremulous. Fine movements often remain surprisingly accurate.	Inappropriate speed and force of movements, overshooting, and clumsy turns. Intention tremors may further impair fine movements.
REFLEXES IN AFFECTED AREAS				
DEEP TENDON	Absent	Hyperactive	Normal, though may be impaired by rigidity	Normal. Knee jerks may be swinging (pendular).
PLANTAR	Absent	Extensor (Babinski response)	Flexor	Flexor
ABDOMINALS	Absent	Absent	Normal	Normal

Table 17-6

Table 17-6 Patterns of Sensory Loss

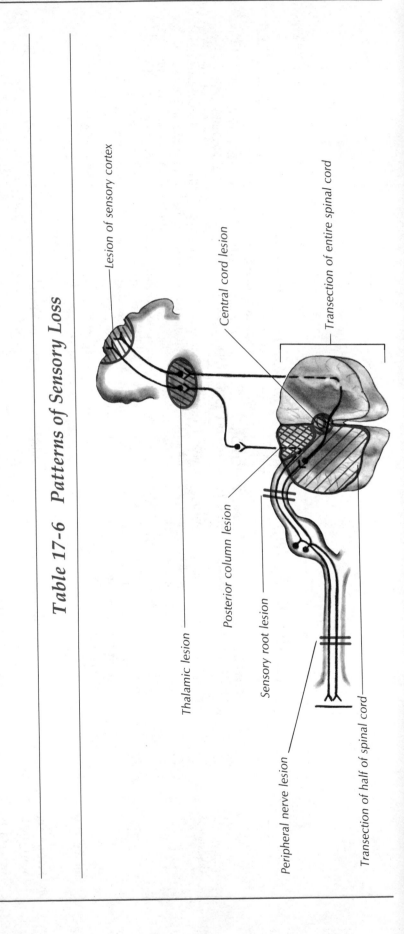

Lesion of sensory cortex

Central cord lesion

Transection of entire spinal cord

Thalamic lesion

Posterior column lesion

Sensory root lesion

Peripheral nerve lesion

Transection of half of spinal cord

Table 17-6

LOCATION OF THE LESION	SENSORY DEFICIT	ASSOCIATED MOTOR CHANGES
PERIPHERAL NERVE	Usually a loss of all sensations in the distribution of a peripheral nerve on the involved side, but different sensations may be affected differently	Often signs of a lower motor neuron lesion in the muscles supplied by the involved nerve
MULTIPLE PERIPHERAL NERVES (*Peripheral Polyneuropathy*)	Usually a loss of all sensations in a distal and symmetrical distribution, with gradual shading from normal to diminished sensation	Often lower motor neuron signs similarly distributed, but a peripheral neuropathy may be purely sensory
SENSORY ROOT(S)	Loss of all sensations in the spinal segments involved and on the same side. More than one root must usually be affected.	None from a sensory root lesion alone
CENTRAL CORD (as in Early *Syringomyelia*)	Loss of pain and temperature sensations in one or several dermatomes. Other sensations are preserved unless sensory tracts in the cord become involved.	Lower motor neuron signs involving the same spinal segments may be present. Later, upper motor neuron signs below the level of the lesion may appear.
POSTERIOR COLUMN	Loss of position and vibration, stereognosis, number-writing, and two-point discrimination, on the involved side. Loss is often bilateral.	None unless upper motor pathways in the cord are also affected
TRANSECTION OF HALF OF THE SPINAL CORD (*Brown–Séquard Syndrome*)	Loss of position and vibration sensations below the level of the lesion on the involved side. Loss of pain and temperature sensations on the opposite side from one or two dermatomes below the level of the lesion downward. Touch is relatively unaffected.	Upper motor neuron signs below the level of the lesion on the involved side
TRANSECTION OF THE ENTIRE SPINAL CORD	Bilateral loss of all sensation below the level of the lesion	Bilateral upper motor neuron signs below the level of the lesion
THALAMUS	Decrease in all sensations over the entire half of the body on the side opposite the lesion. Diffuse pain may be present in the area of sensory loss.	Upper motor neuron signs (hemiparesis) on the side opposite the lesion may occur if the adjacent corticospinal tract is involved.
SENSORY CORTEX	Loss of discriminative sensations on the opposite side of the whole body. There may be some decrease in other sensations but less prominently.	If motor pathways are involved by the lesion, upper motor neuron signs on the side opposite the lesion

Table 17-7

Table 17-7   Abnormal Postures in the Comatose Patient

HEMIPLEGIA (Early)

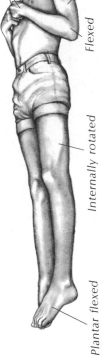

Externally rotated

Flaccid

Sudden unilateral brain damage involving the corticospinal tract may produce a hemiplegia, or one-sided paralysis, which early in its course is flaccid. Spasticity will develop later. The paralyzed arm and leg are slack. They fall loosely and without tone when raised and dropped to the bed. Spontaneous movements or responses to noxious stimuli are limited to the opposite side. The leg may lie externally rotated. One side of the lower face may be paralyzed, and that cheek puffs out on expiration. Both eyes may be turned away from the paralyzed side.

DECORTICATE RIGIDITY

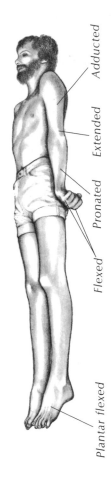

Flexed

Adducted

Flexed

Internally rotated

Plantar flexed

In decorticate rigidity the upper arms are held tight to the sides with elbows, wrists, and fingers flexed. The legs are extended and internally rotated. The feet are plantar flexed. This posture implies a destructive lesion of the corticospinal tracts within or very near the cerebral hemispheres. When unilateral, this is the posture of chronic spastic hemiplegia.

DECEREBRATE RIGIDITY

Flexed   Pronated   Extended   Adducted

Plantar flexed

In decerebrate rigidity the jaws are clenched and the neck extended. The arms are adducted and stiffly extended at the elbows, with forearms pronated, wrists and fingers flexed. The legs are stiffly extended at the knees with the feet plantar flexed. This posture may occur spontaneously or only in response to external stimuli such as light, noise, or pain. It is caused by a lesion in the diencephalon, midbrain, or pons, although severe metabolic disorders such as hypoxia or hypoglycemia may also produce it.

Chapter 18
The Physical Examination of Infants and Children

Robert A. Hoekelman

The anatomy and physiology, the techniques of examination, and the normal and abnormal findings presented in the foregoing sections of this book are focused primarily on the adult patient. Most of what is presented is also applicable to infants and children. In the process of development, however, children are anatomically and physiologically unique. Consequently, many of the techniques of examination, the physical findings, and the significance of the findings are altered in younger patients.

The purpose of this section is to describe how to conduct those parts of the physical examination of infants and children that require different approaches and techniques than those used for the physical examination of adults. No attempt will be made to discuss or describe findings other than the normal, variations of normal, and those accompanying common pathologic conditions of infancy and childhood. Uncommon pathologic conditions will not be presented except for those few that require specific examination techniques for detection. The texts listed in the bibliography should be consulted for complete differential diagnoses of abnormal physical findings.

When assessing an infant or a child, always consider where the patient is on the continuum of growth and development, as well as the age range in which that point is normally reached. You must also reflect upon the different rates of growth of the various systems of the body. For example, growth and development of the central nervous system, the lymphatic system, and the reproductive system parallel neither general somatic growth nor each other. The figure at the right illustrates these differences.

It is essential, therefore, that in examining infants and children you are well acquainted with the normal and abnormal patterns of growth and development. You should be aware, for example, that a physical finding such as a Babinski response is abnormal beyond the age of 2 years, but may be found in as many as 10% of normal subjects prior to that age. The scope of this text does not allow for inclusion of this kind of comprehensive developmental information in any form other than the method used to

GROWTH PATTERNS OF VARIOUS SYSTEMS

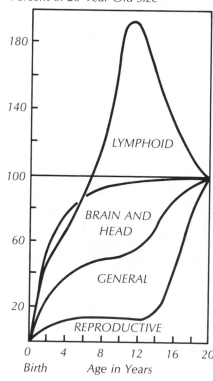

Percent of 20-Year-Old Size

screen for attainment of developmental milestones discussed on page 533 and illustrated on pages 534 and 535—the Denver Developmental Screening Test. Texts dealing with this information in greater depth are listed in the bibliography.

Measurement of length, weight, and head circumference at various ages is very useful in comparing physical growth for individual infants, children, and adolescents with norms in these dimensions. The grids for length and weight on page 528 are used for females and those on page 529 for males. Similar grids are available for head circumference measurements. Entries on these grids should be made at each well-child visit, more frequently scheduled during the first 2 years of life than thereafter (see page 530 for Guidelines for Health Supervision recommended by the American Academy of Pediatrics). More frequent measures should be recorded when a patient is not keeping pace with these physical growth parameters over time or begins to fall behind the expected patterns of growth.

In each part of the pediatric physical examination, beginning with the approach to the patient, it is useful to consider *four developmental levels:* infancy (the first year), early childhood (1 year through 4 years), late childhood (5 years through 12 years), and adolescence (13 years through 20 years). Only the first three of these developmental levels will be discussed in this chapter. The physical examination of the adolescent patient is conducted essentially as that of the adult, described in the preceding chapters of this textbook.

Because treatment of individual systems here is brief, sections on *techniques of examination* are set off in boldface rather than presented separately, as in the earlier chapters.

The reader should return to Chapter 4, *Physical Examination: Approach and Overview,* to recall the methods and sequence of examining an adult patient before proceeding with the descriptions of the methods and sequence of conducting physical examinations on infants and children, as detailed in the rest of this chapter. By and large, the methods used to examine adults can be applied to the examination of infants and children. There are certain exceptions to this, however, which are noted in the various sections that follow. The sequence of examination is different in infants and children in that potentially painful or distressing maneuvers should be performed near the end of the examination and relatively non-disturbing maneuvers performed early on. For example, palpating the head and neck, determining the range of motion of the extremities at each joint, and auscultating the heart and lungs are best done early, since they are less threatening than looking into the ears and mouth or palpating the abdomen, which should be done near the end of the examination. Areas of the body in which the patient, by history, is having pain should be examined last.

In general, neophyte (and some veteran) examiners are intimidated by the thought of approaching a tiny baby or a screaming child, especially if the physical examination is performed under the critical eyes of anxious parents. While it takes a bit of courage to overcome this feeling, one soon comes to accept this challenge easily and to enjoy almost all such encounters.

APPROACH TO THE PATIENT

Infancy

The newborn should be examined briefly, immediately after birth, to determine the general condition of cardiorespiratory, neurologic, and gastrointestinal systems and to detect any gross congenital abnormalities.

Newborn infants may be classified according to their birth weight, their gestational age (maturity), or a combination of these two dimensions.

Classification by Birth Weight
Premature = Birth weight < 2500 grams
Full-term = Birth weight ≥ 2500 grams

Classification by Gestational Age
Pre-term = Gestation ≤ 37 weeks
Term = Gestation 38 to 42 weeks
Post-term = Gestation ≥ 42 weeks

Classification by Birth Weight and Gestational Age
Weight Small for Gestational Age (SGA) = Birth weight < 10th percentile on the intrauterine growth curve

Weight Appropriate for Gestational Age (AGA) = Birth weight within the 10th and 90th percentile on the intrauterine growth curve

Weight Large for Gestational Age (LGA) = Birth weight > 90th percentile on the intrauterine growth curve

(Figures on pages 528–529 adapted from: Hamill PVV, Drizd TA, Johnson CL, Reed RB, Roche AF, Moore AM: Physical growth: National Center for Health Statistics percentiles. AM J CLIN NUTR 32:607–629, 1979. Data from the National Center for Health Statistics [NCHS], Hyattsville, MD. Figures provided through the courtesy of Ross Laboratories, Columbus, OH)

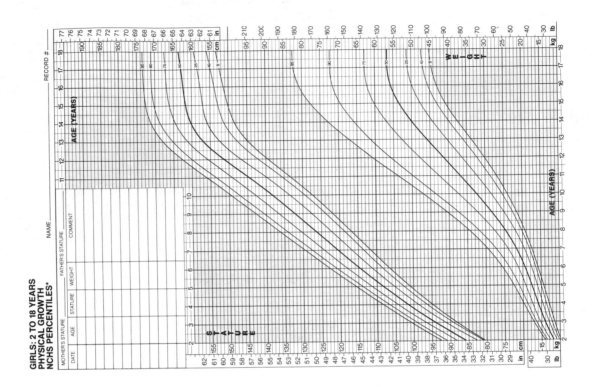

GIRLS: 2 TO 18 YEARS
PHYSICAL GROWTH
NCHS PERCENTILES*

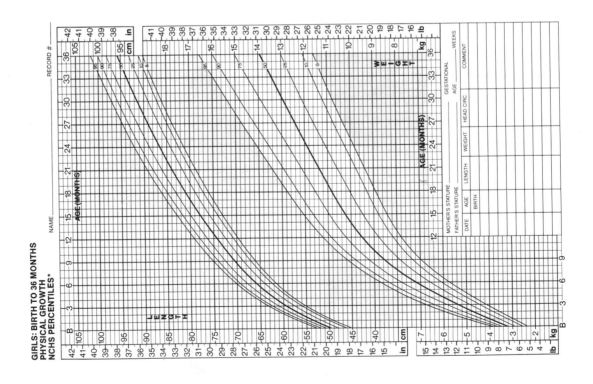

GIRLS: BIRTH TO 36 MONTHS
PHYSICAL GROWTH
NCHS PERCENTILES*

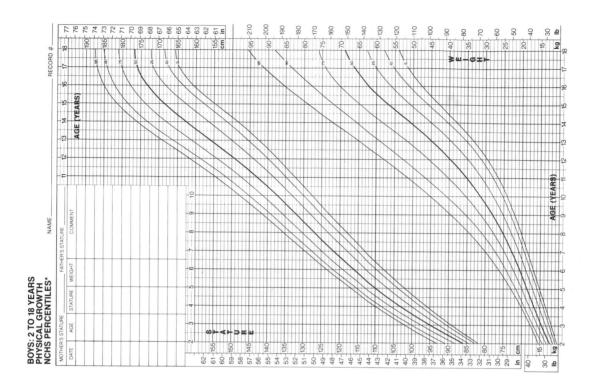

BOYS: 2 TO 18 YEARS
PHYSICAL GROWTH
NCHS PERCENTILES*

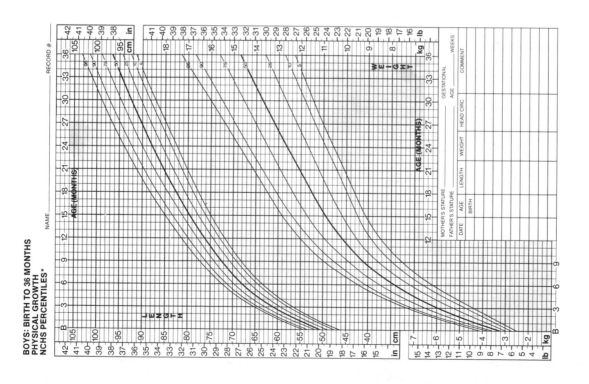

BOYS: BIRTH TO 36 MONTHS
PHYSICAL GROWTH
NCHS PERCENTILES*

GUIDELINES FOR HEALTH SUPERVISION

Each child and family is unique; therefore these **Guidelines for Health Supervision of Children and Youth**[1] are designed for the care of children who are receiving competent parenting, have no manifestations of any important health problems, and are growing and developing in satisfactory fashion. **Additional visits may become necessary** if circumstances suggest variations from normal. These guidelines represent a consensus by the Committee on Practice and Ambulatory Medicine, in consultation with the membership of the American Academy of Pediatrics

through the Chapter Chairmen.

The Committee emphasizes the great importance of **continuity of care** in comprehensive health supervision[2] and the need to avoid **fragmentation of care**[3].

A **prenatal visit** by the parents for anticipatory guidance and pertinent medical history is strongly recommended.

Health supervision should begin with medical care of the newborn in the hospital.

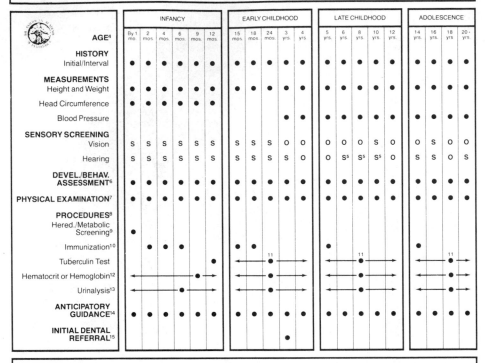

	INFANCY						EARLY CHILDHOOD					LATE CHILDHOOD					ADOLESCENCE			
AGE[4]	By 1 mo.	2 mos.	4 mos.	6 mos.	9 mos.	12 mos.	15 mos.	18 mos.	24 mos.	3 yrs.	4 yrs.	5 yrs.	6 yrs.	8 yrs.	10 yrs.	12 yrs.	14 yrs.	16 yrs.	18 yrs.	20- yrs
HISTORY Initial/Interval	●	●	●	●	●	●	●	●	●	●	●	●	●	●	●	●	●	●	●	●
MEASUREMENTS Height and Weight	●	●	●	●	●	●	●	●	●	●	●	●	●	●	●	●	●	●	●	●
Head Circumference	●	●	●	●	●	●														
Blood Pressure										●	●	●	●	●	●	●	●	●	●	●
SENSORY SCREENING Vision	S	S	S	S	S	S	S	S	S	O	O	O	O	O	S	O	O	S	O	O
Hearing	S	S	S	S	S	S	S	S	S	S	O	O	S[5]	S[5]	S[5]	O	S	S	O	S
DEVEL./BEHAV. ASSESSMENT[6]	●	●	●	●	●	●	●	●	●	●	●	●	●	●	●	●	●	●	●	●
PHYSICAL EXAMINATION[7]	●	●	●	●	●	●	●	●	●	●	●	●	●	●	●	●	●	●	●	●
PROCEDURES[8] Hered./Metabolic Screening[9]	●																			
Immunization[10]		●	●	●			●	●				●					●			
Tuberculin Test						●			●[11]					●[11]				●[11]		
Hematocrit or Hemoglobin[12]		←—————			●			←—————		●				←—————		●		←—————		→
Urinalysis[13]		←—————		●				←—————		●										
ANTICIPATORY GUIDANCE[14]	●	●	●	●	●	●	●	●	●	●	●	●	●	●	●	●	●	●	●	●
INITIAL DENTAL REFERRAL[15]										●										

1. Committee on Practice and Ambulatory Medicine, 1981.
2. Statement on Continuity of Pediatric Care, Committee on Standards of Child Health Care, 1978.
3. Statement on Fragmentation of Pediatric Care, Committee on Standards of Child Health Care, 1978.
4. If a child comes under care for the first time at any point on the Schedule, or if any items are not accomplished at the suggested age, the Schedule should be brought up to date at the earliest possible time.
5. At these points, history may suffice; if problem suggested, a standard testing method should be employed.
6. By history and appropriate physical examination; if suspicious, by specific objective developmental testing.
7. At each visit, a complete physical examination is essential, with infant totally unclothed, older child undressed and suitably draped.
8. These may be modified, depending upon entry point into schedule and individual need.
9. PKU and thyroid testing should be done at about 2 wks. Infants initially screened before 24 hours of age should be rescreened.
10. Schedule(s) per Report of Committee on Infectious Disease, ed. 18, 1982.

11. The Committee on Infectious Diseases recommends tuberculin testing at 12 months of age and every 1-2 years thereafter. In some areas, tuberculosis is of exceedingly low occurrence and the physician may elect not to retest routinely or to use longer intervals.
12. Present medical evidence suggests the need for reevaluation of the frequency and timing of hemoglobin or hematocrit tests. One determination is therefore suggested during each time period. Performance of additional tests is left to the individual practice experience.
13. Present medical evidence suggests the need for reevaluation of the frequency and timing of urinalyses. One determination is therefore suggested during each time period. Performance of additional tests is left to the individual practice experience.
14. Appropriate discussion and counselling should be an integral part of each visit for care.
15. Subsequent examinations as prescribed by dentist.

N.B.: **Special chemical, immunologic, and endocrine testing** are usually carried out upon specific indications. Testing other than newborn (e.g., inborn errors of metabolism, sickle disease, lead) are discretionary with the physician.

Key: ● = to be performed; **S** = subjective, by history; **O** = objective, by a standard testing method.

These guidelines, promulgated in 1982, recommend the frequency with which visits for health supervision of infants, children, and adolescents should occur and the various activities and procedures that should be included during each visit. (Provided through the courtesy of the American Academy of Pediatrics)

The figure on page 531, devised by Battaglia and Lubchenco of the University of Colorado, depicts nine possible categories of maturity for newborn infants based upon birth weight and gestational age: pre-term SGA, AGA, and LGA; term SGA, AGA, and LGA; and post-term SGA, AGA, and LGA.

Each of these categories has a different mortality rate, highest for pre-term SGA and AGA infants and lowest for term AGA infants. Furthermore, pre-

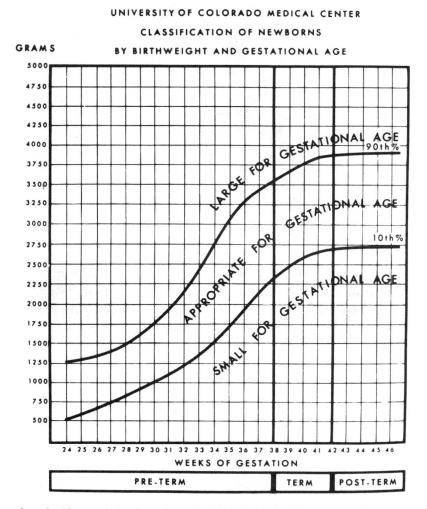

UNIVERSITY OF COLORADO MEDICAL CENTER
CLASSIFICATION OF NEWBORNS
BY BIRTHWEIGHT AND GESTATIONAL AGE

(Reproduced with permission from Battaglia FC, Lubchenko LO: A practical classification of newborn infants by weight and gestational age. J Pediatr 71:161, 1967)

term AGA infants are more prone to hyaline membrane disease, apnea, patent ductus arteriosus with left-to-right shunt, and infection, while preterm SGA infants are more likely to experience asphyxia, hypoglycemia, and hypocalcemia.

Several physical and neurological characteristics of newborns, defined by Dubowitz, Dubowitz, and Goldberger, can also be used to estimate an infant's gestational age fairly accurately. (See the bibliography.)

The infant's immediate adaptation to extrauterine life can be assessed with a set of five clinical signs developed by Dr. Virginia Apgar, each scored on a 3-point scale (0, 1, or 2). The Apgar scores may range from 0 to 10, using the method of scoring shown in Table 18-1. Each infant should be scored at 1 minute and 5 minutes following birth. If at 5 minutes the Apgar score is 8 or more, a more complete examination can then be conducted.

One-minute Apgar scores of 7 or less usually indicate nervous system depression. Scores of 4 or less indicate severe depression requiring immediate resuscitation.

Listen to the anterior thorax with your stethoscope, palpate the abdomen, and inspect the head, face, oral cavity, extremities, genitalia, and perineum. Pass a small tube through the nose, nasopharynx, and esophagus into the stomach to establish their patency. To be sure that the tube is in the stomach, palpate the epigastrium for the tip itself;

Failure to pass the tube through the nasopharynx suggests *posterior nasal (choanal) atresia.*

Table 18-1 The Apgar Scoring System

CLINICAL SIGN	ASSIGNED SCORE		
	0	1	2
HEART RATE	Absent	<100	>100
RESPIRATORY EFFORT	Absent	Slow and irregular	Good and crying
MUSCLE TONE	Flaccid	Some flexion of the arms and legs	Active movement
REFLEX IRRITABILITY*	No responses	Crying	Crying vigorously
COLOR	Blue, pale	Pink body, blue extremities	Pink all over

* Reaction to insertion of a soft rubber catheter into the external nares

alternatively, feel or listen there for the emergence of a bubble of air blown through the tube into the stomach. Aspirate the gastric contents in premature babies and babies born by cesarean section in order to prevent regurgitation and aspiration.

Failure to pass the tube into the stomach suggests *esophageal atresia,* usually with an associated *tracheoesophageal fistula.*

A more extensive examination of the newborn should be conducted within 12 hours of birth, and again at approximately 72 hours of age when the effects of anesthesia and shock of birth have subsided.

Observe the baby, at first lying undisturbed in the bassinet and then completely undressed on an examining table.

Best results, in terms of responsiveness, are obtained 2 or 3 hours after a feeding when the baby is neither too satiated (and therefore less responsive) nor too hungry (and therefore more agitated).

Observe the baby's color, size, body proportions, nutritional status, and posture as well as respirations and movements of the head and extremities.

Normal newborns lie in a symmetrical position with the limbs semiflexed and the legs partially abducted at the hip. The head is slightly flexed and positioned in the midline or turned to one side. In normal newborns there is spontaneous motor activity of flexion and extension alternating between the arms and legs. The forearms supinate with flexion at the elbow and pronate with extension. The fingers are usually flexed in a tight fist, but may be seen to extend in slow athetoid posturing movements. Low amplitude and high frequency tremors of the arms, legs, and body are seen with vigorous crying and even at rest during the first 48 hours of life.

In *breech babies,* the legs and head are extended, and the legs of a *frank breech baby* are abducted and externally rotated.

Most newborn infants are cooperative during the examination unless it is close to a feeding time.

By 4 days after birth, however, tremors occurring at rest signal central nervous system disease. Asymmetrical movements of the arms or legs at any time should alert the clinician to the possibility of central or peripheral neurologic deficits, birth injuries, or congenital anomalies.

Make sure that the baby is quiet when you auscultate the heart and lungs and palpate the abdomen, since these maneuvers are more diffi-

cult to perform if the baby is crying. Place a sugar nipple, a bottle of formula, or the tip of one of your fingers in a crying baby's mouth to silence the baby long enough to complete these portions of the examination.

Beyond this, the order of examination is of little importance except that hip abduction should be performed at the end because it usually causes the baby to cry.

After the newborn period and throughout the rest of infancy, little difficulty should be encountered in the performance of the complete physical examination. The key to success is distraction, since infants seem to be able to attend to only one thing at a time. It is relatively easy to bring the baby's attention to something other than the examination being performed.

Use a moving object, a flashing light, a game of peek-a-boo, tickling, or any sort of noise to distract the baby.

Infants usually do not object to removal of their clothing. Indeed, most seem to prefer the nude state, perhaps because it allows for greater tactile stimulation. It is wise, however, to leave the diaper in place throughout the examination, removing it only to examine the genitalia, rectum, lower spine, and hips.

You can perform much of the examination with the infant lying or sitting in the parent's lap or held in an upright position against the parent's chest, although this is usually not necessary except with tired, hungry, or acutely ill babies. Occasionally almost the entire physical examination can be completed without waking a sleeping infant.

Observation of the parent–infant interaction is important. The parent's affect in talking about the infant, manner of holding, moving, and dressing the baby, and response to situations that may produce discomfort for the child should be noted. A breast or a bottle feeding should be observed.

With older infants, before performing the general physical examination you should test for attainment of developmental milestones, such as the ability to reach for a toy, transfer a cube from one hand to the other, and use the thumb and forefinger pincer grasp in picking up a small object.

The standard for measuring the attainment of developmental milestones throughout infancy and childhood is the Denver Developmental Screening Test (DDST). It was generated by William K. Frankenburg and Josiah B. Dobbs of the University of Colorado, who used a large population of children from Denver, Colorado, to determine the standards of development against which all infants and preschool children are measured. The DDST is designed to detect developmental delays in personal-social, fine motor-adaptive, language, and gross motor dimensions from birth through 6 years of age. It can be administered easily and rapidly and

This may give some indication of maladaptive nurturing patterns on the parent's part. These observations are important in assessing *malnutrition, colic, chronic regurgitation,* and suspected *parental deprivation.*

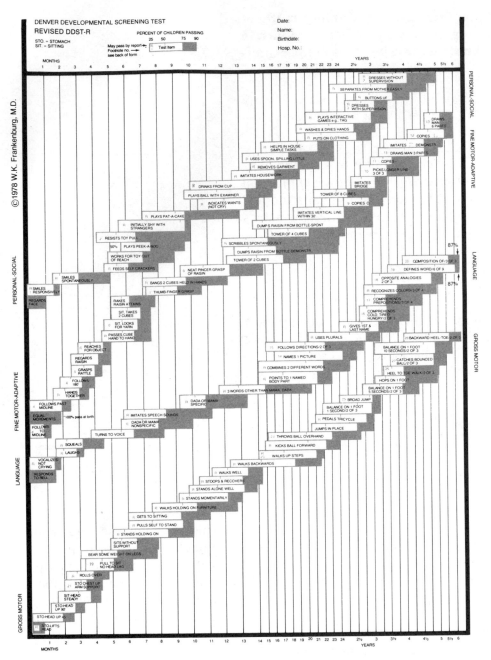

Testing kits, test forms, and reference manuals (which must be used to ensure accuracy in administration of the test) for the DDST-R may be ordered from Ladoca Project and Publishing Foundation, Inc., East 51st Avenue and Lincoln Street, Denver, CO 80216. (Reprinted with permission from William K. Frankenburg, M.D.)

allows monitoring development along these dimensions during these years. The form used for recording the specific observations made is shown above and directions for its use on page 535. Each test item is represented on the DDST form under the appropriate age by a bar, which indicates when 25, 50, 75, and 90 percent of children attain the developmental milestone depicted. It must be emphasized that the DDST is only a

```
                              DATE
                              NAME
        DIRECTIONS            BIRTHDATE
                              HOSP. NO.
```

1. Try to get child to smile by smiling, talking or waving to him. Do not touch him.
2. When child is playing with toy, pull it away from him. Pass if he resists.
3. Child does not have to be able to tie shoes or button in the back.
4. Move yarn slowly in an arc from one side to the other, about 6" above child's face.
   Pass if eyes follow 90° to midline. (Past midline; 180°)
5. Pass if child grasps rattle when it is touched to the backs or tips of fingers.
6. Pass if child continues to look where yarn disappeared or tries to see where it went. Yarn
   should be dropped quickly from sight from tester's hand without arm movement.
7. Pass if child picks up raisin with any part of thumb and a finger.
8. Pass if child picks up raisin with the ends of thumb and index finger using an over hand
   approach.

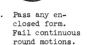 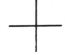

9. Pass any en-   10. Which line is longer?   11. Pass any   12. Have child copy
   closed form.   (Not bigger.) Turn   crossing   first. If failed,
   Fail continuous   paper upside down and   lines.   demonstrate
   round motions.   repeat. (3/3 or 5/6)

   When giving items 9, 11 and 12, do not name the forms. Do not demonstrate 9 and 11.

13. When scoring, each pair (2 arms, 2 legs, etc.) counts as one part.
14. Point to picture and have child name it. (No credit is given for sounds only.)

  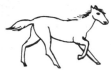

15. Tell child to: Give block to Mommie; put block on table; put block on floor. Pass 2 of 3.
    (Do not help child by pointing, moving head or eyes.)
16. Ask child: What do you do when you are cold? ..hungry? ..tired? Pass 2 of 3.
17. Tell child to: Put block <u>on</u> table; <u>under</u> table; <u>in front</u> of chair, <u>behind</u> chair.
    Pass 3 of 4. (Do not help child by pointing, moving head or eyes.)
18. Ask child: If fire is hot, ice is ?; Mother is a woman, Dad is a ?; a horse is big, a
    mouse is ?. Pass 2 of 3.
19. Ask child: What is a ball? ..lake? ..desk? ..house? ..banana? ..curtain? ..ceiling?
    ..hedge? ..pavement? Pass if defined in terms of use, shape, what it is made of or general
    category (such as banana is fruit, not just yellow). Pass 6 of 9.
20. Ask child: What is a spoon made of? ..a shoe made of? ..a door made of? (No other objects
    may be substituted.) Pass 3 of 3.
21. When placed on stomach, child lifts chest off table with support of forearms and/or hands.
22. When child is on back, grasp his hands and pull him to sitting. Pass if head does not hang back.
23. Child may use wall or rail only, not person. May not crawl.
24. Child must throw ball overhand 3 feet to within arm's reach of tester.
25. Child must perform standing broad jump over width of test sheet. (8-1/2 inches)
26. Tell child to walk forward, ⟋⟍⟋⟍⟶ heel within 1 inch of toe.
    Tester may demonstrate. Child must walk 4 consecutive steps, 2 out of 3 trials.
27. Bounce ball to child who should stand 3 feet away from tester. Child must catch ball with
    hands, not arms, 2 out of 3 trials.
28. Tell child to walk backward, ⟵⟋⟍⟋⟍⟋⟍ toe within 1 inch of heel.
    Tester may demonstrate. Child must walk 4 consecutive steps, 2 out of 3 trials.

<u>DATE AND BEHAVIORAL OBSERVATIONS</u> (how child feels at time of test, relation to tester, attention
span, verbal behavior, self-confidence, etc,):

*Instructions printed on the back of the DDST-R form (p. 534) for administering some of the
items contained in the Denver Developmental Screening Test. (Reprinted with permission
from William K. Frankenburg, M.D.)*

measure of developmental attainment in the dimensions indicated and
not a measure of intelligence.

Early Childhood

One of the most difficult challenges facing the professional who cares for
children in this age group is completing the examination without producing a physical struggle, a crying child, or a distraught parent. When this is

accomplished successfully it provides a great measure of satisfaction to all involved, and comes as close to "art" in the practice of pediatrics as does any other pursuit.

Gaining the confidence and dispersing the fears of the child begin at the moment of encounter and continue throughout the entire visit. The approach may vary with the place and circumstances of the visit; however, a health supervision visit for a well child will in all probability allow greater development of rapport than will a visit at home or in the hospital emergency room when the child is acutely ill.

During the interview, children should usually remain dressed. This may prolong the visit time, but avoids apprehension on their part and affords the opportunity later to observe their response to being undressed or ability to undress themselves. Children are also more apt to play quietly and interact with the parent and examiner more appropriately if fully clothed.

Engage children in conversation appropriate to their ages and ask simple questions concerning their health or illness. Make complimentary remarks about their appearance, dress, or performance, tell a story, or play a simple trick to help "break the ice."

This dialogue will indicate the child's level of receptive and expressive function and will give direction for approach by the examiner.

If children respond to conversation and questions directed to them with silence, shielding of the eyes, or apprehension, it is wise to ignore them temporarily.

Include in your observations during the interview a general assessment of the degree of sickness or wellness, mood, state of nutrition, speech, cry, respiratory pattern, facial expression, apparent chronological and emotional age, posture (particularly as it may reflect discomfort), and developmental skills. In addition, closely observe the parent–child interaction, including the amount of separation tolerated, displays of affection, and response to discipline.

Abusing parents pay little or no attention to their abused child, treating him or her more like a piece of property than a person. By the same token, an abused child usually demonstrates no separation anxiety when physically and environmentally removed from the parents.

Specific developmental testing (such as building towers with blocks, playing ball with the examiner, and performing hop, skip, and jump maneuvers) is best accomplished at the end of the interview, just prior to the formal physical examination. This "fun and games" interlude is likely to improve the child's view of the examiner and enhance cooperation at the time of the examination.

The actual performance of the physical examination, with certain exceptions, need not take place on the examining table. In fact, some parts of the examination can best be accomplished with the child standing, sitting on the parent's lap, or even sitting on the examiner's lap. Also, it is not essential that the child be completely undressed throughout the course of the examination; often, exposing only the part of the body being examined will suffice and most likely avert objection by the child. Occasionally a child's reluctance to undress stems from the coolness of the examining room and the coldness of the examining table and instruments (including the examiner's hands), rather than from apprehension or modesty. When there are two or more siblings to be examined, it is wise to begin with the oldest, who is most likely to be cooperative and set a good example for the younger children.

Actually, only a few children resist undressing. Most will allow themselves to be stripped to their underpants and placed upon the examining table in a sitting position without objection.

During the examination, ask the parent to stand at the head of the examining table, to the right of the child and to your left as you face the examining table. As with infants, distraction is the key to gaining the patient's cooperation. The child in this age group, however, is not as easily distracted as the infant; therefore, approach the patient pleasantly and, whenever possible, explain each step of the examination prior to performing it. Demonstrate the procedure on yourself or on a doll or toy animal. This also helps the child understand what is to be done. For example, you can place the otoscope in your ear, flash the light into your open mouth, or place the stethoscope on your chest. Allow the child to play with the examining instruments prior to their use to create an atmosphere of trust. Play at blowing out the examining light or use the stethoscope bell as a telephone to create attractive diversions.

The initial "laying on of the hands" is the most crucial point of the examination; if resistance is to be encountered, it will most likely be at this point. Therefore the first contact should be in nonvulnerable areas.

Hold the patient's hand, count the fingers, and palpate the wrist and elbow while talking gently in order to place the patient at ease.

Having both of the examiner's hands in contact with the patient's body whenever possible has a comforting effect on the patient and is less apt to produce involuntary withdrawal than is the use of one hand or a few probing fingers.

For example, when examining the heart, place your left hand on the patient's right shoulder while your right hand, holding the stethoscope, makes contact with the chest wall.

In a sense, the left hand acts as both a distracting and a comforting force. The examiner who moves in an unhesitating, firm, and graceful manner and who talks with a friendly, pleasant, reassuring voice throughout the examination is not apt to provoke apprehension.

Use a firm tone of voice and unequivocal instructions when asking a child to perform an act pertaining to the examination. Tell the child what to do rather than asking the child to do it. For example, say "Roll over on your belly" rather than "Will you roll over on your belly for me?"

Some children will cease to resist when spoken to sharply, but usually this will produce increased resistance. Often children will sit or lie passively on the examining table, covering both eyes with their hands, because (to their way of thinking), if they cannot see the examiner, the examiner cannot see them. This posture can certainly be tolerated, since it does not interfere with the examination. The eyes in this instance are easily examined after the child has dressed.

Base the order of your examination on performing the least distressing procedures first and the most distressing last. Thus, perform those parts of the examination that can be accomplished in the sitting position — for example, palpation, percussion, and auscultation of the heart and lungs — before the child lies down. Since lying down may make the child feel more vulnerable and provoke resistance to further examination, accomplish this with great care. Often you can avert apprehension by supporting the head and back with your arm while the child lies down. Once the child is in the supine position, examine the abdomen first, the throat and ears next to last, and the genitalia and rectum last. Examination of the genitalia and perineum, when a rectal examination is not performed, is usually less disturbing to the child than is the examination of the throat. However, in light of the fastidious and perhaps modest nature of some parents, leave these portions of the examination to last.

The child's comfort should be paramount in conducting the examination. Immediately before an examination maneuver the child should be told kindly, but matter-of-factly, of the likelihood of pain or other unpleasant sensations that might result. In instances where the child is extremely apprehensive about one portion of the examination (*e.g.,* the examination of the throat), it is helpful to do this first. Indeed, it may be necessary to complete the entire physical examination before obtaining the history to ensure a reasonable interview. Distasteful portions of the examination should be accomplished quickly so as to minimize the child's discomfort. The examiner should remember, however, that the physical examination is designed to gather essential information, and that the child's comfort may need to be sacrificed to some extent to achieve this end. A completed examination is a comfort and reassurance to the parent and examiner, while an incomplete examination is a frustration and a source of dissatisfaction to both.

Obviously, there will be instances where resistance to the examination will be encountered. Some resisting children will scream and yell throughout the examination but offer no physical resistance. Most, however, will fight the examination and strive to gain an upright position and the comfort and security of a parent's arms. Parents can be helpful here in orally reassuring children and in actually restraining their movements for certain portions of the examination. It is sometimes necessary to ask a parent who is overly sympathetic and ineffective in calming the child to leave the room. Surprisingly, the parent may be happy to leave, but if the request to leave is

Rarely, for the child's sake or the parent's, it is necessary to discontinue the examination

refused the examiner should obtain the assistance of a neutral person to aid in restraining the child, and make the best of it.

before it is completed and return to it another time.

The use of another person, in addition to the parent, to restrain the child is often helpful under ordinary circumstances; however, using other kinds of restraints or mummying methods has no place in the physical examination procedure.

The examiner should not convey feelings of frustration or anger, but should reassure the parent that the child's resistance is not unexpected. Embarrassment may cause the parent to compound the problem by scolding the child. Some parents feel that the examiner is at fault when their child is uncooperative while being examined. Others feel that such resistance is a reflection of the child's level of development of independence.

If this resistance is inappropriate for the child's age, the examiner should consider the possibility of underlying developmental or emotional difficulties.

Neophyte examiners are apt to be less successful in examining very young children than in examining older ones. However, with practice, perseverance, and patience, they should succeed. It is difficult to teach "how to approach a reluctant child." Examiners must learn which techniques work best for them as individuals and which approach they find most comfortable.

Late Childhood

There is usually little difficulty in examining most children after they reach school age. Some, however, may have unpleasant memories of previous encounters with examiners and offer resistance.

Question children to determine their orientation to time and place, their factual knowledge, and their language and number skills. Use intelligence screening tests, such as the Goodenough draw-a-man, the Durrell, and the Bender, when there is some element of doubt concerning the child's intellectual capacity. Keep these tests to a minimum, however, to avoid familiarity-of-content errors should formal psychological testing be necessary. Observe motor skills involved in writing, tying shoelaces, buttoning shirt fronts, and using scissors, and determine right–left discrimination for self (attained at age 6 or 7 years) and for the examiner (attained at age 8 or 9 years).

Modesty on the child's part may be the greatest deterrent to a successful examination. Therefore girls, as early as age 6 or 7, should be gowned. For both boys and girls, leave underpants on until their removal is required, even if the lower half of the body is draped. It is usually wise for examiners who are of the opposite sex from their preadolescent and adolescent patients to leave the room while the patient disrobes. Younger children often request that siblings of the opposite sex depart, and older boys frequently prefer that their mothers leave during the examination.

The order of examination in late childhood can follow that used with adults. At any age it is important to withhold examination of painful areas until last.

THE GENERAL SURVEY

Careful and continuous observation of infants and children is extremely rewarding, as is noting general physical and behavioral signs. This section will cover the measurement of vital signs and body size, which is of particular importance in infants and children because deviations from the normal in this regard are apt to be the first and often the only indicators of the presence of disease.

For example, *parental deprivation, chronic renal disease,* and *hyperthyroidism*

Temperature

For infants and children younger than 7 years, rectal temperatures should be used almost exclusively because accurate oral temperature readings are difficult to obtain. For premature infants, axillary temperatures are satisfactory for close monitoring of temperature regulation, although electronic thermometers for continuous temperature recordings are used in neonatal intensive care units. Otherwise, electronic thermometers are rarely used with infants and children because of their expense and fragility. Temperature recordings should be obtained in any situation in which an infectious, collagen vascular, or malignant disease is suspected. For patients in whom no disease is suspected (*e.g.,* for well-child visits) it is not necessary to determine the body temperature.

The technique of obtaining the rectal temperature is relatively simple. Place the infant or child in a prone position on the examining table, on the parent's lap, or on your own lap. While you separate the buttocks with the thumb and forefinger of one hand, with the other hand gently insert a well lubricated rectal thermometer (inclined approximately 20° from the table or lap) through the anal sphincter approximately one inch into the rectum. One method for holding a child while obtaining the rectal temperature is demonstrated in the illustration on the right.

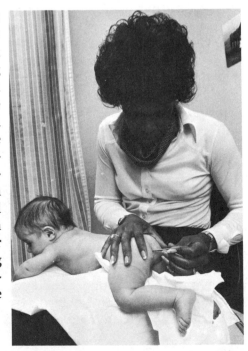

Body temperature in infants and children is less constant than in adults. The average rectal temperature is higher in infancy and early childhood, usually not falling below 99.0° F (37.2° C) until after the third year. At 18 months, 50% of children will have mean rectal temperatures of 100° F (37.8° C) or higher. Ranges in body temperature in individual children may be as much as three or more degrees Fahrenheit during the course of a single day. Rectal temperature recordings may approach 101° F (38.3° C) in normal children, particularly in late afternoon after a full day of activity.

Anxiety may elevate the body temperature, as witnessed by the frequency with which elevated temperatures are found on elective hospital admissions in children.

In the face of overwhelming infection, the temperature in infants may be normal or subnormal. On the other hand, during early childhood extremely high temperature recordings (103° to 105° F, 39.5° to 40.5° C) are common, even with minor infections.

Pulse

The heart rate in infants and children is quite labile and more sensitive to the effects of illness, exercise, and emotion than that in adults. The average heart rates for pediatric patients, according to age, are shown in Table 18-2.

Obtain the heart rate in infants by observing the pulsations of the anterior fontanelle, by palpating the carotid or the femoral arteries, or by directly auscultating the heart if the rate is very rapid. Palpate the radial artery at the wrist in older children and in young children who are cooperative.

Beyond the neonatal period, a pulse greater than 180 usually indicates *paroxysmal auricular tachycardia.*

Table 18-2 Average Heart Rate of Infants and Children at Rest

AGE	AVERAGE RATE	TWO STANDARD DEVIATIONS
Birth	140	50
1st 6 months	130	50
6–12 months	115	40
1–2 years	110	40
2–6 years	103	35
6–10 years	95	30
10–14 years	85	30

Respiratory Rate

As with the heart rate, the respiratory rate in infants and children has a greater range and is more responsive to illness, exercise, and emotion than that in adults. The rate of respirations per minute ranges between 30 and 80 in the newborn, 20 and 40 during early childhood, and 15 and 25 during late childhood, reaching adult levels at age 15 years.

Respiratory rates that exceed 100 per minute are seen in diseases associated with lower respiratory tract obstruction (for example, *bronchiolitis* and *bronchial asthma*).

The respiratory rate may vary appreciably from moment to moment in premature and full-term newborn infants, with periods of rapid breathing alternating with spells of apnea. Therefore the respiratory pattern in these circumstances should be observed for more than the usual 30 to 60 seconds to determine the true rate.

Apnea of greater than 20 seconds duration can occur in both premature infants and seemingly healthy newborns. These infants may be at risk for *Sudden Infant Death Syndrome (SIDS)*.

In infancy and early childhood, diaphragmatic breathing is predominant and thoracic excursion is minimal; therefore, you can more easily ascertain the respiratory rate by observing abdominal rather than chest excursions. Auscultation of the chest and placement of the stethoscope in front of the mouth and external nares are also useful for counting respirations in this age group. In older children, observe the thoracic movement directly or palpate the thorax to determine the respiratory rate.

Blood Pressure

The level of systolic blood pressure increases gradually throughout infancy and childhood. Measured in mm Hg, normal systolic pressures are in the vicinity of 50 (mm Hg) at birth, 60 at 1 month, 70 at 6 months, 95 at 1 year, 100 at 6 years, 110 at 10 years, and 120 at 16 years. The values for infants represent pressures obtained by using the flush method (see description following). The diastolic pressure reaches about 60 mm Hg at 1 year of age and gradually increases throughout childhood to approximately 75 mm Hg.

Measurement of the blood pressure in infants and children is omitted more often than not from the physical examination because it has been erroneously judged to be too difficult to obtain from an active child. When the procedure is explained and demonstrated beforehand, however, most children beyond the age of 3 years are fascinated by the sphygmomanometer and are very cooperative. Obtaining the blood pressure measurement should be part of every examination of every child beyond the age of 4 years and of any infant or toddler whose history or physical examination suggests that the blood pressure may be high or low (rare).

Variations of blood pressure levels in normal individuals are brought on by exercise, crying, and emotional upset. Because children may be anxious

Anxiety may produce elevated systolic blood pressure readings.

about the entire physical examination procedures as well as the blood pressure procedure *per se*, some clinicians prefer to obtain the blood pressure near the end of the examination. Others will repeat the determination at the end of the formal examination if the initial pressure was high. For anxious children with elevated blood pressures in examinations repeated over time, a sedative can be prescribed to allay apprehension, since most sedatives have no primary effect on the blood pressure. The use of sedatives for this purpose is rarely necessary, however.

Use the sphygmomanometer in determining blood pressures of children as you would in an adult. The width of the cuff should be one half to two thirds the length of the upper arm or leg. The width of the inflatable rubber bag should be approximately 40% of the circumference of the arm, while the bag's length should be approximately twice its width. A narrower cuff will elevate the pressure reading, while a wider cuff will lower it and will interfere with the technique of the procedure by partially covering the brachial artery as it traverses the antecubital space.

With children, unlike adults, the point at which the sounds first become muffled (Phase IV) is recorded as the diastolic pressure. At times, especially in early childhood, the heart sounds are not audible due to a narrow or deeply placed brachial artery; in such instances, palpate the radial artery at the wrist to determine the blood pressure. The point at which the pulse is first felt is recorded as the systolic pressure. This is approximately 10 mm Hg lower than the systolic pressure determined by auscultatory means. The diastolic pressure cannot be determined by using the radial pulse method.

In infants and very young children, smallness of the extremity and lack of cooperation preclude the use of auscultatory and palpation techniques to determine the blood pressure. However, a value lying somewhere between the systolic and diastolic pressures can be obtained by using the *flush technique.*

With the cuff in place, wrap an elastic bandage snugly around the elevated arm, proceeding from the fingers to the antecubital space. This essentially empties the capillary and venous network. Inflate the cuff to a pressure above the expected systolic reading, remove the bandage, and place the pallid arm at the patient's side. Allow the pressure to fall slowly until the sudden flush of normal color returns to the forearm, hand, and fingers. The endpoint is strikingly clear. This method may be used in the leg with equally good results.

For infants and young children, a specific cause of hypertension can usually be determined. In older children and adolescents, however, the etiology may be obscure, and in many instances observed elevated blood pressure may be a developmental phenomenon that disappears over time.

Renal disease (78%), renal arterial disease (12%), *coarctation of the aorta* (2%), and *pheochromocytoma* (0.5%) are the most common causes of hypertension in children.

Children who demonstrate hypertension without apparent cause should be monitored on a long-term basis using percentile charts, as shown below. Patients with blood pressure levels sustained above the 95th percentile should have extensive evaluations performed.

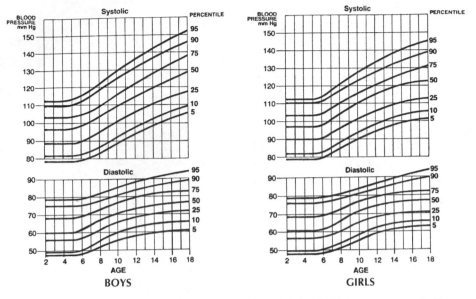

Percentiles of blood pressure measurement in boys and girls (right arm, seated). (Reproduced with permission from the Report of the Task Force on Blood Pressure Control in Children of the National Heart, Lung, and Blood Institute. Pediatrics [Suppl] 59:797–820, 1977)

Somatic Growth

Growth, as reflected in increases in body weight, length, and girth along expected pathways and within certain limits, is probably the best indicator of health (see pp. 528–529). The significance of any measure is determined by relating it to prior measurements of the same dimension, to mean values and standard deviations for that dimension as they occur in other individuals, and to measures of other dimensions in the same patient. Measures of somatic growth in infants and children, therefore, should be plotted on standard growth charts so they can be seen in these relationships.

Measurements of height and weight above the 97th percentile or below the 3rd percentile on standard growth charts may indicate a growth disturbance and require investigation.

HEIGHT. **Measure the body length of infants by placing them in the supine position on a measuring board or in a measuring tray, as illustrated on page 545. If these are not available, determine the length by measuring the distance between marks made on the examining table paper that indicate the crown and the heel of the infant. Direct measurement of the infant with a tape is inaccurate, unless accomplished with an assistant holding the baby still with the legs extended. Measure the height in older children by standing the child with heels, back, and head against a wall marked with a centimeter or inch rule. Hold a small board flat against the top of the child's head and at right angles to the rule to complete the measure.**

Hold a small board flat against the top of the child's head and at right angles to the rule to complete the measure.

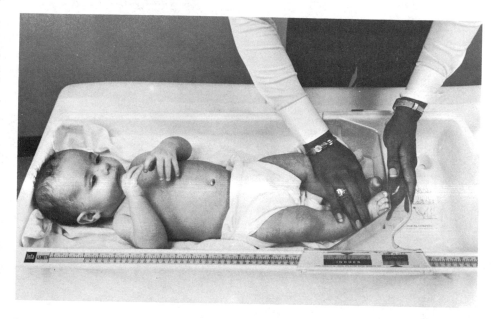

Weighing scales equipped with a height measure are not so satisfactory because children are not so likely to stand erect when not against a wall; many younger children are also fearful of standing on the scale's slightly raised, unsteady base.

WEIGHT. **Weigh infants directly with an infant scale, rather than indirectly by holding them and subtracting your weight from the total weight registered. Remove all clothing, except for underpants in children beyond infancy and dressing gowns provided for girls in late childhood. Use balance rather than spring scales, and whenever possible weigh the child on the same scale at each visit.**

HEAD CIRCUMFERENCE. The head circumference should be determined at every physical examination during the first 2 years of life, at least biennially thereafter, and at any initial examination at whatever age, to determine the rate of growth and absolute growth of the head.

A cloth or soft plastic centimeter tape is preferred for this procedure, but disposable paper tapes are satisfactory.

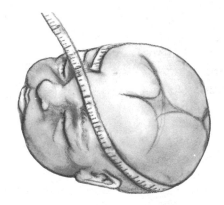

Place the tape over the occipital, parietal, and frontal prominences to obtain the greatest circumference. During infancy and early childhood, this is best done with the patient supine.

The measurement of the head circumference reflects the rate of growth of the cranium and its contents.

Measurements of chest circumference and the abdominal circumference are, in general, inaccurate and have no use in clinical situations.

If growth is delayed, *premature closure of the sutures* or *microcephaly* should be considered. When growth is too rapid, *hydrocephalus, subdural hematoma,* or *brain tumor* should be suspected.

THE SKIN

Infancy

The skin of the newborn infant has many unique characteristics. The texture is soft and smooth. An erythematous flush, giving the entire surface of the skin the appearance of a "boiled lobster" in white infants, is present during the first 8 to 24 hours, after which the normal pale pink coloring predominates. Vasomotor changes in the dermis and subcutaneous tissue—a response to cooling or chronic exposure to radiant heat—produce a mottled appearance *(cutis marmorata)*, particularly on the trunk, arms, and legs. In normal newborns, a striking color change is often seen: one side of the body is red, the other pale, and an abrupt border separates the two sides at the midline. This phenomenon *(harlequin dyschromia)* is transient and of unknown etiology. Blueness of the hands and feet *(acrocyanosis)* is present at birth and may remain for several days. It may recur throughout early infancy under chilling conditions. After 4 or 5 hours the cyanosis in the hands becomes less marked than in the feet.

Melanotic pigmentation of the skin is not intense in most black newborns, with the exception of the nailbeds and the skin of the scrotum. Ill-defined blackish blue areas located over the buttocks and lower lumbar regions are often seen, especially in black, Native American, and oriental babies. These areas, called *Mongolian spots,* are due to the presence of pigmented cells in the deeper layers of the skin. The spots become less noticeable as the pigment in the overlying cells becomes more prominent, and they eventually disappear in early childhood.

There is a fine, downy growth of hair called *lanugo* over the entire body, but mostly on the shoulders and back. The amount and length vary from baby to baby, being unusually prominent in prematures. Most of this hair is shed within 2 weeks. The amount of hair on the head of a newborn varies considerably, being absent entirely in some and abundant in others. All of the original hair is shed within a few months and replaced with a new crop, sometimes of a different color.

Desquamation of the skin may be present normally at birth, varying in degree from a scattered flakiness to complete shedding of entire areas in large sheets of cornified epidermis. Also, a cheesy white material, composed of sebum and desquamated epithelial cells and called *vernix caseosa,*

Generalized pallor indicates either anoxia, in which case the pulse will be slowed, or severe anemia, in which case the pulse will be very rapid.

This marbled, or dappled, reticular pattern is especially prominent in premature infants and *cretins* (congenital hypothyroidism), and in infants with *Down's syndrome.*

If acrocyanosis does not disappear within 8 hours, cyanotic congenital heart disease should be considered.

covers the body in varying degrees at birth. It is always present in the vaginal labial folds and under the fingernails. A certain amount of puffiness and edema, even to the point of pitting over the hands, feet, lower legs, pubis, and sacrum, may be present normally but usually disappears by the second or third day.

Normal "physiologic" jaundice, which occurs in approximately 50% of all babies, appears on the second or third day and usually disappears within a week, but may persist for as long as a month.

Use natural daylight rather than artificial light when evaluating for the presence of jaundice at any age. In borderline cases, press a glass slide against the infant's cheek. This will help you detect the presence of jaundice by producing a blanched background for contrast.

Older infants who are fed yellow vegetables (carrots, sweet potatoes, and squash) may develop a pale, yellow orange color to the skin, which is sometimes mistaken for jaundice. However, the pigmentation in this condition, called *carotenemia*, is limited to the palms, soles, nose, and nasolabial folds.

Three dermatologic conditions are seen in newborns with enough frequency to deserve description. None is of clinical significance. *Milia*, pinhead-sized, smooth, white, raised areas without surrounding erythema, on the nose, chin, and forehead, are caused by retention of sebum in the openings of the sebaceous glands. These areas may be present at birth, but more often appear within the first few weeks of life and disappear spontaneously over the course of several weeks. *Miliaria rubra* consists of scattered vesicles on an erythematous base, usually on the face and trunk, caused by obstruction of the ducts of the sweat glands. This rash also disappears spontaneously, within 1 to 2 weeks. *Erythema toxicum*, which usually appears on the second or third day of life, consists of erythematous macules with central urticarial wheals or vesicles scattered diffusely over the entire body, appearing much like flea bites. Eosinophiles may be seen on smear of the vesicular fluid. The cause is unknown and the lesions disappear spontaneously within a week.

Irregular, reddened areas are frequently found over the nape of the neck ("stork's beak" mark) and on the upper eyelids, the forehead, and the upper lip ("angel kisses"). The redness is due to proliferation of the capillary bed of the skin. These lesions are variously called *capillary hemangioma, nevus flammeus, nevus vasculosus,* and *telangiectatic nevus.* They invariably disappear at about a year of age, although they may occasionally reappear, even in adulthood, when the skin flushes in anger or embarrassment. When such lesions appear on other areas of the skin, they are larger, darker (purplish), more sharply demarcated, and may involve the mucosa of the mouth or vagina. These "port-wine stains" are not likely to fade.

In general, jaundice that appears within 24 hours of birth should alert one to the possible presence of hemolytic disease, and jaundice that persists beyond 2 weeks of age should raise suspicions of biliary obstruction. Jaundice may indicate severe infection at any time in infancy, particularly in the newborn period.

When a port-wine stain affects the skin innervated by the ophthalmic portion of the trigeminal nerve, the vascular network of the meninges and ocular orbit may also be affected. This can result in epicortical or meningeal calcifications, seizures, hemiparesis, mental retardation, and glaucoma — the *Sturge–Weber syndrome.*

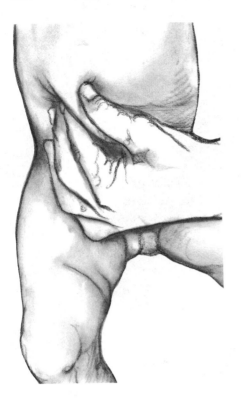

The examination of the skin should go beyond observation and include palpation.

Roll a fold of loosely adherent skin on the abdominal wall between your thumb and forefinger to determine its consistency, the amount of subcutaneous tissue present, and the degree of hydration.

The skin in well hydrated infants and children will return to its normal position immediately upon release.

Delay in return, a phenomenon called *tenting,* usually occurs in dehydrated patients.

Early and Late Childhood

The skin in the normal child beyond the first year does not present any variations worthy of note. The techniques of examination and the general classification of pathologic lesions for this age are as with the adult.

THE HEAD AND NECK

Infancy

The *head* accounts for one fourth of body length and one third of body weight at birth, whereas at full maturity it only accounts for one eighth of body length and, for most, one tenth of body weight. The bones of the skull are separated from one another by membranous tissue spaces called *sutures.* The areas where the major sutures intersect in the anterior and posterior portions of the skull are known as *fontanelles.* The sutures and fontanelles, shown in this figure, form the basis for much of the physical assessment of the head in infancy.

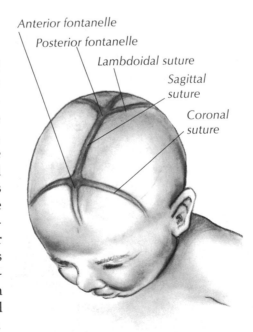

Anterior fontanelle
Posterior fontanelle
Lambdoidal suture
Sagittal suture
Coronal suture

The sutures can be felt as slightly depressed ridges, and the fontanelles as soft concavities. The anterior fontanelle measures 4 cm to 6 cm in its largest diameter at birth, and normally closes between 4 and 26 months of age; 90% close between 7 and 19 months. The posterior fontanelle measures 1 cm to 2 cm at birth, and usually closes by 2 months of age. The intracranial pressure is reflected in the amount of tenseness and fullness seen and felt in the anterior fontanelle. Increased intracranial pressure produces a bulging, full anterior fontanelle. This is normally seen when a baby cries, coughs, or vomits. Pulsations of the fontanelle reflect the peripheral pulse.

Increased intracranial pressure is found in infectious and neoplastic diseases of the central nervous system, and with obstruction to the ventricular circulation. Decreased intracranial pressure, reflected in a depressed fontanelle, is a sign of dehydration in infants.

For best results, examine the anterior fontanelle for tenseness and fullness while the baby is quietly sitting or being held in an upright position.

The degree to which the anterior fontanelle is held to be an indicator of intracranial pressure and a barometer of serious central nervous system illness can be appreciated by noting that seasoned clinicians palpate the anterior fontanelle before proceeding with any other part of the physical examination on an acutely ill baby.

Dilated scalp veins are indicative of longstanding increased intracranial pressure.

The cranial bones of the newly born infant may overlap at the sutures to a certain degree. This phenomenon, called *molding,* results from passage of the head through the birth canal, and disappears within 2 days. It is not seen in babies born by cesarian section.

Newborn babies often have a soft swelling with edema and bruising of the scalp over a portion of the occipitoparietal region. This is the *caput succedaneum,* which is caused by the drawing of that portion of the scalp into the cervical os at the time the amniotic sac ruptures. The negative pressure or vacuum effect caused by the loss of amniotic fluid produces distention of capillaries with extravasation of blood and fluid locally. These findings subside within the first 24 hours of life.

A second type of localized swelling involving the scalp, the *cephalohematoma,* is seen with reasonable frequency in the newborn infant (see Table 18-3, p. 552).

In examining the infant's head, ascertain the shape and symmetry of the skull and face.

Asymmetry of the cranial vault (*plagiocephaly*) will occur when an infant sleeps constantly on one side when in the supine position. Such positioning results in a flattening of the occiput on the dependent side and a prominence of the frontal region on the opposite side. It disappears as the baby becomes more active and spends less time in one position. In almost all instances, symmetry is restored when the position of the head becomes less constant. *In utero* positioning may result in transient facial asymmetries. If the head is flexed on the sternum, this may produce a shortened chin (*micrognathia*); pressure of the shoulder on the jaw may create a temporary lateral displacement of the mandible.

Plagiocephaly is apt to be more prominent in infants with *torticollis* secondary to injury to the sternomastoid muscle at birth, in the mentally and physically handicapped, and in understimulated infants secondary to parental neglect.

The head of the premature infant at birth is relatively long in the occipito-frontal diameter and narrow in the bitemporal diameter. This relationship continues for most of the first year of life. An abnormally large head (*hydrocephaly* or *megacephaly*) and an abnormally small head (*microcephaly*) should be recognized easily in classical presentation, but either condition will initially require frequent observation, including measurements, for early diagnosis and treatment (see Table 18-3, p. 552).

If, in palpating the skull of the newborn, you press your thumb or forefinger firmly over the temporoparietal or parietooccipital areas, you may feel the underlying bone give momentarily, much as a ping-pong ball would respond to similar pressure.

This condition, known as *craniotabes,* is due to osteoporosis of the outer table of the involved membranous bone. It may be found in some normal infants. Elicitation of this finding is not recommended unless craniotabes due to other causes is suspected.

Percuss the parietal bone by tapping your index or middle finger directly against its surface.

This will produce a "cracked-pot" sound (*Macewen's sign*) prior to closure of the cranial sutures in normal infants.

Percuss at the top of the cheek just below the zygomatic bone in front of the ear, using the tip of your index or middle finger.

One or two contractions of the facial muscles in response to percussion are present in many newborn infants and can persist normally throughout infancy and early childhood (Chvostek's sign).

Transillumination of the skull is a useful procedure and should be part of every initial examination of an infant.

In a completely darkened room, place a standard 3-battery flashlight, with a soft rubber collar attached to the lighted end, flush against the skull at various points (see Table 18-3, p. 552). In normal infants, a 2-cm halo of light is present around the circumference of the flashlight

The shape of the head may be altered by premature closure of one or more of the cranial sutures (*craniosynostosis*). The nature of the resultant deformity of the skull depends on the sutures involved. Although palpation of affected sutures may reveal a raised bony ridge in the final stages, early diagnosis is made by roentgenographic means.

Craniotabes may result from increased intracranial pressure, as in *hydrocephaly,* from metabolic disturbances such as *rickets,* and from infection such as *congenital syphilis.*

Macewen's sign can be elicited in older infants and children who have increased intracranial pressure that causes separation of closed cranial sutures, *e.g.,* in *lead encephalopathy* and *brain tumor.*

Chvostek's sign is quite striking and its elicitation may produce prolonged contraction of the facial muscle in *hypocalcemic tetany* and *tetanus* (newborns and older children) and *tetany due to hyperventilation* (children and adolescents).

Uniform transillumination of the entire head occurs when the cerebral cortex is partially absent or thinned. Localized

when it is placed over the frontoparietal area, and a 1-cm halo is present when the flashlight is placed over the occipital area.

Routine auscultation of the skull to detect the presence of a *bruit* is of little use until a child reaches late childhood, since a systolic or continuous bruit may be heard over the temporal areas in normal children until the age of 5. Similar findings may be found in older children who have a significant anemia.

The *neck* of the newborn is relatively short.

While the infant is in the supine position, palpate the neck with your thumb and forefinger, feeling for masses, lymph nodes, cysts, and the position of the thyroid cartilage and the trachea. Move the head through its full range of motion at the neck (extension, forward and lateral flexion, and rotation 90° to the left and right).

The neck is supple and easily mobile in all directions throughout infancy. Its musculature is not sufficiently developed to enable the infant to turn the head from side to side until 2 weeks of age, to lift the head 90° when lying in a prone position until 2 months of age, or to hold the head upright when placed in a sitting position until 3 months of age.

bright spots may be seen with *subdural effusion* and *porencephalic cysts.*

Bruits heard in nonanemic older children suggest increased intracranial pressure or an intracranial arteriovenous shunt or aneurysm.

A *thyroglossal duct fistula* or *cyst* may be seen or felt in the midline immediately superior to the thyroid cartilage. Thyroglossal duct cysts are rarely found at birth but may appear in early infancy. They are usually small, rounded, and firm, and can be differentiated from midline subcutaneous lesions in that they move with swallowing.

Cervical lymphadenopathy is not seen frequently during infancy. When it is, the cause is usually due to viral or bacterial infection.

Remnants of the three lower branchial clefts may be seen as skin tags, cysts, or fistulas along the anterior border of the sternomastoid muscle.

Injury to the sternomastoid muscle with bleeding into the muscle belly as it is stretched during the birth process results in wry neck *(torticollis).* The head is tilted and twisted toward the injured side, and in 2 or 3 weeks a firm fibrous mass may be felt within the muscle. This ordinarily disappears in 3 to 4 months, but occasionally requires excision.

Table 18-3

Table 18-3 Abnormal Enlargement of the Head in Infancy

CEPHALOHEMATOMA

HYDROCEPHALY

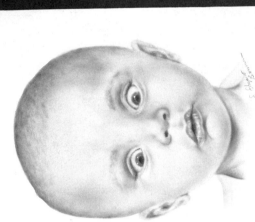

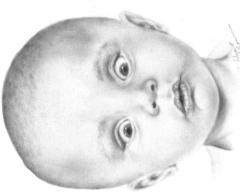

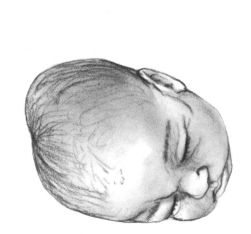

Although not present at birth, cephalohematomas appear within the first 24 hours and are due to subperiosteal hemorrhage involving the outer table of one of the cranial bones. The swelling (see illustration above, which shows a cephalohematoma overlying the left parietal bone), unlike the *caput succedaneum* and hematomas associated with skull fractures, does not extend across a suture. It may be small and well localized or may involve the entire bone. Occasionally bilateral, symmetrical swellings occur after difficult deliveries. Although initially soft, the swellings develop a raised bony margin within 2 to 3 days, due to the rapid deposition of calcium at the edges of the elevated periosteum. The entire process usually disappears within a few weeks, but may remain as a residual osteoma that is not resorbed for a year or two.

In hydrocephaly the eyes are deviated downward, revealing the upper scleras and creating the *"setting sun" sign* as shown in the figure above. The setting sun sign is also seen briefly in some normal newborns. (Redrawn from Paine RS: Neurological examination of infants and children. Pediatr Clin North Am 7:476, 1960)

Transillumination of the skull in advanced cases of hydrocephaly produces a glow of light over the entire cranium, as illustrated above.

Table 18-4

Table 18-4 Diagnostic Facies in Childhood

DOWN'S SYNDROME	CRETINISM	BATTERED-CHILD SYNDROME	PERENNIAL ALLERGIC RHINITIS

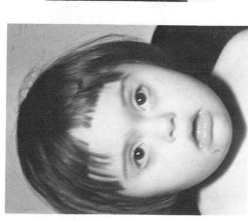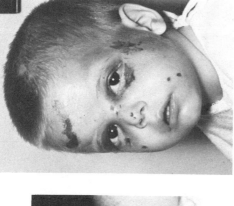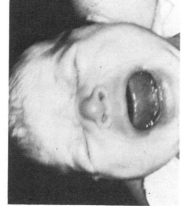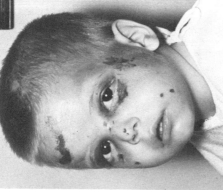

The child who has Down's syndrome (Trisomy 21) usually has a small, rounded head, a flattened nasal bridge, oblique palpebral fissures, prominent epicanthal folds, small, low-set, shell-like ears, and a relatively large tongue. (A black-and-white print of a color photograph, reproduced with permission from Dynski–Klein M: Color Atlas of Pediatrics, p 309. London, Year Book Medical Publishers/Wolfe Medical Publications, 1975)

The child with cretinism (congenital hypothyroidism) has coarse facial features, a low-set hair line, sparse eyebrows, and an enlarged tongue. (A black-and-white print of a color photograph, reproduced with permission from Gellis S, Feingold M: Syndromes in Pediatrics, Part I. In Famous Teachings in Modern Medicine. Medcom, Inc, 1969)

The child who has been physically abused (battered) usually has old and fresh bruises about the head and face as well as a sad, forlorn facial expression.

The child suffering from perennial allergic rhinitis has an open mouth (cannot breath through the nose), and edema and discoloration of the lower orbitopalpebral grooves ("allergic shiners"). Such a child is often seen to push the nose upward and backward with a hand ("allergic salute") and to use facial grimaces (wrinkling of the nose and mouth) to relieve nasal itching and obstruction. (Illustration reproduced with permission from Marks MB: Allergic shiners: Dark circles under the eyes in children. Clin Pediatr 5:656, 1966)

Early and Late Childhood

Beyond infancy the examination of the head and neck, except as previously mentioned, should follow the procedures used in examining the adult. There are diagnostic facies in childhood that reflect chromosomal abnormalities, endocrine defects, social disease, chronic illness, and other categories of disease (see Table 18-4, p. 553, for examples).

Swelling of the parotid gland may be difficult to detect during the early stages of mumps.

Parotid swelling and tenderness strongly suggest *mumps.*

With your index finger, palpate along a line extending from the outer canthus of the eye to the lower tip of the pinna.

Tenderness will be elicited when mumps is present.

Inspect the orifice of the parotid (Stenson's) duct, which emerges from the midportion of the buccal mucosa.

Redness and swelling are usually present with mumps.

Parotid gland swelling, from any cause, extends above and below the mandible at the angle of the jaw, while the swelling due to *cervical adenitis* occurs only below these landmarks.

The lymphatic system for adults, including the lymph nodes, is described on pages 159–160 and 184 (head and neck), 315–316 (axilla and breast), 359 (male genitalia), 375 (female genitalia), and 409–410 (arms and legs).

Cervical lymphadenopathy may occur under a variety of circumstances, including:

As shown in the figure on page 525, the lymphatic system during childhood reaches its zenith of growth at 12 years of age, and the size of its various components (lymph nodes and the tonsils and adenoids in particular) is greater between the ages of 6 and 20 years than at other ages. Because of this, parents and physicians often become concerned about the significance of individual lymph nodes (especially those in the cervical region that may be normally "enlarged" and even visible) in terms of the potential for such nodes to be malignant. Most lymph nodes, cervical or otherwise, that are enlarged in children, however, are either just "normally so" or due to local infections (mostly viral) and are not due to malignant disease. This is particularly the case if the node is less than 2 cm in diameter, if it is not hard or fixed to the skin or underlying tissues, and, in the case of cervical lymph nodes, if the chest x-ray is normal. Concern regarding malignancy is raised when a supraclavicular lymph node is enlarged, when fever lasting more than a week without apparent cause accompanies the lymphadenopathy, and when there has been a weight loss of 5 pounds or more within the past 6 months.

1. *Acute anterior cervical lymphadenitis* of bacterial origin with or without preceding or concomitant acute tonsillitis or pharyngitis. The tonsillar lymph node on the affected side is most often involved and is very swollen and tender.

2. *Acute posterior cervical lymphadenitis* secondary to acute otitis externa, acute or chronic mastoiditis (rare), and scalp lesions (*pediculosis capitis, tinia capitis*)

3. *Infectious mononucleosis* caused by Epstein–Barr

virus. Generalized lymph-adenopathy may occur, but the cervical lymph nodes are most prominently involved and may be quite large and tender.

4. *Kawasaki disease* (mucocu-taneous lymph node syn-drome) of unknown cause. Again, generalized lymph-adenopathy is usual and the cervical lymph nodes are likely to be involved, sometimes to a marked degree and sometimes quite minimally.

5. Malignant disease, includ-ing *leukemia, Hodgkin's disease, non-Hodgkin's lymphoma,* and *metastatic cancer,* may appear with enlarged cervical lymph nodes or enlarged lymph nodes in other regions of the body.

Occipital lymphadenopathy may also occur with scalp lesions and is usually present with rubella.

Neck mobility is an important determinant in considering central nervous system diseases, especially meningitis, because the neck may be less sup-ple than normal when such diseases are present.

With the child in the supine position, cradle the head in your hands so that you provide its complete support (p. 556). Move the head gently in all directions to determine the presence of any resistance to motion, especially to flexion. Normally, the head moves freely.

Nuchal rigidity, or marked resistance to movement of the head in any direction, suggests meningeal irritation, which may be present with central nervous system infections, bleeding, and tumors.

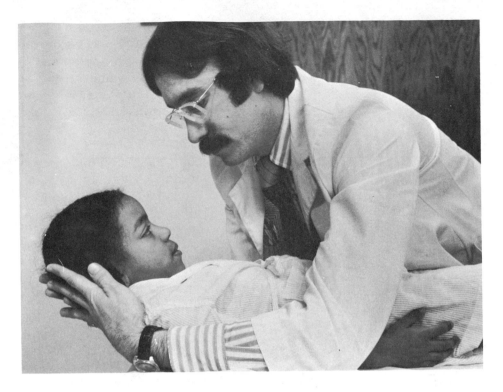

In infancy and early childhood, this is a more reliable test for nuchal rigidity and meningeal irritation than *Brudzinski's sign* or *Kernig's sign* (see pp. 506–507). The neck may retain its mobility in infants, even at times when meningeal irritation, as with meningitis, is present.

To detect nuchal rigidity in early and late childhood, ask the child to sit with legs extended on the examining table. Normally children should be able to sit upright and voluntarily touch their chins to their chests. Younger children may be persuaded to flex their necks forward by getting them to look at a small toy or a light beam placed on their upper sternum.

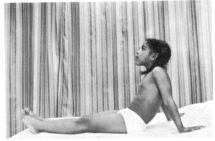

When meningeal irritation is present, the child assumes the *tripod position* and is unable to assume a full upright position to perform the chin-to-chest maneuver.

THE EYE

Infancy

It is somewhat difficult to examine the eyes of the newborn because the lids are ordinarily held tightly closed. Attempts at separating the lids usually increase the contraction of the orbicularis oculi muscles. Since bright light causes the infant to blink the eyes, the newborn's eyes should be examined in subdued lighting.

Hold the baby upright in your extended arms, fixing the head in the midline with your thumbs as illustrated below. Rotate slowly in one direction. This usually causes the eyes to open, providing a clear view of the scleras, pupils, irises, and extraocular movements. The eyes look

in the direction you are turning. When the rotation stops, the eyes look in the opposite direction, following a few unsustained nystagmoid movements.

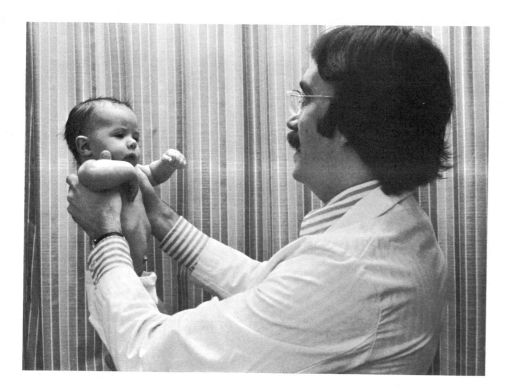

Conjugate eye movements develop rapidly after birth, but definitive following movements are not seen for a few weeks. Nystagmus in one or many directions is common immediately after birth. During the first 10 days of life the eyes do not move but remain fixed, staring in one direction, as the head is slowly moved through the full range of motion *(doll's eye test).* Intermittent alternating convergent strabismus is frequently seen or reported by parents during the first 6 months of life.

Nystagmus present after a few days may be indicative of blindness.

Should alternating convergent strabismus persist beyond 6 months or become unilateral sooner, or if divergent strabismus is observed at any time, the baby should be referred to an ophthalmologist because this may indicate ocular muscle weakness or diminished visual acuity.

Small subconjunctival, scleral, and retinal hemorrhages are common in newborns. Because the pupillary reactivity to light is poor during the first 4 to 5 months, reactions are best observed by first shading one eye and then uncovering it. The *optical blink reflex,* wherein the infant blinks the eyes and dorsiflexes the head in response to a bright light, is normally present in all newborns and may be used to test light perception. Inequality of the size of the pupils in both bright and subdued light is common, but should be considered significant if it is constant over time and associated with

If retinal hemorrhages are extensive, severe anoxia, *subdural hematoma,* or subarachnoid hemorrhage should be suspected.

other ocular or central nervous system findings. The corneal reflex is present at birth in all babies.

The irides should be inspected for the presence of a cleft *(coloboma)* and for *Brushfield's spots.* The latter appear as white specks scattered in a linear fashion, usually around the entire circumference of the iris; although present in some normal infants, they strongly suggest *Down's syndrome.* The presence of prominent inner epicanthal folds along with an upward outer slant to the eyelids is also suggestive of this malady (see Table 18-4). Chemical conjunctivitis, due to placement of silver nitrate in the eyes at birth as a prophylaxis against gonorrheal conjunctivitis *(ophthalmia neonatorum),* occurs frequently in normal infants and is characterized by edema of the lids and inflammation of the conjunctivas with a purulent discharge.

Dacryocystitis and *nasolacrimal duct obstruction* with ocular discharge and tearing may follow chemical conjunctivitis due to silver nitrate instillation.

Demonstrate the red retinal (or fundus) reflex by setting the ophthalmoscope at "0" diopters and viewing the pupil at a distance of approximately 10 inches. Normally a red or orange color is reflected from the fundus through the pupil.

A *funduscopic examination* should be performed on all infants. Normally the examination can be postponed until between 2 and 6 months of age, when the infant is most cooperative, unless the ocular or neurologic examination indicates that it should be done immediately. Such examinations are not difficult to perform if patience and persistence are exercised. However, a mydriatic solution may be required.

Instill a mydriatic (10% phenylephrine with 1% mydriacyl — 2 drops in each eye every 15 minutes over a 45-min period) for proper visualization. Place the baby in a supine position on the examining table or on the parent's lap, or have the parent hold the baby upright over the shoulder. If the baby needs calming, use a sugar nipple. Lid retraction can be accomplished, if necessary, with your thumb and first finger. The method of funduscopic examination is otherwise the same as with adults. The cornea can ordinarily be seen at + 20 diopters, the lens at + 15 diopters, and the fundus at "0" diopters.

Both retinal anomalies and opacities of the cornea, anterior chamber, or lens will interrupt the light pathway and give a partial red reflex or a completely dark reflex. In infants, *cataracts,* a *persistent posterior lenticular fibrovascular sheath,* and *retrolental fibroplasia* may cause a dark light reflex. Beyond infancy, *retinal detachment, chorioretinitis,* and *retinoblastoma* should be suspected when an abnormal retinal reflex is encountered.

The optic disc is paler in infants, the peripheral vessels are not well developed, and the foveal light reflection is absent. *Papilledema* is rarely seen, even with markedly increased intracranial pressure, because the fontanelles and open sutures absorb the increased pressure, sparing the optic discs. Until age 3 years the sutures will separate sufficiently to prevent papilledema. If vascular or optic disc anomalies are found, the parents' fundi should be examined to determine a possible genetic origin and prognosis for the findings.

Retinal hemorrhages associated with intracranial bleeding are accompanied by dilated, congested, tortuous retinal veins. Pigmentary changes occur in the retina in newborns with congenital *toxoplasmosis, cytomegalic inclusion disease,* and *rubella* infections.

The development of central vision progresses from birth, when only light perception is thought to be present, to adult visual levels attained at approximately 6 years of age.

The assessment of vision in the newborn is based on the presence of visual reflexes—direct and consensual pupillary constriction in response to light, and blinking in response to bright light and to movement of an object quickly toward the eyes.

Those visual reflexes imply that both light perception and some degree of visual acuity are present shortly after birth. Opticokinetic nystagmus (produced by the rapid movement of vertical black lines across the visual fields), used as a test of vision on one group of newborns 1½ to 5 days after birth, demonstrated a visual acuity of at least 20/670 in 93% of the group. That this acuity improves is evident even without refractive measurement references. At 2 to 4 weeks of age, fixation on objects occurs; at 5 to 6 weeks, coordinated eye movements in following an object are seen; at 3 months the eyes converge and the baby begins to reach for various sized objects at various distances as eye–hand coordination and the ability to focus are accomplished. At the age of 1 year, normal visual acuity is in the range of 20/200.

Failure to progress along these lines may indicate mental deficiency as well as diminished or absent vision.

Early Childhood

When examining a child in this age group, the most important condition the examiner must detect is *amblyopia ex anopsia*. This is not the most serious ophthalmologic disease, but in comparison with others of significance it is the most prevalent and offers, with early intervention, the best prognosis. Improvement in this condition is unlikely if treatment is instituted after the sixth year of life. Amblyopia means reduced vision in an otherwise normal eye, and the reduced vision in this situation is caused by disuse. In essence, because of disconjugate fixation, one of the two images received by the optic cortex is suppressed to avoid diplopia or images of unequal clarity. One eye then becomes "lazy" and stops functioning to its full capacity; visual acuity in that eye is reduced markedly by suppression of central (foveal) vision. Since the two most common causes of amblyopia exanopsia are *strabismus* and *anisometropia* (an eye with a refractive error 1.5 diopters or more greater than its pair), it is important to be able to test for muscle weakness and visual acuity accurately.

Obstructive amblyopia is secondary to a *cataract, corneal opacity,* or severe *ptosis.*

Muscle weakness causing deviation of one eye inwardly *(esotropia)* or outwardly *(exotropia)* may be detected by the *Hirschberg test,* the *prism test,* or the *cover test.*

The *Hirschberg test* ascertains the location of the reflection of a light on the cornea of each eye. Attract the patient's attention to a light held at your midforehead. While the patient's eyes are fixed upon the light, note the light's reflection on each cornea. First, hold the patient's head fixed in the midline and then turn it to the left and right while ocular fixation on the light is maintained.

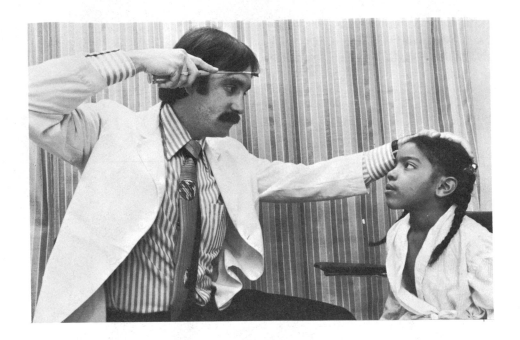

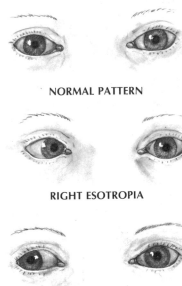

NORMAL PATTERN

RIGHT ESOTROPIA

RIGHT EXOTROPIA

To detect esotropia and exotropia, look for a change in the corneal reflection pattern of lateral gaze. The reflections on each cornea should be symmetrically placed; the type and degree of tropia can be determined by noting the pattern of asymmetrical placement of the reflections. The normal pattern and those with esotropia and exotropia are shown to the right. The light patterns should also be noted with upward, downward, and upper-outer and downward-outer movements of the eyes, although these are much less likely to reveal muscle imbalances.

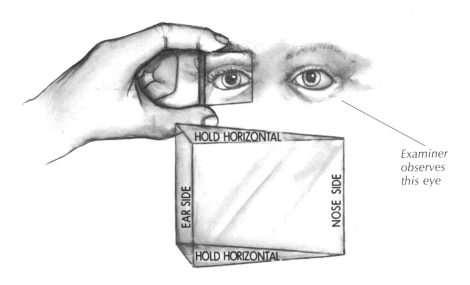

HOLD HORIZONTAL

EAR SIDE

NOSE SIDE

HOLD HORIZONTAL

Examiner observes this eye

The *prism test* is conducted in much the same way as the Hirschberg test.

Again, attract the patient's attention to a light held at your midforehead. While the patient's eyes are fixed upon the light, hold a 4-diopter

prism, base out, in front of one eye while observing the other eye (see figure to the right). If the observed eye moves inward or outward and remains in whichever position it has moved, strabismus is present. The opposite eye is tested in the same way. An amblyopic (lazy) eye will not move when the prism is placed in front of it.

The *cover test* is the most sophisticated of the three tests for strabismus because it detects frank strabismus, differentiates the type of deviation, and determines the characteristics of any latent deviation.

Attract the patient's attention once more to the midforehead light. Place your hand on the top of the child's head and your thumb in front of one eye while observing the other for movement. Then remove your thumb and observe both eyes for movement. If either or both eyes move, a strabismus is present. Repeat the test, covering and uncovering the other eye with your thumb.

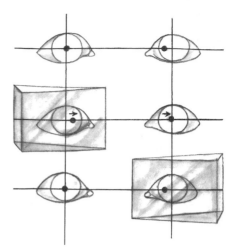

PRISM TEST IN LEFT ESOTROPIA

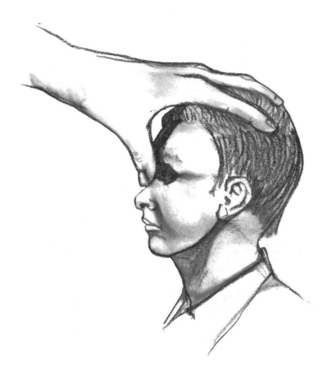

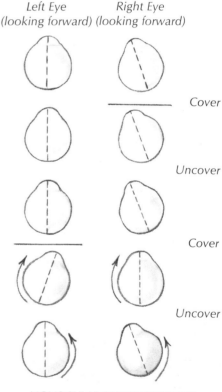

MONOCULAR RIGHT ESOTROPIA

The combination of movements observed allows for differential diagnosis of the strabismus in question. The results of using the cover test, more properly called the cover–uncover test, in monocular right esotropia are shown at the right.

Testing visual acuity in early childhood is not a simple matter. The variables of the child, the examiner, the testing environment, and the test itself all contribute significantly to the outcome and should be given careful attention if valid results are to be obtained. Unfortunately, there is no testing method that accurately measures visual acuity in children under the age of 3 years. Since each eye must be tested separately to detect amblyopia, one eye must be covered by an elastoplast bandage to ensure complete occlusion. Resistance to placement of the patch may be overcome by calling it a "pirate's patch." A child with amblyopia might accept the patch on the amblyopic eye, but not on the good eye.

Opticokinetic testing is the most accurate method for testing visual acuity in this age group; however, this method requires too much technical equipment to use in most settings. Two other simpler *tests of visual acuity* are of some worth.

The *miniature toy test* uses identical sets of small toys representing familiar objects. Give the child one set and keep the other. Ask the child to match each toy as it is shown at a distance of 10 feet. *Worth's test* uses five balls ranging from ½ to 1 ½ inches in diameter. Beginning with the largest, throw each on the floor and ask the child to retrieve it. These tests, at best, detect only grossly impaired vision rather than the degree of such impairment.

In children over the age of 3 years, the *Snellen E chart* (a form of direct visual testing) is very adequate. Most youngsters will cooperate in indicating, either orally or by positioning of the fingers, in which direction the E is pointing. For those who initially have difficulty with this test, a single E card can be sent home with the child for practice purposes. Charts with pictures instead of Es are often used but have no special advantage, nor do any other testing methods generally available. The normal visual acuity at age 3 years is $\pm 20/40$, at age 4 to 5 years, $\pm 20/30$, and at 6 to 7 years, 20/20.

Visual field examination in infants and young children can be done with the child sitting on the parent's lap.

Hold the head in the midline while bringing a dangling object, such as a measuring tape case or a small toy, into the child's field of vision from several points behind, above, and below. Deviation of the eyes in its direction indicates that the child has seen the object.

Late Childhood

The eye problems and methods of examining the eye for this age group have been covered in the adult section. In general, vision testing machines used for mass screening in schools tend to underrate visual acuity and produce over-referrals.

You can distinguish a simple refractive error from organic causes of diminished vision by asking the child to take the vision test looking through a pinhole punched in a card. Visual acuity improves using the pinhole card when refractive errors are present, but not when organic ocular disease exists.

THE EAR

Infancy

Note the position of the ears in relation to the eyes. Normally the ear joins the scalp on or above the extension of a line drawn across the inner and outer canthus of the eye.

Examination of the ear in the immediate neonatal period only establishes the patency of the ear canal, because the tympanic membranes are obscured by accumulated vernix caseosa for the first 2 or 3 days of life. In infancy the ear canal is directed downward from the outside; therefore, **the pinna should be pulled gently downward** for the best visualization of the ear drum. The light reflex on the tympanic membrane is diffuse and does not assume the cone shape for several months.

Inspect the ear and surrounding skin. Test the hearing in infants by eliciting the *acoustic blink reflex*. **This is positive (and indicates that the infant can hear) when one observes a blinking of the eyes in response to a sudden sharp sound produced at a distance of about 12 inches from the ear by snapping the fingers, clapping the hands, or using a bell or other kinds of mechanical noisemaking devices. Be sure that in generating the sound you do not produce an airstream that could cause the baby to blink.**

The acoustic blink reflex is difficult to elicit during the first 2 or 3 days of life, and may disappear temporarily after it is elicited a few times. This is a crude test at best, and the absence of blinking in response to sound is not diagnostic of deafness nor does its presence assure normal hearing. At 2 weeks of age the infant may jump in response to a sudden noise; at 10 weeks the response may be momentary cessation of body movements. Between 3 and 4 months of age, the eyes and head will turn toward the source of sound. Even before this, an increase in respiratory rate may occur when familiar sounds are heard and generate anticipation of forthcoming pleasures. Most hospital newborn nurseries test the hearing of all babies on their second or third day of life with a warbled pure-tone screening device.

Early Childhood

The examination of the ear becomes more difficult as the child grows older. Greater resistance is encountered because the ear canals are sensitive and the child cannot observe the procedure.

Often it is helpful if you initially place the otoscopic speculum gently into the external auditory canal of one ear, removing it instantly and repeating the procedure on the other. Then you can begin again, taking

Small, deformed, or low-set auricles may indicate associated congenital defects, especially renal agenesis or anomalies.

A small skin tab, cleft, or pit is frequently found just forward of the tragus and represents a remnant of the first branchial cleft.

Because the parents' impression of the baby's auditory acuity is usually correct, when parents believe that their baby cannot hear it should be assumed that they are correct until proven otherwise.

the necessary time in the actual examination with a child whose apprehensions have been allayed.

The ears can be successfully examined even in struggling children if care is taken in restraining them and in manipulating both ear and otoscope gently.

Place the patient in the supine position. Ask the parent or an assistant to hold the child's arms extended, close to the sides of the head, thus limiting movement from side to side. Make your approach from the child's right side and lean across the lower chest and upper abdomen to restrict movements of the trunk. A third person may be required to hold the feet and legs if the child struggles unduly; however, this is rarely necessary.

This same restraining procedure may be used in examining the eyes, nose, and throat, as illustrated below.

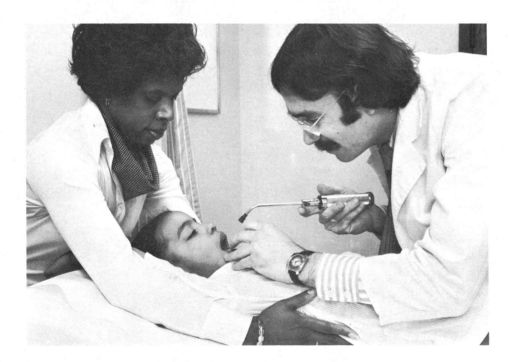

When examining the right ear, turn the child's head to the left and hold it firmly in this position with the lateral aspect of your right hand and wrist. Hold the otoscope in your right hand in an inverted position and manipulate the auricle with your left hand, the lateral aspect of which can be used to help restrain movement of the child's head. In this age group, the external auditory canal is directed upward and backward from the outside, and the pinna must be pulled upward, outward, and backward to afford the best visualization. The thumb and forefinger of your right hand, which holds the otoscope, should be buffered from

sudden movements of the child's head by your restraining right hand and your forearm, which rests firmly on the examining table. See the illustration below.

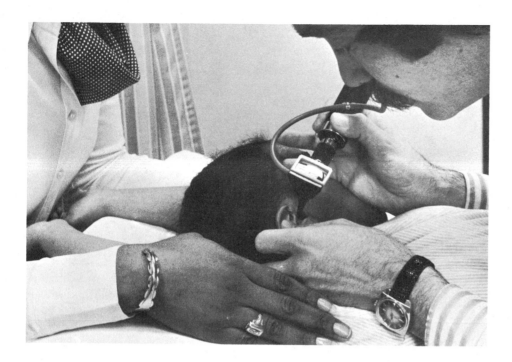

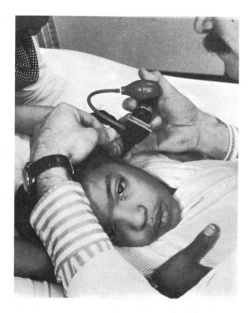

When examining the left ear, turn the patient's head to the right and hold it firmly in this position with the lateral aspect of your left hand and wrist. The thumb and forefinger of your left hand should manipulate the auricle, and your right hand should hold the otoscope in an inverted position. The lateral aspect of the fifth finger of your right hand is held against the patient's head to provide a buffer against sudden movement by the patient. This procedure is demonstrated in this figure.

The speculum of the otoscope should be as large in diameter as will allow for comfortable ¼- to ½-inch penetration into the external auditory canal. This provides maximum visualization of the canal and drum and a reasonable seal to observe the effects of pneumatic otoscopy. Some examiners attach a rubber tip to the end of the speculum to gain a tighter, more comfortable seal.

Pneumatic otoscopy should be part of every otoscopic examination; it is accomplished by observing the tympanic membrane as the pressure in the external auditory canal is increased or decreased. You can do this by introducing and removing air from the canal—by applying positive and negative pressures with a rubber squeeze bulb (as shown in the figure here and the second figure on p. 565), or by blowing and sucking on a rubber tube attached to the otoscope (shown in the first figure on p. 565).

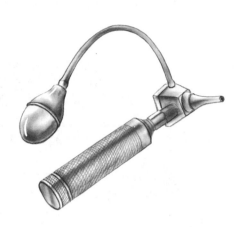

When air is introduced into the normal ear canal, the tympanic membrane and its light reflex are seen to move inward. When air is removed, the tympanic membrane moves outward, toward the examiner. This to and fro movement of the tympanic membrane has been likened to the luffing of a sail.

This movement is absent in chronic middle ear infection *(serous otitis media)*, and diminished in some cases of *acute otitis media.*

Cerumen accumulation within the ear canal commonly obscures the view of the tympanic membrane in children. Very often this is unilateral. There are several instruments and ear washing techniques that may be used to remove ear wax comfortably, but they will not be described here.

Accumulation of purulent material and debris in the ear canal is found both in *otitis externa* and in *otitis media* with a ruptured tympanic membrane. Washing out the ear canal is contraindicated, in the first instance because of the pain created by the procedure, and in the second instance because the cleansing fluid and canal debris will be forced into the middle ear through the perforated tympanic membrane.

Otitis media and *otitis externa* may be differentiated clinically by gentle movement of the pinna, which will cause exquisite pain in otitis externa but no discomfort in purulent otitis media.

Simple auditory screening in this age group can be accomplished by whispering at a distance of 8 feet.

Ask the child questions or give commands, taking care that lip reading is not allowable. In addition you can use a tuning fork to screen for hearing, using your own auditory acuity as the control.

Acute *mastoiditis* in children is accompanied by a forward protrusion of the pinna of the ear on the affected side, in addition to the redness, swelling, and tenderness overlying the mastoid bone.

If these screening methods reveal any diminution of hearing, full audiometric testing should be performed. Furthermore, all children should be given a full-scale acoustic screening test with an audiometer prior to beginning school, as should any child, at whatever age, with delayed speech development. Because of their complexity, audiometric screening devices

Significant, temporary hearing loss for as long as 4 months may follow an episode of otitis media.

used for older children are often unsatisfactory for use in early childhood; when delayed or defective speech is present, direct referral to a hearing and speech center may be more appropriate.

Late Childhood

As the child grows older, the ease and techniques of examining the ears and testing the hearing approach the levels and methods for adults. There are no unique abnormalities, or variations from the normal, concerning the ear and its function in this age group, as compared with older age groups, including the "selective deafness" some children and adolescents demonstrate in hearing only what they choose when spoken to in either soft or loud voices by their parents and teachers.

THE NOSE AND THROAT

Infancy

Test the patency of the nasal passages by occluding each nostril alternately while holding the infant's mouth closed. This will not cause stress in a normal baby, since most newborns are nasal breathers. On the other hand, occluding both nares simultaneously and allowing the mouth to open will cause considerable distress. Indeed, some infants are unable to breathe through their mouths at all (*obligate nasal breathers*). Obstruction of the posterior nasal passage(s) can be confirmed by attempting to pass a number 14 French catheter through each nostril into the posterior nasopharynx.

Obstruction of the nasal passages in newborn infants occurs with *choanal atresia* and with displacement of the nasal cartilage during delivery.

The *mouth* of the newborn is edentulous. The gums are smooth with a raised, 1-mm, serrated fringe of tissue on the buccal margins. Occasionally, pearllike retention cysts are seen along the ridges and are often mistaken for teeth—they disappear spontaneously within a month or two.

Rarely, *supernumerary teeth* are found. These are soft, have no enamel, and shed within a few days. They should be removed, however, to prevent their aspiration into the lower respiratory tract.

Petechiae are commonly found on the soft palate after birth.

The frenulum of the upper lip may be quite thick and extend from the superior aspect of the inner lip to the posterior portion of the upper gum, creating a deep notch in the midline of the gum. The frenulum of the tongue varies in consistency from a thin, filamentous membrane to a thick, fibrous cord. Its length varies, such that it may attach midway on the undersurface of the tongue or at its very tip. A heavy fibrous frenulum that extends to the tip of the tongue may interfere with its protrusion (*tongue tie*). There will be no difficulties encountered with nursing or speech, however, if the tongue can be extended as far as the alveolar ridge, which is possible in almost all instances.

Epstein's pearls, pinhead-sized, white or yellow, rounded elevations that are located along the midline of the hard palate near its posterior border, are caused by retained secretions and disappear within a few weeks or months.

Visualization of the *pharynx* is best accomplished while a baby is crying. This is true throughout infancy and early childhood. A tongue blade produces strong reflex elevation of the base of the tongue and obstructs the view of the infant's pharynx. Tonsillar tissue is not seen in the newborn.

Oral moniliasis *(thrush)* is a common malady in infants, usually contracted from mothers with vaginal moniliasis. In thrush, a lacy white material with an erythematous base is seen on the surface of the oral mucous membranes. Difficulty in removing it distinguishes it from milk curds, which wipe away.

There is little saliva produced during the first 3 months of life. As the infant begins to produce saliva, drooling occurs, because there are no lower teeth to provide a dam for retention.

The presence of large amounts of saliva in the newborn suggests a *tracheoesophageal fistula.*

Listen to the infant's *breathing* and the *quality of the cry.*

A shrill or high-pitched cry in infancy may indicate increased intracranial pressure. A hoarse cry should make one suspect hypocalcemic *tetany* or *cretinism,* while absence of any cry suggests severe illness or profound mental retardation. A continuous inspiratory and expiratory stridor may be caused by a relatively small larynx *(infantile laryngeal stridor),* or by delay in the development of the cartilage in the tracheal rings *(tracheomalacia).*

Early and Late Childhood

Visualize the anterior portion of the *nose* by pushing up its tip. Use a large-bored speculum attached to the otoscope to look deeper into the nostrils.

Examination of the *mouth* may present difficulties in early childhood, and restraints are usually needed (see figure on page 564). The young child may be more comfortable sitting in the parent's lap, as shown on page 569.

The presence of *Koplik's spots,* although a diagnostic sign now rarely seen, deserves description. Their appearance on the buccal mucosa opposite the first and second molars in a child with fever, coryza, and cough is proof positive of prodromal measles *(rubeola),* and the appearance of a generalized

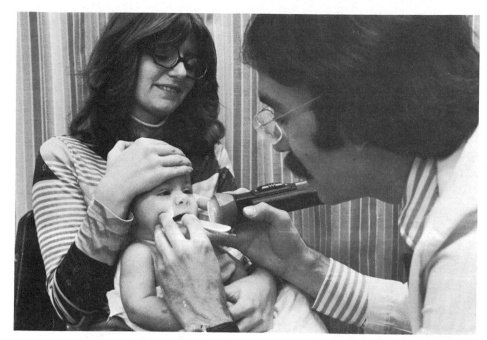

maculopapular rash within 24 hours can be predicted with certainty. Koplik's spots appear as grains of salt on individual erythematous bases. Their number varies according to when in the course of the illness they are observed. When three or more appear in a particular spot, they should be easily recognized.

When children clamp their teeth and purse their lips, gently push the tongue blade through the lips along the buccal mucosa and between the alveolar ridges behind the molars. This produces a gag reflex and, with it, complete visualization of the *pharynx*.

A direct assault on the front teeth will only meet with failure and a splintered tongue blade. Most children, however, are not that resistant and can be easily enticed to open their mouths, especially if they do not see a throat stick in the examiner's hand. Children who can stick out their tongues and say "ahhh!" do not require further manipulation for complete visualization of the pharynx. A good examiner can determine all that needs to be known with one quick look. Older children will permit placement of the tongue blade on one side of the base of the tongue and then the other. A transilluminator attachment to the oto–ophthalmoscopic handle is more useful than the standard penlight or flashlight in that its giraffe-like configuration allows for delivery of concentrated light in the recesses of the oral cavity and the pharynx.

The transilluminator may also be used, of course, to transilluminate the sinuses when sinusitis is suspected. This requires a completely dark room and a cooperative child.

***Transilluminate the frontal sinuses* by firmly placing the tip of the light above each eye against the inner aspect of the supraorbital ridge of the frontal bone.**

Normally, one sees a faint glow of light transmitted through the bone outlining the frontal sinus on the same side.

Transillumination is absent or diminished when sinusitis is present.

Transilluminate the maxillary sinuses **by placing the neck and head of the light in the patient's mouth and pressing the tip against first one side and then the other of the hard palate. Instruct the patient to seal both lips around the shaft of the transilluminator attachment while you look for the maxillary sinus glow on the corresponding side of the face. Cleanse the transilluminator before and after using it for this purpose.**

The appearance of the *tongue* may indicate disease. The *coated* tongue is nonspecific, the *smooth* tongue is found in avitaminosis, and the *strawberry* and *raspberry* tongues are seen at specific stages of scarlet fever. The *scrotal* and *fissured* tongues have no significance (see Table 7-20, p. 218).

The *teeth* should be examined for timing and sequence of eruption, number, character, condition, and position. Abnormalities of the enamel may reflect past or present, general or localized disease. Malocclusion should be looked for in late childhood. Most malocclusion and misalignment of teeth due to thumb sucking in early childhood are reversible if the habit is substantially arrested by age 6 or 7 years. When examining for maxillary protrusion *(overbite)* or mandibular protrusion *(underbite)*, one should be careful not to fall into the trap of asking the child to "show your teeth," because the upper and lower teeth are aligned reflexly when they are presented for inspection.

Dental caries are caused by bacterial activity and reflect poor nutrition and oral hygiene. Extensive decay of the primary teeth may be associated with prolonged bottle feeding ("nursing-bottle caries"), especially in children who take their bottles to bed at night and during naps.

Green coloration of the teeth is seen following severe *erythroblastosis fetalis;* grayish mottling of the enamel may result from the administration of tetracycline in infancy and early childhood; and black lines along the gingival margins signal the ingestion of heavy metals.

Rather, ask the child to bite down as hard as possible. Upon parting the lips you will observe the true bite. In normal children the upper teeth slightly override the lower teeth.

Malocclusion is most often due to hereditary predisposition, but may be due to chronic mouth breathing secondary to obstruction of the nasal airway. Maxillary overgrowth is associated with *chronic hemolytic anemia.* Mandibular overgrowth occurs rarely in the initial stages of *juvenile rheumatoid arthritis,* affecting the temporomandibular joint; micrognathia eventually ensues, however, in chronic cases.

The *primary teeth* erupt in a more predictable fashion than when they are shed or when the secondary teeth arrive. At age 7 months, most infants have two upper and two lower central incisors. From that point on, four teeth are added every 4 months, so there are eight at 11 months, 12 at 15 months, 16 at 19 months, and a full complement of 20 at 23 months. Normally, the shedding of primary teeth begins at about age 5 years; it precedes the eruption of corresponding *secondary teeth,* which begins at the end of early childhood between 6 and 7 years of age and ends in early adulthood at age 17 to 22 years.

When the *throat* is examined, the size and appearance of the *tonsils* should be noted. In both early and late childhood the tonsils are relatively larger than in infancy and adolescence, as demonstrated by the abundance of lymphoid tissue at this time of life (see figure on p. 525). They appear even larger as they move out of their fossae toward the midline and forward when the gag reflex is elicited or when the tongue is voluntarily protruded and the traditional "ahhh!" is sounded. The tonsils usually have deep crypts on their surfaces, which often have white concretions or food particles protruding from their depths. This is no indication of disease current or past.

A white exudate over the surface of the tonsils suggests *streptococcal tonsillitis;* a thick, gray, adherent exudate suggests *diphtheritic tonsillitis;* and necrosis (a grayish discoloration of the tonsillar tissue itself, rather than an exudate or a membrane overlying it) suggests *infectious mononucleosis.* All three conditions produce a fetid odor, but no one odor is distinguishable from the others. When one tonsil appears inflamed and unilaterally protrudes toward the midline and forward, *peritonsillar abscess* is an almost certain diagnosis.

The *adenoids* are not ordinarily visible unless extremely enlarged or unless the soft palate is elevated with the tongue blade to expose them in the nasopharynx. Adenoidal size can be determined indirectly by noting the degree of posterior nasal obstruction present when the patient sniffs through each nostril, and by the nasal quality they produce in the voice. Their size may also be determined directly by palpation. Adenoidal palpation should be carried out when there is a history of recurrent fever, headaches, and cough, and thus the diagnoses of *chronic adenoiditis* and *adenoidal abscess* are entertained.

During this examination, position the child and restrain as for examination of the throat (see p. 564). Tape three tongue blades together, place them, with your left hand, between the molars, and turn them on edge to ensure wide exposure. Place your plastic-gloved right index finger through the mouth into the nasopharynx behind the soft palate, and very rapidly palpate and thoroughly massage the adenoidal and surrounding lymphoid tissue. The procedure is accomplished with three or four quick strokes of the finger.

In cases of chronic adenoiditis and adenoidal abscess, palpation will reveal enlarged and boggy adenoidal tissue, and massage will produce copious amounts of bloody mucus and purulent material.

The child and parents should be warned that this procedure is uncomfortable and is likely to be followed by vomiting.

The same method may be used to palpate a peritonsillar abscess to determine the presence or absence of fluctuation and the posterior

pharyngeal wall to determine the presence and state of a retropharyngeal abscess.

Absence or asymmetry of movement of the soft palate in response to gagging and phonation, which is indicative of paralysis or weakness, should be noted. Asymmetry and corresponding voice change are often observed for varying periods following tonsillectomy.

Often overlooked in the examination of the throat is the presence of a submucosal cleft palate in which the muscles of the medial portion of the soft palate are missing. The mucosa is intact, however, and the underlying defect is easily missed. This condition is usually associated with notching of the posterior margin of the hard palate and a bifid uvula. Children with this anatomic variation may have hypernasal speech, but many have no voice changes. Adenoidectomy should be avoided, since difficulties with regurgitation of liquids and food into the nasal passages and nasality of speech will surely occur.

The child who has a croupy cough, hoarseness, difficulty swallowing, and signs of upper respiratory tract obstruction may have acute *epiglottitis.* In such a case, the epiglottis is markedly swollen and cherry red. Invoking the gag reflex in this instance could produce complete laryngeal obstruction and a fatal outcome. Therefore, great care must be taken in examining the throat. It should be done only once, if at all, and then deftly and gently with the child in the upright position, with a tracheostomy set at hand for use in the event that complete upper airway obstruction results from the examination procedure. The danger of such obstruction is sufficiently great that many clinicians prefer to omit direct examination of the throat in suspected cases of acute epiglottitis, and to rely on lateral x-rays of the neck to establish the diagnosis.

THE THORAX, BREASTS, AND LUNGS

Infancy

The configuration of the infant's *thorax* is rounded, with the anteroposterior diameter being equal to the transverse diameter. The *thoracic index,* which is the ratio of the transverse diameter to the anteroposterior diameter, is 1 at birth. At 1 year of age it is 1.25, and it reaches 1.35 at 6 years without much change thereafter.

The chest wall in infancy is thin with little musculature, and the bony and cartilaginous rib cage is very soft and pliant. The tip of the xiphoid process is often seen protruding anteriorly immediately beneath the skin at the apex of the costal angle.

Pectus excavatum may be manifested in early infancy by marked midline sternal retractions with normal inspiration, but it and other thoracic defor-

The *breasts* of the newborn in both male and female are often enlarged and engorged with secretion of a white liquid called "witch's milk." This is due to maternal estrogen effect and usually lasts only a week or two.

mities such as *pectus carinatum* ("chicken breast" deformity) do not ordinarily become evident until early childhood (see p. 246).

The respiratory rate and patterns in infancy and early childhood are discussed on page 542. The predominantly diaphragmatic breathing produces a simultaneous drawing in of the lower thorax and protrusion of the abdomen on inspiration and the reverse on expiration — termed *paradoxical breathing.*

When paradoxical breathing changes to predominantly thoracic breathing, intraabdominal or intrathoracic pathology, which restricts the use of the diaphragm, should be suspected. On the other hand, an *increase* in abdominal breathing suggests pulmonary disease.

Newborn infants, especially those born prematurely, exhibit irregular breathing. This is characterized by alternating periods of breathing at normal rates (30 to 40 per minute) with "periodic breathing" during which the respiratory rate slows markedly and may even cease 3 or more times for 3 seconds or longer. These alternating respiratory patterns have been observed in 30% to 95% of premature babies during sleep, but less frequently in full-term infants. The short apneic periods are not accompanied by bradycardia.

Periods of apnea lasting longer than 20 seconds and accompanied by bradycardia may indicate the presence of cardiopulmonary or central nervous system disease, or that the infant is at high risk for *Sudden Infant Death Syndrome (SIDS).*

Feel for tactile fremitus in infants by placing your hand on the chest when the baby cries. Place your whole hand, palm and fingertips, over the anterior, lateral, or posterior thorax to detect gross changes in transmission of sound through the parenchyma of the lung, pleura, and chest wall. Percuss the infant's chest directly by tapping the thoracic wall with one finger, or indirectly by using the finger-on-finger method.

Dullness may be elicited in infants when consolidation of the lung, an intrathoracic mass, or pleural fluid is present.

The percussion note is normally hyperresonant throughout. Any decrease in hyperresonance detected over the lung fields has the same significance as dullness in the adult.

Use the bell or small diaphragm stethoscope when auscultating the infant's chest, to allow for maximum localization of findings.

The breath sounds are louder and harsher than in adults because the stethoscope is closer to the origin of the sounds. Breathing in newborns is usually intermittently slow and shallow, then rapid and deep, so the examiner must be both patient and opportunistic. Breath sounds will often be diminished on the side of the chest opposite the direction in which the head is turned. There may be fine crackles at the end of deep inspiration in normal newborns and older infants. Crying, fortunately, will produce all of the deep breaths one could want and actually enhances auscultation, except in the unusual baby who cries on inspiration as well as expiration.

Extension or other movement of the head with inspiration indicates use of accessory muscles of respiration, and usually accompanies severe respiratory disease.

Because of the smallness of the thoracic cage and the ease of sound transmission within it, breath sounds are rarely entirely absent. Even with atelectasis, effusion, empyema, and pneumothorax, breath sounds are diminished rather than absent. In infants, pure bronchial breathing is rarely heard, even when consolidation is present. Wheezes, which are palpable and audible vibrations caused by air rushing through a narrowed segment of the lumen, occur more frequently in infancy and early childhood than in older children and adults because the small lumen of the tracheobronchial tree is easily narrowed by slight swelling of the mucous membrane or by small amounts of mucus.

An inspiratory wheeze is indicative of narrowing high in the tracheobronchial tree, while an expiratory wheeze indicates narrowing lower down.

Early and Late Childhood

Breast development for girls may begin normally as early as 8 years of age. Asymmetrical growth with resulting differences in size of the breasts during preadolescence is the rule; symmetrical breast growth is the exception. Completion of growth through adolescence corrects these inequalities in most instances. It is often helpful to explain this both to parents and to the young person herself, even if no mention of the subject is made by them.

The breath sounds on auscultation of the lungs in early and late childhood, as in infancy, are louder and harsher than in adults because of the continued relative lack of musculature and subcutaneous tissue overlying the thorax. Respiratory patterns are more regular than in infancy, and increasing cooperation in taking deep breaths and conducting other breathing maneuvers during auscultation of the lungs is obtained with increasing age.

The stethoscope may be a threatening instrument to the very young child; therefore, your success in placing it upon the chest will be enhanced if you say what it is and if you allow the child to manipulate it or even listen through it.

You can usually generate tactile fremitus easily by feeling the chest wall while carrying on a conversation with the child. A surprising number will say "99" or "1, 2, 3" when asked to, which will help you elicit tactile fremitus. You can usually gain the child's cooperation in deep breathing and breath holding by demonstrating each maneuver. If this is not successful, ask the child to blow out a match held too far away for immediate success. This seldom fails to produce full inspiration.

THE HEART

The examination of the heart in infants and children is, with few exceptions, conducted in the same manner as with the adult. The femoral pulses assume greater importance, since their diminution (as compared with the radial pulse) or their absence may be the only findings to raise suspicion of *coarctation of the aorta* in infancy and early childhood.

Feel along the inguinal ligament midway between the iliac crest and the symphysis pubis for the femoral pulse.

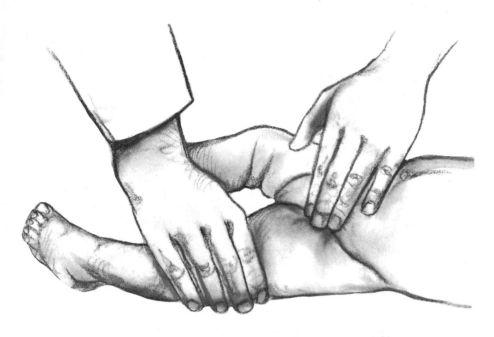

Because the respiratory rate may approximate the heart rate in infancy, breath sounds may be thought to be murmurs.

Occlude the nares momentarily to interrupt the respirations long enough to clarify this issue.

There are some distinct characteristics of the cardiac findings in normal infants and children that are not found in adults. The apical impulse (PMI), which is often visible, is at the level of the 4th interspace until age 7 years, when it drops to the 5th interspace. It is to the left of the midclavicular line until age 4 years, is at the midclavicular line between ages 4 and 6, and moves to the right of it at age 7. On percussion the heart appears larger than it actually is because of its more horizontal position and the overlying thymus gland at its base. *Sinus arrhythmia* is almost always present, and *premature ventricular contractions* are quite common. The heart sounds are louder than in adults because the chest wall is thinner, and they are of higher pitch and shorter duration. S_1 is louder than S_2 at the apex. Splitting of S_2 at the apex is found in 25% to 33% of children. S_2 is louder than S_1 in the pulmonic area.

The physical indications of severe heart disease include those not found with the stethoscope. Poor weight gain, delayed development, tachypnea, tachycardia, a prominent, active, heaving or thrusting precordium, cyanosis, and clubbing of the fingers and toes all signal cardiac disease. Heart failure is marked by venous engorgement, pulsus alternans, gallop rhythm, and hepatic enlargement. Pulmonary and peripheral edema appear late in the course of heart failure. (Peripheral edema, when it occurs in children, is more likely to be caused by renal failure.)

When S_2 is equal to or greater than S_1 at the apex, prolongation of the P–R interval on the electrocardiogram should be suspected. Splitting of S_2 in the pulmonic area may be found normally, but is frequently present in *mitral stenosis* and *right bundle branch block*.

In the pediatric cardiac examination the *murmur* assumes great significance in differential diagnosis, because more than 50% of all children (indeed, some say all) develop an innocent murmur at some time during childhood, and because significant heart disease in the pediatric age group is infrequent in the absence of a murmur. The examiner must therefore distinguish between the innocent and the organic murmur. The intensity of murmurs is graded on a scale of 1 to 6, as shown on page 289.

The *innocent murmur* has received over 120 labels indicative of its benign or functional nature, its origin, or its auscultatory characteristics. It is systolic in timing, is usually of short duration and of grade 3 or less in intensity, and has an empty, low-pitched, vibratory, musical groaning quality to its sound. It is usually loudest along the left sternal border, either in the 2nd or 3rd intercostal spaces or in the 4th or 5th intercostal spaces medial to the apex. It is poorly transmitted and is heard best with the patient in the supine position. Its intensity may vary with change in position, with the phase of respiration, with exercise, and from day to day. The most important characteristic of the innocent murmur is that it is heard in the absence of any other demonstrable evidence of cardiovascular disease.

A *venous hum* (see Table 9-15, p. 310) is heard commonly during childhood.

The noninnocent or *organic murmurs* are caused by congenital or acquired heart disease. Almost all acquired heart disease productive of murmurs in childhood is caused by acute rheumatic fever. An organic murmur first appearing before 3 years of age is almost always caused by a congenital cardiac defect, and one first appearing after that age is usually caused by rheumatic valvulitis.

The murmurs of congenital cardiac defects are caused either by abnormal communications between the arterial and venous circuits of the heart and great vessels or by valvular deformities. For the most part they are coarse in character, systolic in timing, and usually heard best at the base of the heart. The murmurs of *ventricular septal defect* and of *patent ductus arteriosus* have been described on pages 307 and 310. Those of *aortic stenosis* and *pulmonic stenosis* are described on page 305.

The presence or absence of cyanosis may be helpful to the examiner in differentiating the various types of congenital heart disease that have similar murmurs (see Table 18-5).

More often than not, the final diagnostic impression must await the results of electrocardiograms, chest x-rays, cardiac catheterization, echocardiograms, and more sophisticated studies.

The murmurs associated with acquired rheumatic heart disease include those of mitral stenosis (see p. 309), mitral regurgitation (see p. 307), aortic stenosis (see p. 305), and aortic regurgitation (see p. 309). Stenosis and

Murmurs of grade 3 or higher usually indicate the presence of heart disease.

In *atrial septal defect,* a grade 1 to 3 coarse systolic murmur is heard at the 2nd and 3rd left interspaces. It is less coarse than the murmur of a ventricular septal defect, is rarely accompanied by a thrill, and is not widely distributed. The murmur of *coarctation of the aorta* (adult type) is heard in the same area, is louder, is transmitted to the back medial to the scapula, and may be accompanied by a visible pulsation and palpable thrill at the suprasternal notch. It is also associated with decreased to absent femoral pulses and elevated blood pressure in the upper extremities. The murmurs associated with *tetralogy of Fallot, pure pulmonic stenosis, tricuspid atresia, transposition of the great vessels,* and *Eisenmenger's syndrome* are grades 3 to 5 in intensity, are systolic in timing, may be heard best at the left 2nd and 3rd interspaces, are not well transmitted, may or may not be accompanied by a thrill, and have no individual distinguishing characteristics. These murmurs may be absent in infancy. In addition, palpable liver pulsations may be present with tricuspid atresia and pure pulmonic stenosis.

regurgitation of the same valve usually occur concomitantly. Mitral val-vular disease occurs in 90% of children who develop heart disease follow-ing acute rheumatic carditis, either alone or in combination with aortic valvular disease. Aortic valve involvement occurs in approximately 25% of cases. The tricuspid and pulmonic valves are rarely involved in the rheumatic process.

The examiner of a child's heart should be able to differentiate normal from abnormal findings. Final decisions regarding specific abnormalities must often be left to the pediatric cardiologist, whose experience and access to special diagnostic tools will be more likely to bring accurate diagnoses and appropriate management. Therefore, early referral of the infant or child found to have evidence of congenital or acquired heart disease should be made to a pediatric cardiologist.

Table 18-5 Cyanosis and Congenital Heart Disease

NO CYANOSIS	Septal defects—small
	Patent ductus arteriosus
	Pure pulmonic stenosis— mild
	Coarctation of the aorta
	*Right coronary artery
	*Subendocardial fibroelas- tosis
	*Glycogen storage disease
EARLY CYANOSIS	Tetralogy of Fallot—severe
	Tricuspid atresia
	Transposition of the great vessels
	Two- and three-chambered hearts
	Severe pulmonic stenosis with intact ventricular septum
LATE CYANOSIS	Eisenmenger complex
	Pure pulmonic stenosis— mild
	Tetralogy of Fallot
	Septal defects—large

* Present with cardiac enlargement, tachycardia, and tachypnea, but without a heart murmur

THE ABDOMEN

Infancy

The abdomen in infants is protuberant, due to poorly developed abdomi-nal musculature.

A newborn with a concave abdomen should be immedi-ately investigated for *diaphrag-matic hernia* with displacement of some of the abdominal organs into the thoracic cavity.

The *umbilical cord* should be checked routinely at birth for the number of vessels present. Normally, two thick-walled umbilical arteries and one thin-walled umbilical vein are present. The arteries are of smaller diameter than is the vein, and the vein is usually found at the 12 o'clock position at the level of the abdominal wall.

A high correlation exists be-tween the presence of only a *single umbilical artery* and a variety of congenital anomalies.

The umbilicus in the newborn may have a relatively long cutaneous por-tion (*umbilicus cutis*), which is covered with skin, or a relatively long amniotic portion (*umbilicus amnioticus*), which is of firm gelatinous sub-stance. The amniotic portion dries up within a week and falls off within

Failure of the *navel* to heal, with granulomatous tissue for-mation at its base, occurs frequently.

two. The cutaneous portion retracts to become flush with the abdominal wall during the same period.

Infants are prone to *umbilical hernias* (see p. 351), *ventral hernias*, and *diastasis recti*. However, these are not usually discernible until 2 or 3 weeks of age. All are easily detected with crying.

The presence of diastasis recti may reflect a congenital weakness of the abdominal musculature (rare), or result from a chronically distended abdomen. Most, however, are normal variants and disappear in early childhood.

The defect in the abdominal wall at the umbilicus may be as large as 1½ inches in diameter, and the hernia itself may protrude 3 to 4 inches from the abdominal wall when intraabdominal pressure is increased. Most umbilical hernias disappear by 1 year of age.

A superficial abdominal venous pattern is observable until puberty. Abdominal reflexes are usually absent until after the first year of life.

Dilated veins may indicate portal vein obstruction. In veins below the umbilicus the direction of venous flow in *portal hypertension* is downward.

Palpation of the infant's abdomen is relatively easy.

Obtain relaxation by holding the infant's legs flexed at the knees and hips with one hand, and palpate with the other.

The *liver edge* and *spleen tip* are more often palpable than not, and frequently both *kidneys* can be felt by using the technique described for adults. The *bladder* is often felt and normally percussed to the level of the umbilicus. The *descending colon* is easily felt and may appear as a sausage-like mass in the left lower quadrant. Any abdominal masses of other origin are easily outlined.

In *Hirschsprung's disease* (congenital megacolon), a midline suprapubic mass representing a feces-filled rectosigmoid is often found.

Differentiate *cysts*, which occur rarely, from solid *tumors* by transillumination.

Avoid the spasm and rigidity encountered in palpating the abdomen of a crying infant with the administration of a bottle feeding or a sugar nipple.

Percussion of the infant's abdomen is accomplished as in the adult, but the examiner must allow for a greater amount of air within the stomach and the intestinal lumen because infants frequently swallow air when feeding and crying.

Auscultation of the abdomen should be accomplished before palpation. During auscultation, metallic tinkling every 10 to 30 seconds is heard normally.

An increase in pitch or frequency of bowel sounds, or marked diminution, is indicative of *intestinal obstruction* and *ileus*, respectively. A venous hum is a sign of *portal hypertension*.

The abdominal examination technique is altered when *pyloric stenosis* is suspected.

Place the infant, unclothed, in the supine position and stand at the foot of the table. Direct a bright light at table height across the abdomen from the patient's right side. Feed the infant a bottle of sugar water or milk and observe the abdomen closely. When pyloric stenosis is present, peristaltic waves are seen to go across the upper abdomen from left to right. These become increasingly large and frequent as the feeding progresses, as shown in the figure below.

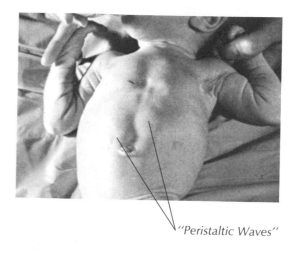

"Peristaltic Waves"

Inevitably the baby will vomit with projectile force. At this point, palpate deeply in the right upper quadrant. This will most likely reveal the presence of an olive-sized pyloric mass. Similar palpation with the baby in the prone position may prove more successful.

Early and Late Childhood

Protuberance of the abdomen, apparent when the child is in the upright position and disappearing when the child lies down, is noted in most children until adolescence.

Children are almost universally ticklish when you first place your hand on the abdominal wall. This reaction disappears in most cases, particularly if you distract the child by conversation and by placing your whole hand flush on the surface for a few moments without making initial probing movements with your fingers. With children whose sensitivity persists, placement of the child's hand under yours, as shown in the illustration on page 580, will reduce apprehension and increase relaxation of the abdominal musculature. Precede deep palpation with light superficial palpation of all quadrants. The last area you should examine is that which the history suggests as the site of pathology.

Tenderness may be determined by direct response of the child or may be detected by a change in the facial expression or in the pitch of the child's cry.

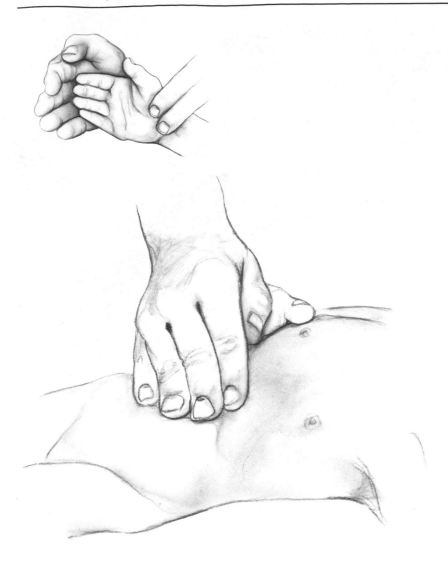

The *liver* and *spleen* are easily palpated in most children. The edge of the liver is normally felt 1 cm to 2 cm below the right costal margin. It is sharp and soft and moves easily when pushed from below upward during deep inspiration. The size of the liver is better determined by percussion than by palpation. Table 18-6 shows the expected liver span by percussion in the right midclavicular line for male and female patients by age.

A pathologically enlarged liver is usually palpable at more than 2 cm below the costal margin and has a rounded, firm edge.

As a rule the spleen, like the liver, is felt easily in most children. It too is soft with a sharp edge, and appears as a downward, tonguelike projection at the left costal margin.

You can often palpate the spleen between the thumb and forefinger of your right hand, and will find it to be freely moveable.

Pulsations in the epigastrium caused by the aorta are seen normally.

The pulsations of an enlarged right ventricle may be transmitted through the diaphragm and be visible in the epigastrium.

Table 18-6	Expected Liver Span of Infants, Children, and Adolescents by Percussion				
	MEAN ESTIMATED LIVER SPAN (cm)			MEAN ESTIMATED LIVER SPAN (cm)	
AGE IN YRS	MALES	FEMALES	AGE IN YRS	MALES	FEMALES
6 (mos)	2.4	2.8	8	5.6	5.1
1	2.8	3.1	10	6.1	5.4
2	3.5	3.6	12	6.5	5.6
3	4.0	4.0	14	6.8	5.8
4	4.4	4.3	16	7.1	6.0
5	4.8	4.5	18	7.4	6.1
6	5.1	4.8	20	7.7	6.3

Deeply palpate the abdomen to the left of the midline to feel the *aorta* **and its pulsations.**

Because the omentum is poorly developed in early childhood, localization of intraabdominal infection or other inflammatory reaction is less apt to occur than in late childhood and adolescence.

Tenderness and spasm of the abdominal musculature are usually diffuse whenever serious pathology occurs within the abdomen; *generalized peritonitis* should be suspected.

Ask the child to sit up from a supine position while you push down against the forehead with your hand.

This maneuver will elicit pain in the right lower quadrant in *acute appendicitis* when the appendix is lying anteriorly. When the appendix lies retrocecally over the psoas and obturator muscles, positive *psoas* and *obturator signs* are present (see p. 349).

THE GENITALIA AND RECTUM

Infancy

Examining the genitalia in the male infant presents no difficulties. The *foreskin* adheres to the *glans penis,* covers it completely, and has a tiny orifice at its distal end. It does not retract over the glans until the infant is several months old, and then only if it has been stretched on a regular basis.

Hypospadias is present when the urethral orifice appears at some point along the ventral surface of the glans or the shaft of the penis. The foreskin in

Many male infants in our society are still circumcised in the immediate neonatal period, so that the glans penis is exposed to its base. However, the number so circumcised has diminished in recent years.

The *testes* are normally found in the scrotum, or in the inguinal canal from which they can easily be milked down into the scrotum.

In the newborn female the *labia minora* are prominent. They quickly atrophy and become almost nonexistent until puberty. More often than not there is a bloody, mucoid vaginal discharge during the first week of life, due to the maternal estrogen influence on the cervix and vaginal mucosa. A serosanguinous vaginal discharge may supplant this for a week or two more.

Visualize the perineal structures, the urethral orifice, the hymen, and the vaginal mucosa by separating the labia with the thumb and forefinger of one hand while you press forward and downward from within the rectum with the index finger of your other hand. The rectoperineal portion of this examination should be used only when intravaginal pathology is suspected.

The genitalia of both male and female breech babies may be markedly edematous and bruised for several days following delivery.

The *rectal examination* of infants (and of patients in early and late childhood) should be performed whenever intraabdominal, pelvic, or perirectal disease is suspected. It should be performed with the patient in the supine position. This allows for deeper penetration of the examining finger and for combined abdominal and rectal examination maneuvers.

Hold the feet together and flex the knees and hips upon the abdomen with one of your hands while the index finger of your other hand is introduced into the rectum. Once this is done, place your first hand upon the abdomen to conduct a bimanual examination. The index finger is preferred for the rectal examination, even in infancy, because of its greater tactile sensitivity. Regardless of the size of your examining finger, slight bleeding and protrusion of the rectal mucosa will occur upon its removal.

Early and Late Childhood

The size of the *penis* in early childhood and prepubescence is of little significance unless it is very large. In obese boys the fat pad over the symphysis pubis may envelop the penis, obscuring it completely. The testes in young boys are quite retractile and are often found in the inguinal canal rather than in the scrotum.

these instances is incompletely formed ventrally.

Hydroceles of the testes and the spermatic cord are common in infancy and often associated with actual or potential *inguinal hernias.* Hydroceles may be differentiated easily from hernias in that the former transilluminate and are not reducible.

Enlargement of the penis to adolescent or adult size occurs in *precocious puberty,* due to an excess in circulating androgens of adrenal or testicular origin.

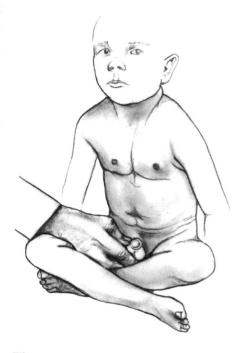

This occurs with tumors of these organs or of the pituitary gland. Other signs of virilization —pubic and axillary hair, increased testicular size, increased somatic growth and muscle mass, hirsutism, and deepening of the voice— usually accompany the penile enlargement.

You can overcome testicular retractibility by having the child sit in a crosslegged squatting position on the examining table, as illustrated here. A diagnosis of undescended testicle should not be made until you have palpated the inguinal canal and scrotum with the patient in this position.

Cryptorchidism, or undescended testicle, may occur unilaterally or bilaterally, with the testicle remaining in the abdomen or within the inguinal canal.

The examination for *inguinal hernia* in this age group is similar to that performed on the adult and should be done with the patient standing.

Because the child's cough may be of insufficient strength to demonstrate a reduced hernia, the hernia can sometimes be demonstrated if the child attempts to lift a heavy object, such as the end of the examining table or the chair in which you are sitting.

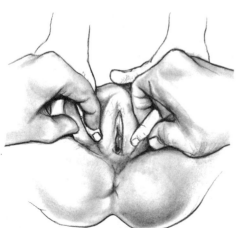

You can often make the examination of the female genitalia in this age group easier for yourself and more comfortable for the child by using the child's own hands to distract and reassure her, as shown here.

Fusion of the labia minora is commonly seen. It may be partial, with only the posterior portion of the labia fused, or it may be complete. A thin membrane that joins the labial edges is easily lysed with a cotton swab or a probe. The labia will also separate if an estrogen-containing cream is applied to the labia once or twice daily for several days.

You can obtain greater relaxation and cooperation during the rectal examination in this age group if you first demonstrate and then ask the child to try breathing in and out rapidly "like a puppy dog."

Perianal skin tabs are common and have no significance. Bimanual rectoabdominal palpation in females will reveal a small midline mass, which is the *cervix*. Any other mass that is palpable on this examination should be considered abnormal, since none of the other anatomical structures are normally palpable until adolescence. Vaginoabdominal palpation as a method of examining the pelvic structures, and direct visualization of the vagina and cervix, are not considered part of the ordinary physical examination in childhood. When visualization of the vagina and cervix is indicated on the basis of the history or abdominal or perineal findings, it is best accomplished with an otoscope equipped with a vaginal speculum.

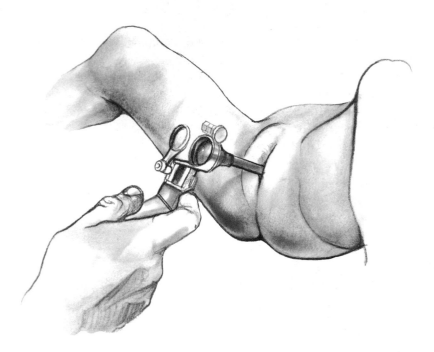

Secondary sexual *hair growth* parallels the development of other secondary sexual characteristics. Pubic hair may appear sparsely as early as the eighth year. Axillary, facial, body, arm, and leg hair proliferate in sequence before and during puberty.

THE MUSCULOSKELETAL SYSTEM

Infancy

The *range of motion* at all joints is greatest in infancy and gradually lessens throughout childhood to adult levels.

At birth, the *feet* may appear deformed if they retain their intrauterine positioning. Such positional deformities can be distinguished by the ease with which the affected foot can be manipulated to neutral and over-corrected positions. Scratching or stroking along the outer edge of the positionally deformed foot will cause it to assume a normal position.

True deformities do not return to even the neutral position through manipulation.

When examining the feet, look for inversion of the foot and note the relationship of the forefoot to the hindfoot. Is the forefoot adducted at the metatarsal–tarsal line (a line across the junctions of the tarsal and metatarsal bones)?

Normally, a straight line drawn from the center of the heel forward through the center of the metatarsal–tarsal line bisects either the second toe or the space between the second and third toes. When this line crosses the toes more laterally, the forefoot is adducted. Adduction of the forefoot distal to the metatarsal–tarsal line *(metatarsus adductus deformity)* is common. Spontaneous correction occurs within the first 2 years of life.

When the forefoot is twisted inward on its longitudinal axis (inverted) in addition to being adducted, *metatarsus varus* exists, as shown in the figures below.

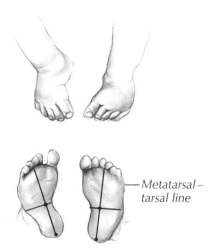

Metatarsal–tarsal line

In metatarsus varus the line drawn through the center of the metatarsal–tarsal line is displaced laterally, as shown above.

Talipes varus is present when the forefoot is adducted and the entire foot is inverted. Both of these foot deformities require orthopedic correction.

During infancy there is a distinct *bowlegged growth pattern.* This begins to disappear at 18 months of age, when a transition from bowlegs to knock-knees occurs. The *knock-knee pattern* usually persists from 2 until 6 to 10 years of age, when a balancing takes place and, for most, the legs straighten. Some babies exhibit a twisting or torsion of the tibia inwardly or outwardly on its longitudinal axis. This invariably corrects itself during the second year of life.

When infants stand, their legs are set wide apart and the weight is borne on the inside of the feet. When walking is accomplished, a wide-based gait is used for the first year or two. This causes a certain degree of *pronation of the feet* and incurving of the Achilles tendons (viewed from behind).

The longitudinal arch in infancy is obscured by adipose tissue, giving the foot the appearance of being flat. This is accentuated by pronation of the foot so that the infant is often misdiagnosed as being flatfooted.

The *hips* of all infants should be examined for signs of dislocation.

Place the baby in the supine position with the legs pointing toward you. Flex the legs to right angles at the hips and knees, placing your middle fingers over the greater trochanter of each femur and your thumbs over the lesser trochanter, as shown in the figures below. Abduct both hips simultaneously until the lateral aspect of each knee touches the examining table. This maneuver is known as the *Ortolani* test.

When a *congenitally dislocated hip* is present, you will see, feel, and sometimes hear a "click" as the femoral head, which in this condition lies posterior to the acetabulum, enters the acetabulum at some point in the 90° abduction arc. This finding is known as the *Ortolani sign.*

Beyond the newborn period, as the muscles surrounding the hip increase in strength, the "click" of the Ortolani sign is less obtainable; then decreased abduction of the flexed legs (at the hip, on one or both sides) becomes the significant finding in detecting unilateral or bilateral *congenital dislocation of the hip.*

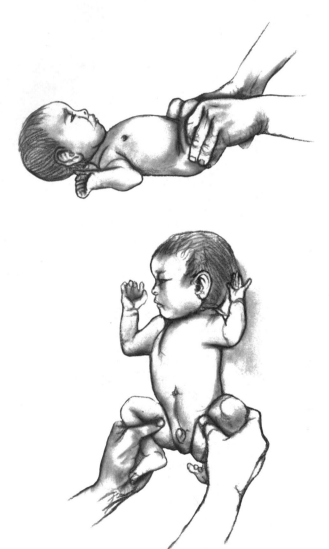

To detect an unstable (nondislocated but potentially dislocatable) hip, place your thumb medially over the lesser trochanter and your index or middle finger laterally over the greater trochanter as shown in the figure on page 587; press your thumb backward and outward. Feel for movement of the head of the femur laterally against some resistance as it slips out onto the posterior lip of the acetabulum. Normally no movement is felt. Then, with your index or middle finger, press the

greater trochanter forward and inward. Feel for a sudden movement of the femoral head inward as it returns to the hip socket. Again, movement is not normally felt. Movement in both directions constitutes *Barlow's sign.*

The presence of Barlow's sign is not diagnostic of a congenital dislocated hip, but it indicates the need to observe the baby very carefully for this possibility.

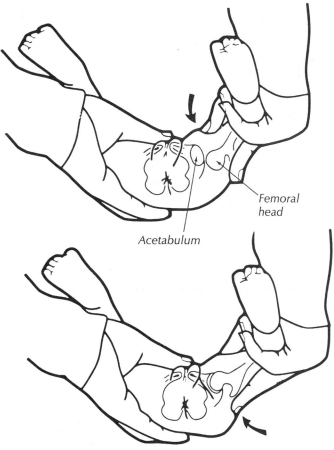

Femoral head

Acetabulum

(Reproduced with permission from Burnside JW: Physical Diagnosis: An Introduction to Clinical Medicine, 16th ed, p 246. Baltimore, Williams & Wilkins, 1981)

Early and Late Childhood

From both in front of and behind, watch the child standing upright. You can often detect the presence of musculoskeletal difficulties in this age group by closely observing the child in various postures (*e.g.,* from the front and rear while the child is standing upright with the feet together, walking, stooping to obtain an object from the floor, rising from the supine position, and touching the toes or shins while standing).

In childhood, the thoracic convexity is decreased and the lumbar concavity is increased. Lordosis is common and rarely causes symptoms.

Test for severe hip disease with its associated weakness of the gluteus medius muscle by observing the child from behind as the weight is shifted from one leg to the other. **The pelvis is seen to remain level when the weight is borne on the unaffected side and to tilt toward the unaffected hip when weight is borne on the affected side** (*Trendelenburg's sign*).

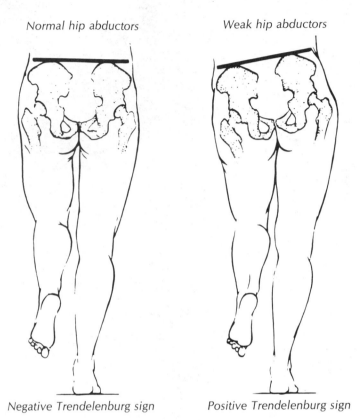

Normal hip abductors   Weak hip abductors

Negative Trendelenburg sign   Positive Trendelenburg sign

(Reproduced with permission from Chung SMR: Hip Disorders in Infants and Children, p 65. Philadelphia, Lea & Febiger, 1981)

Determine *shortening of the leg* in hip disease by comparing the distance from the anterior superior spine of the ilium with the medial malleolus on each side (see p. 457).

When you suspect *scoliosis* (see p. 467), ask the child to bend forward. Mark the spinous processes with a felt tip pen. After the child stands erect, look for a curve in the line of ink dots.

THE NERVOUS SYSTEM

Infancy

Neurologic screening to include assessment of positioning, spontaneous and induced movements, cry, knee and ankle jerk responses, and elicitation of the rooting, grasp, tonic neck, and Moro automatisms should be performed on all newborns. Babies showing abnormalities in these areas and those at risk for central nervous system disease should have repeated complete neurologic assessments.

The findings during the neurologic examination in infancy, especially in the newborn period, differ markedly from those present in children and adults.

The central nervous system at birth is underdeveloped and functions at subcortical levels. Cortical function develops slowly after birth and cannot be tested in its entirety until early childhood. Thus, in the newborn period and early infancy, findings of normal brainstem and spinal functioning do not ensure an intact cortical system, and abnormalities of the brainstem and spinal cord may exist without concomitant cortical abnormalities. There are a number of specific reflex activities (*infantile automatisms*) found in the normal newborn that disappear in early infancy.

The absence of infantile automatisms in the neonate or the persistence of some beyond their expected time of disappearance may indicate severe central nervous system dysfunction.

The neurologic examination in infancy will enable the clinician to detect extensive disease of the central nervous system, but will be of little use in pinpointing minute lesions and specific functional deficits.

The general appearance, positioning, activity, cry, and alertness of the newborn baby should be noted, as these observations are an important part of the neurologic assessment of this age group.

Test for *motor function* by putting each major joint through its range of motion to determine whether normal muscle tone, spasticity, or flaccidity is present.

Beyond the newborn period, throughout infancy, specific *gross and fine motor coordination testing* can be accomplished by using an age-appropriate protocol, such as the *Denver Developmental Screening Test* (see pp. 533–535). This test also assesses social and language development. Discrepancies in achievement in the motor and communication areas may suggest whether the deficit is in the motor, sensory, or intellectual spheres. Knowledge of when developmental landmarks are normally achieved is essential in assessing the function of the infant's nervous system.

Postural indications of severe intracranial disease include persistent asymmetries, predominant extension of the extremities, and constant turning of the head to one side. Marked retroflexion of the head, stiffness of the neck, and extension of the arms and legs (*opisthotonus*) indicate severe meningeal or brainstem irritation, seen in intracranial infection or hemorrhage (see figure below).

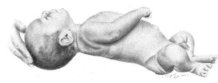

(Redrawn from Paine RS: Neurological examination of infants and children. Pediatr Clin North Am 7:477, 1960)

The *sensory examination* for infants is rather limited in terms of defining neurologic disease. Thresholds of touch, pain, and temperature are higher than in older children, and reactions to these stimuli are relatively slow.

Absence of withdrawal when a painful stimulus is applied to an extremity indicates anesthesia

Gently touch the baby's arms and legs with a pin, and observe movement of the stimulated extremity or change in the facial expression. If the pin is used vigorously enough, crying will result.

or paralysis. If a change in facial expression or a cry is elicited in the absence of withdrawal, paralysis is indicated rather than anesthesia. With spinal cord lesions, the extremity will withdraw reflexly in response to pain but there will be no concomitant change in the baby's facial expression or cry.

The *cranial nerves* are tested in infancy as in the adult. The difficulties encountered in assessing the function of the 2nd and 8th nerves have already been mentioned.

The 12th nerve is easily tested. Pinch the nostrils of the infant. This produces a reflex opening of the mouth and raising of the tip of the tongue.

If *12th nerve paresis* is present, the tongue tip will deviate toward the affected side.

Because the corticospinal pathways are not fully developed in infants, the *spinal reflex mechanisms* (deep tendon reflexes and plantar response) are variable in infancy. Their presence in exaggerated form, or their absence, has very little diagnostic significance unless there is asymmetry of response or change in response from a previous testing.

The technique for eliciting these reflexes is similar to that used with adults, except that your semiflexed index or middle finger can substitute for the neurologic hammer, its tip acting as the striking point. Your thumbnail may be used to elicit the plantar response.

The *Babinski response* to plantar stimulation can be elicited in some normal infants, and until 2 years of age in a few of these. However, a flexion response to plantar stimulation is elicited in more than 90% of normal newborns. The *triceps reflex* is usually not present until after 6 months of age. Rapid, rhythmic plantar flexion of the foot in response to eliciting the ankle reflex *(ankle clonus)* is a common finding in newborns; as many as eight to ten such contractions in response to one stimulus may occur normally *(unsustained ankle clonus)*.

When the contractions are continuous *(sustained ankle clonus)*, severe central nervous system disease should be suspected.

You can also elicit ankle clonus by pressing the thumb over the ball of the infant's foot and abruptly dorsiflexing the foot.

The *abdominal reflexes* are absent in the newborn but appear within the first 6 months of life. The *anal reflex,* however, is normally present in newborns and is important to elicit when spinal cord lesions are present or suspected.

With the baby in a supine position, straighten and raise the lower legs, scratch the perianal region with a pin, and observe contracture of the external anal sphincter.

An absent anal reflex strongly suggests loss of innervation of the external sphincter muscle due to a spinal cord lesion at the level of the lower sacral segments or higher, such as a congenital anomaly *(spina bifida)*, a tumor, or an injury.

INFANTILE AUTOMATISMS

The infantile automatisms are reflex phenomena that are present at birth or appear shortly thereafter. Some remain only a few weeks while others persist well into the second year of life. Automatisms have prognostic value for central nervous system integrity. Attempts to elicit any of them (except the rooting, grasp, tonic neck, and Moro responses) should be made only when central nervous system function is in question. Each automatism is listed here with the method of elicitation and the prognostic significance of its presence or absence. All are present at birth unless otherwise indicated. The time of disappearance is also listed.

Blinking (Dazzle) Reflex. Disappears after first year. The eyelids close in response to bright light.

Absence may indicate blindness.

Acoustic Blink (Cochleopalpebral) Reflex. Disappearance time is variable. Both eyes blink in response to a sharp loud noise.

Absence may indicate decreased hearing.

Palmar Grasp Reflex. Disappears at 3 or 4 months.

With the baby's head positioned in the midline and the arms semi-flexed, place your index fingers from the ulnar side into the baby's hands and press against the palmar surfaces. A positive response is one of flexion of all of the baby's fingers to grasp your fingers. This method allows for comparison of both hands. If the reflex is absent or weak you can enhance it by offering the baby a bottle, since sucking facilitates grasping.

Persistence of the grasp reflex beyond 4 months suggests cerebral dysfunction. It should be noted that babies normally hold their hands clenched during the first month of life. Persistence of the fisted hand beyond 2 months also suggests central nervous system damage.

Light stroking of the ulnar surface of the hand and fifth finger will produce extension of the thumb and other fingers *(digital response reflex).*

Rooting Reflex. Disappears at 3 or 4 months; may be present longer during sleep.

Absence of this reflex indicates severe generalized or central nervous system disease.

With the baby's head positioned in the midline and the hands held against the anterior chest, stroke with your forefinger the perioral skin at the corners of the baby's mouth and at the midline of the upper and lower lips.

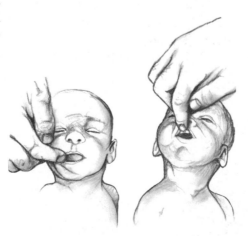

In response, the mouth will open and turn to the stimulated side. When the upper lip is stimulated, the head will retroflex; when the lower lip is stimulated, the jaw will drop. This response will also occur with stimulation of the infant's cheek at some distance from the corners of the mouth.

Trunk Incurvation (Galant's) Reflex. Disappears at 2 months.

Transverse spinal cord lesions may be detected by testing for the presence of this reflex. It is absent in transverse spinal cord lesions or injuries.

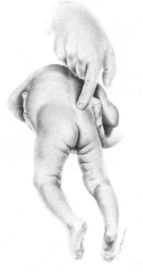

Hold the baby horizontally and prone in one of your hands. Stimulate one side of the baby's back approximately 1 cm from the midline along a paravertebral line extending from the shoulder to the buttocks. This produces a curving of the trunk toward the stimulated side, with shoulders and pelvis moving in that direction.

(Redrawn from Paine RS: Neurological examination of infants and children. Pediatr Clin North Am 7:490, 1960)

Vertical Suspension Positioning. Disappears after 4 months.

While you support the baby upright with your hands under the axillae, the head is normally maintained in the midline and the legs are flexed at the hips and knees.

Fixed extension and adduction of the legs (scissoring) indicates *spastic paraplegia* or *diplegia.*

Placing Response. Best after the first 4 days. Disappearance time is variable.

Hold the baby upright from behind by placing your hands under the baby's arms with your thumbs supporting the back of the head, and allow the dorsal surface of one foot to touch the undersurface of a table top. This procedure is demonstrated in the four illustrations on page 593.

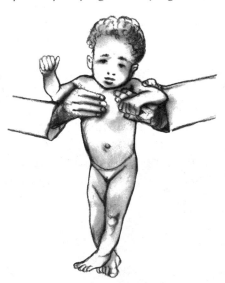

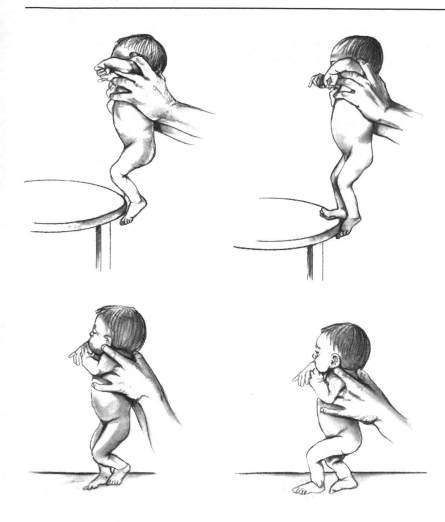

Take care not to plantar flex the foot. The baby responds by flexing the hip and knee and placing the stimulated foot on the table top. Repeat the process stimulating the other foot. With one foot placed on the table top, the opposite leg will step forward and a series of alternate stepping movements of both legs will occur as you move the baby gently forward.

These responses are absent when paresis is present and in babies born by breech delivery.

Rotation Test. Disappearance time is variable.

Hold the baby under the axillae, at arm's length facing you, and turn him or her in one direction and then the other. The head turns in the direction in which you turn the baby. If you restrain the head with your thumbs, the baby's eyes will turn in the direction in which you turned (see figure on p. 557).

The head and eyes do not move, as noted, in the presence of vestibular dysfunction. Early detection of *strabismus* may be accomplished with this maneuver.

Tonic Neck Reflex. May be present at birth but usually appears at 2 months and disappears at 6 months.

With the baby in the supine position, as shown on page 594, turn the head to one side, holding the jaw over the shoulder. The arm and leg on

When this reflex is elicited each time it is evoked it should be

the side to which the head is turned extend, while the opposite arm and leg flex. **This response does not normally occur each time this maneuver is performed.**

considered abnormal, at any age. It will persist beyond the time of expected disappearance in major cerebral damage.

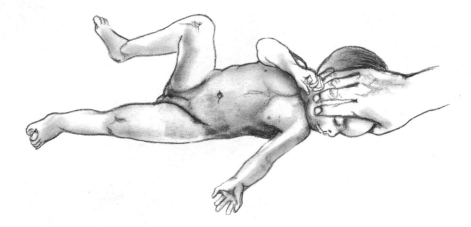

Two *mass reflexes* occur in the presence of normal subcortical mechanisms that are not yet under significant inhibitory control from higher cerebral centers. They are present at birth and disappear by the third month.

Perez Reflex. **Hold the baby in a suspended prone position in one of your hands. Place the thumb of your other hand on the baby's sacrum and move it firmly toward the head along the entire length of the spine. A positive response is usually one of extension of the head and spine, flexion of the knees on the chest, a cry, and emptying of the bladder.**

The last occurs with sufficient frequency to make this reflex useful in the collection of urine specimens from neonates.

Absence of either reflex during the first 3 months of life indicates severe cerebral insult, injury to the upper cervical cord, advanced anterior horn cell disease, or severe myopathy.

Moro Response (Startle Reflex). **You can produce the Moro response in several ways: by lifting the supine baby's head to an angle approximately 30° from the examining table and suddenly releasing your grip and allowing the head to fall backward, catching it before it hits the table (as shown in the figure on page 595); by holding the baby in the supine position, supporting the head, back, and legs, and then suddenly lowering the entire body about 2 feet and stopping abruptly; by holding the baby in the supine position, supporting the back and pelvis with one hand and arm and the head with the other hand, and allowing the head to drop several centimeters with a sudden, rapid, not too forceful movement; or by producing a sudden loud noise (*e.g.,* striking the examining table with the palms of your hands on either side of the baby's head).**

The response itself is one in which the arms briskly abduct and extend with the hands open and fingers extended, and the legs flex slightly and abduct (but less so than the arms). The arms then return forward over the body in a clasping maneuver and the baby emits an audible cry.

Persistence of the Moro response beyond 4 months may indicate neurologic disease; persistence beyond 6 months is almost conclusive evidence of such. An asymmetric response in the upper extremities suggests hemiparesis, injury to the brachial plexus, or fracture of the clavicle or humerus. Low spinal injury and congenital dislocation of the hip may produce absence of the response in one or both legs.

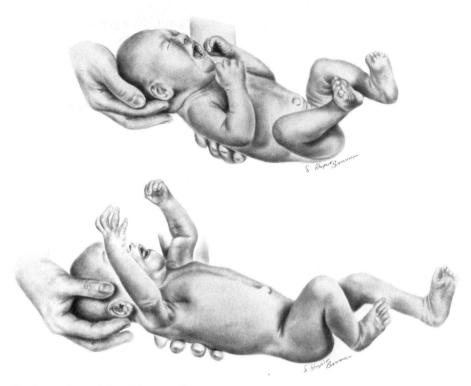

(Redrawn from Paine RS: Neurological examination of infants and children. Pediatr Clin North Am 7:494, 1960)

GENERAL INDICATORS OF CENTRAL NERVOUS SYSTEM DISEASE

The following *general findings in infancy* should suggest to the clinician the presence of central nervous system disease:

1. Abnormal localized neurological findings

2. Failure to elicit expected responses

3. Asymmetry of normal responses

4. Late persistence of normal responses

5. Reemergence of vanished responses

6. Developmental delays

Certain combinations of findings in infancy suggest specific diagnoses. The presence of the setting sun sign, opisthotonos, and a disappearing or absent Moro response suggest *kernicterus.*

In *congenital hemiplegia,* absent or diminished movement of the extremities involved, along with abnormal posturing, is seen rather than any changes in reflexes and muscle tone.

Bilateral cerebral injury produces hypotonia with normal or brisk deep tendon reflexes, delay in reaching motor milestones, and persistence of the tonic neck reflex.

Early and Late Childhood

Beyond infancy, when the infantile automatisms have disappeared, the neurologic examination is conducted in much the same manner as with the adult. Samples of handwriting and figure drawing with both hands are useful in detecting fine motor defects. Stereognosis, vibration, position, two-point discrimination, number identification, and extinction are not usually testable in the child under 3 years of age, and in many under 5 years. The gait should be observed with the child both walking and running. Asymmetric movements of the arms in walking or running may indicate a hemiparesis, as may unequal wear of the soles and heels on the child's shoes (although there are localized neurologic and orthopedic conditions that may produce unequal shoe wear).

Observe the child rising from the floor from a supine position so that you can note the manner in which the muscles of the neck, trunk, arms, and legs are used to assume first the sitting position and then the standing position (see figures below and on facing page).

Evidence of neurologic deficits, muscular weaknesses, and orthopedic defects may be detected here that would not be noted otherwise.

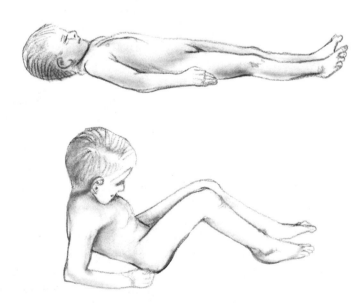

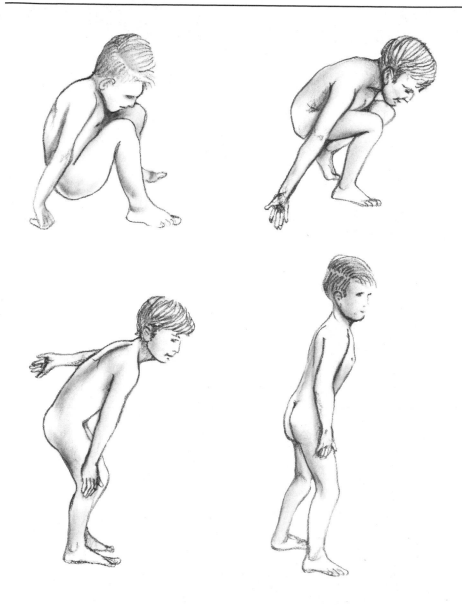

In certain forms of *muscular dystrophy* with pelvic girdle weaknesses, rising from a supine to a standing position is accomplished as shown below (*Gowers's sign*).

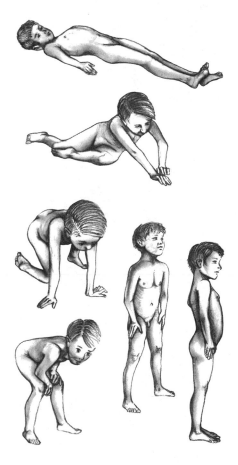

When nystagmus, unsteady gait, or history of streptomycin therapy is present, *vestibular function* should be tested. This is accomplished with the *cold caloric test*.

Inject water at 65° F temperature into the external auditory canal with an ear syringe. Observe for nystagmus, which should occur within 30 seconds.

The absence of nystagmus occurs with 8th nerve damage from *drug toxicity, meningitis* or *brain tumor*, or *labyrinthitis*.

At All Ages

In essence, the complete neurologic examination in infancy and childhood includes elements of all the parts of the general physical examination as well as the specific components of the neurologic examination outlined here. The clinician is constantly assessing neurologic functioning throughout the course of every patient encounter. All of the observations made and impressions gained are used to determine the integrity of the central and peripheral nervous systems. This is equally true in the examination of adults.

Chapter 19
Clinical Thinking: From Data to Plan

Like colors on an artist's palette, clinical data lack form and meaning. The clinician must not only gather data through interviewing and examination; he or she must also analyze them, identify the patient's problems, evaluate the patient's responses to the illness, and, together with the patient, formulate a plan. This chapter describes this sequence of activities and focuses on the clinical thinking that underlies it.

FROM DATA BASE TO PLAN

Since Lawrence L. Weed introduced the problem-oriented system of recordkeeping, certain terms have gained wide acceptance. Information given by the patient, or possibly by family members or significant others, is called *subjective data*. *Objective data* include two kinds of information: physical findings and laboratory reports. Since both physical examination and laboratory work are human activities, they too, admittedly, involve subjective elements, and, as we shall see later, all kinds of data are subject to error. A comprehensive set of subjective and objective data, such as you might gather in evaluating a new patient, makes up a *data base* for that patient.

In recording the data base you should describe your findings as accurately as possible, whether they deal with what the patient tells you or with what you observe. Although inference and interpretation inevitably affect the organization of your materials, statements in the data base should describe, not interpret. Thus, "late inspiratory crackles at the bases of both lungs" is appropriate, while "signs of congestive heart failure" is not.

In the *assessment* process, however, you go beyond perception and description to analysis and interpretation. Here you select relevant pieces of your data, think about their possible meanings, and try to explain them logically. For example, a patient's complaint of a "scratchy throat" and "stuffy nose," together with your observations of a swollen nasal mucosa and slight redness of the pharynx, give you the subjective and objective data on which to base a presumptive diagnosis of viral nasopharyngitis.

In order to understand a patient's problems and work out an appropriate plan, you will usually need to evaluate not only the health problem but also the patient's responses to it. What does the patient understand about the illness and about your diagnosis? What are the patient's feelings about them, and why? What are the patient's goals in seeing you? Even in a situation as apparently simple as the patient with nasopharyngitis, consider the implications of the following possibilities: (1) patient A is a student with a very important examination tomorrow; (2) patient B has just heard news of a locally severe epidemic of meningococcal meningitis; (3) patient C's 8-year-old daughter has acute lymphatic leukemia and is scheduled to come home from the hospital in 2 days. Probably no single plan can meet the needs of all three of these patients.

Once you have tentatively defined the problems and gained at least a preliminary understanding of the patient's responses to them, you are ready to work out a *plan* with the patient. In Weed's terminology a plan has three parts: diagnostic, therapeutic, and educational. For example, you might decide on a throat culture, a decongestant for the patient's stuffy nose, cautionary advice against overfatigue, and a brief review of upper respiratory infections, their causes, and their modes of transmission.

Defining part of the plan as "educational" has one misleading connotation — that the process of communication is unidirectional. It should not be. The patient should participate in making the plan. Appropriate "education" depends on what the patient already knows and wants to know. Give the patient an opportunity to tell you. Other parts of the plan may well be influenced by the patient's goals, economic means, competing responsibilities, and the opinions of family or friends — to name just a few variables. Establishing a successful plan requires interviewing skills and interpersonal sensitivity, not just knowledge of diagnostic and therapeutic techniques.

The diagram below summarizes the sequence from data base to plan. The effects of the assessment process on the data base, as implied by the bidirectional arrows between them, will be discussed later in the chapter.

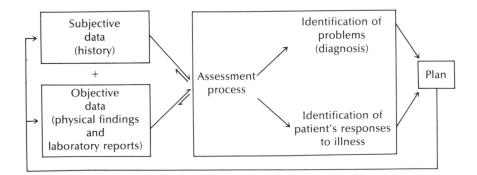

After a plan has been implemented, the process recycles. The clinician gathers more data, assesses the patient's progress, modifies the problem list if indicated, and adjusts the plan appropriately.

ASSESSMENT: THE PROCESS OF CLINICAL THINKING

Since assessment takes place in the clinician's mind, its processes often seem inaccessible, even mysterious, to the beginning student. Experienced clinicians, moreover, think so quickly, with little overt or conscious effort, that they sometimes have difficulty in explaining their own logic. They also think in different ways, with different, individualistic personal styles. Some general principles underlie this analytic process, however, and certain explicit steps may help you think constructively and purposefully about your data. The thinking process starts at the beginning of your patient encounter, not at the end, but assume for the moment that you already have a data base to consider. You must answer the questions, "What is wrong with the patient? What are the problems?" To do so, try the following steps:

1. *Identify the abnormal findings* in the patient's data base. Make a list of the *symptoms* noted by the patient, the *signs* that you observed on physical examination, and any *laboratory reports* that are available to you.

2. *Localize these findings anatomically.* This step may be easy. The symptom of scratchy throat and the sign of a reddened pharynx, for example, clearly localize a problem in the pharynx. Other data, however, present greater difficulty. Chest pain, for example, might originate in the heart, the pleural surfaces, the esophagus, or the musculoskeletal system. If the pain consistently occurs with exercise and disappears with rest, either the heart or possibly the musculoskeletal system is probably involved. If the patient notes pain only when carrying groceries with the left arm, the musculoskeletal system becomes the likely culprit. Be as explicit in your localization as your data allow, but no more so. You may have to settle for a body region (*e.g.*, the chest) or a body system (*e.g.*, musculoskeletal system), or you may be able to define the exact structure involved (*e.g.*, left pectoral muscle). Some symptoms and signs, such as fatigue or fever, have no localizing value but may be useful in the next step, interpreting probable process.

3. *Interpret the findings in terms of the probable process.* A patient's problem may stem from a *pathological* process involving a bodily structure. There are a number of such processes, variably classified, including congenital, inflammatory, immunologic, neoplastic, metabolic, nutritional, degenerative, vascular, traumatic, and toxic. Other problems are *pathophysiological*, such as increased gastrointestinal motility or congestive heart failure, while others still are *psychopathological*, such as a disorder of mood or of thought processes. Redness and pain are two of the four classic signs of inflammation, and a red, painful throat, even without the other two signs — heat and swelling — strongly suggests an inflammatory process in the pharynx.

4. *Make a hypothesis about the nature of the patient's problem.* Here you will have to draw on all the knowledge and experience you can muster, and it is here that reading will be most helpful in learning about

abnormalities and diseases. Until your experience and knowledge broaden you may not be able to reach highly explicit hypotheses, but proceed as far as you can with the data and knowledge you have. The following steps should help:

a. *Select the most specific and central findings* around which to construct your hypothesis. If a patient reports loss of appetite, nausea, vomiting, fatigue, and fever, for example, and if you find a tender, somewhat enlarged liver and mild jaundice, build your hypothesis around jaundice and hepatomegaly rather than fatigue and fever. Although the other symptoms are useful diagnostically, they are much less specific.

b. Using your inferences about the structures and processes involved, *match your findings against all the conditions you know that can produce them.* For example, you can match your patient's red throat with a list of inflammatory conditions affecting the pharynx; or you can compare the symptoms and signs of the jaundiced patient with the various inflammatory, toxic, and neoplastic conditions that might produce this kind of clinical picture.

c. *Eliminate those diagnostic possibilities that fail to explain the findings.* You might consider conjunctivitis as a cause of the patient's red eye, for example, but eliminate this possibility because it does not explain the dilated pupil or decreased visual acuity.

d. *Weigh the competing possibilities* and *select the most likely diagnosis* from among those conditions that might be responsible for the patient's findings. You are looking, of course, for a *close match* between the patient's clinical presentation and a typical case of a given condition. Other clues help in this selection too. The *statistical probability* of a given disease in a patient of this age, sex, race, habits, lifestyle, and locality should have major impact on your selection. You should consider the possibilities of osteoarthritis and metastatic prostatic cancer in a 70-year-old man with back pain, for example, but not in a 25-year-old woman with the same complaint. The *timing of the patient's illness* also makes a difference. Productive cough with purulent sputum, fever, and chest pain that develops acutely over 24 hours suggests quite a different problem than do identical symptoms that develop over 3 or 4 months. In making a tentative diagnosis, unfortunately, you can seldom reach certainty but must often settle for the most probable explanation. Such is the real world of applied science.

e. Finally, in considering possible explanations for a patient's problem, give special attention to conditions that are *potentially life-threatening,* such as myocardial infarction and subdural hematoma, or *potentially treatable,* such as drug-induced delirium. Here you are trying to minimize the risk of missing conditions that may occur less frequently or be less probable but that, if present, would be particularly important.

5. Once you have made a hypothesis about a patient's problem, you will usually want to *test that hypothesis.* You may need further history, additional maneuvers on physical examination, or laboratory studies

to confirm or rule out your tentative diagnosis. When the diagnosis seems clear-cut—a simple upper respiratory infection, for example, or a case of hives—this step may not be necessary.

6. You should then be ready to *establish a working definition of the problem.* Make this at the highest level of explicitness and certainty that the data allow. You may be limited here to a symptom, such as "pleuritic chest pain, cause unknown." At other times you can define a problem explicitly in terms of structure, process, and cause. Examples include "pneumococcal pneumonia, right lower lobe," and "hypertensive cardiovascular disease with left ventricular enlargement, congestive heart failure, and sinus tachycardia."

The assessment process is not yet complete. You must next *consider the patient's responses to the illness,* together with *present and potential responses to your diagnoses.* What are the patient's understandings, feelings, and goals? You are then ready to *work out a plan* with the patient for that problem.

DIFFICULTIES AND VARIATIONS

LIMITATIONS OF THE MEDICAL MODEL. Although medical diagnosis is based primarily on identifying abnormal structures, disturbed processes, and specific causes, you will frequently see patients whose complaints do not fall neatly into these categories. Some symptoms defy analysis, and you may never be able to move beyond simple descriptive categories such as "fatigue" or "anorexia." Other problems relate to the patient's life rather than to the body. Loss of a job or loved one threatens a person, for example, and probably increases the risk of subsequent illness. Identifying such life events, evaluating a person's responses to them, and working out a plan to help the person cope with them are just as appropriate as dealing with the pharyngitis or duodenal ulcer. Some people, moreover, seek health care to maintain their health, not to detect and correct a disease. For them, and most others, in fact, "health maintenance" becomes a legitimate item on a list of "problems," and plans may include, for example, immunizations, nutritional advice, explorations of feelings about an important life event, and recommendations for seat belts or exercise.

SINGLE VERSUS MULTIPLE PROBLEMS. One of the greatest difficulties faced by the student is deciding whether to cluster the patient's symptoms into one or into several problems. The patient's *age* may help, since young people are more likely to have single diseases while older people tend to have multiple ones. Sometimes the *timing* of symptoms helps. An episode of pharyngitis 6 weeks ago is probably unrelated to fever, chills, chest pain, and cough today. Involvement of different *body systems* may be useful. While symptoms and signs within a single system can often be explained by one disease, manifestations in different, apparently unrelated systems frequently require more than one explanation. You might decide, for example, to group a patient's high blood pressure and sustained thrusting apical impulse with the flame-shaped retinal hemorrhages, place them in the cardiovascular system, and label the constellation "hypertensive cardiovascular disease with hypertensive retinopathy." You will likely develop another problem around the diarrhea and left lower quadrant tenderness.

Some diseases, on the other hand, affect more than one body system. As you gain in knowledge and experience, you will become increasingly adept at recognizing such *multisystem conditions* and at building plausible explanations that link together their seemingly unrelated manifestations. In trying to explain the productive cough, hemoptysis, and weight loss reported by a 60-year-old man who has smoked cigarettes for 40 years, you probably even now would postulate lung cancer as a probable cause. You might even support this hypothesis by your observation of clubbed fingernails. With time you will also recognize that his other symptoms and signs can be linked to the same diagnosis. The dysphagia is caused by extension of the cancer to the esophagus; the pupillary inequality is a Horner's syndrome caused by pressure on the cervical sympathetic chain; and the jaundice results from metastases to the liver.

AN UNMANAGEABLE ARRAY OF DATA. In trying to understand a patient's problems, the clinician is often confronted with a relatively long list of symptoms and signs and an equally long list of potential explanations or labels. As already suggested, you can tease out separate clusters of observations and deal with them one cluster at a time.

You can also analyze a given group of observations by asking key questions, the answers to which steer your thinking in one direction and allow you to ignore others temporarily. For example, you may ask what produces and relieves a person's chest pain. If the answer is exercise and rest respectively, you can concentrate on the cardiovascular system (and possibly the musculoskeletal system as well) and put aside the gastrointestinal tract. If the pain results from eating quickly and is relieved by regurgitating the food, you logically concentrate on the upper gastrointestinal tract. A series of such discriminating questions forms a branching logic tree or algorithm and is helpful in collecting data, analyzing them, and reaching conclusions that probably explain them.

QUALITY OF THE DATA. Virtually all the information with which the clinician works is subject to error. Patients forget symptoms, misremember the sequence in which they occurred, hide important but embarrassing facts, and shape their stories toward what interviewers seem to want to hear. Clinicians misunderstand their patients, overlook some relevant information, fail to ask the one key question, jump to premature diagnostic conclusions, or forget to examine the genitals of a patient with asymptomatic testicular carcinoma. You can avoid some of these errors by being thorough, by keeping an open mind as you gather data, and by analyzing any mistakes that you might make. Clinical data, however, including laboratory work, are inherently imperfect. The quality of information may be judged by its accuracy, precision, sensitivity, specificity, and predictive value.

Accuracy refers to the closeness with which a measurement reflects the true value of an object. *Precision*, on the other hand, refers to the reproducibility of a measurement.* These terms are illustrated below by four attempts to hit a target, at the center of which lies "truth."

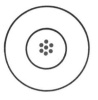   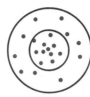

Accurate
and
precise

Inaccurate
but
precise

Inaccurate
and
imprecise

Note that a measurement may be quite precise and inaccurate at the same time, as shown in the second example. In the example on the far right the average of a large number of measurements would be accurate, but because of the imprecision an individual measurement cannot be so considered. In the usual clinical setting both of the imprecise examples, therefore, would have to be considered inaccurate.

Estimates of liver size by percussion illustrate these principles. The fact that such estimates vary between 2 cm and 3 cm depending on the force of percussion demonstrates that liver percussion is not an especially precise technique. The fact that percussion leads to smaller estimates of liver size than do radioisotope liver scans suggests that it is not very accurate either. Even so, percussion provides a better estimate than palpation alone.

Sensitivity of an observation or test refers to its ability to identify persons with a certain disease or condition among a group of people all of whom have that particular condition. When an observation fails to identify the abnormality in a person who has it, the result is called falsely negative. A highly sensitive test or observation detects most of the people with a given condition (the true positives) and has few false negatives.

Specificity of an observation or test refers to its ability to identify correctly those people who do *not* have the condition. A test that is 95% specific correctly identifies 95 out of 100 normal people. The other 5 are false positives.

---

* Definitions of these and similar terms vary with the discipline in which they are used. Accuracy, as used here, might also be considered as validity, precision as reliability.

Heart murmurs provide good examples of sensitivity and specificity. The vast majority of patients with significant valvular aortic stenosis have systolic murmurs audible in the aortic area. A systolic murmur is, therefore, quite a sensitive criterion for valvular aortic stenosis. When auscultation for an aortic systolic murmur is used to detect this condition, it finds most of the cases and misses only a few. The false negative rate is low. Such a murmur, however, sorely lacks specificity. Many other conditions, such as increased blood flow across a normal valve or the sclerotic changes associated with aging, may also produce this kind of murmur. If you were to use an aortic systolic murmur as your sole criterion for aortic stenosis, you would falsely label many patients as having it, thus producing many false positives. In contrast, the high-pitched decrescendo diastolic murmur heard best along the left sternal border is a murmur quite specific for aortic regurgitation. Normal people virtually never have such a murmur, and other conditions that might cause a similar sound are uncommon. The specificity of this murmur is very high.

The *positive predictive value* of an observation or test is the characteristic that is most relevant to the clinical setting. It refers to the proportion of positive observations that accurately predict the presence of a condition in a given population. In a group of women found to have suspicious breast nodules in a cancer screening program, for example, the proportion later determined to have breast cancer would constitute the positive predictive value of "suspicious nodules."

The *negative predictive value* of an observation or test refers to the proportion of negative observations that accurately predict the absence of a condition in a population. In a screening program for breast cancer, the proportion of women without suspicious nodules who really have no breast cancer constitutes the negative predictive value of the observation.

Unlike sensitivity and specificity (where populations by definition are all affected or unaffected respectively), predictive values depend heavily upon the prevalence of the condition within that population. Given unchanging sensitivity and specificity, the positive predictive value of an observation rises with prevalence while the negative predictive value falls.

These terms are often illustrated with the help of a 2 × 2 table that shows the results of an observation, both positive and negative, in a group of people some of whom have the disease and some of whom do not. Shown on page 607 is an observation with a sensitivity of 95% and a specificity of 90%, used in a group of 200 people, only half of whom have the disease.

Two examples further illustrate these principles and show how predictive values vary with prevalence. Consider first an imaginary population A with 1000 people. The prevalence of disease X in this population is high —40%. You can quickly calculate that 400 of these people have X. You then set out to detect these cases with an observation that is 90% sensitive and 80% specific. Of the 400 people with X, the observation detects

Disease

	Present	Absent	
+	95 true positive observations	10 false positive observations	105 total positive observations
−	5 false negative observations	90 true negative observations	95 total negative observations
	100 total persons with the disease	100 total persons without the disease	200 total persons

Observation (label on left side between + and −)

$$\text{Sensitivity} = \frac{\text{true positive observations (95)}}{\text{total persons with disease (95 + 5)}} \times 100 = 95\%$$

$$\text{Specificity} = \frac{\text{true negative observations (90)}}{\text{total persons without disease (90 + 10)}} \times 100 = 90\%$$

$$\text{Positive predictive value} = \frac{\text{true positive observations (95)}}{\text{total positive observations (95 + 10)}} \times 100 = 90.5\%$$

$$\text{Negative predictive value} = \frac{\text{true negative observations (90)}}{\text{total negative observations (90 + 5)}} \times 100 = 94.7\%$$

.90 × 400, or 360 (the true positives). It misses the other 40 (400 − 360, the false negatives). Out of the 600 people without X, the observation proves negative in .80 × 600, or 480. These people are truly free of X, as the observation suggests (the true negatives). But the observation misleads you in the remaining 120 (600 − 480). These people are falsely labelled as having X when they are really free of it (the false positives). These figures are summarized below:

Disease X

	Present	Absent	
+	360 true positive observations	120 false positive observations	480 total positive observations
−	40 false negative observations	480 true negative observations	520 total negative observations
	400 persons with X	600 persons without X	1000 total persons

Observation (label on left side between + and −)

As a clinician who does not have perfect knowledge of who really does or does not have disease X, you are faced with a total of 480 people with positive observations. You must try to distinguish between the true and the false positives and will undoubtedly use additional kinds of data to help you in this task. Given only the sensitivity and specificity of your observation, however, you can determine the probability that a positive observation is a true positive, and you may wish to explain it to the concerned patient. This probability is calculated as follows:

$$\text{Positive predictive value} = \frac{\text{true positives (360)}}{\text{total positives (360 + 120)}} \times 100 = 75\%$$

Thus 3 out of 4 of the persons with positive observations really have the disease and 1 out of 4 does not.

By a similar calculation you can determine the probability that a negative observation is a true negative. The results here are reasonably reassuring to the involved patient:

$$\text{Negative predictive value} = \frac{\text{true negatives (480)}}{\text{total negatives (480 + 40)}} \times 100 = 92\%$$

As prevalence of the disease in a population diminishes, however, the predictive value of a positive observation diminishes remarkably while the predictive value of a negative observation, already fairly good in population A, rises further. Consider a second population, B, of 1000 people, only 1% of whom have disease X. Now there are only 10 cases of X and 990 people without X. If this population is screened with the same observation, which has a 90% sensitivity and an 80% specificity, here are the results:

	Disease X		
	Present	Absent	
+	9 true positive observations	198 false positive observations	207 total positive observations
−	1 false negative observations	792 true negative observations	793 total negative observations
	10 persons with X	990 persons without X	1000 total persons

(Observation on the left spanning the + and − rows)

$$\text{Positive predictive value} = \frac{9}{207} \times 100 = 4\%$$

$$\text{Negative predictive value} = \frac{792}{793} \times 100 = 99+\%$$

You are now confronted with possibly upsetting 207 people (all those with positive observations) in order to detect 9 out of the 10 real cases. The predictive value of a positive observation is only 4%. Improving the specificity of your observation without diminishing its sensitivity would be very helpful, if it were possible. For example, if you could increase the specificity of the observation from 80% to 98% (given the same prevalence of 1% and sensitivity of 90%), the positive predictive value of the observation would improve from 4% to 31%—scarcely ideal but certainly better.

THE INTERPLAY OF ASSESSMENT AND DATA COLLECTION

The concepts of sensitivity and specificity help in both the collection and the analysis of data. They even underlie some of the basic strategies of interviewing. A question that is characterized by high sensitivity, if answered in the affirmative, may be particularly useful for screening and for gathering evidence to support a hypothesis. For example, "Have you had any discomfort or unpleasant feelings in your chest?" is a highly sensitive question for angina pectoris and in patients with this condition would yield few falsely negative responses. It is a good first screening question, but because there are many other causes of chest discomfort it is not at all specific. With additional directed questions about location, quality, and duration of the discomfort you can further test your hypothesis of angina pectoris. A pain that is retrosternal, pressing, and less than 10 minutes in duration—each a reasonably sensitive attribute of angina pectoris but not by itself specific—would add importantly to your growing evidence for the diagnosis. To confirm a hypothesis, a more specific question, if answered in the affirmative, is especially helpful. Precipitation of the pain by exercise and its prompt relief by rest are answers that serve this purpose.

Data with which to test a hypothesis come from the physical examination as well as from the history, and from both you can often screen, build your case, and clinch a diagnosis, even before obtaining further diagnostic tests. Consider the following list of evidence: cough, fever, a shaking chill, left-sided chest pain that is aggravated by breathing, and dullness throughout the left lower posterior lung field with crackles, bronchial breathing, and increased voice sounds. Cough and fever are good screening items for pneumonia, the next items support the hypothesis, and bronchial breathing with increased voice sounds in this distribution is very specific for lobar pneumonia. A chest x-ray would confirm the diagnosis.

Negative responses to a question or the absence of physical signs are also diagnostically useful, especially when the symptoms or signs are usually positive in a certain condition, *i.e.*, when they have a high sensitivity. For example, if a patient with cough and left-sided pleuritic chest pain does not have fever, bacterial pneumonia becomes much less likely (except possibly in infancy and old age). Likewise, in a patient with severe dyspnea, the absence of orthopnea makes left ventricular failure a less probable explanation for the shortness of breath.

Skilled clinicians use this kind of logic in making assessments whether or not they are conscious of its statistical underpinnings. They often start to generate tentative hypotheses from the patient's identifying data and the chief complaint, and then build evidence for one or more of these hypotheses and discard others as they ask questions and look for physical signs. In developing a present illness they borrow items from other parts of the history, such as the family history, the past history, and the review of systems. If a middle-aged patient complains of chest pain, the skilled clinician does not stop after determining the attributes of the pain. If the pain suggests coronary artery disease, further questions probe the risk factors for this condition such as smoking, high blood pressure, diabetes mellitus, and a family history of the disease. In both history and physical examination the clinician also focuses explicitly on other possible manifestations of coronary artery disease, such as congestive heart failure, and on evidence of atherosclerosis elsewhere in the body, such as intermittent claudication and diminished or absent pulses in the legs. By generating hypotheses early and by testing them sequentially, experienced clinicians improve their efficiency and enhance the relevance and value of the data they collect. They dig and collect less ore but they find more gold.

Because prevalence strongly affects the predictive value of an observation, prevalence too influences the assessment process. Because coronary artery disease is much more common in middle-aged men than in young women, you should pursue angina as a cause of chest pain more actively in the former group. The effect of prevalence on predictive value explains why your odds of making a correct assessment are better when you hypothesize a common condition as opposed to a rare one. The combination of fever, headache, myalgias, and cough probably has the same sensitivity and specificity for influenza throughout the year, but your chances of making this diagnosis correctly by using this cluster of symptoms is much greater during a winter flu epidemic than it is during a quiet August.

Prevalence varies importantly with clinical setting as well as with season. Chronic bronchitis is probably the most common cause of hemoptysis among patients seen in a general medical clinic. In the oncology clinic of a tertiary medical center, however, lung cancer might head the list, while in a group of postoperative patients on a general surgical service irritation from an endotracheal tube or pulmonary infarction might be most likely. In certain parts of the Far East, in contrast, one should think first of a worm called a lung fluke. When you hear hoofbeats in the distance, according to the familiar saying, bet on horses, not on zebras, unless of course you're visiting the zoo.

While there are enormous values in structuring your data collection so as to test hypotheses, there are also risks. First, initial judgments are often wrong. They allow you to overlook important data and may prevent you from entertaining other, possibly sounder hypotheses. Second, premature formulation of hypotheses may lead you to the premature asking of direct questions, and thus you may miss important parts of the patient's story. Third, focusing in on a single problem may lead you to incomplete assessment. Not every patient needs a complete evaluation, of course, but some have hypertension, some are seriously depressed, and some have cervical cancer. You cannot detect these problems unless you make the proper observations; to do so you have to be reasonably complete.

DEVELOPING A PROBLEM LIST AND PLAN

Turn now to the history and physical examination recorded for Mrs. N. in Chapter 20. Make a list of her symptoms and signs. Group these items together in a clinically rational way. Note that much of this clustering has already been done in constructing Mrs. N.'s present illness, since headache, nausea, vomiting, and psychological stress have all been placed together. You may or may not agree with this organization. Identify the problems to the degree that you can, and assess the patient's response to her illness.

Make a tentative problem list. In the Weed system two parallel columns are used: active problems go on the left, inactive ones on the right. The problem list is placed at the front of the patient's clinical record, and all notes refer to these problems by name and number.

Date problem entered	No.	Active problems	Inactive problems
	1		

For each active problem, develop an initial plan insofar as you can. Some problems, of course, may need no immediate attention. Undoubtedly you will want more information in some areas. Make getting it part of your plan.

Chapter 20
The Patient's Record

The clinical record documents the patient's history and physical findings. It shows how clinicians assessed the problems, what plans they made on the patient's behalf, what actions they took, and how the patient responded to their efforts. An accurate, clear, well organized record reflects and facilitates sound clinical thinking. It leads to good communication among the many professionals who participate in caring for the patient, and helps to coordinate their activities. It also serves to document the patient's problems and health care for medicolegal purposes.

When creating a record you do more than simply make a list of what the patient has told you and what you have found on examination. You must review your data, organize them, evaluate the importance and relevance of each item, and construct a clear, concise, yet comprehensive report. If you are a beginner, organizing the present illness will probably constitute one of the most difficult problems because considerable knowledge is needed to recognize which symptoms and signs are related to each other. That muscular weakness, heat intolerance, excessive sweating, diarrhea, and weight loss all constitute a present illness, for example, may not be apparent to either the patient or the student who is unfamiliar with hyperthyroidism. Until your knowledge and judgment grow, the patient's story itself and the seven key attributes of symptoms listed on pages 3 and 14 are helpful guides.

Regardless of your experience, certain principles will help you organize a good record. Order is imperative. Use it consistently and obviously so that future readers, including yourself, can easily find specific points of information. Keep items of history in the history, for example, and do not let them stray into the physical examination. Make your headings clear, use indentations and spacing to accentuate your organization, and asterisk or underline important points. Arrange the present illness in chronological order, starting with the current episode and then filling in the relevant background information. If a patient with longstanding diabetes is hospitalized in coma, for example, start with the events leading up to the coma, and then summarize the past history of the diabetes.

The amount of detail to record often poses a vexing problem. As a student, you may wish (or you may be required) to be quite detailed, since doing so is one way to build your descriptive skills, vocabulary, and speed — admittedly a painful, tedious process. Pressures of time, however, will ultimately force some compromises. The following guidelines may be useful in choosing what to record and what to omit:

1. *Record all the data* — both positive and negative — *that contribute directly to your assessment.* No diagnosis should be made, no problem identified, unless you have clearly spelled out the data upon which your assessment is based.

2. *Describe specifically any pertinent negative information* (i.e., the absence of a symptom or a sign) when other portions of the history or physical examination suggest that an abnormality might exist or develop in that area. For example, if the patient has large and unexplained bruises, you should specifically note the negative history for other kinds of bleeding, for injury and physical violence, for medications and nutritional deficits that might lead to bruising, and for familial bleeding disorders. If a patient feels depressed but not suicidal, state both facts. If the patient has no emotional problems, on the other hand, a comment on suicide is clearly unnecessary.

3. *Data not recorded are data lost.* No matter how vividly you can recall a detail today, you will probably not remember it in a few months. The phrase "neurologic exam negative," even in your own handwriting, may leave you wondering a few months hence: "Did I really do a sensory exam?"

4. On the other hand, information can be buried in a mass of excessive detail, to be discovered by only the most persistent reader. *Omit most of your negative findings* unless they relate directly to the patient's complaints or to specific exclusions in your diagnostic assessment. Do not try to list all the abnormalities that you did *not* observe. Instead, concentrate on a few major ones (such as "no heart murmurs") and try to describe structures in a concise, positive way. "Cervix pink and smooth" indicates that you saw no redness, ulcers, nodules, masses, cysts, or other suspicious lesions, but the description is shorter and much more readable. You can even omit certain bodily structures despite the fact that you examined them. You may thus leave out normal eyebrows and eyelashes even though you looked at them.

5. Save valuable time and space by omitting superfluous words. *Avoid redundancies* such as those in parentheses in the following examples: pink (in color), resonant (by percussion), tender (to palpation), both (right and left) ears, (audible) murmur, and (bilaterally) symmetrical thorax. Repetitive introductory phrases such as "The patient reports no . . ." are also redundant and may be omitted. Unless you have indicated otherwise, readers will assume that the patient gave you the history. *Use short words* instead of long and probably fancier ones when they mean the same thing: "seen" for "visualized," and "heard" for "auscultated." Try to *describe what you observed, not what you did.* "Optic discs seen" may mark an exciting moment in your career when you first glimpsed them, and it may be all you can claim during your first few tries at an ophthalmoscopic examination. "Disc

margins sharp," however, adds important information with only two additional letters.

6. *Be as objective as possible.* Hostility, moralizing comments, disgust, and disapproval have no place in the patient's record, whether conveyed in words, penmanship, or punctuation. Notes such as "PATIENT DRUNK AND LATE TO CLINIC AGAIN!!" tell more about the writer than about the patient and, furthermore, might prove embarrassing in court.

Because records are scientific and legal documents, they should be understandable. Employ abbreviations and symbols only if they are commonly used and understood. Some clinicians may wish to develop an elegant style and should certainly be encouraged to do so. Time is usually scarce, however, and style may be sacrificed in favor of concise completeness. In the sample record that follows, for example, words and brief phrases substitute for whole sentences. Legibility, of course, is always a virtue. Diagrams add greatly to the speed and ease with which a record communicates its message. Two examples follow:

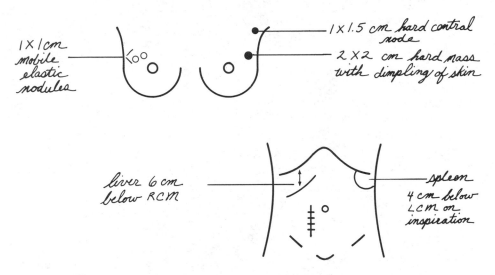

Make measurements in centimeters, not in fruits, vegetables, or nuts. "Pea-sized," "lemon-sized," and "walnut-sized" lesions vaguely convey an idea but make accurate evaluations and future comparisons impossible. How big were the lemons or peas? Did the walnut have a shell?

You should write the record as soon as possible, before the data fade from your memory. In your initial attempts at interviewing, you will probably prefer just to take notes when talking with a patient. As you gain experience, however, work toward recording in final form the past medical history, family history, and review of systems as you take them. Leave spaces for filling in later the present illness, the psychosocial history, and any other complex areas. During a physical examination it is wise to record immediately such specific measurements as the blood pressures in three positions. Recording a large number of items and descriptions interrupts the flow of the examination, however, and you will soon learn to remember your findings until you have finished.

Recording the history and physical examination is simplified, of course, by printed forms. If your institution or agency provides them, you may be expected to use them. You should also, however, be able to create a record without using a form. The example that follows offers one moderately complete guide. Although it is longer than most you may see in patients' charts, it still does not reflect every question and technique that you have learned to use. Note the difference in the statements that introduce the history and the physical examination. The basic identifying data start the history, while a descriptive paragraph that summarizes your general survey begins the physical examination.

Mrs. Audrey N., 1463 Maple Blvd., Capital City
12/13/86
Mrs. N. is a 54-year-old, widowed, white saleswoman.

REFERRAL. None.

SOURCE. Self, seems reliable.

CHIEF COMPLAINT. Headaches.

PRESENT ILLNESS. For about 3 mo Mrs. N. has been increasingly troubled by headaches: bifrontal, usually aching, occasionally throbbing, mild to moderately severe. She has missed work only once because of headaches, when she felt nauseated and miserable and vomited several times. Otherwise, nausea is associated only occasionally. Headaches now average once a wk, usually are there when she wakes up, and last all day. Little relief from aspirin. It helps to lie down, be quiet, use cold wet towel on head. No other related symptoms, no local weakness, no numbness or visual symptoms.

Mrs. N. first began to have headaches at age 15. "Sick headaches" recurred through her mid-20s, then diminished to one every 2 or 3 mo and finally almost disappeared.

Has recently had increased pressure at work, is also worried about daughter (see psychosocial). Thinks headaches may be like those in the past, but wants to be sure because mother died of a stroke. Is concerned that they make her irritable with her family.

PAST HISTORY

General Health. Good.

Childhood Illnesses. Only measles and chickenpox.

Adult Illnesses. None serious.

Psychiatric Illness. None.

Injuries. Stepped on glass at beach, 1983, laceration, sutured, healed.

Operations. Tonsillectomy, age 6; appendectomy, age 13.

Hospitalizations. St. Mary's, acute kidney infection, 1974.

CURRENT HEALTH STATUS

Allergies. Generalized skin rash with itching from <u>sulfa</u>.

Immunizations. Oral polio vaccine, yr uncertain; tetanus shots × 2 in 1983, followed by a booster 1 yr later; flu vaccine, 11/85, no reaction.

Screening Tests. Pap smear 1983, "normal." No mammograms.

Environmental Hazards. Medicines kept in unlocked medicine cabinet. Cleaning solutions, furniture polish, and Drano kept in unlocked cabinet below sink.

Safety Measures. Seat belt regularly.

Exercise/Leisure. "No time."

Sleep. Generally good, average 7 hr, sometimes has trouble falling asleep, is waked by alarm.

Diet. Breakfast—Orange juice, 2 sweet rolls, black coffee
      Mid-morning—Doughnut, coffee
      Lunch—Hamburger and bun or fish sandwich, coffee
      Dinner—Meat or fish, vegetable, potato, sometimes fruit, sometimes cookies
      Snacks in evening (*e.g.,* chips, cola)
      Has almost no milk or cheese

Current Medications. Aspirin for headaches, multivitamins. Has taken "water pill" for ankle swelling, but none in past several mo.

Tobacco. About 1 pack cigs per day from age 18 (36 pack yr).

Alcohol/Drugs. Rare drink (wine) only, doesn't like it. No drugs.

FAMILY HISTORY

(There are two methods of recording the family history. The diagrammatic format is more helpful than the narrative in tracing genetic disorders. The negative family information follows either format.)

* Asterisk or underline important points.

1. Diagrammatic

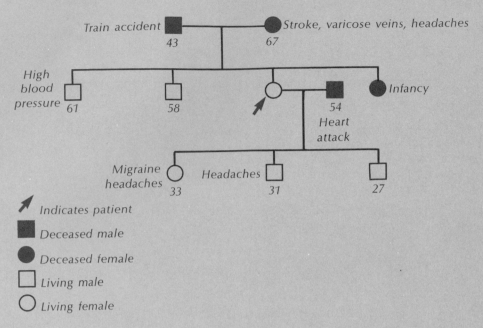

Train accident — 43 (Deceased male)
Stroke, varicose veins, headaches — 67 (Deceased female)

High blood pressure — 61
58
Patient (arrow)
54 — Heart attack (Deceased male)
Infancy (Deceased female)

Migraine headaches — 33
Headaches — 31
27

↗ Indicates patient
■ Deceased male
● Deceased female
□ Living male
○ Living female

2. Narrative Outline

Father died, 43, train accident
Mother died, 67, stroke, had had varicose veins, headaches
One brother, 61, has high blood pressure, otherwise well
One brother, 58, apparently well but for mild arthritis
One sister, died in infancy, ? cause
Husband died, 54, heart attack
One daughter, age 33, "migraine headaches," otherwise well
One son, 31, headaches
One son, 27, well

No family history of diabetes, tuberculosis, heart or kidney disease,
cancer, anemia, epilepsy, or mental illness

*PSYCHOSOCIAL. Born and raised in Lake City, finished high school,
married at age 19. Worked in store for 2 yr, then moved with husband to
Capital City, had 3 children. Mr. N. had steady factory job but to help with
income Mrs. N. went back to work 10 yr ago. Children have all married.
4 yr ago Mr. N. died suddenly of a heart attack. Finances now tight. Has
moved to small apartment to be near daughter, Dorothy. Dorothy's husband has a drinking problem and Mrs. N.'s apartment serves as a haven
for Dorothy and her 2 young children. Mrs. N. feels responsible for helping the family, is tense and nervous, but denies depression.

Typically up at 7:00 a.m., works 9:00 to 5:30, eats dinner alone. Dorothy or children visit most evenings and weekends. Moderate number of squabbles and considerable strain.

REVIEW OF SYSTEMS

*General. Has gained about 10 lb in the past 4 yr.

Skin. No rashes or other changes.

Head. No head injury. See present illness.

Eyes. Reading glasses for 5 yr, last checked 1 yr ago. No other symptoms.

Ears. Hearing good. No tinnitus, vertigo, infections.

Nose, Sinuses. Occasional mild cold. No hay fever, sinus trouble.

*Mouth and Throat. Some bleeding of gums recently. Last to dentist 2 yr ago. Occasional canker sore, has had one for 4 days.

Neck. No lumps, goiter, pain.

Breasts. No lumps, pain, discharge. Does breast self exams sporadically.

Respiratory. No cough, wheezing, pneumonia, tuberculosis. Last chest x-ray 1974, St. Mary's Hospital, normal.

Cardiac. No known heart disease or high blood pressure; last blood pressure taken in 1983. No dyspnea, orthopnea, chest pain, palpitations. No EKG.

*GI. Appetite good; no nausea, vomiting, indigestion. Bowel movement about once daily though sometimes has hard stools, q 2–3 d, when especially tense; no diarrhea or bleeding. No pain, jaundice, gallbladder or liver trouble.

*Urinary. Acute kidney infection, 1974, with fever and right flank pain; treated with pills, including sulfa; no recurrence. No frequency, dysuria, hematuria; nocturia × 1, large volume; occasionally loses some urine when coughs hard.

Genitoreproductive. Menarche at 13, regular periods, tapered off in late 40s and stopped at 49; no bleeding since; mild hot flashes and sweats then, none now.

Gravida 3, para 3, living children 3. Prolonged labor during first pregnancy, otherwise normal. Little sexual interest now, not sexually active.

Musculoskeletal. Mild *aching low back pain* often after a long day's work; no radiation down legs; used to do back exercises, but not now. No other joint pain.

Peripheral Vascular. *Varicose veins* appeared in both legs during first pregnancy. Has had swollen ankles after prolonged standing for 10 yr; wears light elastic panty hose; tried "water pill" 5 mo ago but it didn't help much; no history of phlebitis or leg pain.

Neurologic. No faints, seizures, motor or sensory loss. Memory good.

Hematologic. Except for bleeding gums, no easy bleeding. No anemia.

Endocrine. No known thyroid trouble, temperature intolerance. Sweating average. No symptoms or history of diabetes.

Psychiatric. See present illness and psychosocial.

PHYSICAL EXAMINATION

Mrs. N. is a short, moderately obese, middle-aged woman who walks and moves easily and responds quickly to questions. She wears no makeup but her hair is neatly fixed and her clothes immaculate. Although her ankles are swollen, her color is good and she lies flat without discomfort. She talks freely but is somewhat tense, with moist, cold hands.

P 94, regular   R 18   BP 164/98 right arm, lying
                          160/96 left arm, lying
                          152/88 right arm, lying (wide cuff)

                        Ht (without shoes) 157 cm (5'2")
Temp 37.1° C (oral)   Wt (dressed) 65 kg (143 lb)

Skin. Palms cold and moist, but color good. Scattered cherry angiomas over the upper trunk.

Head. Hair of average texture. Scalp and skull normal.

Eyes. Vision 20/30 in both eyes. Fields full by confrontation. Conjunctivas pink. Scleras clear. Pupils round, regular, equal, react to light. Extraocular movements intact. Disc margins sharp. No arteriolar narrowing, A–V nicking, hemorrhages, or exudates.

Ears. Wax partially obscures right drum. Left canal clear and drum negative. Acuity good (to whispered voice). Weber midline. AC > BC.

Nose. Mucosa pink, septum midline. No sinus tenderness.

Mouth. Mucosa pink. Several interdental papillae red and slightly swollen. Teeth in good repair. Tongue midline, negative but for a small (3 × 4 mm), shallow, white <u>ulcer</u> on an erythematous base, located on the undersurface near the tip; it is slightly tender but not indurated. Tonsils absent. Pharynx negative.

Neck. Trachea midline. Thyroid isthmus barely palpable, lobes not felt.

Nodes. Small (less than 1 cm), soft, nontender, and mobile tonsillar and posterior cervical nodes bilaterally. No axillary or epitrochlear nodes. Several small inguinal nodes bilaterally—soft and nontender.

Thorax and Lungs. Thorax symmetrical. Good expansion. Lungs resonant. Breath sounds normal with no added sounds.

Cardiovascular. Jugular venous pressure at level of sternal angle, with patient elevated at 30°. Carotid pulses normal and symmetrical. Apical impulse barely palpable in the 5th left interspace 8 cm from the midsternal line. Physiologic splitting of S_2. No S_3 or S_4. A grade 2/6 medium-pitched midsystolic <u>murmur</u> heard at the aortic area; does not radiate to the neck.

Breasts. Large, pendulous, symmetrical. No masses. Nipples erect and without discharge.

Abdomen. Obese, but symmetrical. Well-healed right lower quadrant scar. Bowel sounds normal. Except for a slightly tender sigmoid colon, no masses or tenderness. Liver, spleen, and kidneys not felt. Liver span 7 cm in right midclavicular line. No CVA tenderness.

Genitalia. Vulva normal. On straining, a mild <u>cystocele</u> appears. Vagina negative. Parous, smooth, pink cervix, nontender. Uterus anterior, midline, smooth, not enlarged. Adnexa difficult to delineate because of obesity and poor relaxation, but there is no tenderness. Pap smears taken. Rectovaginal examination confirms above.

Rectal. Negative. Brown stool, negative for occult blood.

Peripheral Vascular

Pulses (4+ = normal)

	RADIAL	FEMORAL	POPLITEAL	DORSALIS PEDIS	POSTERIOR TIBIAL
RT	4+	4+	4+	4+	4+
LT	4+	4+	4+	4+	4+

2+ edema of feet and ankles with 1+ edema extending up to just below knees. Moderate varicosities of saphenous veins bilaterally from midthigh to ankles, with venous stars on both lower legs. No stasis pigmentation or ulcers. No calf tenderness.

Musculoskeletal. No joint deformities. Range of motion, including hands, wrists, elbows, shoulders, spine, hips, knees, ankles, is normal.

Neurologic

Cranial Nerves. See head and neck. Also—

N5—Sensation intact, strength good

N7—Facial movement good

N11—Sternomastoids and trapezii strong

Motor. No atrophy or involuntary movements. Gait, heel-to-toe, heel and toe walking, knee bends, hops well done. Romberg negative. Grip and arms strong.

Sensory. Pain, vibration, light touch, and stereognosis screened and intact.

Reflexes. (Two methods of recording may be used, depending upon personal preference: a tabular form or a stick figure diagram, as shown below and at right.)

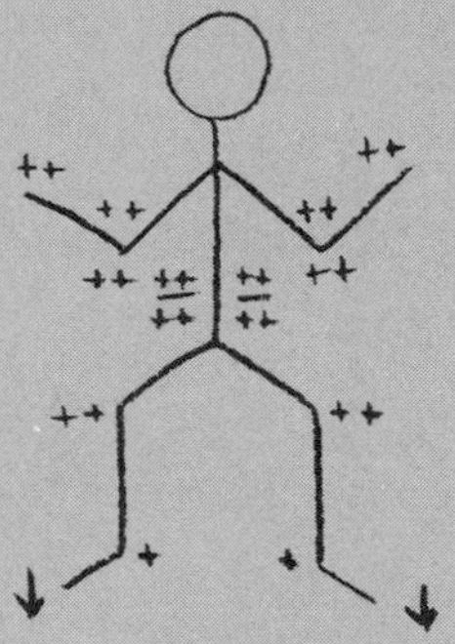

	BICEPS	TRICEPS	SUP	ABD	KNEE	ANKLE	PL
RT	2+	2+	2+	2+/2+	2+	1+	↓
LT	2+	2+	2+	2+/2+	2+	1+	↓

Mental Status. Tense but alert and cooperative. Thought coherent. Oriented. Cognitive testing not done in detail.

Before looking at the next page, assess Mrs. N.'s symptoms and physical findings. Then construct your own problem list for Mrs. N., as suggested in Chapter 19. You may choose to list the problems in order of their relative importance. In the Weed system, however, problems retain their same numbers over time while their relative importance often changes.

One way to organize Mrs. N.'s problem list is shown on the following page.

The clinician constructed the following problem list for Mrs. N. and placed it at the front of the chart.

Date problem entered	No.	Active problems	Inactive problems
12/13/86	1	Migraine headaches	
12/13/86	2		Acute kidney infection
12/13/86	3	Allergy to sulfa	
12/13/86	4	Tensions secondary to family situation, finances, and stress at work	
12/13/86	5	Gingivitis	
12/13/86	6	Low back pain	
12/13/86	7	Varicose veins with venous insufficiency	
12/13/86	8	Cystocele with occasional stress incontinence	
12/13/86	9	Borderline blood pressure	
12/13/86	10	Diet high in calories, fat, and carbohydrates, low in calcium	

Different clinicians often organize somewhat different problem lists for the same patient, and yours probably does not agree exactly with this one. Good lists vary in their emphases, length, and detail according to many factors, including the clinicians' philosophies, specialties, and perceptions of their appropriate roles in the care of the patient. The list illustrated here includes problems that need some attention now (such as the headaches) or may need further observation or possible future attention (such as the blood pressure and cystocele). The allergy is listed as an active problem to warn against inadvertent future prescriptions of sulfa drugs.

A few items noted in the history and physical examination, such as canker sores and constipation, do not appear in this problem list because they are relatively common phenomena that do not seem to demand attention. Such judgments are occasionally wrong, of course. Problem lists that are cluttered with relatively insignificant items, however, diminish in value. Some clinicians would undoubtedly judge this list too long; others would bring greater explicitness to problems such as "tensions," "diet," and "gingivitis." No one can specialize in everything.

The patient's record included notes on two of Mrs. N.'s problems:

1. Migraine headaches

   Assessment. Supporting this diagnosis are "sick headaches" in earlier life, recurrent course of headaches, their duration, their relief by cold and quiet, associated nausea and vomiting (once at least), and positive family history. Further, no related neurologic symptoms or signs. Headaches may be somewhat more frequent than typical migraine headaches, pain is usually aching rather than throbbing, and there are obvious tensions at work and at home. Tension headaches should also be considered, therefore, but the headaches fit this pattern less well.

Plan
    Diagnostic. Observation only. Mrs. N. to look for possible precipitating factors.
    Therapeutic. Continue aspirin as needed.
    Education. Nature of migraine discussed. Patient pleased and relieved.

9. Borderline blood pressure

Assessment. Some of apparent elevation clearly related to obese arms, and some may be related to anxiety of a first visit. No evidence of target organ damage.

Plan
    Diagnostic. Repeat BP in one month. Use wide cuff. Urinalysis.
    Therapeutic. None now. Consider diet change on next visit.
    Education. Need for BP checks explained.

A month later Mrs. N. returned for a second visit. Part of the progress notes read as follows:

1. Migraine headaches

Subjective (S). Has had only 2 headaches, both mild, without associated symptoms. No longer worried about them. Cannot detect any precipitating factors.
Objective (O). Not reexamined.
Assessment (A). Improved.
Plan (P). Return as needed.

9. Borderline blood pressure

S. None.
O. BP 146/84 right arm, lying (wide cuff).
    Urinalysis normal.
A. Borderline isolated systolic hypertension.
P. Repeat BP in 3 months.

Although you have insufficient information about most of Mrs. N.'s other problems, including her own priorities, try to develop an approach to them. What further data do you need?

What information do you need and how do you obtain it? These are the questions with which the book began and which continue throughout it—and long afterward. The process of learning about a patient continues far beyond the first encounter, and understanding grows in depth, complexity, and fascination. Although your knowledge of Mrs. N. is incomplete, you know a great deal about her and have the tools with which to expand your knowledge further. Needed now is repetitive practice, with supervision, in using your newly acquired tools.

Bibliography

GENERAL REFERENCES

Anatomy and Physiology

Anderson JE: Grant's Atlas of Anatomy, 8th ed. Baltimore, Williams & Wilkins, 1983

Basmajian JV: Grant's Method of Anatomy, 10th ed. Baltimore, Williams & Wilkins, 1980

Guyton AC: Textbook of Medical Physiology, 7th ed. Philadelphia, WB Saunders, 1986

Moore KL: Clinically Oriented Anatomy, 2nd ed. Baltimore, Williams & Wilkins, 1985

West JB (ed): Best and Taylor's Physiological Basis of Medical Practice, 11th ed. Baltimore, Williams & Wilkins, 1985

Williams PL, Warwick R (eds): Gray's Anatomy, 36th ed. Philadelphia, WB Saunders, 1980

Physical Examination

Burnside JW: Physical Diagnosis: An Introduction to Clinical Medicine, 16th ed. Baltimore, Williams & Wilkins, 1981

Clain A: Bailey's Demonstrations of Physical Signs in Clinical Surgery, 16th ed. Chicago, Year Book Medical Publishers, 1980

DeGowin EL, DeGowin RL: Bedside Diagnostic Examination, 4th ed. Philadelphia, WB Saunders, 1981

Delp MH, Manning RT: Major's Physical Diagnosis, 9th ed. Philadelphia, WB Saunders, 1981

Dunphy JE, Botsford TW: Physical Examination of the Surgical Patient, 4th ed. Philadelphia, WB Saunders, 1975

Judge RD, Zuidema GD, Fitzgerald FT: Clinical Diagnosis: A Physiologic Approach, 4th ed. Boston, Little, Brown & Co, 1982

Prior JA, Silberstein JS, Stang JM: Physical Diagnosis: The History and Examination of the Patient, 6th ed. St. Louis, CV Mosby, 1981

Walker HK, Hall WD, Hurst JW (eds): Clinical Methods: The History, Physical and Laboratory Examinations. Boston, Butterworth, 1980

Walker WF: Color Atlas of General Surgical Diagnosis. Chicago, Year Book Medical Publishers, 1976

Zatouroff M: Color Atlas of Physical Signs in General Medicine. Chicago, Year Book Medical Publishers, 1976

Changes with Age

ADOLESCENTS

Hofmann AD, Greydanus DE: Adolescent Medicine. Menlo Park, CA, Addison-Wesley, 1983

Rapp CE Jr: The adolescent patient. Ann Intern Med 99:52, 1983

Tanner JM: Growth at Adolescence, 2nd ed. Oxford, Blackwell Scientific Publications, 1962

OLDER PERSONS

Andres R, Bierman EL, Hazzard WR: Principles of Geriatric Medicine. New York, McGraw-Hill, 1985

Brocklehurst JC (ed): Textbook of Geriatric Medicine and Gerontology, 3rd ed. Edinburgh, Churchill Livingstone, 1985

Cassel CK, Walsh JR: Geriatric Medicine. New York, Springer, 1984

Finch CE, Schneider EL (eds): Handbook of the Biology of Aging, 2nd ed. New York, Van Nostrand Reinhold, 1985

Kamal A, Brocklehurst JC: Color Atlas of Geriatric Medicine. Oradell, NJ, Medical Economics Books, 1984

Libow LS, Sherman FT (eds): The Core of Geriatric Medicine: A Guide for Students and Practitioners. St Louis, CV Mosby, 1981

Mezey MD, Rauckhorst LH, Stokes SA: Health Assessment of the Older Individual. New York, Springer-Verlag, 1980

Rowe JW, Besdine RW (eds): Health and Disease in Old Age. Boston, Little, Brown & Co, 1982

Samiy AH: Clinical manifestations of disease in the elderly. Med Clin North Am 67:333, 1983

Steinberg FU (ed): Care of the Geriatric Patient, in the Tradition of EV Cowdry, 6th ed. St Louis, CV Mosby, 1983

Medicine and Surgery

Andreoli TE, Carpenter CCJ, Plum F et al: Cecil Essentials of Medicine. Philadelphia, WB Saunders, 1986

Blacklow RS: MacBryde's Signs and Symptoms: Applied Pathologic Physiology and Clinical Interpretation, 6th ed. Philadelphia, JB Lippincott, 1983

Branch WT Jr: Office Practice of Medicine, Philadelphia, WB Saunders, 1982

Fishman MC, Hoffman AR, Klausner RD et al: Medicine, 2nd ed. Philadelphia, JB Lippincott, 1985

Harvey AM, Johns RJ, McKusick VA et al (eds): The Principles and Practice of Medicine, 21st ed. East Norwalk, CT, Appleton-Century-Crofts, 1984

Petersdorf RG, Adams RD, Braunwald E et al (eds): Harrison's Principles of Internal Medicine, 10th ed. New York, McGraw-Hill, 1983

Sabiston DC Jr: Textbook of Surgery: The Biological Basis of Modern Surgical Practice, 13th ed. Philadelphia, WB Saunders, 1986

Schwartz SI (ed): Principles of Surgery, 4th ed. New York, McGraw-Hill, 1984

Wyngaarden JB, Smith LH Jr (eds): Cecil Textbook of Medicine, 17th ed. Philadelphia, WB Saunders, 1985

CHAPTER 1. INTERVIEWING AND THE HEALTH HISTORY

Baron RJ: An introduction to medical phenomenology: I can't hear you while I'm listening. Ann Intern Med 103:606, 1985

Benjamin A: The Helping Interview, 3rd ed. Boston, Houghton Mifflin, 1981

Butler RN, Lewis MI: Aging and Mental Health: Positive Psychosocial and Biomedical Approaches. St Louis, CV Mosby, 1982

Cassel EJ: The nature of suffering and the goals of medicine. N Eng J Med 306:639, 1982

Enelow AJ, Swisher SN: Interviewing and Patient Care, 3rd ed. New York, Oxford University Press, 1986

Engel GL, Morgan WL Jr: Interviewing the Patient. Philadelphia, WB Saunders, 1973

Friel PB: Death and dying. Ann Intern Med 97:767, 1982

Garcia WJ: Medical Sign Language: Easily Understood Definitions of Commonly Used Medical, Dental and First Aid Terms. Springfield, IL, Charles C Thomas, 1983

Hackett TP, Cassem NH (eds): Massachusetts General Hospital Handbook of General Hospital Psychiatry. St Louis, CV Mosby, 1978

Havens LL: Taking a history from the difficult patient. Lancet 1:138, 1978

Korsch BM, Freemon B, Negrete VF: Practical implications of doctor–patient interaction analysis for pediatric practice. Am J Dis Child 121:110, 1971

Levinson D: A Guide to Clinical Interviewing. Philadelphia, WB Saunders, 1987

The Occupational and Environmental Health Committee of the American Lung Association of San Diego and Imperial Counties: Taking the occupational history. Ann Intern Med 99:641, 1983

Sapira JD: Reassurance therapy: What to say to symptomatic patients with benign diseases. Ann Intern Med 77:603, 1972

Starfield B, Borkowf S: Physicians' recognition of complaints made by parents about their children's health. Pediatrics 43:168, 1969

Three Contrasting Views on Using First Names

Angelou M: I Know Why the Caged Bird Sings, pp 21–27. New York, Bantam Books, 1971 *(The memories of a black woman)*

Conant EB: Addressing patients by their first names. N Eng J Med 308:226, 1983 *(A patient's view)*

Heller ME: Addressing patients by their first names. N Eng J Med 308:1107, 1983 *(Short report of a survey of obstetrical outpatients)*

CHAPTER 2. AN APPROACH TO SYMPTOMS

General References

For most symptoms in this chapter please see the relevant references in later chapters and the texts listed under *Medicine and Surgery.* Among the latter the following three are especially helpful:

Blacklow RS: MacBryde's Signs and Symptoms: Applied Pathologic Physiology and Clinical Interpretation, 6th ed. Philadelphia, JB Lippincott, 1983

Branch WT Jr: Office Practice of Medicine. Philadelphia, WB Saunders, 1982

Petersdorf RG, Adams RD, Braunwald E et al (eds): Harrison's Principles of Internal Medicine, 10th ed. New York, McGraw-Hill, 1983

Sexual History and Related Topics

Cassens BJ: Social consequences of the acquired immunodeficiency syndrome. Ann Intern Med 103:768, 1985

Felman YM, Nikitas JA: Obtaining history of patient's sexual activities. NY State J Med 79:1879, 1979

Holland JC, Tross S: The psychosocial and neuropsychiatric sequelae of the acquired immunodeficiency syndrome and related disorders. Ann Intern Med 103:760, 1985

Kaplan HS: Evaluation of Sexual Disorders: Psychological and Medical Aspects. New York, Brunner/Mazel, 1983

Kolodny RC, Masters WH, Johnson VE: Textbook of Sexual Medicine. Boston, Little, Brown & Co, 1979

Nichols SE; Psychosocial reactions of persons with the acquired immunodeficiency syndrome. Ann Intern Med 103:765, 1985

Ostrow DG, Obermaier A: Sexual practices history. In Ostrow DG, Sandholzer TA, Felman YM (eds): Sexually Transmitted Diseases in Homosexual Men. New York, Plenum 1983

Roberts SJ: Gay health issues. In Jarvis LL (ed): Community Health Nursing: Keeping the Public Healthy. Philadelphia, FA Davis, 1985

Woods NF: Human Sexuality in Health and Illness, 3rd ed. St Louis, CV Mosby, 1984

Urinary Incontinence

Brink C: Promoting urine control in older adults: Assessing the problem. Geriatric Nursing 1:241, 1980

Wells T: Promoting urine control in older adults: Scope of the problem. Geriatric Nursing 1:236, 1980

Williams ME, Pannill FC III: Urinary incontinence in the elderly: Physiology, pathophysiology, diagnosis, and treatment. Ann Intern Med 97:895, 1982

Miscellaneous

Fox GN: Restless legs syndrome. Am Fam Physician 33:147, 1986

Harris RT: Bulimarexia and related serious eating disorders with medical complications. Ann Intern Med 99:800, 1983

Herzog DB, Copeland PM: Eating disorders. N Eng J Med 313:295, 1985

Kapoor WN, Karpf M, Wieand S et al: A prospective evaluation and follow-up of patients with syncope. N Eng J Med 309: 197, 1983 (The letters responding to this article, N Eng J Med 309:1650, 1983, suggest the difficulties of classifying patients with syncope.)

Komaroff AL: Acute dysuria in women. N Eng J Med 310:368, 1984

Lennard-Jones JE: Functional gastrointestinal disorders. N Eng J Med 308:431, 1983

Lipsitz LA: Syncope in the elderly. Ann Intern Med 99:92, 1983

CHAPTER 3. MENTAL STATUS

American Psychiatric Association: Diagnostic and Statistical Manual of Mental Disorders, 3rd ed. Washington, DC, American Psychiatric Association, 1980

Birren JE, Schaie KW (eds): Handbook of the Psychology of Aging, 2nd ed. New York, Van Nostrand Reinhold, 1985

Busse EW, Blazer DG (eds): Handbook of Geriatric Psychiatry. New York, Van Nostrand Reinhold, 1980

Drugs that cause psychiatric symptoms. Med Lett Drugs Ther 28:81, 1986 (Useful listing)

Kaplan HI, Sadock BJ: Modern Synopsis of Comprehensive Textbook of Psychiatry/IV, 4th ed. Baltimore, Williams & Wilkins, 1985

Nicholi AM Jr (ed): The Harvard Guide to Modern Psychiatry. Cambridge, Belknap Press of Harvard University Press, 1978

Strub RL, Black FW: The Mental Status Examination in Neurology, 2nd ed. Philadelphia, FA Davis, 1985

Thaler O, Engel I, Goldstein R: Mental status examination. Unpublished. Department of Psychiatry, University of Rochester Medical Center

CHAPTER 5. THE GENERAL SURVEY

McFadden JP, Price RC, Eastwood HD et al: Raised respiratory rate in elderly patients: A valuable physical sign. Br Med J 284:626, 1982 (*A rate over 25 per min suggests lower respiratory infection.*)

National Institutes of Health Consensus Development Conference: Health Implications of Obesity. Ann Intern Med 103 (6, pt 2), 1985 (*Twenty articles — an excellent source for the measurement and health risks of obesity*)

Nichols GA: Taking adult temperatures: Rectal measurements. Am J Nurs 72:1092, 1972

Nichols GA, Kucha DH: Taking adult temperatures: Oral measurements. Am J Nurs 72:1091, 1972

Tandberg D, Sklar D: Effect of tachypnea on the estimation of body temperature by an oral thermometer. N Eng J Med 308:945, 1983

Tanner JM: Growing up. Sci Am 229(3):34, 1973

CHAPTER 6. THE SKIN

Beaven DW, Brooks SE: Color Atlas of the Nail in Clinical Diagnosis. Chicago, Year Book Medical Publishers, 1984

Chanda JJ: The clinical recognition and prognostic factors of primary cutaneous malignant melanoma. Med Clin North Am 70:39, 1986

Fitzpatrick TB, Polano MK, Suurmond D: Color Atlas and Synopsis of Clinical Dermatology. New York, McGraw-Hill, 1983

Jeghers H, Edelstein LM: Skin color in health and disease. In Blacklow RS: MacBryde's Signs and Symptoms: Applied Pathologic Physiology and Clinical Interpretation, 6th ed. Philadelphia, JB Lippincott, 1983

McLaury P: Head lice: Pediatric social disease. Am J Nurs 83:1300, 1983

Moschella SL, Hurley HJ: Dermatology, 2nd ed. Philadelphia, WB Saunders, 1985

Rassner G: Atlas of Dermatology with Differential Diagnoses, 2nd ed. Baltimore, Urban & Schwarzenberg, 1983

Rosen T, Martin S: Atlas of Black Dermatology. Boston: Little, Brown & Co, 1981

Sauer GC: Manual of Skin Diseases, 5th ed. Philadelphia, JB Lippincott, 1985

CHAPTER 7. THE HEAD AND NECK

Eyes

Havener WH: Synopsis of Ophthalmology: The Ophthalmoscopy Book, 6th ed. St Louis, CV Mosby, 1984

Michaelson IC: Textbook of the Fundus of the Eye, 3rd ed. Edinburgh, Churchill Livingstone, 1980

Miller NR: Walsh and Hoyt's Clinical Neuro-Ophthalmology, 4th ed. Baltimore, Williams & Wilkins, 1982

Newell FW: Ophthalmology: Principles and Concepts, 5th ed. St Louis, CV Mosby, 1982

Straatsma BR (moderator): Aging-related cataract: Laboratory investigation and clinical management. Ann Intern Med 102:82, 1985

Vaughan D, Asbury T: General Ophthalmology, 10th ed. Los Altos, CA, Lange Medical Publications, 1983

Ears, Nose, and Throat

Aronson MD, Komaroff AL, Pass TM et al: Heterophil antibody in adults with sore throat: Frequency and clinical presentation. Ann Intern Med 96:505, 1982 (Infectious mononucleosis)

Bluestone CD, Stool SE: Pediatric Otolaryngology. Philadelphia, WB Saunders, 1983

Branch WT Jr, Weinstein L: Diseases of the upper respiratory tract. In Branch WT Jr: Office Practice of Medicine, Philadelphia, WB Saunders, 1982

Chole RA: Color Atlas of Ear Disease. New York, Appleton-Century-Crofts, 1982

Hawke M, Keene M, Alberti PW: Clinical Otoscopy: A Text and Colour Atlas. Edinburgh, Churchill Livingstone, 1984

Turner JS Jr, McConnel FMS: Disorders of the Ears, Nose and Throat. In Hurst JW (ed): Medicine for the Practicing Physician. Stoneham, MA, Butterworths, 1983

Mouth

Lynch MA, Brightman VJ, Greenberg MS (eds): Burket's Oral Medicine: Diagnosis and Treatment, 8th ed. Philadelphia, JB Lippincott, 1984

McCarthy PL, Shklar G: Diseases of the Oral Mucosa, 2nd ed. Philadelphia, Lea & Febiger, 1980

Pindborg JJ: Atlas of Diseases of the Oral Mucosa, 4th ed. Philadelphia, WB Saunders, 1985

Shafer WG, Hine MK, Levy BM: A Textbook of Oral Pathology, 4th ed. Philadelphia, WB Saunders, 1983

Neck

Ingbar SH: The thyroid gland. In Wilson JD, Foster DW: Williams Textbook of Endocrinology, 7th ed. Philadelphia, WB Saunders, 1985 (See pp. 742–743 for inspection and palpation of the gland.)

Jeghers H, Clark SL Jr, Templeton AC: Lymphadenopathy and disorders of the lymphatics. In Blacklow RS (ed): MacBryde's Signs and Symptoms: Applied Pathologic Physiology and Clinical Interpretation, 6th ed. Philadelphia, JB Lippincott, 1983

Linet OI, Metzler C: Practical ENT: Incidence of palpable cervical nodes in adults. Postgrad Med 62(4):210, 1977

CHAPTER 8. THE THORAX AND LUNGS

Baum GL, Wolinsky E: Textbook of Pulmonary Diseases, 3rd ed. Boston, Little, Brown & Co, 1983 (Comprehensive textbook)

Forgacs P: The functional basis of pulmonary sounds. Chest 73:399, 1978

Forgacs P: Lung Sounds. London, Baillière Tindall, 1978

Lal S, Ferguson AD, Campbell EJM: Forced expiratory time: A simple test for airways obstruction. Br Med J 1:814, 1964

Lehrer S: Understanding Lung Sounds (with audiocassette). Philadelphia, WB Saunders, 1984

Loudon R, Murphy RL: Lung sounds. Am Rev Respir Dis 130:663, 1984 (Review of the literature)

Snider GL: Clinical Pulmonary Medicine. Boston, Little, Brown & Co, 1981 (See pp. 63–85 for the pulmonary history and physical examination.)

Williams TJ, Ahmad D, Morgan WKC: A clinical and roentgenographic correlation of diaphragmatic movement. Arch Intern Med 141:878, 1981

CHAPTER 9. THE CARDIOVASCULAR SYSTEM

Cardiovascular Medicine

Braunwald E (ed): Heart Disease: A Textbook of Cardiovascular Medicine, 2nd ed. Philadelphia, WB Saunders, 1984 (Comprehensive textbook)

Hurst JW, Logue RB, Rackley CE et al (eds): The Heart, 6th ed. New York, McGraw-Hill, 1986 (Comprehensive textbook)

Huston TP, Puffer JC, Rodney WM: The athletic heart syndrome. N Eng J Med 313:24, 1985

Schlant RC, Felner JM, Miklozek CL et al: Mitral valve prolapse. DM 26:1, 1980

Physical Examination

Perloff JK: Physical Examination of the Heart and Circulation. Philadelphia, WB Saunders, 1982

Rothman A, Goldberger AL: Aids to cardiac auscultation. Ann Intern Med 99:346, 1983 (Critical review of the diagnostic efficacy of special auscultatory aids)

Tilkian AG, Conover MB: Understanding Heart Sounds and Murmurs: With an Introduction to Lung Sounds, 2nd ed. Philadelphia, WB Saunders, 1984 (with audiocassette)

Measuring and Interpreting Blood Pressure

The 1984 Report of the Joint National Committee on Detection, Evaluation, and Treatment of High Blood Pressure. Bethesda, MD, US Department of Health and Human Services, Public Health Service, National Institutes of Health, 1984

Adams CE, Leverland MB: Environmental and behavioral factors that can affect blood pressure. Nurse Pract 10(11):39, 1985

Kaplan NM: Hypertension: Prevalence, risks, and effect of therapy. Ann Intern Med 98 (Part 2):705, 1983 (*Argument against overdiagnosis and premature treatment*)

Kirkendall WM, Feinleib M, Freis ED et al: Recommendations for human blood pressure determination by sphygmomanometers. Circulation 62:1146A, 1980

O'Brien ET, O'Malley K: ABC of blood pressure measurement. Br Med J 2:795, 851, 920, 982, 1048, 1124, 1201, 1979

Pickering G: Normotension and hypertension: The mysterious viability of the false. Am J Med 65:561, 1978 (*The false dichotomy between normal and abnormal*)

Blood Pressure and the Elderly

Lipsitz LA, Nyquist RP Jr, Wei JY et al: Postprandial reduction in blood pressure in the elderly. N Eng J Med 309:81, 1983

Rowe JW: Systolic hypertension in the elderly. N Eng J Med 309:1246, 1983

CHAPTER 10. THE BREASTS AND AXILLAE

Pubertal Changes

Harlan WR, Harlan EA, Grillo GP: Secondary sex characteristics of girls 12 to 17 years of age. The US Health Examination Survey. J Pediatr 96:1074, 1980

Marshall WA, Tanner JM: Variations in pattern of pubertal changes in girls. Arch Dis Child 44:291, 1969

Tanner JM: Growth at Adolescence, 2nd ed. Oxford, Blackwell Scientific Publications, 1962

Diagnosis

Donegan WL: Diagnosis. In Cancer of the Breast, 2nd ed. Major Problems in Clinical Surgery 5, 1979

Haagensen CD, Bodian C, Haagensen DE Jr: Breast Carcinoma: Risk and Detection. Philadelphia, WB Saunders, 1981

Love SM, Gelman RS, Silen W: Fibrocystic "disease" of the breast—a nondisease? N Eng J Med 307:1010, 1982

Mushlin AI: Diagnostic tests in breast cancer: Clinical strategies based on diagnostic probabilities. Ann Intern Med 103:79, 1985

Breast Self-Examination — Techniques and Efficacy

Eggertsen SC, Bergman JJ: Breast self-examination: Historical perspective and current progress. J Fam Pract 16:713, 1983

Holtzman D, Celentano DD: The practice and efficacy of breast self-examination: A critical review. Am J Public Health 73:1324, 1983

Stromberg M: Screening for early detection. Am J Nurs 81:1652, 1981

Gynecomastia

Niewoehner CB, Nuttall FQ: Gynecomastia in a hospitalized male population. Am J Med 77:633, 1984 (*A surprisingly high prevalence that needs to be confirmed in other groups*)

CHAPTER 11. THE ABDOMEN

Textbooks

Cope's Early Diagnosis of the Acute Abdomen, 16th ed (revised by Silen W). New York, Oxford University Press, 1983

Sleisenger MH, Fordtran JS: Gastrointestinal Disease: Pathophysiology, Diagnosis, Management, 3rd ed. Philadelphia, WB Saunders, 1983

Issues and Problems in Estimating Liver Size

Castell DO, O'Brien KD, Muench H et al: Estimation of liver size by percussion in normal individuals. Ann Intern Med 70:1183, 1969

Sapira JD, Williamson DL: How big is the normal liver? Arch Intern Med 139:971, 1979

Castell DO: How big is the normal liver, indeed! Arch Intern Med 139:968, 1979

Ralphs DNL, Venn G, Khan O et al: Is the undeniably palpable liver ever "normal"? Ann R Coll Surg Engl 65:159, 1983

Splenic Percussion

Castell DO: The spleen percussion sign: A useful diagnostic technique. Ann Intern Med 67:1265, 1967 (*This study, based on 10 cases of splenomegaly and 10 controls, still needs replication. Although the sign may be useful, false positives have been reported.*)

Problems in Diagnosing Appendicitis

Bonello JC, Abrams JS: The significance of a "positive" rectal examination in acute appendicitis. Dis Colon Rectum 22:97, 1979

Berry J Jr, Malt RA: Appendicitis near its centenary. Ann Surg 200:567, 1984 (*Among patients operated on for appendicitis, symptoms, signs, and laboratory tests cannot identify the roughly 1 out of 5 who do not have the disease. As diagnostic accuracy increases, so do the chances of perforation.*)

CHAPTER 12. MALE GENITALIA AND HERNIAS

Pubertal Changes

Harlan WR, Grillo GP, Cornoni-Huntley J et al: Secondary sex characteristics of boys 12 to 17 years of age. The US Health Examination Survey. J Pediatr 95:293, 1979

Marshall WA, Tanner JM: Variations in the pattern of pubertal changes in boys. Arch Dis Child 45:13, 1970

Tanner JM: Growth at Adolescence, 2nd ed. Oxford, Blackwell Scientific Publications, 1962

Texts of Urology

Smith DR: General Urology, 11th ed. Los Altos, CA, Lange Medical Publications, 1984 *(See pp. 36–43 for examination of the genitourinary tract.)*

Walsh PC, Gittes RF, Perlmutter AD et al: Campbell's Urology, 5th ed. Philadelphia, WB Saunders, 1986 *(See vol 1, pp. 280–285, for examination of the genitourinary tract.)*

Hernias

Morton JH: Abdominal wall hernias. In Schwartz SI: Principles of Surgery, 4th ed. New York, McGraw-Hill, 1984

Nyhus LM, Bombeck CT: Hernias. In Sabiston DC Jr: Textbook of Surgery: The Biological Basis of Modern Surgical Practice, 13th ed. Philadelphia, WB Saunders, 1986

Sexually Transmitted Diseases

Bingham JS: Sexually Transmitted Diseases. Baltimore, Williams & Wilkins, 1984 *(A well illustrated pocket guide)*

Corey L, Adams HG, Brown ZA et al: Genital herpes simplex virus infections: Clinical manifestations, course, and complications. Ann Intern Med 98:958, 1983

Corey L, Holmes KK: Genital herpes simplex virus infections: Current concepts in diagnosis, therapy, and prevention. Ann Intern Med 98:973, 1983

DeVita VT Jr, Hellman S, Rosenberg SA (eds): AIDS: Etiology, Diagnosis, Treatment, and Prevention. Philadelphia, JB Lippincott, 1985

Jaffe HW, Hardy AM, Morgan WW et al: The acquired immunodeficiency syndrome in gay men. Ann Intern Med 103:662, 1985

Stamm WE, Koutsky LA, Benedetti JK et al: *Chlamydia trachomatis* urethral infections in men: Prevalence, risk factors, and clinical manifestations. Ann Intern Med 100:47, 1984

Ostrow DG, Altman NL: Sexually transmitted diseases and homosexuality. Sex Transm Dis 10:208, 1983

Wolbert J: Sexually transmitted diseases in homosexual men. Nurse Pract 8(9):35, 1983

CHAPTER 13. THE FEMALE GENITALIA

Pubertal Changes

See the three references listed in the *Pubertal Changes* section under Chapter 10.

Texts of Obstetrics and Gynecology

Bongiovanni AM: Adolescent Gynecology: A Guide for Clinicians. New York, Plenum, 1983

Danforth DN, Dignam WJ, Hendricks CH et al (eds): Obstetrics and Gynecology, 4th ed. Philadelphia, Harper & Row, 1982

Jones GS, Jones HW Jr: Gynecology, 3rd ed. Baltimore, Williams & Wilkins, 1982

Kistner RW: Gynecology: Principles and Practice, 4th ed. Chicago, Year Book Medical Publishers, 1986

Romney SL, Gray MJ, Little AB et al: Gynecology and Obstetrics: The Health Care of Women, 2nd ed. New York, McGraw-Hill, 1981

The Pelvic Examination — Three Sets of Suggestions

Hein K: The first pelvic examination and common gynecological problems in adolescent girls. Women Health 9(2/3):47, 1984

Magee J: The pelvic examination: A view from the other end of the table. Ann Intern Med 83:563, 1975

Primrose RB: Taking the tension out of pelvic exams. Am J Nurs 84:72, 1984

Sexually Transmitted Diseases

Brunham RC, Paavonen J, Stevens CE et al: Mucopurulent cervicitis—the ignored counterpart in women of urethritis in men. N Eng J Med 311:1, 1984

See also the references listed under Chapter 12, above.

CHAPTER 14. THE ANUS AND RECTUM

Lieberman DA: Common anorectal disorders. Ann Intern Med 101:837, 1984

Quinn TC: Gay bowel syndrome: The broadened spectrum of nongenital infection. Postgrad Med 76(2):197, 1984

Schrock TR: Diseases of the anorectum. In Sleisenger MH, Fordtran JS: Gastrointestinal Disease: Pathophysiology, Diagnosis, Management, 3rd ed. Philadelphia, WB Saunders, 1983

Tests for occult blood. Med Lett Drugs Ther 28:5, 1986

Thomson JPS, Nicholls RJ, Williams CB (eds): Colorectal Disease. New York, Appleton-Century-Crofts, 1981

CHAPTER 15. THE PERIPHERAL VASCULAR SYSTEM

Jeghers H, Clark SL Jr, Templeton AC: Lymphadenopathy and disorders of the lymphatics. In Blacklow RS (ed): MacBryde's Signs and Symptoms: Applied Pathologic Physiology and Clinical Interpretation, 6th ed. Philadelphia, JB Lippincott, 1983

Juergens JL, Spittell JA Jr, Fairbairn J II (eds): Allen-Barker-Hines Peripheral Vascular Diseases, 5th ed. Philadelphia, WB Saunders, 1980

Spittell JA Jr (ed): Clinical Vascular Disease. Cardiovasc Clin 13 (2), 1983

CHAPTER 16. THE MUSCULOSKELETAL SYSTEM

Bluestone R: Symptoms and signs of articular disease. In Resnick D, Niwayama G: Diagnosis of Bone and Joint Disorders, Vol 1. Philadelphia, WB Saunders, 1981

Hoppenfeld S: Physical Examination of the Spine and Extremities. East Norwalk, CT, Appleton-Century-Crofts, 1976

Kelley WN, Harris ED Jr, Ruddy S et al: Textbook of Rheumatology, 2nd ed. Philadelphia, WB Saunders, 1985

McCarty DJ (ed): Arthritis and Applied Conditions: A Textbook of Rheumatology, 10th ed. Philadelphia, Lea & Febiger, 1985

Polley HF, Hunder GG: Rheumatologic Interviewing and Physical Examination of the Joints, 2nd ed. Philadelphia, WB Saunders, 1978

Rodnan GP, Schumacher HR (eds): Primer on the Rheumatic Diseases, 8th ed. Atlanta, GA, Arthritis Foundation, 1983

CHAPTER 17. THE NERVOUS SYSTEM

Anatomy and Physiology

Chusid JG: Correlative Neuroanatomy and Functional Neurology, 18th ed. Los Altos, CA, Lange Medical Publications, 1982

Gilman S, Winans SS: Manter and Gatz's Essentials of Clinical Neuroanatomy and Neurophysiology, 6th ed. Philadelphia, FA Davis, 1982

Neurology

Adams RD, Victor M: Principles of Neurology, 3rd ed. New York, McGraw-Hill, 1985

Plum F, Posner JB: The Diagnosis of Stupor and Coma, 3rd ed. Contemporary Neurology Series 19, 1980

Rowland LP (ed): Merritt's Textbook of Neurology, 7th ed. Philadelphia, Lea & Febiger, 1984

The Neurologic Examination

Aids to the Examination of the Peripheral Nervous System: Medical Research Council Memorandum No. 45. London, Her Majesty's Stationery Office, 1976

Bickerstaff ER: Neurological Examination in Clinical Practice, 4th ed. Oxford, Blackwell Scientific Publications, 1980

DeJong RN: The Neurologic Examination: Incorporating the Fundamentals of Neuroanatomy and Neurophysiology, 4th ed. Hagerstown, Harper & Row, 1979

Mancall EL: Alpers and Mancall's Essentials of the Neurologic Examination, 2nd ed. Philadelphia, FA Davis, 1981

Mayo Clinic Department of Neurology: Clinical Examinations in Neurology, 5th ed. Philadelphia, WB Saunders, 1981

Van Allen MW, Rodnitzsky RL: Pictorial Manual of Neurologic Tests: A Guide to the Performance and Interpretation of the Neurologic Examination, 2nd ed. Chicago, Year Book Medical Publishers, 1980

CHAPTER 18. THE PHYSICAL EXAMINATION OF INFANTS AND CHILDREN

Battaglia FC, Lubchenco LO: A practical classification of newborn infants by weight and gestational age. J Pediatr 71:159, 1967

Burnside JW: Physical Diagnosis: An Introduction to Clinical Medicine, 16th ed. Baltimore, Williams & Wilkins, 1981

Caceres CA, Perry W: The Innocent Murmur: A Problem in Clinical Practice. Boston, Little, Brown & Co, 1967

Capraro VJ: Gynecological examination in children and adolescents. Pediatr Clin North Am 19:511, 1972

Chung SM: Hip Disorders in Infants and Children. Philadelphia, Lea & Febiger, 1981

Dubowitz LV, Dubowitz C, Goldberger C: Clinical assessment of gestational age in the newborn infant. J Pediatr 77:1, 1970

Frankenburg WK, Camp BW (eds): Pediatric Screening Tests. Springfield, IL, Charles C Thomas, 1975

Gorman JJ, Cogan DG, Gellis SS: An apparatus for grading the visual acuity of infants on the basis of opticokinetic nystagmus. Pediatrics 19:1088, 1957

Hoekelman RA et al (eds): Primary Care Pediatrics. St Louis, CV Mosby, 1986

Illingworth RS: An Introduction to Developmental Assessment in the First Year. London, National Spastics Society Medical Education and Information Unit, 1962

Lawson EE, Grand RJ, Neff RK, Cohen LF: Clinical estimation of liver span in infants and children. Am J Dis Child 132:474, 1978

Lowrey GH: Growth and Development of Children, 7th ed. Chicago, Year Book Medical Publishers, 1978

Lubchenco LO, Searls DT, Brazie JV: Neonatal mortality rate: Relationship to birth weight and gestational age. J Pediatr 81:814, 1972

Nadas AS, Fyler DC: Pediatric Cardiology, 3rd ed. Philadelphia, WB Saunders, 1972

Newell FW: Ophthalmology: Principles and Concepts, 5th ed. St Louis, CV Mosby, 1982

Paine RS: Neurological examination of infants and children. Pediatr Clin North Am 7:471, 1960

Sweet AY: Classification of the low-birth-weight infant. In Klaus MH, Fanaroff AA (eds): Care of the High-Risk Neonate, 2nd ed. Philadelphia, WB Saunders, 1979

Tachdjian MO: Diagnosis and treatment of congenital deformities of the musculoskeletal system in the newborn and the infant. Pediatr Clin North Am 14:307, 1968

Thomas A, Chesni Y, Dargassies SS: The Neurological Examination of the Infant. London, National Spastics Society Medical Education and Information Unit, 1960

Van Allen MW: Pictorial Manual of Neurological Tests: A Guide to the Performance and Interpretation of the Neurologic Examination, 2nd ed. Chicago, Year Book Medical Publishers, 1980

CHAPTER 19. CLINICAL THINKING: FROM DATA TO PLAN

Brody DS: The patient's role in clinical decision-making. Ann Intern Med 93:718, 1980

Clinical disagreement: I. How often it occurs and why. II. How to avoid it and how to learn from one's mistakes. Can Med Assoc J 123:499, 613, 1980

Cutler P: Problem Solving in Clinical Medicine: From Data to Diagnosis, 2nd ed. Baltimore, Williams & Wilkins, 1985

Engel GL, Morgan WL Jr: The diagnostic process. In Interviewing the Patient. London, WB Saunders, 1973

Feinstein AR: Clinical Judgment. Baltimore, Williams & Wilkins, 1979

Feinstein AR: A bibliography of publications on observer variability. J Chron Dis 38:619, 1985

Griner, PF, Mayewski RJ, Mushlin AI et al: Selection and interpretation of diagnostic tests and procedures: Principles and applications. Ann Intern Med 94:553, 1981

Hart FD: French's Index of Differential Diagnosis, 12th ed. Bristol, John Wright and Sons, 1985 *(An illustrated encyclopedia)*

Seller RH: Differential Diagnosis of Common Complaints. Philadelphia, WB Saunders, 1986

Seward C, Mattingly D: Bedside Diagnosis, 12th ed. Edinburgh, Churchill Livingstone, 1985

CHAPTER 20. THE PATIENT'S RECORD

Hurst JW, Walker HK: The Problem-Oriented System. New York, Medcom Press, 1972

Index

Numbers followed by an *f* indicate a figure; *t* following a page number indicates tabular material. Page numbers in boldface denote material found on color plates. Numbers followed by *n* indicate material found in footnote.

alcohol consumption
  asking about, 16
  liver disease related to, 45
Allen test, 413
allergic rhinitis, 212*t*
amblyopia, 561, 562
amblyopia ex anopsia, 559
amenorrhea, 49, 50, 378
amnestic syndrome, distinguishing
    features, 116*t*
anal canal, 398
anal fissure, 403*t*
analgesia, 497
anal reflex, 590
anarthria, 110*t*
anemia, hemolytic, 570
anesthesia, 497
aneurysm, dissecting aortic, 66*t*–67*t*
"angel kisses," 547
anger, dealing with, during
    interview, 22–23
angina pectoris, chest pain, 66*t*–67*t*
angioma(s), cherry, 136
angioneurotic edema, 214*t*
angle, sternal, 222
angular stomatitis, 213*t*
anisocoria, 193*t*
anisometropia, 559
ankle(s)
  anatomy and physiology, 433
  clonus, 506, 590
  dorsiflexion, 493
  examination technique, 447–448
  motions at, 433
  range of motion, 448
  reflex, 471, 504–505
  ulcers, 421*t*
ankylosing spondylitis, 454–455
ankylosis, 442
anorectal fistula, 403*t*
anorectal junction, 398
anorexia, 42
anoxia, 546, 557
antihypertensive medication, 274
anus
  abnormalities, 403*t*–404*t*
  anatomy and physiology, 398–399
  examination technique
    for female, 402
    lesions, 77*t*, 401
    for male, 400–402
anxiety(ies)
  abnormal, 103

blood pressure and, 542
chest pain and, 36, 66*t*–67*t*
during health history interview,
    22
with hyperventilation, dyspnea,
    68*t*–69*t*
irrational, 112*t*–113*t*
temperature elevation with, 541
aorta
  abdominal, 330
  anatomy and physiology, 255,
    257, 258
  coarctation, 543, 575
    murmur of, 576
  palpation, 346–347, 581
  tortuous, 268
aortic regurgitation, 274, 309*t*
aortic stenosis, 92*t*–93*t*, 305*t*–306*t*,
    576
aortic systolic murmurs, 267
aortic valve, 258, 262
Apgar scoring system, 531, 532*t*
aphasia, 100–101, 110*t*
aphonia, 110*t*
aphthous ulcer, 215*t*
apical impulse, 254*n*, 267, 281–282,
    575
apnea, 542
apocrine glands, 134
appearance of patient, as clinical
    tool, in mental status
    examination, 99–100
appendicitis
  abdominal pain and tenderness
    of, 41, 74*t*–75*t*, 355*t*
  assessment of, 348–350
  in children, 581
appetite, 42
apprehensive patient, blood
    pressure measurement with,
    275
aqueous humor, 149
arcus senilis, 161
areola, 311, 323, 326*t*
Argyll Robertson pupils, 194*t*
arm(s)
  examination techniques, 412–413
  inspection of, 412
  pain in, 54
arrhythmia(s)
  assessment of, 276
  differentiation of, 296*t*
  sinus, 575

syncope and, 92*t*–93*t*
arterial pulse, 264, 269–271
  abnormalities of, 297*t*
arterioles, in eye, 174
arteriosclerosis, 268
arteriosclerosis obliterans, 86*t*–87*t*,
    415
artery(ies)
  anatomy and physiology, 406–407
  insufficiency, 418–419, 420*t*, 421*t*
  occlusion, 86*t*–87*t*, 412
arthralgias, 55
arthritis. *See also specific types*
  acromioclavicular, 463*t*
  of elbow, 461*t*
  gouty, 88*t*–89*t*, 464*t*
  pain and inflammation of, 442
  skin symptoms, 56
ascites
  assessment of, 347–348
  protuberant abdomen from, 352*t*
assessment process. *See also under
    specific organs*
  from data base to plan, 599–600
  description of, 601–603
  interplay with data collection,
    609–611
asteatosis, 136
astereognosis, 499
asterixis, 518*t*
asthma, bronchial
  cough of, 70*t*
  dyspnea of, 68*t*–69*t*
  pediatric, 542
astigmatism, 171
ataxia, 485, 517*t*
atelectasis, 252*t*
athetosis, 519*t*
atresia, 531, 532, 537
atrial septal defect, 576
atrioventricular node, 262
atrium, 254, 257
atrophic vaginitis, 393*t*
atrophy
  hands, 440–441
  muscular, 488–489
  optic, 197*t*
  skin, 143*t*
attention
  assessment of, 96
  tests of, 104–105
attrition of teeth, 217*t*
auricle, 153, 176

mammary souffle, 267n
manual compression test, 418
manubrium, 430
Marfan's syndrome, 130
mass(es), abdominal, 339–340, 345, 350
mastoiditis, 566
mastoid process, 153
mediastinal crunch, 249t
megacephaly, 550
megacolon, congenital, 578
melanin, 135, 217t
melanoma, malignant, **208**
melanotic pigmentation, 546
melena, 43, 76t
memory, 96, 105
menarche, 314, 376
Meniere's disease, 64t
meningeal irritation, 62t–63t, 556
meningeal signs, 506–507
meningitis, 32, 597
menisci, 435
menopause, 50, 385
menorrhagia, 49–50
menstruation, 49, 378
mental function, components of, 96–97
mental retardation, 24–25
mental status
  assessments, 108, 123
  changes in, with age, 97
  screening for, 65
  techniques of examination, 98–108
metacarpophalangeal joint, 428
metal ingestion, signs of, 570
metastases, peritoneal, 404t
metatarsalgia, 447
metatarsals, 433
metatarsophalangeal joint(s), 433, 447
metatarsus adductus deformity, 585
metatarsus varus, 585
metrorrhagia, 50
microaneurysms, 199t
microcephaly, 550
micrognathia, 549
micturition syncope, 92t–93t
midclavicular line, 224
milia, 547
miliaria rubra, 547
miniature toy test, 562
miosis, 169

mitral valve
  aging, 268
  anatomy, 255–256, 259
  regurgitation
    causes, 267, 268
    in infants and children, 576–577
    murmurs, 307t
  sounds, 260, 261
  stenosis, 259, 286, 575, 576
    cough from, 70t
    hemoptysis from, 71t–72t
    murmurs of, 309t
molding, 549
Mongolian spots, 546
moniliasis, 215t, 568
monilia vaginitis, 392t
mononucleosis, infectious, 219t, 554–555, 571
mons pubis, 373
mood, assessment of, as clinical tool, 96, 101, 102
Moro response, 594–595
motion, limitation of, 55
motor function
  behavior and appearance of, 99, 131
  coordination testing, 589
  deficits, 473
  disorders, dysphagia of, 73t
  testing during infancy, 589
motor neuron
  anatomy, 470
  disorders
    lower, 514t, 521t
    upper, 515t, 521t
motor pathways, 471–473
motor system
  dysfunctions, differentiation of, 521t
  examination technique, 485–496
mouth
  abnormalities of buccal mucosa, 215t
  aging and, 161
  anatomy, 156–157
  examination techniques, 121, 182–183
  of newborn, 567
  symptoms, 35–36
movement(s). See also specific movements
  of hip, 437
  involuntary, 58, 518t–520t

at neck, 438
mucocele, 214t
multiple symptoms, patients with, 22
mumps, 187t, 554
murmur(s)
  aging and, 267
  in children, 575–576
  continuous, 288
  description, 260–261
  diastolic, 287, 288n, 308t–309t
  innocent, 290, 306t, 576
  intensity, 288–289
  listening for, 287
  mechanisms, 304t
  midsystolic, 305t–306t
  organic, 576
  origination, 285
  pansystolic or holosystolic, 307t
  pulmonic systolic, 267
  relation to chest wall location, 261–262
  shape, 288–289
  systolic, 287, 288n, 290
Murphy's sign, 350
muscle(s). See also specific muscles
  eye, 148
  of limbs and trunk, inspection of, 488–489
  strength, testing of, 490–493
  tone, assessment of, 489
muscular dystrophy, 597
musculoskeletal system
  anatomy and physiology, 426–439
  assessing coordination, 494–496
  assessment of, 54–56
  changes with age, 440–441
  examination techniques, 123
    general approach, 442–443
  further motor assessment, 488–496
  infancy, 584–587
  special maneuvers, 455–457
myalgias, 55
myasthenia gravis, 481
mydriasis, 169, 171
mydriatic drug, 171
myocardial contractility, 263
myocardial infarction
  chest pain, 66t–67t
  syncope, 92t–93t
myoclonus, 520t
myomas, 385, 395t

indications, 378
position, 380
technique, 378–380
pelvic inflammatory disease, 384, 397t
pelvis
anatomy, 436–437
diseases, causing abdominal tenderness, 354t
examination. *See* pelvic examination
referred pain from, 90t
penis
abnormalities of, 368t
anatomy, 359
carcinoma of, 368t
development, 360–362
discharge from, 51–52
inspection of, 363–364
palpation, 364
size in childhood, 582
peptic ulcer, abdominal pain with, 74t–75t
percussion
abdomen, 336–339, 578
chest, 234–238, 241–242
heart, 284
liver, 580, 581t
notes
in bronchi and lung abnormalities, 250t–252t
characteristics of, 237
Perez reflex, 594
perforating veins, 408
pericardial friction rub, 310t
pericarditis, chest pain with, 66t–67t
perineum, 373
periodic breathing, 573
periodontitis, 216t
periorbital edema, 189t
peristalsis, 334
peristaltic waves, 579
peritoneum
inflammation, tenderness associated with, 355t
irritation, assessment for, 340
metastases, 404t
peritonitis, 581
peritonsillar abscess, 219t, 571–572
periurethral inflammation, 364
petechiae, 59, 144t, 567
Peutz-Jeghers syndrome, 214t
Peyronie's disease, 368t

Phalen's test, 456
pharynx
abnormalities, 219t
anatomy, 156–157
examination techniques, 121, 183
visualization in child or infant, 568, 569
pheochromocytoma, 543
phimosis, 364
phlebitis, signs, 417
phlegm. *See* sputum
phobias, 103
physical examination. *See also specific organs*
approach, 118–121
general survey, 121
overview, 121–124
physical violence, discussion of, in health history interview, 16–17
pigmentation, melanotic, 546
pilonidal cyst and sinus, 403t
pinguecula, 190t
pitcher's elbow, 461t
placing response, 592–593
plagiocephaly, 549
plantar flexion, 433
plantar responses, 471, 505–506
plantar wart, 465t
plaque, skin, 142t
platelet disorder, 59
pleural effusion, 237, 238
pleural fluid, 250t
pleural pain, 66t–67t
pleurisy, abdominal tenderness, 354t
PMS. *See* premenstrual tension syndrome
pneumonia
cough in, 70t
dyspnea in, 68t–69t
hemoptysis in, 71t–72t
lobar, 234, 242, 251t
pneumothorax, 68t–69t, 252t
point localization, 500
point-to-point testing, 495–496
polydipsia, 47, 59
polymenorrhea, 49–50
polymyalgia rheumatica, 88t–89t
polyneuropathy, 496–497
polyphagia, 59
polyp(s)
cervical, 391t

nasal, 212t
rectal, 404t
polyuria, 47, 59, 82t
popliteal artery, 407
popliteal pulse, 415
porencephalic cysts, 551
portal hypertension, 578
port-wine stain, 547
position, sense of, 474, 496–497, 498
positioning, vertical suspension, 592
postconcussion syndrome, headaches associated with, 62t–63t
posterior root, 470
posterior tibial pulse, 416
posttraumatic stress disorder, 113t
postural tremors, 518t
posture
abnormalities, 516t–517t
assessment of, 99, 131
color changes of chronic arterial insufficiency and, 418–419
of comatose patient, 524t
for intracranial disease, 589
pouch, rectouterine, 374
precision, data, 605
precocious puberty, 582
precordial bulge, 280
predictive value, 606–609, 610
pregnancy
abdominal protuberance, 352t
breast changes, 315
changes in, 394t
questions related to, 50
ruptured tubal, 397t
uterus position, 330
preload, 263
premenstrual tension syndrome (PMS), 50
prepatellar bursa, 435
prepuce, 364
presbyopia, 161, 164
pressure overload, 263–264
pressure sores, 419
prism test, 560–561
problem list, development, 611
prolapse
of rectum, 404t
of uterus, 395t
pronation
of elbows, 446
of feet, 585
of forearm, 429